MW01030302

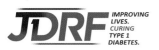

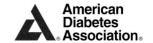

AMERICAN DIABETES ASSOCIATION / JDRF

TYPE 1 DIABETES
SOURCEBOOK

Anne Peters, MD, and Lori Laffel, MD, MPH, editors

Jane Lee Chiang, MD, managing editor

This publication was funded through
a grant from The Leona M. and Harry B. Helmsley
Charitable Trust.

Director, Book Publishing, Abe Ogden; *Managing Editor*, Greg Guthrie; *Acquisitions Editor*, Victor Van Beuren; *Production Manager*, Melissa Sprott; *Copyediting and Composition Services*, Cenveo; *Cover Design*, Jody Billert; *Printer*, Versa Press.

Printed in the United States of America
1 3 5 7 9 10 8 6 4 2

The suggestions and information contained in this publication are generally consistent with the *Clinical Practice Recommendations* and other policies of the American Diabetes Association, but they do not represent the policy or position of the Association or any of its boards or committees. Reasonable steps have been taken to ensure the accuracy of the information presented. However, the American Diabetes Association cannot ensure the safety or efficacy of any product or service described in this publication. Individuals are advised to consult a physician or other appropriate health care professional before undertaking any diet or exercise program or taking any medication referred to in this publication. Professionals must use and apply their own professional judgment, experience, and training and should not rely solely on the information contained in this publication before prescribing any diet, exercise, or medication. The American Diabetes Association—its officers, directors, employees, volunteers, and members—assumes no responsibility or liability for personal or other injury, loss, or damage that may result from the suggestions or information in this publication.

♾ The paper in this publication meets the requirements of the ANSI Standard Z39.48-1992 (permanence of paper).

ADA titles may be purchased for business or promotional use or for special sales. To purchase more than 50 copies of this book at a discount, or for custom editions of this book with your logo, contact the American Diabetes Association at the address below, at booksales@diabetes.org, or by calling 703-299-2046.

American Diabetes Association
1701 North Beauregard Street
Alexandria, Virginia 22311

DOI: 10.2337/9781580404785

Library of Congress Cataloging-in-Publication Data

The American Diabetes Association/JDRF
type 1 diabetes sourcebook / Anne Peters and Lori Laffel, editors.
    p. ; cm.
  Type 1 diabetes sourcebook
  Includes bibliographical references and index.
  ISBN 978-1-58040-478-5 (hardback)
  I. Peters, Anne L. II. Laffel, Lori. III. American Diabetes Association. IV. Juvenile
Diabetes Foundation International. V. Title: Sourcebook for type 1 diabetes.
  [DNLM: 1. Diabetes Mellitus, Type 1. WK 810]

616.462—dc23
                                 2012041724

For Morgan, who inspired this project and provides hope for the future of people living with type 1 diabetes.

Contents

Preface

The aim of the *Type 1 Diabetes (T1D) Sourcebook* is to survey the existing landscape and compile an authoritative document that assesses the current state of T1D and guides the practicing diabetes professional in providing state-of-the-art T1D care. This volume relies on the expertise and knowledge of a cross-disciplinary team of diabetes experts and seeks to go beyond clinical handbooks, consensus statements, and research articles in its scope and depth. The compilation of the *Sourcebook* required a multidisciplinary effort, just like that needed to care for people with diabetes. The *Sourcebook* provides a unique focus on T1D across the lifespan. It offers perspectives from both pediatric and adult providers with the primary goal of differentiating itself from previous publications that apply to patients with type 2 diabetes. The increased occurrence of T1D across the lifespan, the ongoing need to uncover preventive approaches or interventions to preserve β-cell function, and the burgeoning availability of advanced intensive treatment options, coupled with the ongoing challenges to maintain adherence and prevent diabetes burnout require this focused effort.

Each section or chapter offers an up-to-date literature review along with fundamental approaches to management of T1D patients of all ages. Finally, each section provides a realistic view of current shortcomings or gaps in care or research. The *Sourcebook* begins with a review of the diagnostic criteria for diabetes and provides review chapters on epidemiology, pathogenesis, and research related to the prevention and reversal of T1D. Subsequent chapters discuss the establishment of glycemic goals for patients and explore evaluation and patient education with a focus on empowering patients and families to engage in intensive self-care. These are followed by extensive chapters dealing with treatment and therapies, with a focus not only on glycemic control, but also on behavioral issues, nutrition, exercise, adjunctive therapies, management of related complications, and specific scenario treatment guidance for issues such as sick days and diabetic ketoacidosis. In addition, this book contains sections devoted specifically to men's health and women's health as well as reproductive concerns. The *Sourcebook* concludes with a section addressing specific settings and populations, specifically inpatient management, pediatric care in schools, employment, geriatrics, special population groups, and developing countries.

The ultimate aims of this *Sourcebook* are twofold: first, to provide the beginning of a new set of care standards specifically for the patient with type 1 diabetes and, second, to promote a research agenda directed at basic investigation, clinical and translational research, and health care delivery in efforts to improve overall health, prevent the occurrence of acute and chronic complications, preserve quality of life, and protect the futures for all individuals, pediatric and adult, living with type 1 diabetes. We want providers to know that T1D patients are not the same as patients with type 2 diabetes; thus, we describe the specific approaches for T1D individuals across the lifespan.

Anne Peters, MD
Lori Laffel, MD, MPH
Jane Lee Chiang, MD

Acknowledgments

The editors have many people to thank for their efforts on this publication, since no book is a solo effort. First, thanks to the Helmsley Charitable Trust and specifically to David Panzirer for his wisdom, his unrelenting passion toward improving the lives of people with diabetes, and his drive to move us forward. The ADA and JDRF both believed in this project and supported our efforts; in particular thanks to Dr. Sue Kirkman, without whose sanity and careful edits this book would never have been completed. Additionally, the publications staff at the ADA have been consummate professionals, and we are very grateful to their patience. We thank the members of the steering committee for their guidance and help pulling all of the pieces together.

Without the tireless efforts of Dr. Jane Lee Chiang, this project would have never seen the light of day. She did a fantastic job. We thank Dr. David Kendall for starting us off on this process. Special thanks to our husbands and children (of all ages) for putting up with our obsessive work habits. And most of all we thank our friends and patients with type 1 diabetes for sharing their struggles and successes as we work together to treat and hopefully someday cure this disorder.

Anne Peters, MD
Lori Laffel, MD, MPH

Members of the Steering Committee

CO-CHAIRS

Anne Peters, MD
Director, USC Clinical Diabetes Programs
Professor of Medicine, Keck School of Medicine
University of Southern California
Los Angeles, CA

Lori Laffel, MD, MPH
Chief, Pediatric, Adolescent and Young Adult Section
Investigator, Genetics and Epidemiology Section
Joslin Diabetes Center
Associate Professor of Pediatrics
Harvard Medical School
Boston, MA

MEMBERS

Belinda Childs, APRN, MN, BC-ADM, CDE
Diabetes Nurse Specialist
MidAmerica Diabetes Associates, PA
Wichita, Kansas

Richard A. Insel, MD
Chief Scientific Officer
Juvenile Diabetes Research Foundation
New York, NY

M. Sue Kirkman, MD
Senior Vice President, Medical Affairs and
    Community Information
American Diabetes Association
Alexandria, VA

Margaret A. Powers, PhD, RD, CDE
Research Scientist
International Diabetes Center
Park Nicollet Health System
Minneapolis, MN

Richard Rubin, PhD, CDE
Professor in Medicine and in Pediatrics
School of Medicine
Johns Hopkins University
Baltimore, MD

Desmond Schatz, MD
Professor and Associate Chairman of Pediatrics
Medical Director, Diabetes Center
University of Florida College of Medicine
Gainesville, FL

Linda Siminerio, RN, PhD, CDE
Executive Director
University of Pittsburgh Diabetes Institute
Pittsburgh, PA

List of Contributors

Nora Alghothani, MD
Fellow
Division of Endocrinology, Diabetes, and
 Metabolism
The Ohio State University
Columbus, OH

Pamela Allweiss, MD, MPH
Medical Officer
Centers for Disease Control and
 Prevention
Division of Diabetes Translation
Atlanta, GA

Barbara J. Anderson, PhD
Professor of Pediatrics
Associate Head, Psychology Section
Baylor College of Medicine
Houston, TX

Florence M. Brown, MD
Assistant Professor of Medicine
Harvard Medical School, Beth Israel
 Deaconess Medical Center
Co-Director
Joslin Diabetes Center, Adult Diabetes,
 Diabetes in Pregnancy Program
Boston, MA

H. Peter Chase, MD
Professor of Pediatrics
Barbara Davis Center for Childhood
 Diabetes
University of Colorado School of
 Medicine
Aurora, CO

Jane Lee Chiang, MD
Adjunct Clinical Assistant Professor
Division of Endocrinology, Department
 of Pediatrics

Stanford University
Stanford, CA

William L. Clarke, MD
Robert M. Blizzard Professor of Pediatric
 Endocrinology
Chief, Division of Pediatric
 Endocrinology
University of Virginia Health Sciences
 Center
Charlottesville, VA

Sheri R. Colberg, PhD, FACSM
Professor of Exercise Science
Human Movement Sciences Department
Old Dominion University
Norfolk, VA

Kathleen Dungan, MD, MPH
Assistant Professor of Medicine
Division of Endocrinology, Diabetes, and
 Metabolism
The Ohio State University
Columbus, OH

Steven Edelman, MD
Founder and Director, Taking Control of
 Your Diabetes 501(c)3
Professor of Medicine
University of California San Diego
Veterans Affairs Medical Center
San Diego, CA

Martha M. Funnell, MS, RN, CDE
Associate Research Scientist
Department of Medical Education
Michigan Diabetes Research and Training
 Center
Ann Arbor, MI

Stephen E. Gitelman, MD
Mary B. Olney, MD / KAK Distinguished
  Professorship in Pediatric
  Diabetes and Clinical Research
Professor of Clinical Pediatrics
Director, Pediatric Diabetes Program
Division of Pediatric Endocrinology
University of California at San Francisco
San Francisco, CA

Ann E. Goebel-Fabbri, PhD
Assistant Professor of Psychiatry
Harvard Medical School
Psychologist
Behavioral and Mental Health Unit
Joslin Diabetes Center
Boston, MA

Jeffrey S. Gonzalez, PhD
Assistant Professor
Ferkauf Graduate School of Psychology,
  Yeshiva University
Diabetes Research Center, Albert Einstein
  College of Medicine
Bronx, NY

Carla J. Greenbaum, MD
Director, Diabetes Program
Benaroya Research Institute
Seattle, WA

Michael J. Haller, MD
Associate Professor
Pediatric Endocrinology
University of Florida
Gainesville, FL

Kara Hawkins, MD
Staff Physician
VA Pittsburgh Healthcare System
Clinical Assistant Professor of Medicine
University of Pittsburgh Department of
  Medicine, Division of Endocrinology
Pittsburgh, PA

Laurie A. Higgins, MS, RD, LDN, CDE
Coordinator of Pediatric Nutrition
  Education & Research
Pediatrics, Adolescent and Young Adult
  Section
Joslin Clinic
Boston, MA

Irl B. Hirsch, MD
Professor of Medicine
University of Washington School of
  Medicine
Seattle, WA

William C. Hsu, MD
Assistant Professor of Medicine
Joslin Diabetes Center
Harvard Medical School
Boston, MA

Heba Ismail, MB BCh, MSc
Pediatric Endocrine Fellow
Division of Pediatric Endocrinology
Seattle Children's Hospital
Seattle, WA

Crystal Crismond Jackson
Director, Safe at School
Government Affairs & Legal Advocacy
American Diabetes Association
Alexandria, VA

Tamarra James-Todd, PhD, MPH
Associate Epidemiologist/Instructor in
  Medicine
Division of Women's Health, Department
  of Medicine
Brigham and Women's Hospital, Harvard
  Medical School
Boston, MA

Georgeanna J. Klingensmith, MD
Professor of Pediatrics
Barbara Davis Center for Childhood
  Diabetes
University of Colorado School of
  Medicine
Aurora, CO

David C. Klonoff, MD, FACP
Medical Director, Diabetes Research
  Institute
Mills-Peninsula Health Services
San Mateo, CA

Mary Korytkowski, MD
Interim Chief, Professor of Medicine
Division of Endocrinology
University of Pittsburgh
Pittsburgh, PA

Lori Laffel, MD, MPH
Chief, Pediatric, Adolescent and
  Young Adult Section
Investigator, Genetics and Epidemi-
  ology Section
Joslin Diabetes Center
Associate Professor of Pediatrics
Harvard Medical School
Boston, MA

David Maahs, MD, PhD
Associate Professor of Pediatrics
Barbara Davis Center for Childhood
  Diabetes
Children's Hospital Colorado
University of Colorado Denver
  School of Medicine
Aurora, CO

Hussain Mahmud, MD
Clinical Assistant Professor of
  Medicine
Division of Endocrinology and
  Metabolism
University of Pittsburgh School of
  Medicine
Pittsburgh, PA

Medha N. Munshi, MD
Director of Joslin Geriatric Diabetes
  Programs
Beth Israel Deaconess Medical
  Center
Assistant Professor of Medicine,
  Harvard Medical School
Boston, MA

Trevor Orchard, MD, M Med Sci,
  FAHA, FACE
Professor of Epidemiology, Medicine
  & Pediatrics
Department of Epidemiology
GSPH, University of Pittsburgh
Pittsburgh, PA

Bruce A. Perkins, MD, MPH,
  FRCP(C)
Associate Professor and Clinician
  Scientist
Department of Medicine, Division of
  Endocrinology and Metabolism

University Health Network—
  Toronto General Hospital
University of Toronto
Toronto, Ontario, Canada

Anne Peters, MD
Director, USC Clinical Diabetes
  Programs
Professor of Medicine, Keck School
  of Medicine
University of Southern California
Los Angeles, CA

Jeremy Hodson Pettus, MD
Endocrinology Fellow
University of California, San Diego
San Diego, CA
Co-director of Type 1 Track
Taking Control of Your Diabetes
Del Mar, CA

Andrew M. Posselt, MD, PhD,
  FACS
Associate Professor in Residence
Division of Transplantation
Department of Surgery
University of California–San
  Francisco
San Francisco, CA

Michael C. Riddell, PhD
Associate Professor & Graduate
  Program Director
School of Kinesiology and Health
  Science
Muscle Health Research Centre
York University
Toronto, Ontario, Canada

Elizabeth R. Seaquist, MD
Professor
Division of Endocrinology and
  Diabetes
Department of Medicine
Pennock Family Chair in Diabetes
  Research
University of Minnesota Medical
  School
Minneapolis, MN

Janet Silverstein, MD
Professor and Chief of Pediatric
  Endocrinology
University of Florida
Gainesville, FL

Linda M. Siminerio, RN, PhD, CDE
Executive Director
University of Pittsburgh Diabetes Institute
Pittsburgh, PA

Peter Stock, MD, PhD
Professor of Surgery
University of California, San Francisco,
  Department of Surgery, Division of
  Transplant Surgery
University of California, San Francisco
San Francisco, CA

William V. Tamborlane, MD
Professor and Chief
Pediatric Endocrinology
Yale School of Medicine
New Haven, CT

Guillermo E. Umpierrez, MD
Professor of Medicine
Emory University School of Medicine
Section Head, Endocrinology & Diabetes
Grady Health System
Atlanta, GA

Raynard Washington, PhD, MPH
University of Pittsburgh Graduate School
  of Public Health
Pittsburgh, PA

Joseph I. Wolfsdorf, MB BCh
Clinical Director and Associate Chief
Director, Diabetes Program
Division of Endocrinology, Children's
  Hospital Boston
Boston Children's Hospital Chair in
  Endocrinology
Professor of Pediatrics, Harvard Medical
  School
Boston, MA

Howard Wolpert, MD
Senior Physician
Director, Insulin Pump Program
Section of Adult Diabetes
Joslin Diabetes Center
Boston, MA

Jennifer Ann Wyckoff, MD
Assistant Professor
Division of Metabolism, Endocrinology,
  and Diabetes
University of Michigan, Department of
  Internal Medicine
Ann Arbor, MI

Mary Ziotas Zacharatos, RD, CDE,
  CDN, LD
Certified Diabetes Educator
Adult Endocrinology
Park Nicollet—International Diabetes
  Center
Minneapolis, MN

Consortia Studying
Type 1 Diabetes

Consortia Studying Type 1 Diabetes

Consortium	Full name of consortium	Consortium activities	Consortium website
T1DGC	Type 1 Diabetes Genetics Consortium	T1DGC was established with the primary goal of organizing international efforts to identify genes that determine an individual's risk of T1D.	www.t1dgc.org
TEDDY	The Environmental Determinants of Diabetes in the Young	The primary objective(s) of TEDDY is the identification of infectious agents, dietary factors, or other environmental exposures that are associated with increased risk of autoimmunity and T1D.	teddy.epi.usf.edu
nPOD	Network for Pancreatic Organ Donors with Diabetes	The mission of nPOD is to characterize pancreata and related tissues from organ donors with T1D or who are islet autoantibody positive and utilize the tissues to address key immunological, histological, viral, and metabolic questions related to how T1D develops.	www.jdrfnpod.org
SEARCH	Search for Diabetes in Youth	SEARCH identifies cases of diabetes in children/youth <20 years of age in six geographically dispersed populations that encompass the ethnic diversity of the United States.	www.searchfordiabetes.org
TrialNet	Type 1 Diabetes TrialNet	TrialNet is an international network conducting studies that will improve the understanding of T1D disease development and test interventions to interdict the T1D disease process, particularly strategies for T1D prevention.	www.diabetestrialnet.org

Continued

Consortia Studying Type 1 Diabetes (continued)

Consortium	Full name of consortium	Consortium activities	Consortium website
ITN	Immune Tolerance Network	ITN is an international consortium dedicated to the clinical evaluation of novel tolerogenic approaches for the treatment of autoimmune diseases (including T1D), asthma, and allergic diseases, and the prevention of graft rejection.	www.immune tolerance.org
TRIGR	Trial to Reduce IDDM in the Genetically at Risk	TRIGR is testing whether weaning to a casein hydrolysate formula during the first 6–8 months of life—in place of cow's milk-based formula—reduces the incidence of autoimmunity and T1D in genetically susceptible newborn infants.	trigr.epi.usf.edu
DirecNet	Diabetes Research in Children Network	DirecNet is investigating the potential use of glucose monitoring technology and its impact on the management of T1D in children.	public.direc.net

Source: Skyler JS, Ricordi C: Stopping type 1 diabetes: attempts to prevent or cure type 1 diabetes in man. *Diabetes* 60:1–8, 2011. Reprinted with permission.

1

Type 1 Diabetes in the 21st Century: A Review of the Landscape

Michael J. Haller, MD

INTRODUCTION

In the almost 100 years since the discovery of insulin, the landscape of type 1 diabetes (T1D) has changed dramatically. From the initial use of impure insulin preparations described by Banting, Best, Collip, and McCloud as "thick brown muck" to the use of recombinant insulin analogues, insulin pumps, and continuous glucose monitors, our evolving capacity to aggressively manage T1D has improved the lives of millions living with the disease.[1] In the U.S., it is estimated that 5–10% of people with diagnosed diabetes have T1D, with 1–2 million Americans living with the disease.[2] T1D remains the major type of diabetes in youth, accounting for almost all cases in children under 10 and the vast majority of diabetes cases among teens. Although the incidence of type 2 diabetes (T2D) is increasing in American youth aged 10 to 19 years, particularly in certain high-risk racial and ethnic groups, the incidence of T1D remains higher than the incidence of T2D in this age group. The overall incidence of T1D is more than four times higher than that of T2D in American youth, with 15,600 youth newly diagnosed with T1D annually versus 3,600 diagnosed with T2D.[2] Although T1D is associated with childhood, and was formerly called *juvenile diabetes*, it can be diagnosed at any age. Unfortunately, most of the available citations about incidence in adulthood are problematic: they are either very old, in select populations, or are reviews that do not have original sources of data. There is no authoritative source for the incidence of T1D in adults in the U.S. population. However, it is important to note that T1D is not a childhood disease and may be diagnosed into adulthood with an additional peak in the sixth and seventh decades of life.[3]

T1D is a presumed autoimmune disease mediated by a complex interplay of environmental and genetic factors. Although more than 80–90% of T1D cases occur in those without a family history, genetic factors strongly influence the disease.[4] The most important genetic determinants of T1D are the human leukocyte antigen (HLA) complex on chromosome 6; specifically, two HLA class II haplotypes (DR3 and DR4, DQA0302/501 and DQB0301/0201) have been implicated in T1D development. Over 90% of young children with T1D carry either one or both haplotypes, though less than 5% of the population with HLA-conferred genetic susceptibility develops the disease.[5] If genetic factors alone determined T1D risk, the concordance rate in identical twins would be expected to be 100%. Long-term studies have demonstrated concordance rates as high as 65% up to age 60. However, rates never reach 100%. The age at which concordant twins develop diabetes can differ by decades, providing additional evidence of both the genetic and environmental factors affecting T1D risk.[6] Similarly, the general U.S.

DOI: 10.2337/9781580404785ch01

population risk for T1D is 1 in 300 (0.3%) and as high as 1 in 100 (1%) by age 70 but climbs to 1 in 20 (5%) in those with a first-degree relative affected by T1D.[7]

While a complex combination of genetic and environmental determinants is responsible for autoimmunity, the final common pathway in T1D appears to be the activation of CD8 T-cells armed with a unique specificity for β-cell destruction. The initial phases of β-cell death remain enigmatic but result in the release of intracellular antigens. These permit naïve mature B-lymphocytes and naïve CD4 T-cells access to typically sequestered self-antigens. Sampling of these auto-antigens by β-cells leads to the production of islet-specific autoantibodies (ICA, GAD, ICA512, IAA, and ZnT8) and may result in further activation of autoreactive T-cells through epigenetic spreading, the process whereby T-cells become increasingly activated to additional β-cell antigens.[8] T1D-specific autoantibodies are not believed to be directly pathological, but along with genetic and metabolic information have been instrumental in allowing the development of highly accurate T1D prediction algorithms (see chapter 2).

During the largely silent preclinical phase of the disease, β-cell mass decline may continue for weeks, months, or even years until waning insulin supplies are no longer able to preserve normal glucose metabolism (see Fig. 1.1).[9] Due to the inherent heterogeneity of β-cell autoimmunity, no single model of β-cell decline can be used to describe every patient who develops T1D. That said, the final common pathway of severe insulin deficiency ultimately results in an inability to inhibit fatty acid metabolism and in the development of diabetic ketoacidosis (DKA). Despite improved awareness of T1D, between 25–30% of newly diagnosed U.S. patients present with DKA at diagnosis. Approximately 0.5–1% of those who present in DKA will develop cerebral edema, and 50% of those children will die or have long-term neurological sequelae. Because the incidence of T1D is continuing to increase worldwide at a rate of nearly 3% per year, appreciation of the early signs and symptoms of T1D remains the most effective strategy to prevent DKA-related morbidity and mortality.[10]

Once diagnosed, patients with T1D are subjected to a lifetime of multiple daily insulin injections or continuous subcutaneous insulin infusion (CSII), frequent self-monitoring of blood glucose (SMBG), the unpredictable nature of blood glucose excursions, the potential for microvascular and macrovascular complications, and the incredible economic and psychological burdens associated with managing a disease that requires management 24 h a day, 365 days a year. The tools available to predict and manage T1D continue to improve at a remarkable pace. In addition, an improved understanding of the etiopathogenesis of T1D suggests we will one day succeed in our ultimate goal of preventing and reversing the disease. Until then, we must continuously drive the field forward to provide therapies that are not only safe and effective but that also reduce the very real physical, psychological, and economic burdens of living with T1D.

CLINICAL PRESENTATION OF T1D

Insulin deficiency resulting in prolonged hyperglycemia and ketoacidosis explains the classic presenting symptoms of polyuria, polydipsia, and polyphagia. In children, the third member of the classic diabetes triad, polyphagia, is often

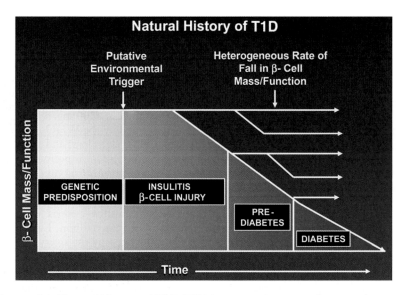

Figure 1.1 Natural history of T1D. T1D is an autoimmune disease characterized by the T-cell–mediated destruction of β-cells. The classic model suggests patients with a genetic predisposition are exposed to putative environmental factors that initiate autoimmunity. Once initiated, autoimmunity may wax and wane but typically results in the loss of β-cell mass and function until the patient ultimately develops signs and symptoms associated with diabetes. Owing to the highly heterogeneous nature of T1D, some patients will be diagnosed in severe DKA and with virtually no remaining β-cell function while others will be diagnosed when entirely asymptomatic and with a robust surviving β-cell mass.

absent because ketosis can cause anorexia. Perhaps most importantly, nonspecific symptoms such as vomiting, abdominal discomfort, constipation, and headache (common presenting complaints in the outpatient setting) should not be overlooked as possible signs of new-onset T1D. Additionally, enuresis in a previously toilet-trained child, nocturia, pyogenic skin infections, recurrent Candidal rash in babies and toddlers, monilial vaginitis in women, or tinea cruris in men also require consideration of diabetes. Moreover, the heterogeneous nature of T1D, and its capacity to affect patients of all ages and ethnicities, requires constant consideration when evaluating patients. As but one example, more than 30% of American youth and 50% of adults are now overweight or obese, requiring clinicians to resist the temptation to exclude T1D from the differential diagnosis simply because a patient is overweight.[11] Adults developing T1D may follow a less precipitous course with few or no symptoms and an elevated glucose level identified incidentally on routine blood work. These individuals may be treated (unsuccessfully) with oral agents before it is determined that they are actually patients with evolving T1D who need treatment with insulin.

DIAGNOSING DIABETES

Standards of care endorsed by the American Diabetes Association (ADA) and the World Health Organization (WHO) provide a number of overlapping criteria for the diagnosis of diabetes. Based largely on data linked to risk of retinopathy in T2D patients, all subtypes of diabetes (with the exception of gestational diabetes) are currently diagnosed by any one of the following: *1*) fasting plasma glucose ≥126 mg/dl (7.0mmol/L), *2*) a 2-h plasma glucose ≥200 mg/dl during a formal oral glucose tolerance test (OGTT) as described by the WHO, *3*) classic symptoms of hyperglycemia (polyuria, polydipsia, and weight loss) and a random plasma glucose ≥200mg/dl, or *4*) hemoglobin A1c (A1C) ≥6.5% performed and confirmed in a National Glycohemoglobin Standardization Program (NGSP)–certified assay standardized to the Diabetes Control and Complications Trial (DCCT) (see Table 1.1).[12] In the absence of unequivocal hyperglycemia, results should be confirmed by repeat testing of the initially positive criteria as discordance between the different diagnostic criteria is not uncommon. Further, as the ADA/WHO diagnostic criteria are heavily influenced by the overwhelming burden of T2D worldwide (>90% of diabetes cases), clinicians must recall that these criteria are not T1D-specific and do not always provide optimal sensitivity for the diagnosis of T1D.

An NGSP method, standardized or traceable to the DCCT reference assay, for A1C should be used at diagnosis and for ongoing monitoring. The recent assimilation of A1C as a diagnostic standard for diabetes exemplifies the challenges of the diagnostic criteria when evaluating patients. Because A1C can be performed in the nonfasting state, has less day-to-day variability, and does not require stringent patient participation when measured for diagnostic purposes, A1C has several desirable qualities of a diagnostic tool. However, A1C may not provide optimal sensitivity when evaluating patients with diverse disease processes culminating in hyperglycemia. In patients who rapidly develop the disease, A1C may not rise above current diagnostic criteria despite marked hyperglycemia. Similarly, in patients known to be at increased risk for T1D, serial fasting and OGTT-stimulated glucose concentrations are likely a more sensitive diagnostic test than A1C when using a cutoff of 6.5%[13]. Given the need to prevent the serious morbidity and mortality of DKA at diagnosis, ongoing efforts to develop cost-effective screening or case-finding strategies in high-risk patients may eventually lead to diagnostic criteria more specific to T1D.[13]

Table 1.1 Diagnostic Criteria of Diabetes

Fasting plasma glucose	>126 mg/dl (7.0 mmol/L) *or*
2-h plasma glucose	>200 mg/dl (11 mmol/L) during OGTT *or*
Clinical symptoms	Polyuria, polydipsia, weight loss, and random plasma glucose >200 mg/dl *or*
Hemoglobin A1C	>6.5%*

*A1C should be performed using a method that is NGSP-certified and standardized to the DCCT assay.

DIABETES SUBTYPES

ADA and WHO criteria are used to broadly diagnose diabetes, however, a combination of immunologic, genetic, and phenotypic features must be used to differentiate among the different forms of diabetes. A brief review of other forms of diabetes is necessary to frame our ongoing discussion of T1D. (See chapter 2 for further discussion of T1D diagnosis.)

T1D has at least two broad subcategories: type 1a diabetes and type 1b diabetes. Type 1a diabetes, the primary focus of the *T1D Sourcebook*, refers to diabetes that is autoimmune in its etiopathogenesis. Type 1b diabetes results from nonimmune-mediated β-cell loss (pancreatic agenesis, pancreatectomy, etc.). In addition to these broad subtypes, the inherent heterogeneity of T1D has necessitated additional monikers for patients within the broad framework of T1D. Some patients, classified as having fulminant T1D, experience rapid β-cell destruction; they present with DKA despite near normal A1C. Conversely, patients labeled as Latent Autoimmune Diabetes of Adulthood (LADA) develop T1D over many years, with gradual β-cell decline that may not be recognized as immune-mediated for years (and sometimes decades) after the development of hyperglycemia.

Given the growing epidemic of obesity, physicians must also remember that autoimmune diseases do not spare those who are overweight or obese. As such, when an obese patient presents with polyuria, polydipsia, and hyperglycemia, careful consideration should be given to making a diagnosis of T1D versus T2D. A missed or delayed diagnosis of T1D could result in rapid development of DKA. Moreover, because patients with T2D can develop glucose toxicity and a severe enough β-cell deficiency to cause DKA, clinicians must also be careful not to label all new-onset patients who present with DKA as having T1D. Ketonemia and ketonuria are not typically seen in T2D, but may be present. They more commonly occur in teens with new-onset T2D than in adults with T2D. Pancreatic islet autoantibodies are generally absent in T2D but have been reported in patients with a T2D phenotype. These cases emphasize the heterogeneity and crossover of these two distinct diseases. Some groups have used labels such as *double diabetes* or *type 1.5 diabetes* to describe children with characteristics of both diseases. Our preference is to not use such terms. Instead, we consider all patients with evidence of autoimmunity to have T1D, while acknowledging the presence of a T2D phenotype (also thought of as T1D plus the metabolic syndrome) and emphasizing the importance of monitoring for and treating associated comorbidities. In such cases, the presence of autoantibodies can be helpful. Definitive classification of diabetes as type 1 or type 2 can be delayed, but treatment with insulin should always be initiated.

Beyond our focus on T1D we must acknowledge that T2D accounts for the overwhelming majority of the world's diabetes. In the U.S. alone, over 25 million people have T2D and more than 7 million of them are unaware of their diagnosis. Characterized by obesity, insulin resistance, dyslipidemia, hypertension, microvascular and macrovascular complications, and a predisposition in African Americans, Hispanics, and Native Americans, T2D indirectly accounts for nearly 1 in every 10 health care dollars.[14] Given the tremendous burden T2D places on the U.S. health care system, it is not surprising that patients, health care providers, and researchers often use the nonspecific term *diabetes* when referring to

T2D. However, the practice of referring to T2D as simply diabetes cultivates numerous dangerous misconceptions regarding the etiology, pathophysiology, and treatment of other subtypes of diabetes.

In addition to T1D and T2D, a growing number of Americans are diagnosed with diabetes during pregnancy. Gestational diabetes mellitus (GDM) currently affects ~7% of pregnancies (200,000 cases annually) with 5–10% of affected women diagnosed with T2D after delivery (and some are diagnosed with auto-immune T1D, as well).[15] (See chapter 17 for more details.) Even for those who return to normal postpartum glucose metabolism, the 20-year risk of developing T2D approaches 60% once GDM has been diagnosed. Notably, the screening and diagnostic criteria for GDM are unique from other forms of diabetes.

Cystic fibrosis–related diabetes (CFRD) is another subtype of diabetes requiring a unique therapeutic approach. Named for the characteristic *cyst* and *fibrosis* formation noted in the exocrine pancreas of affected patients, cystic fibrosis (CF) is an autosomal recessive disorder caused by a mutation in a chloride transporter known as the cystic fibrosis transmembrane conductance regulator. While the primary complication in CF is chronic pulmonary disease, up to 75% of adults with CF develop glucose intolerance and nearly 15% have CFRD. CFRD is unique in that it shares some pathophysiology with both T1D and T2D. Namely, patients with CFRD have a combination of *1)* reduced β-cell mass (a feature typically associated with T1D) secondary to the chronic pancreatic inflammation and *2)* severe insulin resistance (a feature associated with T2D) as a result of chronic and often subclinical pulmonary infections. Given the unique hypermetabolic state associated with CF, patients with CFRD require high-calorie diets and tight glycemic control to avoid a catabolic state. As such, current CFRD guidelines discourage the use of oral hypoglycemics or calorie restriction and focus instead on the use of insulin to manage glucose abnormalities.[16]

Finally, clinicians should be aware of the monogenic forms of diabetes. Accounting for only 1–5% of all diabetes cases, monogenic diabetes results from single gene mutations that are inherited in an autosomal dominant fashion. These mutations do not result in insulin resistance or autoimmunity but instead induce diabetes by blunting the capacity of otherwise normal β-cells to release insulin. The two main forms of monogenic diabetes are neonatal diabetes mellitus (NDM) and maturity-onset diabetes of the young (MODY). NDM is a rare condition and occurs in 1/100,000 to 1/500,000 newborns and is often mistaken for T1D due to its association with ketoacidosis and its requirement for insulin therapy. However, T1D is exceedingly rare before 6 months of age and any child diagnosed with T1D before 9 months of age should be screened for monogenic diabetes. There are two forms of NDM, transient NDM, which resolves within weeks to months, and permanent NDM, which is associated with a lifelong dependence on insulin. Testing for known diagnostic mutations allows accurate differentiation of the two subtypes of NDM and emphasizes the need for clinicians to be aware of rare forms of diabetes. In contrast to NDM, MODY is a mild form of diabetes that is commonly, but not always, diagnosed in adulthood. Patients initially diagnosed with T1D who fail to demonstrate autoantibody positivity or who persist with near normal glycemic control on minimal insulin should be screened for MODY. Diagnosis of MODY is especially important as some forms of MODY may be controlled with oral hypoglycemic agents. For a subset of patients, the appropriate diagnosis can mean the difference between a lifetime of insulin injections or effective glycemic control with a sulfonylurea.[17]

EPIDEMIOLOGY OF T1D: INCIDENCE AND PREVALENCE

Epidemiologic patterns of T1D provide insight into the etiology, natural history, and complications of the disease. Findings from large T1D registry studies, such as the WHO Multinational Project for Childhood Diabetes (DIAMOND Project), the SEARCH for Diabetes in Youth (SEARCH), and the Epidemiology and Prevention of Diabetes (EURODIAB), show global variation in the incidence, prevalence, and temporal trends in T1D (see Fig. 1.2).

In the U.S., more than 215,000 children <20 years of age have diabetes, with the overwhelming number of cases afflicted with T1D.[2] The prevalence of T1D in U.S. children is 1.7–2.5/1000 individuals, while the incidence is between 15 and 17/100,000/year.[18] Recent data from the SEARCH study confirm a 23% increase in the prevalence of T1D between 2001 and 2009 and an increase in

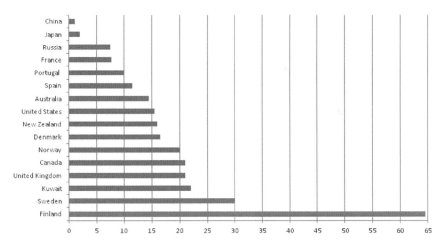

Figure 1.2 Global incidence rates of T1D. Incidence of T1D is affected by a combination of genetic and environmental factors. This is exemplified in the marked differences in T1D incidence when comparing rates across countries. The incidence of T1D in China is extremely low at 0.1/100,000/year while the rate in the U.S. is considered intermediate at >24/100,000/ year.[19,81,82] Finland has one of the highest incidence rates globally at >64.2 cases/100,000/year.[58]

incidence among non-Hispanic whites from 24.1 to 27.2/100,000 from 2002 to 2009.[19] This amounts to a 2.6% (95% CI 1.03–4.28) relative increase in T1D per year in American youth <20 years of age. Ongoing research will address changing incidence rates in racial and ethnic minority groups.

Over 15,000 new cases of T1D are diagnosed each year in the U.S. Recent data are needed regarding the incidence of T1D in adults. Notably, nearly 85% of people living with T1D are adults.[19] Two peaks of T1D presentation occur in childhood: one between 5 and 7 years of age, and the other at puberty. However, the incidence and prevalence of T1D varies dramatically around the world with more than a 400-fold variation in incidence among reporting countries.[11] T1D is uncommon in China, India, and Venezuela, where the incidence is only 0.1/100,000. The disease is far more common in Sardinia and Finland, with the incidence >50/100,000 individuals per year. Rates of >20/100,000 are observed in Sweden, Norway, Portugal, Great Britain, Canada, and New Zealand.[11] Wide variations have been observed between neighboring areas in Europe and North America. Estonia, separated from Finland by less than 75 miles, has a T1D incidence less than one-third that of Finland. Puerto Rico has an incidence similar to the mainland U.S. (17/100,000), while neighboring Cuba has an incidence of <3/100,000.[20]

With few exceptions, population-based T1D registries show an increasing incidence of T1D over time. These observations emphasize the urgent need to increase efforts aimed at identifying causative environmental agents and gene-environment interactions responsible for T1D. The DIAMOND Project, initiated by the WHO in 1990 to describe the incidence and trends of T1D in children worldwide for the period of 1990–1999, analyzed children aged ≤14 years of age from 114 populations in 112 centers in 57 countries. A total of 43,013 cases were diagnosed in the study populations of 84 million children. The age-adjusted incidence of T1D varied from 0.1/100,000/year in China and Venezuela to 40.9/100,000/year in Finland. The average annual increase in incidence calculated from 103 centers was 2.8% (95% CI 2.4–3.2%). The increase in incidence was 2.4% (95% CI 1.3–3.4%) during the years 1990–1994 and slightly higher at 3.4% (95% CI 2.7–4.3%) during the second study period of 1995–1999. The trends in incidence grouped by continents showed statistically significant increases all over the world (4.0% in Asia, 3.2% in Europe, and 5.3% in North America), except in Central America and the West Indies, where the trend was a decrease of 3.6%. Only among the European populations did the trend in incidence diminish with age.[21]

The DIAMOND registry showed that the highest incidence rates were among European and North American populations, varying from 4 to 64.2/100,000/year in Europe and from 11 to 25/100,000/year in North America. In Oceania, the incidence of T1D was also high at 14 to 22/100,000/year, reflecting ethnic diversity within this region. Among African populations, incidence ranged between 1 to 9/100,000/year. The incidence among South American populations varied between <1 to 10/100,000/year. In Central America and the West Indies, the range of variation was from 2 to 17/100,000/year. The majority of Asian populations had a very low incidence of <1/100,000/year, with the exception of Kuwait, which had a very high incidence of 22/100,000/year.[21]

The U.S. populations included in the DIAMOND study, drawn from Pennsylvania, Alabama, and Illinois, reported incidences of 10 to 20/100,000/year.

Approximately half of the European populations reported incidences of 5 to 10/100,000/year. In most populations, the incidence increased with age and was highest among children 10–14 years of age. Due to public health concerns about the increasing incidence of diabetes (both T1D and T2D), the Centers for Disease Control and Prevention (CDC) and the National Institute of Diabetes and Digestive and Kidney Diseases (NIDDK) funded the SEARCH for Diabetes in Youth Study in the U.S. in 2001. SEARCH is an ongoing multiethnic, observational study conducted in six centers that encompass the racial/ethnic diversity of the U.S. The goals are: *1)* estimate the prevalence and incidence of T1D and T2D in youth <20 years of age, according to age, gender, and race/ethnicity, *2)* characterize risk factors and complications of diabetes, and *3)* evaluate health care quality and quality of life of children living with diabetes in the U.S. Youth with diabetes are identified in geographically defined populations in Ohio, Washington, South Carolina, Colorado, Hawaii, and southern California, and among Indian Health Service beneficiaries in selected American Indian populations.

In 2001, ~3.5 million children <20 years of age were under surveillance at the SEARCH research centers, and the overall prevalence of diabetes (T1D, T2D, or unspecified) was 1.8/1,000. SEARCH data estimated that 154,369 youth had physician-diagnosed diabetes in 2001.[22] Since 2002, the number of children <20 years of age under surveillance to estimate diabetes incidence has been ~5.5 million. The overall incidence of diabetes in 2002 and 2003 was estimated to be 24.3/100,000/year. SEARCH estimated that 15,000 youths are diagnosed with T1D annually.[23] Using U.S. data from the Colorado Insulin-Dependent Diabetes Mellitus (IDDM) study registry and the SEARCH study, T1D incidence was shown to increase in the past 3 decades.[10] The incidence was 14.8/100,000/year (95% CI 14.0–15.6) in 1978 to 1988, and increased to 23.9/100,000/year (95% CI 22.2–25.6) in 2002 to 2004 for the state of Colorado. During this 26-year period, the incidence of T1D increased by 2.3% (95% CI 1.6–3.1) per year, with significant increases for both non-Hispanic white and Hispanic youth. The EURODIAB Study reported that the incidence of T1D was increasing fastest among the very young, those <5 years of age, with increases of 5.4%, 4.3%, and 2.9% in the age groups 0–4 years, 5–9 years, and 10–14 years, respectively.[24]

Despite the historical focus on children when discussing the epidemiology of T1D, it is critical to consider that adults make up 25–50% of newly diagnosed patients and represent the overwhelming majority of patients living with T1D. Importantly, adults with LADA may represent an additional 10% of those adults incorrectly diagnosed with T2D. As these patients are far more likely to progress rapidly to requiring insulin therapy, clinicians treating adults must be aware of the need to screen for LADA, particularly in their patients with relatively low BMI.

ENVIRONMENT

T1D results from the interaction of genes, the environment, and the immune system. Indeed, the disparate geographic prevalence, rising worldwide incidence, and 50% or greater discordance rate in identical twins provide evidence that environmental agents are operative.[25] The aforementioned islet-specific autoantibodies can frequently be detected within the first few years of life,[26–28] and it appears that triggering environmental encounters may occur very early in development. Because there is invariably a latent period between the appearance of T1D-associated autoantibodies and disease onset, additional environmental factors—probably interacting with genetic factors—also appear to modulate the progression of the disease.[29]

Early nutrition or infection have been the most frequently implicated early environmental influences of β-cell autoimmunity.[30] There is no direct evidence to date that either nutrition or infection plays a major role in causation; however, one example, prenatal rubella infection, is often cited as providing such evidence.[31,32] Prenatal rubella infection is associated with β-cell autoimmunity in up to 70% and diabetes in up to 40% of children infected, though postnatal infection is not associated with increased risk.[31,33–37] The introduction of universal rubella vaccination has virtually abolished the disease and the occurrence of this form of diabetes, proving that T1D may be prevented by modification of environmental factors.

A relationship between β-cell autoimmunity and exposure to enteroviral infections *in utero* has also been proposed.[32,38,39] Studies from both Finland and Sweden suggest that maternal enterovirus infection may increase the likelihood of subsequent T1D development in the offspring.[32,38] Higher levels of antibodies to procapsid enterovirus antigens were found in the pregnant sera of mothers of the children developing diabetes. The presence of antibodies against enteroviruses in people with autoimmunity does not, however, prove a causal relationship. It should also be noted that the number of women exposed to enteroviral infection during pregnancy is decreasing and that infection in early childhood has become less common.[40] Islet-related autoantibodies have also been detected after mumps, measles, chickenpox, and rotavirus infections.[41–43] These considerations do not exclude arguments based on changing antigenicity of foods or viruses or timing of exposure to them. Persons with autoimmunity may also be more prone to enteroviral infection, may have a stronger humoral response to infection due to their particular HLA genotype, or may be in a nonspecific hyperimmune state marked by elevation of antibody levels to a variety of exogenous antigens.[30] With this background, it is clear that well-planned prospective studies in larger populations are essential.

As one example of potentially noninfectious influences on the natural history of T1D, we will discuss the potential protective effect of breast-feeding versus early exposure to cow's milk on the incidence of autoimmunity.[44–49] This area of research remains controversial, though an extensive meta-analysis confirmed a small but statistically significant association (odds ratio ~1.5) between T1D, a shortened period of breast-feeding, and cow's milk exposure before 3 to 4 months of age.[50] Another suspect is bovine serum albumin (BSA). It has been shown that antibodies to BSA, immunologically distinct from human serum albumin, were present in 100% of Finnish children with new-onset T1D but were absent in controls.[47] Structural similarities between BSA and an islet protein (ICA$_{69}$) were proposed as an appealing pathogenic concept of molecular mimicry, by which the early introduction of cow's milk would allow absorption of the intact protein before gut maturation, thus immunizing the infant and directing an immune response to the islets through its ICA$_{69}$ mimic.[51] However, there is strong evidence to counter each argument advancing the cow's milk hypothesis.[44]

No association between early exposure to cow's milk and ß-cell autoimmunity in young siblings and offspring of diabetic patients has been shown in several other studies.[52] Despite increased breast-feeding in developed countries, the incidence of childhood diabetes continues to rise.[53] We and others were unable to show any link between the presence of antibodies to BSA and T1D.[46,54] Finally, ICA[69] has been found in several organs besides the pancreas and cross-reactivity of these antibodies with BSA has not been confirmed.

The ingestion of nutrients containing plant elements such as soy and wheat may have an effect on diabetes development, at least as defined in NOD mice studies.[55] In humans, two recent studies, the Diabetes Autoimmunity Study in the Young (DAISY) and the German study of offspring of T1D parents (BABYD-IAB) provided evidence that susceptibility to T1D is associated with the timing of cereal and gluten exposure.[56,57] In the DAISY study, initial exposure to cereal between birth and 3 months of age and after 7 months of age imparted risk of autoimmunity. The German BABYDIAB study demonstrated an increased risk for autoimmunity in infants initially exposed to gluten before 3 months of age and found no increased risk in those initially exposed to gluten after 6 months of age. Although both studies provide interesting findings, their conclusions are in some ways contradictory and demonstrate the need for larger collaborative investigations in order to determine how early dietary exposures affect autoimmunity risk.

As previously discussed, the highest incidence of T1D worldwide occurs in Finland (now ~64.2/100,000/year with an anticipated increase in incidence rate to 128/100,000 by the year 2020).[58] Sun exposure in northern Finland is extremely limited and presumably results in low serum vitamin D concentrations among Finns. It has been suggested that ensuring adequate vitamin D supplementation for infants may reverse the increasing incidence of T1D.[59] It has been proposed that vitamin D compounds may act as selective immunosuppressants, as illustrated by their ability to either prevent or markedly suppress development of autoimmune disease in animal models of T1D.[60] Vitamin D has been shown to stimulate transforming growth factor (TGF) β-1 and interleukin 4 (IL-4), which may suppress inflammatory T-cell (Th1) activity.[61] Unfortunately, interventions using the activated form of vitamin D (1,25(OH)2 vitamin D) have been ineffective in preserving residual β cell function following the diagnosis of T1D.[62]

Toxic doses of nitrosamine compounds may also cause diabetes due to free radical generation.[63,64] The effects of dietary nitrate, nitrite, or nitrosamine exposure on human T1D risk are less clear.[65,66] Several perinatal risk factors for childhood diabetes are also associated with T1D development.[67] The effect of maternal–child blood group incompatibility is fairly strong (both ABO and Rh factor with ABO > Rh) and needs to be further explored. Other perinatal factors conferring increased risk include preeclampsia, neonatal respiratory distress, neonatal infections, caesarian section, birth weight, gestational age, birth order, and maternal age.[68–72] It will be important to determine whether these factors really do contribute and the interaction of these with other unknown risk factors. Rodent studies also suggested that administration of diphtheria-tetanus-pertussis (DPT) vaccine at 2 months of age increases the incidence of diabetes compared with that of unvaccinated individuals or of individuals vaccinated at birth. However, prospective studies have not identified any associations between early childhood immunizations and β-cell autoimmunity.[73,74]

Finally, it has been argued that the *loss* of protective environmental factors could account for the rising incidence of T1D.[75] One model that supports this concept is the *hygiene hypothesis*. The hygiene hypothesis suggests that exposure to infective agents in early childhood is necessary for maturation of the normal neonatal immune response. In the absence of such exposures, and in combination with genetic susceptibilities, immunoregulatory pathways may be permanently shifted towards autoimmunity (Th1) or allergic (Th2) disease.[76,77] Supporting this theory is the parallel rise in the rates of asthma, allergy, and T1D. The hygiene hypothesis model is consistent with the fact that NOD mice are far less likely to develop diabetes in the presence of pinworms and other infections.

Despite our growing understanding of the natural history of T1D, our knowledge of the complex interplay between environment and genetics remains inadequate to fully understand the etiopathogenesis of T1D. The Environmental Determinants of Diabetes in Youth (TEDDY) consortium is attempting to perform a more definitive analysis. TEDDY is a consortium of six international centers (four in the U.S. and two in Europe) that seeks to identify infectious agents, dietary exposures, and other environmental factors associated with the development of β-cell autoimmunity in genetically susceptible children.[78,79] Correlations of islet autoimmunity with environmental exposure will presumably help identify the environmental factors that trigger the autoimmune cascade and permit specific preventive intervention. To achieve the power needed for the TEDDY analyses, >200,000 newborns were initially HLA screened and >20,000 high-risk children were identified. A cohort of >8,000 children with increased genetic risk consented to participate in the 15-year follow-up study. These children (median age, 3 years in 2012) are being intensively followed with frequent blood, hair, nail, stool, and urine sampling. In addition, families keep records of dietary intake, immunizations, and illnesses. Those who develop T1D autoantibodies receive additional metabolic follow-up to further characterize the natural history of T1D. To date, >100 children from this cohort have developed T1D. Our hope is that the dedicated families and children participating in TEDDY will ultimately help determine the combination of environmental factors associated with β-cell autoimmunity. With an improved understanding of the factors affecting T1D, we should then be better prepared to develop rational prevention strategies.

The health care and quality of life costs of living with T1D remain daunting. Recent estimates suggest that the current cohort of 1.4 million T1D patients will incur direct and indirect costs > $400 billion in their lifetime.[80] We would be wise to admit the many deficiencies in our understanding of T1D. Honest appraisals of the gaps in our knowledge base should improve care for patients living with T1D, while speeding us toward the achievement of our ultimate goal, the prevention and reversal of T1D.

EDITORIAL COMMENTS: FILLING THE GAPS

1. There is a need to understand the changing incidence of T1D across all ages.
2. There is a need to investigate the unique contributions of genetic susceptibility and environmental exposures on the processes that trigger or promote β-cell autoimmunity.

3. There is a need to understand possible contributions of the gut and the microbiome on the development of β-cell autoimmunity.
4. Ongoing studies are needed to prevent, interrupt, and reverse the autoimmunity that leads to T1D.

REFERENCES

1. Bliss M: *The Discovery of Insulin*, University of Chicago Press, 1984
2. Centers for Disease Control and Prevention. National Diabetes Fact Sheet: National Estimates and General Information on Diabetes and Prediabetes in the United States, 2011. Atlanta, GA, U.S. Department of Health and Human Services, Centers for Disease Control and Prevention, 2011
3. National Diabetes Data Group, National Institute of Diabetes and Digestive and Kidney Diseases, National Institutes of Health: *Diabetes in America*. 2nd ed. Available from http://diabetes.niddk.nih.gov/dm/pubs/america/contents.aspx. Accessed 20 October 2012
4. Haller MJ, Atkinson MA, Schatz DA: Efforts to prevent and halt autoimmune beta cell destruction. *Endocrinol Metab Clin North Am* 39:527–539, 2010
5. Virtanen SM, Knip M: Nutritional risk predictors of beta cell autoimmunity and type 1 diabetes at a young age. *Am J Clin Nutr* 78:1053–1067, 2003
6. Redondo MJ, Jeffrey J, Fain PR, Eisenbarth GS, Orban T: Concordance for islet autoimmunity among monozygotic twins. *N Engl J Med* 359:2849–2850, 2008
7. Bonifacio E, Ziegler AG: Advances in the prediction and natural history of type 1 diabetes. *Endocrinol Metab Clin North Am* 39:513–525, 2010
8. Bonifacio E, Lampasona V, Bernasconi L, Ziegler AG: Maturation of the humoral autoimmune response to epitopes of GAD in preclinical childhood type 1 diabetes. *Diabetes* 49:202–208, 2000
9. Atkinson MA, Eisenbarth GS: Type 1 diabetes: new perspectives on disease pathogenesis and treatment. *Lancet* 358:221–229, 2001
10. Vehik K, Hamman RF, Lezotte D, Norris JM, Klingensmith G, Bloch C, Rewers M, Dabelea D: Increasing incidence of type 1 diabetes in 0- to 17-year-old Colorado youth. *Diabetes Care* 30:503–509, 2007
11. Haller MJ, Atkinson MA, Schatz D: Type 1 diabetes mellitus: etiology, presentation, and management. *Pediatr Clin North Am* 52:1553–1578, 2005
12. American Diabetes Association. Standards of medical care in diabetes: 2012. *Diabetes Care* 35 (Suppl. 1):S11–S63, 2012
13. Vehik K, Cuthbertson D, Boulware D, Beam CA, Rodriguez H, Legault L, Hyytinen M, Rewers MJ, Schatz DA, Krischer JP: Performance of HbA$_{1c}$ as an early diagnostic indicator of type 1 diabetes in children and youth. TEDDY, TRIGR, Diabetes Prevention Trial–Type 1, and Type 1 Diabetes TrialNet Natural History Study Groups. *Diabetes Care* 35:1821–1825, 2012
14. Economic costs of diabetes in the U.S. in 2007. *Diabetes Care* 31:596–615, 2008
15. American Diabetes Association. Standards of medical care in diabetes: 2010. *Diabetes Care* 33 (Suppl. 1):S11–S61, 2010
16. Moran A, Brunzell C, Cohen RC, Katz M, Marshall BC, Onady G, Robinson KA, Sabadosa KA, Stecenko A, Slovis B: Clinical care guidelines for

cystic fibrosis–related diabetes: a position statement of the American Diabetes Association and a clinical practice guideline of the Cystic Fibrosis Foundation, endorsed by the Pediatric Endocrine Society. *Diabetes Care* 33:2697–2708, 2010

17. Shields BM, McDonald TJ, Ellard S, Campbell MJ, Hyde C, Hattersley AT: The development and validation of a clinical prediction model to determine the probability of MODY in patients with young-onset diabetes. *Diabetologia* 55:1265–1272, 2012

18. Karvonen M, Viik-Kajander M, Moltchanova E, Libman I, LaPorte R, Tuomilehto J: Incidence of childhood type 1 diabetes worldwide. Diabetes Mondiale (DiaMond) Project Group. *Diabetes Care* 23:1516–1526, 2000

19. American Diabetes Association abstracts. *Diabetes* 61 (Suppl. 1):A52, 2012

20. LaPorte RE, Matsushima M, Chang Y-F: *Prevalence and Incidence of Insulin-dependent Diabetes.* Bethesda, MD, NIH, 1995

21. DIAMOND Project Group: Incidence and trends of childhood type 1 diabetes worldwide 1990-1999. *Diabetic Med* 23:857–866, 2006

22. Liese AD, D'Agostino RB, Jr, Hamman RF, Kilgo PD, Lawrence JM, Liu LL, Loots B, Linder B, Marcovina S, Rodriguez B, Standiford D, Williams DE: The burden of diabetes mellitus among US youth: prevalence estimates from the SEARCH for Diabetes in Youth Study. *Pediatrics* 118:1510–1518, 2006

23. Dabelea D, Mayer-Davis EJ, Imperatore G: The value of national diabetes registries: SEARCH for Diabetes in Youth Study. *Curr Diabetes Rev* 10:362–369, 2010

24. Patterson CC, Dahlquist GG, Gyürüs E, Green A, Soltész G: Incidence trends for childhood type 1 diabetes in Europe during 1989–2003 and predicted new cases 2005–20: a multicentre prospective registration study. EURODIAB Study Group. *Lancet* 373:2027–2033, 2009

25. Olmos P, A'Hern R, Heaton DA, Millward BA, Risley D, Pyke DA, Leslie RD: The significance of the concordance rate for type 1 (insulin-dependent) diabetes in identical twins. *Diabetologia* 31:747–750, 1988

26. Ziegler AG, Hummel M, Schenker M, Bonifacio E: Autoantibody appearance and risk for development of childhood diabetes in offspring of parents with type 1 diabetes: the 2-year analysis of the German BABYDIAB study. *Diabetes* 48:460–468, 1999

27. Rewers M, Bugawan TL, Norris JM, Blair A, Beaty B, Hoffman M, McDuffie RS, Jr, Hamman RF, Klingensmith G, Eisenbarth GS, Erlich HA: Newborn screening for HLA markers associated with IDDM: diabetes autoimmunity study in the young (DAISY). *Diabetologia* 39:807–812, 1996

28. Akerblom HK, Knip M, Simell O: From pathomechanisms to prediction, prevention and improved care of insulin-dependent diabetes mellitus in children. *Ann Med* 29:383–385, 1997

29. Leslie RD, Elliott RB: Early environmental events as a cause of IDDM. Evidence and implications. *Diabetes* 43:843–850, 1994

30. Graves PM, Norris JM, Pallansch MA, Gerling IC, Rewers M: The role of enteroviral infections in the development of IDDM: limitations of current approaches. *Diabetes* 46:161–168, 1997

31. Menser MA, Forrest JM, Bransby RD: Rubella infection and diabetes mellitus. *Lancet* 1:57–60, 1978

32. Dahlquist GG, Ivarsson S, Lindberg B, Forsgren M: Maternal enteroviral infection during pregnancy as a risk factor for childhood IDDM: a population-based case-control study. *Diabetes* 44:408–413, 1995
33. Ginsberg-Fellner F, Witt ME, Yagihashi S, Dobersen MJ, Taub F, Fedun B, McEvoy RC, Roman SH, Davies RG, Cooper LZ, et al.: Congenital rubella syndrome as a model for type 1 (insulin-dependent) diabetes mellitus: increased prevalence of islet cell surface antibodies. *Diabetologia* 27 (Suppl.):87–89, 1984
34. Bodansky HJ, Grant PJ, Dean BM, McNally J, Bottazzo GF, Hambling MH, Wales JK: Islet-cell antibodies and insulin autoantibodies in association with common viral infections. *Lancet* 2:1351–1353, 1986
35. Blom L, Nystrom L, Dahlquist G: The Swedish childhood diabetes study: vaccinations and infections as risk determinants for diabetes in childhood. *Diabetologia* 34:176–181, 1991
36. Clarke WL, Shaver KA, Bright GM, Rogol AD, Nance WE: Autoimmunity in congenital rubella syndrome. *J Pediatr* 104:370–373, 1984
37. Karounos DG, Wolinsky JS, Thomas JW: Monoclonal antibody to rubella virus capsid protein recognizes a beta-cell antigen. *J Immunol* 150:3080–3085, 1993
38. Hyoty H, Hiltunen M, Knip M, Laakkonen M, Vahasalo P, Karjalainen J, Koskela P, Roivainen M, Leinikki P, Hovi T, et al.: A prospective study of the role of coxsackie B and other enterovirus infections in the pathogenesis of IDDM. Childhood Diabetes in Finland (DiMe) Study Group. *Diabetes* 44:652–657, 1995
39. Clements GB, Galbraith DN, Taylor KW: Coxsackie B virus infection and onset of childhood diabetes. *Lancet* 346:221–223, 1995
40. Viskari HR, Koskela P, Lonnrot M, Luonuansuu S, Reunanen A, Baer M, Hyoty H: Can enterovirus infections explain the increasing incidence of type 1 diabetes? *Diabetes Care* 23:414–416, 2000
41. Helmke K, Otten A, Willems WR, Brockhaus R, Mueller-Eckhardt G, Stief T, Bertrams J, Wolf H, Federlin K: Islet cell antibodies and the development of diabetes mellitus in relation to mumps infection and mumps vaccination. *Diabetologia* 29:30–33, 1986
42. Champsaur HF, Bottazzo GF, Bertrams J, Assan R, Bach C: Virologic, immunologic, and genetic factors in insulin-dependent diabetes mellitus. *J Pediatr* 100:15–20, 1982
43. Honeyman MC, Coulson BS, Stone NL, Gellert SA, Goldwater PN, Steele CE, Couper JJ, Tait BD, Colman PG, Harrison LC: Association between rotavirus infection and pancreatic islet autoimmunity in children at risk of developing type 1 diabetes. *Diabetes* 49:1319–1324, 2000
44. Schatz DA, Maclaren NK: Cow's milk and insulin-dependent diabetes mellitus. Innocent until proven guilty. *JAMA* 276:647–648, 1996
45. Norris JM, Beaty B, Klingensmith G, Yu L, Hoffman M, Chase HP, Erlich HA, Hamman RF, Eisenbarth GS, Rewers M: Lack of association between early exposure to cow's milk protein and beta-cell autoimmunity: Diabetes Autoimmunity Study in the Young (DAISY). *JAMA* 276:609–614, 1996
46. Atkinson MA, Bowman MA, Kao KJ, Campbell L, Dush PJ, Shah SC, Simell O, Maclaren NK: Lack of immune responsiveness to bovine serum albumin in insulin-dependent diabetes. *N Engl J Med* 329:1853–1858, 1993

47. Karjalainen J, Martin JM, Knip M, Ilonen J, Robinson BH, Savilahti E, Akerblom HK, Dosch HM: A bovine albumin peptide as a possible trigger of insulin-dependent diabetes mellitus. *N Engl J Med* 327:302–307, 1992
48. Martin JM, Trink B, Daneman D, Dosch HM, Robinson B: Milk proteins in the etiology of insulin-dependent diabetes mellitus (IDDM). *Ann Med* 23:447–452, 1991
49. Borch-Johnsen K, Joner G, Mandrup-Poulsen T, Christy M, Zachau-Christiansen B, Kastrup K, Nerup J: Relation between breast-feeding and incidence rates of insulin-dependent diabetes mellitus. A hypothesis. *Lancet* 2:1083–1086, 1984
50. Gerstein HC: Cow's milk exposure and type I diabetes mellitus. A critical overview of the clinical literature. *Diabetes Care* 17:13–19, 1994
51. Pietropaolo M, Castano L, Babu S, Buelow R, Kuo YL, Martin S, Martin A, Powers AC, Prochazka M, Naggert J, et al.: Islet cell autoantigen 69 kD (ICA69). Molecular cloning and characterization of a novel diabetes-associated autoantigen. *J Clin Invest* 92:359–371, 1993
52. Couper JJ, Steele C, Beresford S, Powell T, McCaul K, Pollard A, Gellert S, Tait B, Harrison LC, Colman PG: Lack of association between duration of breast-feeding or introduction of cow's milk and development of islet autoimmunity. *Diabetes* 48:2145–2149, 1999
53. Wright AL: The rise of breastfeeding in the United States. *Pediatr Clin North Am* 48:1–12, 2001
54. Ivarsson SA, Mansson MU, Jakobsson IL: IgG antibodies to bovine serum albumin are not increased in children with IDDM. *Diabetes* 44:1349–1350, 1995
55. Scott FW, Marliss EB: Conference summary: diet as an environmental factor in development of insulin-dependent diabetes mellitus. *Can J Physiol Pharmacol* 69:311–319, 1991
56. Norris JM, Barriga K, Klingensmith G, Hoffman M, Eisenbarth GS, Erlich HA, Rewers M: Timing of initial cereal exposure in infancy and risk of islet autoimmunity. *JAMA* 290:1713–1720, 2003
57. Ziegler AG, Schmid S, Huber D, Hummel M, Bonifacio E: Early infant feeding and risk of developing type 1 diabetes-associated autoantibodies. *JAMA* 290:1721–1728, 2003
58. Harjutsalo V, Sjöberg L, Tuomilehto J: Time trends in the incidence of type 1 diabetes in Finnish children: a cohort study. *Lancet* 371:1777–1782, 2008
59. Hypponen E, Laara E, Reunanen A, Jarvelin MR, Virtanen SM: Intake of vitamin D and risk of type 1 diabetes: a birth-cohort study. *Lancet* 358:1500–1503, 2001
60. Saggese G, Federico G, Balestri M, Toniolo A: Calcitriol inhibits the PHA-induced production of IL-2 and IFN-gamma and the proliferation of human peripheral blood leukocytes while enhancing the surface expression of HLA class II molecules. *J Endocrinol Invest* 12:329–335, 1989
61. Mathieu C, Casteels K, Waer M, Laureys J, Valckx D, Bouillon R: Prevention of diabetes recurrence after syngeneic islet transplantation in NOD mice by analogues of 1,25(OH)2D3 in combination with cyclosporin A: mechanism of action involves an immune shift from Th1 to Th2. *Transplant Proc* 30:541, 1998

62. Bizzarri C, Pitocco D, Napoli N, Di Stasio E, Maggi D, Manfrini S, Suraci C, Cavallo MG, Cappa M, Ghirlanda G, Pozzilli P: No protective effect of calcitriol on beta-cell function in recent-onset type 1 diabetes: the IMDIAB XIII trial. IMDIAB Group. *Diabetes Care* 33:1962–1963, 2010

63. Pont A, Rubino JM, Bishop D, Peal R: Diabetes mellitus and neuropathy following Vacor ingestion in man. *Arch Intern Med* 139:185–187, 1979

64. Schein PS, Alberti KG, Williamson DH: Effects of streptozotocin on carbohydrate and lipid metabolism in the rat. *Endocrinology* 89:827–834, 1971

65. Kostraba JN, Gay EC, Rewers M, Hamman RF: Nitrate levels in community drinking waters and risk of IDDM. An ecological analysis. *Diabetes Care* 15:1505–1508, 1992

66. Dahlquist GG, Blom LG, Persson LA, Sandstrom AI, Wall SG: Dietary factors and the risk of developing insulin dependent diabetes in childhood. *BMJ* 300:1302–1306, 1990

67. Dahlquist GG, Patterson C, Soltesz G: Perinatal risk factors for childhood type 1 diabetes in Europe. The EURODIAB Substudy 2 Study Group. *Diabetes Care* 22:1698–1702, 1999

68. McKinney PA, Parslow R, Gurney K, Law G, Bodansky HJ, Williams DR: Antenatal risk factors for childhood diabetes mellitus: a case-control study of medical record data in Yorkshire, UK. *Diabetologia* 40:933–939, 1997

69. Patterson CC, Carson DJ, Hadden DR, Waugh NR, Cole SK: A case-control investigation of perinatal risk factors for childhood IDDM in Northern Ireland and Scotland. *Diabetes Care* 17:376–381, 1994

70. Flood TM, Brink SJ, Gleason RE: Increased incidence of type I diabetes in children of older mothers. *Diabetes Care* 5:571–573, 1982

71. Blom L, Dahlquist G, Nystrom L, Sandstrom A, Wall S: The Swedish childhood diabetes study: social and perinatal determinants for diabetes in childhood. *Diabetologia* 32:7–13, 1989

72. Dahlquist G, Kallen B: Maternal-child blood group incompatibility and other perinatal events increase the risk for early-onset type 1 (insulin-dependent) diabetes mellitus. *Diabetologia* 35:671–675, 1992

73. Hummel M, Ziegler AG: Vaccines and the appearance of islet cell antibodies in offspring of diabetic parents: results from the BABY-DIAB study. *Diabetes Care* 19:1456–1457, 1996

74. Classen JB: The timing of immunization affects the development of diabetes in rodents. *Autoimmunity* 24:137–145, 1996

75. Todd JA: A protective role of the environment in the development of type 1 diabetes? *Diabet Med* 8:906–910, 1991

76. Singh B: Stimulation of the developing immune system can prevent autoimmunity. *J Autoimmun* 14:15–22, 2000

77. Black P: Why is the prevalence of allergy and autoimmunity increasing? *Trends Immunol* 22:354–355, 2001

78. Available at http://www.niddk.nih.gov/patient/TEDDY/TEDDY.htm Accessed 20 October 2012

79. Available at http://archives.niddk.nih.gov/patient/teddy/teddy.aspx. Accessed 20 October 2012

80. Tao BT, Taylor DG: Economics of type 1 diabetes. *Endocrinol Metab Clin North Am* 39:499–512

81. Writing Group for the SEARCH for Diabetes in Youth Study Group, Dabelea D, Bell RA, D'Agostino RB Jr, Imperatore G, Johansen JM, Linder B, Liu LL, Loots B, Marcovina S, Mayer-Davis EJ, Pettitt DJ, Waitzfelder B: Incidence of diabetes in youth in the United States. *JAMA* 297:2716–2724, 2007
82. Bell RA, Mayer-Davis EJ, Beyer JW, D'Agostino RB, Lawrence JM, Linder B, Liu LL, Marcovina SM, Rodriguez BL, Williams D, Dabelea D, SEARCH for Diabetes in Youth Study Group: Diabetes in non-Hispanic white youth: prevalence, incidence, and clinical characteristics: the SEARCH for Diabetes in Youth Study. *Diabetes Care* 32 (Suppl. 2):S102–S111, 2009

2

Natural History and Prediction of Type 1 Diabetes

Heba Ismail, MB BCh, and Carla J. Greenbaum, MD

INTRODUCTION

In the U.S., 25% of newly diagnosed patients with type 1 diabetes (T1D) present in ketoacidosis, which carries significant morbidity and even mortality, and incurs high cost.[1,2] The psychological trauma for the patient and family confronted with a startling and severe clinical presentation of an incurable disease is often overwhelming. Yet the disease process begins long before the clinical scenario described above. Moreover, the onset of clinical disease can be predicted and a diagnosis made while individuals are still asymptomatic. Someday, we hope to build on this knowledge and have treatments that will halt disease progression and prevent T1D. Until then, understanding the natural history of T1D can provide insights relevant to patients and families living with the disease. In this chapter, we will discuss how risk is determined in populations, using genetic, immunologic, and metabolic measures. In addition, we will discuss the clinical relevance of using these tests in people with diabetes.

OVERVIEW

Initial pathological specimens from those with T1D featured an absence of pancreatic β-cells and distorted islet structure. Lymphocytic infiltrates were found within the damaged islets' architecture, better known as *insulitis*. Pivotal studies have since found T1D associated with the human leukocyte antigen (HLA) genes important in the adaptive immune response.[3] The discovery of islet cell autoantibodies (ICA) in a small group of patients with polyendocrine disorders,[4] and subsequently in those with typical T1D, led to the concept of an autoimmune disease in which the adaptive immune system mistakenly identifies self (i.e., β-cells) as foreign and thus destroys the cells.

Clinical studies in T1D family members and subsequent studies in those without relatives with T1D demonstrated that the disease process starts long before clinical diagnosis. These studies led to a model of the natural history of disease (see Fig. 1.1) postulating that, over time, genetic risk combined with autoimmunity (measured as autoantibodies) led to β-cell destruction (measured as a loss of insulin secretion). In this model, a clinical diagnosis is made when insufficient insulin secretion cannot maintain glucose homeostasis, triggering hyperglycemia, and the classically described symptoms of polyuria, polydipsia, weight loss, polyphagia, and visual changes.

DOI: 10.2337/9781580404785ch02

Figure 1.1 also illustrates that autoimmune-mediated β-cell destruction continues after diagnosis. Many aspects of this model have proven remarkably accurate over the past quarter century. It is the basis for clinical studies aimed at identifying both disease etiology and those individuals at risk. Additionally, it serves as the foundation for clinical trials aimed at disease preservation and prevention (see chapters 3 and 4).

Conceptually, prediction relies upon genetic, immune, and metabolic markers, each conferring its own level of risk. Usually, individuals are first identified as being at genetic risk by virtue of having a family history or undergoing genetic typing. Those identified as being at genetic risk then undergo autoantibody testing. Those with autoantibodies are then followed with metabolic testing.

Genetic Risk

Description. The overall prevalence for T1D is about 0.3% and the risk among those with a sibling with diabetes is about 5%. Thus the proportionate increase in risk (λs) is about 15, indicating that genetic factors are important in disease (Fig. 2.1).[5] Though recent large-scale studies have identified other genetic associations such as the protein tyrosine phosphatase PTPN22 on chromosome 1, the insulin gene on chromosome 11, and many others[6], by far the strongest genetic association is with the HLA region on chromosome 6. The HLA associations are strongest with the class II region involving both HLA DRB1 and HLA DQB1.[6,7] Individuals usually inherit groups of HLA class II genes together; thus specific DR genes are often inherited with specific DQ genes. This inherited grouping is termed a haplotype.

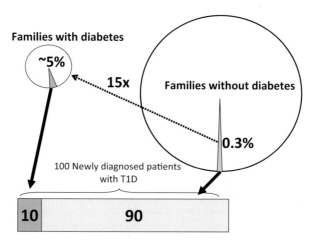

Figure 2.1 Though most individuals with T1D do not have a family member with disease, the risk for other family members is markedly increased as compared to the general population.

A common DR3 haplotype is DRB1*0301-DQA1*0501-DQB1*0201. Similarly, a common DR4 haplotype is DRB1*0401-DQA1*0301-DQB1*0302. Each individual has two haplotypes (one from each parent), which together describe the individual's genotype. Unfortunately for screening programs, HLA class II genotype is neither necessary nor sufficient for development of T1D. While 90% of T1D individuals have either HLA DR3 or HLA DR4 haplotypes, one of these high-risk DR haplotypes is also present in almost 20% of Caucasians without diabetes. About 35% of people with T1D have the genotype DR3/4 (meaning both haplotypes are present) as compared to about 2.4% of those without disease.[8]

Examining the individual HLA DR subtypes and DQ genes provides more information about risk. For example, the DR2 haplotype often carries the DQB1*0602 gene, often described as protective against T1D. Only 1% of those with T1D have this gene as compared with about 20% of the nondiabetic Caucasian population.[8] Thus, while the risk is markedly lower in individuals with this gene, it is not fully protective. Similarly, DRB1*0405 is highly associated with T1D while DRB1*0403 is not. Moreover, there appears to be a shift in HLA type in the T1D population. In concert with rising disease incidence, recent studies suggest that increasing numbers of T1D individuals have HLA class II genotypes other than DR3/4.[9–11]

Using genes to test for diabetes risk. HLA class II screening has been employed particularly in screening at-risk neonates, aimed at better understanding both the natural history and the potential triggers of the disease.[12–17] Another genetic screening approach is to limit testing to the T1D relatives for antibodies. While the vast majority of individuals with T1D have no family member with disease, having a relative with disease increases the risk about 15 fold (Fig. 2.1). Using family history as the genetic screening has the theoretical advantage that genes other than HLA that influence disease risk are likely present within a family, thus obviating the need to test for them. Recent global efforts have identified non-HLA genes associated with T1D and other autoimmune diseases. These studies provide important clues to the mechanisms underlying autoimmunity and suggest new therapeutic approaches.

While beyond the scope of this book, the concept of genetic contribution to disease is moving beyond the presence or absence of DNA-encoded genetic alleles to genetically and environmentally determined variations in the function of genes and their protein products. Technological advances now allow for studies of the transcriptome and proteinome, which assess the function of genes. New therapeutic directions will likely emerge from such studies.

Genetic testing in those with T1D. Is there a role for genetic testing once individuals have diabetes? Currently, outside the cases of monogenic diabetes (see chapter 1), clinical decisions in those diagnosed with T1D do not depend upon an individual's genetic results. It has been reported that individuals with HLA DR3/4 have more rapid β-cell deterioration compared with other HLA types, but there may be other genes that influence the variable natural history of disease postdiagnosis. Work is underway to evaluate the relationships of other genes with the rate of β-cell deterioration in T1D. Similarly, large-scale studies have identified links between immune genes and autoimmune disease and may identify individuals likely to respond to immune therapies. These advances lie in the future.

Autoantibodies

Description. Like HLA typing and family associations, autoantibodies also confer risk for T1D. Currently five diabetes-associated autoantibodies have been validated: islet cell antibodies (ICA), insulin autoantibodies (mIAA), antibodies to glutamic acid decarboxylase (GADab), antibodies to a tyrosine phosphatase (IA-2ab; also known as ICA512ab), and antibodies to the zinc transporter protein (ZnT8ab). The historical aspect of antibodies is important in order to understand their role in disease.

ICAs were the first diabetes-related autoantibodies described, being first reported in individuals with autoimmune polyendocrinopathies (T1D in combination with other autoimmune conditions such as Hashimoto's thyroiditis, Addison's disease, and others).[4] Subsequent studies noted ICAs present in about 80% of individuals with T1D at diagnosis.[18] ICAs are measured by placing the subject's serum on a cadaver pancreas and observing antibody reactivity to islet cells. Since the precise antigenic targets remain unknown and the measurement is labor intensive, it is not routinely available in clinical laboratories. However, the presence of ICA confers additional risk for development of T1D in individuals who have other antibodies. Thus, it is often still incorporated into risk assessments for clinical trials.

Soon after the description of ICA, insulin antibodies were described not only in those with T1D who were treated with insulin (and might expect to develop antibodies in response to injected protein), but also in relatives of T1D individuals who had never received insulin.[19] Insulin antibodies in those never having received insulin are termed insulin *auto*antibodies. It was the discovery of insulin and islet cell autoantibodies in individuals prior to disease onset that laid the foundations for prediction algorithms and clinical trials to prevent or delay disease onset.

Subsequent autoantibodies were described in individuals with T1D and those at risk for disease and duly subjected to validation and standardization. These include antibodies to glutamic acid decarboxylase (GAD) and protein tyrosine phosphatase (IA2 or ICA512). In early studies, about 87% of newly diagnosed individuals had ICA with or without GADabs, and 4% had GADabs alone.[20] Autoantibodies to a protein tyrosine phosphatase, originally termed ICA512 and currently named IA-2 (insulinoma-associated antigen-2), were then described and found to be present in about 32% to 75% of those clinically diagnosed with T1D, dependent on age.[21] Most recently, autoantibodies to the zinc transporter protein were described, validated, and found to be present in 60–80% of recently diagnosed subjects. It was also demonstrated that the inclusion of the ZnT8 assays to combined measurement of GADA, IA2A, and IAA reduced the number of autoantibody-negative individuals with recent T1D diagnosis from 5.8% to 1.8%.[22]

Two important practical concepts thus emerge: First, to assure validity of autoantibody testing results, the clinician should ensure that the clinical laboratory assays perform well in standardization programs by inquiring of the laboratory. Second, if all five antibodies are tested, about 2% of individuals clinically diagnosed with T1D will be autoantibody negative. If one tests only GAD and IA2, as many as 15% may be autoantibody negative. As gleaned from the progression described above, being autoantibody negative does not necessarily mean that individuals do not have immune-mediated β-cell destruction. Their immune systems may not have formed antibodies to an islet protein that we currently measure.

Antibody testing in those with T1D. After diagnosis, antibodies are known to gradually decline over time.[23] Figure 2.2 illustrates the progressive decline in IA-2, GAD, and ZnT8 (illustrated as CWCR) antibodies over time.[24] The reason is not fully understood but may be related to the disappearance of islet tissue (or antigens) over time. Thus, the absence of autoantibodies in an individual who is years from diagnosis provides no insight into the pathophysiology of that individual's disease.

Studies have indicated that having two or more antibodies or high titers is associated with more rapid loss of β-cell function after clinical diagnosis. This information may be helpful for the clinician caring for those with diabetes.[25] Distinguishing between immune-mediated (type 1) diabetes and other forms of diabetes may be challenging. There is a *population* of individuals who clinically appear to have type 2 diabetes (T2D), who possess one or more antibodies, and whose clinical course quickly deteriorates to requiring insulin for glycemic control. These characteristics define LADA (Latent Autoimmune Diabetes of Adults), or type 1.5 diabetes, which has been estimated to occur as frequently as 10% of adults with clinical T2D[26]. However, for the recently diagnosed patient who clinically appears to have T2D, a single autoantibody (usually GAD65) will occur 1–3% of the time by definition. Thus, a single antibody measured once may not be clinically meaningful. In contrast, for those with a repeatedly positive single antibody or the presence of multiple antibodies, the clinician can reliably convey that the patient will need insulin for glycemic control sooner

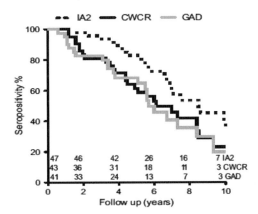

Figure 2.2 Kaplan-Meier analysis of declining autoantibody prevalence in the first 12 years of diabetes. Statistical significance was determined by the Gehan-Breslow-Wilcoxon $\chi2$ test, scored as reversion to antibody-negative status on two sequential samples. IA2A is represented by the dotted line, ZnT8 CWCR (measured with dimeric probes combining multiple epitopes) is represented by the black line, and GAD is represented by the gray line. Reproduced with permission from Wenzlau et al.[24]

rather than later. Measuring autoantibodies in clinical practice to distinguish immune-mediated from nonimmune-mediated diabetes is controversial. While there is considerable expert and clinical opinion on the matter, there is little data that the mere presence of an autoantibody should dictate care.

One Japanese pilot study randomly assigned subjects with antibody-positive T2D to early insulin treatment or oral agents and reported that the serum C-peptide response improved significantly within 6 and 12 months in the insulin group, but decreased progressively in the oral agent treatment group.[27] Moreover, intensive insulin therapy in the Diabetes Control and Complications Trial (DCCT) demonstrated both preservation of β-cell function and reduced complications in those with T1D.[28] Though the DCCT demonstrated that glycemic control was helpful in preserving β-cell function, it did not compare whether insulin therapy was better than other agents in achieving glycemic control. Both studies are often cited to support early insulin treatment in antibody-positive T2D patients.

It may be useful to identify those with immune-mediated diabetes versus T2D, so that providers will be wary of other autoimmune diseases and appropriately screen those relatives at risk for the disease. Non-insulin therapies will fail more rapidly in these individuals as compared to those without immune-mediated diabetes regardless of changes in diet and activity. Thus, the patient and practitioner need to vigilantly monitor the effect of therapies (diet, exercise, non-insulin agents) on glycemic control in such individuals. Failure to control glucose should rapidly lead to insulin therapy rather than allowing months to years of experimenting with non-insulin approaches.

Using antibodies to test for diabetes risk. Prior to clinical diagnosis, autoantibodies are extremely useful in identifying individuals at risk for T1D. Both in relatives of T1D patients as well as in the general population, having two or more antibodies conveys a 27–80% risk for clinical disease over a five-year period.[29,30] Gradations in this risk depend on the associated metabolic state as described below. In single-antibody–positive subjects, the five-year risk is less than 5% and does not appear to increase with time.[31] Moreover, recent incorporation of ZnT8Ab screening suggests that those previously thought to have one antibody who progressed to disease may have also had ZnT8abs.

Large population-based studies looking at babies identified at genetic risk due to HLA type but with no family members with disease have shown that about 2% will confirm positive for at least one autoantibody.[32,33] The frequency of autoantibodies in first- and second-degree family members not genetically typed is about 5%.[34] Interestingly, multiple studies following subjects from birth have found that insulin autoantibodies are almost always detected first with a mean age of seroconversion of about 1 year.[33,35,36] Additional autoantibodies may subsequently develop.

Though antibodies most often occur in early childhood, T1D disease onset occurs throughout adulthood, and it is estimated that up to 60% of individuals will develop disease after the age of 20 years[37]. This provides the rationale for the testing algorithm employed in the Diabetes TrialNet Pathway to Prevention study. Relatives under age 45 are tested for antibodies; those with no antibodies under the age of 18 years are retested annually. Intensive bi-yearly monitoring for diabetes development and eligibility for prevention clinical trials is limited to those with two or more antibodies, with more limited annual monitoring for those with a single antibody.

Decades of research support the use of autoantibody testing as disease predictors. The disease is not felt to be caused by autoantibodies; rather, they serve as markers that the immune system has been activated against the β-cells. Despite decades of work, we have no comparably robust measure of the other arm of the adaptive immune system, namely T-cell activation. Multiple alterations in T-cell number and function have been reported, but the reproducibility, sensitivity, and specificity of these tests are inadequate to incorporate into clinical trials or care.

The model that T1D and other autoimmune diseases are simply an imbalance in effector T or regulatory T-cells (cells that turn the immune response on or off) toward self-antigens cannot be reliably demonstrated in humans. To date, these T-cell measures have neither predictive value nor clinical relevance. Multiple explanations have been suggested for this problem. One theory is that the cells of interest are sequestered in the islet or nearby lymphoid tissue and not readily captured in circulating blood. Another idea is that the immune system is merely reacting to β-cell damage from another cause: death from suicide by the immune system rather than a homicide in response to an environmental pathogen, e.g., a virus. Recent work has also highlighted the role of inflammation in response to injury. Ongoing studies are exploring whether more sensitive measures of β-cell damage and innate immune system activity can aid in disease prediction.

Metabolic Testing

The third major tool for predicting the onset of clinical disease and understanding the clinical course is metabolic testing. This involves measurements of glycemic state or insulin secretion before or after diagnosis. With β-cell destruction as the sine qua non of the disease, a measurement of β-cell mass or function that accurately reflects the clinical picture would be ideal.

Metabolic testing to assess risk for diabetes. Prior to diagnosis, this can be done through measurement of insulin in response to IV glucose administration. The early insulin (<10 min) response after an IV glucose bolus is termed the first phase insulin release (FPIR). Antibody-positive individuals with low FPIR are at increased risk of subsequent clinical disease. Measurement of glucose or insulin during an oral glucose tolerance test with sampling at baseline and at 30, 60, 90, and 120 min provides additional information. Any abnormal glucose tolerance in antibody-positive relatives (fasting glucose >110 mg/dl; 2-h glucose >140 mg/dl; or 30, 60, or 90 min values >200 mg/dl) is strongly predictive of clinical onset, with up to 90% diagnosed with diabetes within five years.

Metabolic testing in those with T1D. After diagnosis, β-cell function is measured by C-peptide. In the pancreatic β-cell, insulin is made as pre-pro-insulin and then cleaved to pro-insulin. The final cleavage is to insulin and C-peptide (C = carboxy-terminus). C-peptide and insulin are secreted in equimolar quantities. Since insulin assays cannot distinguish between endogenous and exogenous insulin postdiagnosis, C-peptide is used as a marker of endogenous β-cell secretion in those being treated with insulin.

Measurement of β-cell function is critically dependent upon the antecedent metabolic state. For example, acute hyperglycemia will suppress insulin secretion. At diagnosis, during metabolic decompensation (hyperglycemia, metabolic acidosis, and ketosis), inflammation or glucose toxicity may lead to low insulin secretion and C-peptide levels. Once patients are stabilized on exogenous insulin, β-cell function may transiently improve as measured by increased C-peptide levels and reduced insulin requirement (*honeymoon phase*). This improvement in function does not represent new β-cells. Moreover, other evidence suggests that changes in peripheral insulin sensitivity account for the honeymoon phase. Most likely, both play a role. Regardless of the pathophysiology, many experts recommend continued insulin treatment while avoiding hypoglycemia during the honeymoon phase.

Endogenous β-cell secretion can be measured using the standard mixed meal tolerance test (MMTT). For this test, a liquid formulation of fats, carbohydrates, and protein is consumed over 5 min and C-peptide is measured at 30-min intervals for 2 or 4 h post ingestion. Under standardized conditions, including time of day and controlled exogenous insulin administration, this test is highly reproducible and suitable for clinical trial use. A C-peptide response may also be elicited by administering glucagon intravenously, known as a glucagon stimulation test (GST). Interestingly however, the C-peptide values are lower with the GST than with the MMTT, which can be partially attributed to the incretin effects of oral administration of a mixed meal.

A random C-peptide value, particularly obtained several hours after a meal, has been used in some studies.[38] This method may be helpful for large, population-based studies. However, random C-peptide values followed over time are not usually considered clinically helpful, as observing gradual changes in individual values is imprecise. Further, the absence of C-peptide in a random sample may be caused by hyperglycemia or high levels of exogenous insulin. Early studies measured 24-h urinary C-peptide levels, a process that was abandoned for many years once serum C-peptide and other tests became available. However, recent studies suggest that urinary C-peptide may provide useful qualitative information in those with diabetes and with a method that is noninvasive.[39] Work in this area is ongoing.

In recent years, some clinicians have measured C-peptide levels in order to distinguish the different diabetes types at the time of diagnosis. It is often unappreciated that many individuals with T1D will have significant amounts of C-peptide, representing residual β-cell function. The standard teaching that T1D is defined as complete absence of β-cells is inaccurate and is a disservice to both patients and providers. We know that at onset and within the first year of diagnosis, one-third of youth with antibody-positive diabetes have C-peptide values in the normal range of healthy adolescents.[40] Moreover, it is not uncommon for those with longstanding T1D to have clinically significant and detectable levels of C-peptide years after diagnosis.[41] The DCCT demonstrated that intensively treated subjects who had residual insulin secretion (as measured by C-peptide response to a mixed meal) >0.2 nmol/L had less hypoglycemia and fewer complications than those with comparable glycemic control but without endogenous secretion.[28] This level is therefore thought to be clinically significant or meaningful. We do not yet know whether even higher levels would result in better clinical outcomes.

In a recent analysis of those in the placebo and control arms of clinical trials to preserve β-cell function, two-thirds of individuals had clinically significant β-cell function at 2 years from diagnosis and 93% had detectable C-peptide levels.[42] Moreover, among 411 participants in the Joslin Medalists study (those with T1D ≥50 years), 67.4% still had detectable C-peptide.[43] Thus, while an absent C-peptide level under properly conducted conditions does indicate absence of β-cell activity, the presence of C-peptide should not exclude the diagnosis of ongoing immune mediated β-cell destruction.

Should C-peptide thus be measured in clinical practice? Like measuring antibodies, this area is controversial. C-peptide presence can be reassuring, but hypo- and hyperglycemia, including diabetic ketoacidosis (DKA), may still occur in a given individual. The C-peptide trend over time may help inform patients of their progressing disease, but in the absence of therapies to preserve β-cell function, this information is unlikely to affect therapeutic approaches.

The current definition of diabetes depends upon glucose values. The American Diabetes Association (ADA) defines diabetes as fasting values of ≥126 mg/dl or 2-h postprandial values of ≥200 mg/dl. The current definitions come from epidemiologic studies that noted inflection points for development of complications in T2D subjects.[44] It is now known that disease progression in T1D involves progressively abnormal postprandial glucose tolerance while fasting glucose values remain relatively stable. Using the ADA definition of diabetes onset, over time, many individuals meet the criteria at a time when they have no symptoms, have normal A1C (indicative of average blood glucose values over the past 2–3 months), and normal fasting glucose but cross the threshold of 200 mg/dl on an OGTT. Hyperglycemic symptoms do not generally occur until individuals have increased fasting glucose. At that point, most will also have an abnormal A1C. Thus, the recent ADA guideline that allows for abnormal A1C as a diagnostic criterion is a very insensitive measure of diabetic glucose tolerance in those on the path for T1D. Defining the onset of T1D by a threshold of glucose is not rooted in science in this population. As with many definitions, the diagnostic threshold should depend on the reason one is creating the definition. To take an extreme case, since essentially all individuals with two confirmed autoantibodies will likely eventually progress to overt clinical disease, perhaps two confirmed autoantibodies should define T1D onset. Sliding further through progression of disease, the presence of abnormal glucose tolerance in antibody-positive individuals could be a definition point for disease onset. The opposite extreme could be to use an abnormal A1C to define disease. As noted above, this would leave a group of individuals with diabetic glucose tolerance and normal A1C values. Most investigators prefer an earlier diagnosis as it may prevent the disease symptoms and the potential morbidity and (rarely) mortality.

More challenging is the treatment for those individuals with silent T1D, those with asymptomatic diabetic oral glucose tolerance tests (OGTTs). Since diabetes treatment guidelines are targeted at an A1C <7% for adolescents and adults, the treatment goal for those with a normal A1C is to prevent individuals from developing metabolic dysregulation and to reduce β-cell demand by providing exogenous insulin. For those with early T1D, expert opinion (i.e., not data driven) recommends either low doses of basal insulin to prevent DKA or prandial insulin to prevent postprandial hyperglycemia. Concerns regarding hypoglycemia are largely unfounded because individuals tolerate these regimens well. Moreover, this approach allows for individuals to learn about the relationship of glucose levels with meals and activities, as well as how to monitor glucose and administer insulin.

CONCLUSION

In conclusion, we can predict T1D onset through measurement of antibodies, and through genetic and metabolic testing. Clinicians should inform individuals that such testing is available for their family members through clinical trials. The use of these measures in those with overt diabetes is controversial and the thoughtful clinician should be aware of the limitations of these measures for individual patients.

REFERENCE LIST

1. Maldonado MR, Chong ER, Oehl MA, Balasubramanyam A: Economic impact of diabetic ketoacidosis in a multiethnic indigent population: analysis of costs based on the precipitating cause. *Diabetes Care* 26:1265–1269, 2003
2. Rewers A, Klingensmith G, Davis C, Petitti DB, Pihoker C, Rodriguez B, Schwartz ID, Imperatore G, Williams D, Dolan LM, Dabelea D: Presence of diabetic ketoacidosis at diagnosis of diabetes mellitus in youth: the SEARCH for Diabetes in Youth Study. *Pediatrics* 121:e1258–e1266, 2008
3. Cudworth AG, Woodrow JC: HL-A system and diabetes mellitus. *Diabetes* 24:345–349, 1975
4. Bottazzo GF, Florin-Christensen A, Doniach D: Islet-cell antibodies in diabetes mellitus with autoimmune polyendocrine deficiencies. *Lancet* 2:1279–1283, 1974
5. Risch N: Assessing the role of HLA-linked and unlinked determinants of disease. *Am J Hum Genet* 40:1–14, 1987
6. Concannon P, Rich SS, Nepom GT: Genetics of type 1A diabetes. *N Engl J Med* 360:1646–1654, 2009
7. Sheehy MJ, Scharf SJ, Rowe JR, Neme de Gimenez MH, Meske LM, Erlich HA, Nepom BS: A diabetes-susceptible HLA haplotype is best defined by a combination of HLA-DR and -DQ alleles. *J Clin Invest* 83:830–835, 1989
8. Redondo MJ, Eisenbarth GS: Genetic control of autoimmunity in type I diabetes and associated disorders. *Diabetologia* 45:605–622, 2002
9. Varney MD, Valdes AM, Carlson JA, Noble JA, Tait BD, Bonella P, Lavant E, Fear AL, Louey A, Moonsamy P, Mychaleckyj JC, Erlich H: HLA DPA1, DPB1 alleles and haplotypes contribute to the risk associated with type 1 diabetes: analysis of the type 1 diabetes genetics consortium families. *Diabetes* 59:2055–2062, 2010
10. Gillespie KM, Bain SC, Barnett AH, Bingley PJ, Christie MR, Gill GV, Gale EA: The rising incidence of childhood type 1 diabetes and reduced contribution of high-risk HLA haplotypes. *Lancet* 364:1699–1700, 2004
11. Fourlanos S, Varney MD, Tait BD, Morahan G, Honeyman MC, Colman PG, Harrison LC: The rising incidence of type 1 diabetes is accounted for

by cases with lower-risk human leukocyte antigen genotypes. *Diabetes Care* 31:1546–1549, 2008

12. The Environmental Determinants of Diabetes in the Young (TEDDY) Study. *Ann N Y Acad Sci* 1150:1–13, 2008
13. Barker JM, Goehrig SH, Barriga K, Hoffman M, Slover R, Eisenbarth GS, Norris JM, Klingensmith GJ, Rewers M: Clinical characteristics of children diagnosed with type 1 diabetes through intensive screening and follow-up. *Diabetes Care* 27:1399–1404, 2004
14. Gullstrand C, Wahlberg J, Ilonen J, Vaarala O, Ludvigsson J: Progression to type 1 diabetes and autoantibody positivity in relation to HLA-risk genotypes in children participating in the ABIS study. *Pediatr Diabetes* 9:182–190, 2008
15. Hummel M, Bonifacio E, Schmid S, Walter M, Knopff A, Ziegler AG: Brief communication: early appearance of islet autoantibodies predicts childhood type 1 diabetes in offspring of diabetic parents. *Ann Intern Med* 140:882–886, 2004
16. Kukko M, Virtanen SM, Toivonen A, Simell S, Korhonen S, Ilonen J, Simel O, Knip M: Geographical variation in risk HLA-DQB1 genotypes for type 1 diabetes and signs of beta-cell autoimmunity in a high-incidence country. *Diabetes Care* 27:676–681, 2004
17. Walter M, Albert E, Conrad M, Keller E, Hummel M, Ferber K, Barratt BJ, Todd JA, Ziegler AG, Bonifacio E: IDDM2/insulin VNTR modifies risk conferred by IDDM1/HLA for development of Type 1 diabetes and associated autoimmunity. *Diabetologia* 46:712–720, 2003
18. Irvine WJ, McCallum CJ, Gray RS, Campbell CJ, Duncan LJ, Farquhar JW, Vaughan H, Morris PJ: Pancreatic islet-cell antibodies in diabetes mellitus correlated with the duration and type of diabetes, coexistent autoimmune disease, and HLA type. *Diabetes* 26:138–147, 1977
19. Palmer J, Asplin C, Clemons P: Insulin autoantibodies in insulin-dependent diabetes before insulin treatment. *Science* 222:1337–1339, 1983
20. Borg H, Fernlund P, Sundkvist G: Protein tyrosine phosphatase-like protein IA2-antibodies plus glutamic acid decarboxylase 65 antibodies (GADA) indicates autoimmunity as frequently as islet cell antibodies assay in children with recently diagnosed diabetes mellitus. *Clin Chem* 43:2358–2363, 1997
21. Winter W, Harris N, Schatz D: Immunological markers in the diagnosis and prediction of autoimmune type 1a diabetes. *Clin Diabetes* 20:183–191, 2002
22. Wenzlau JM, Juhl K, Yu L, Moua O, Sarkar SA, Gottlieb P, Rewers M, Eisenbarth GS, Jensen J, Davidson HW, Hutton JC: The cation efflux transporter ZnT8 (Slc30A8) is a major autoantigen in human type 1 diabetes. *Proc Natl Acad Sci U S A* 104:17040–17045, 2007
23. Tridgell DM, Spiekerman C, Wang RS, Greenbaum CJ: Interaction of onset and duration of diabetes on the percent of GAD and IA-2 antibody-positive subjects in the type 1 diabetes genetics consortium database. *Diabetes Care* 34:988–993, 2011
24. Wenzlau JM, Walter M, Gardner TJ, Frisch LM, Yu L, Eisenbarth GS, Ziegler AG, Davidson HW, Hutton JC: Kinetics of the post-onset decline in zinc transporter 8 autoantibodies in type 1 diabetic human subjects. *J Clin Endocrinol Metab* 95:4712–4719, 2010

25. Borg H, Gottsater A, Fernlund P, Sundkvist G: A 12-year prospective study of the relationship between islet antibodies and beta-cell function at and after the diagnosis in patients with adult-onset diabetes. *Diabetes* 51:1754–1762, 2002

26. Palmer JP, Hampe CS, Chiu H, Goel A, Brooks-Worrell BM: Is latent autoimmune diabetes in adults distinct from type 1 diabetes or just type 1 diabetes at an older age? *Diabetes* 54 Suppl 2:S62–S67, 2005

27. Kobayashi T, Nakanishi K, Murase T, Kosaka K: Small doses of subcutaneous insulin as a strategy for preventing slowly progressive beta-cell failure in islet cell antibody-positive patients with clinical features of NIDDM. *Diabetes* 45:622–626, 1996

28. Steffes MW, Sibley S, Jackson M, Thomas W: Beta-cell function and the development of diabetes-related complications in the diabetes control and complications trial. *Diabetes Care* 26:832–836, 2003

29. Verge CF, Gianani R, Kawasaki E, Yu L, Pietropaolo M, Jackson RA, Chase HP, Eisenbarth GS: Prediction of type I diabetes in first-degree relatives using a combination of insulin, GAD, and ICA512bdc/IA-2 autoantibodies. *Diabetes* 45:926–933, 1996

30. Bingley PJ, Bonifacio E, Williams AJ, Genovese S, Bottazzo GF, Gale EA: Prediction of IDDM in the general population: strategies based on combinations of autoantibody markers. *Diabetes* 46:1701–1710, 1997

31. Orban T, Sosenko JM, Cuthbertson D, Krischer JP, Skyler JS, Jackson R, Yu L, Palmer JP, Schatz D, Eisenbarth G: Pancreatic islet autoantibodies as predictors of type 1 diabetes in the Diabetes Prevention Trial-Type 1. *Diabetes Care* 32:2269–2274, 2009

32. Yu J, Yu L, Bugawan TL, Erlich HA, Barriga K, Hoffman M, Rewers M, Eisenbarth GS: Transient antiislet autoantibodies: infrequent occurrence and lack of association with "genetic" risk factors. *J Clin Endocrinol Metab* 85:2421–2428, 2000

33. Kimpimaki T, Kulmala P, Savola K, Kupila A, Korhonen S, Simell T, Ilonen J, Simell O, Knip M: Natural history of beta-cell autoimmunity in young children with increased genetic susceptibility to type 1 diabetes recruited from the general population. *J Clin Endocrinol Metab* 87:4572–4579, 2002

34. Krischer JP, Cuthbertson DD, Yu L, Orban T, Maclaren N, Jackson R, Winter WE, Schatz DA, Palmer JP, Eisenbarth GS: Screening strategies for the identification of multiple antibody-positive relatives of individuals with type 1 diabetes. *J Clin Endocrinol Metab* 88:103–108, 2003

35. Ziegler AG, Hummel M, Schenker M, Bonifacio E: Autoantibody appearance and risk for development of childhood diabetes in offspring of parents with type 1 diabetes: the 2-year analysis of the German BABYDIAB study. *Diabetes* 48:460–468, 1999

36. Kimpimaki T, Kupila A, Hamalainen AM, Kukko M, Kulmala P, Savola K, Simell T, Keskinen P, Ilonen J, Simell O, Knip M: The first signs of beta-cell autoimmunity appear in infancy in genetically susceptible children from the general population: the Finnish Type 1 Diabetes Prediction and Prevention Study. *J Clin Endocrinol Metab* 86:4782–4788, 2001

37. Rewers M, Norris J, Kretowski A: Epidemiology of Type I Diabetes *in* Type 1 Diabetes: Cellular, Molecular and Clinical Immunology [article online], 2010. Available from http://www.barbaradaviscenter.org/. Accessed 9 July 2012

38. Berger B, Stenstrom G, Sundkvist G: Random C-peptide in the classification of diabetes. *Scand J Clin Lab Invest* 60:687–693, 2000

39. Besser RE, Ludvigsson J, Jones AG, McDonald TJ, Shields BM, Knight BA, Hattersley AT: Urine C-peptide creatinine ratio is a noninvasive alternative to the mixed-meal tolerance test in children and adults with type 1 diabetes. *Diabetes Care* 34:607–609, 2011

40. Greenbaum CJ, Anderson AM, Dolan LM, Mayer-Davis EJ, Dabelea D, Imperatore G, Marcovina S, Pihoker C: Preservation of beta-cell function in autoantibody-positive youth with diabetes. *Diabetes Care* 32:1839–1844, 2009

41. Wang L, Lovejoy NF, Faustman DL: Persistence of prolonged C-peptide production in type 1 diabetes as measured with an ultrasensitive C-peptide assay. *Diabetes Care* 35:465–470, 2012

42. Greenbaum CJ, Beam CA, Boulware D, Gitelman SE, Gottlieb PA, Herold KC, Lachin JM, McGee P, Palmer JP, Pescovitz MD, Krause-Steinrauf H, Skyler J, Sosenko JM: Fall in C-peptide during first 2 years from diagnosis: evidence of at least two distinct phases from Composite TrialNet data. *Diabetes* 61:2066–2073, 2012

43. Keenan HA, Sun JK, Levine J, Doria A, Aiello LP, Eisenbarth G, Bonner-Weir S, King GL: Residual insulin production and pancreatic beta-cell turnover after 50 years of diabetes: Joslin Medalist Study. *Diabetes* 59:2846–2853, 2010

44. Report of the expert committee on the diagnosis and classification of diabetes mellitus. *Diabetes Care* 26 Suppl 1:S5–S20, 2003

45. Eisenbarth G: Chapter 11. Prediction of type 1A diabetes: the natural history of the prediabetic period *in* Type 1 Diabetes: Cellular, Molecular and Clinical Immunology [article online], 2012. Available from http://www.barbaradaviscenter.org/. Accessed 9 July 2012

3

Interdiction: Prevention of β-cell Destruction and Preservation for Those with Existing Type 1 Diabetes

Jane Lee Chiang, MD, and Stephen E. Gitelman, MD

INTRODUCTION

Current therapies and technologies offer a means to live with type 1 diabetes (T1D), but daily management remains imperfect and tedious. To avoid long-term complications from diabetes, individuals must maintain near normal glycemic control. Recapitulating the critical function of the β-cell, namely a closed-loop system in which glucose sensing is tethered to insulin delivery, has yet to be achieved. Thus, the definitive treatment for T1D is to insure that the necessary functional β-cell mass remains. In theory, one could intervene at three different places in the course of T1D to effect a cure:

1. *Prevention*, before the development of diabetes
2. *Preservation*, after the diagnosis, while functional β-cells remain
3. *β-Cell replacement*, for those with preexisting diabetes for an extended period of time and who have no endogenous β-cell function (see chapter 4)

There are important philosophical issues to consider for intervention at each of these stages. In designing such studies, investigators are mindful that T1D is very different from a life-threatening condition such as cancer and therefore must carefully balance the potential risks of the proposed therapy vs. possible benefits. Promising efforts are now underway at all three of these stages, and will be discussed in further detail herein (see chapter 1, Figure 1.1, Natural history of diabetes).

I. RESEARCH CONSIDERATIONS

General

T1D may occur at any age, but children are at highest risk (see chapter 1) and may have a more rapid process of β-cell destruction than found in adults. However, due to potential safety concerns, the Food and Drug Administration (FDA) often mandates that clinical studies start in adults or older youth, unless there is past experience with the proposed therapeutic in a younger age-group. Clinical

DOI: 10.2337/9781580404785ch03

studies may proceed in progressively younger age-groups upon an acceptable safety review and approval from regulatory authorities. However, the studies often require long recruitment times, and ultimately many trials may not be conducted in the youngest age-groups due to lack of efficacy in the older cohorts, presence of safety signals, or feasibility. A lack of efficacy in adults could lead to dismissal of possible therapies that could benefit children, the highest-risk population.

Study End Points

One limitation has been defining early surrogate markers that predict long-term, clinically meaningful end points. The pancreas is inaccessible to routine biopsy, and thus there is no direct means to visualize islets. Currently, there is no imaging modality for routine clinical use nor surrogate immunological measures that correlate with preservation of β-cell mass. Most new-onset trials rely on a stimulated measure of endogenous insulin production as the primary measure, such as response to a mixed-meal tolerance test with C-peptide area under the curve (AUC) at 2 or 4 h.[1] This outcome reflects β-cell function, and may not necessarily correlate with β-cell mass. Others have adopted a composite end point that may have more robust clinical significance, such as A1C <6.5% coupled with <0.5 units/kg/day of exogenous insulin.[2] For prevention trials, the primary outcome may be development of autoantibodies, or change in metabolism, from euglycemia to impaired glucose tolerance or progression to frank diabetes.

Animal Models

Preclinical models of T1D are very limited, with greatest reliance on the nonobese diabetic (NOD) mouse.[3] Agents that have demonstrated efficacy in preclinical models of T1D, such as the NOD mouse, have often been considered for clinical trials. Over 300 agents have been shown to prevent T1D in the NOD mouse, but such results have generally not translated to man. Thus, there has been widespread criticism of this model as a means of informing investigators about potential therapies in humans. Further thought may need to be given for the particular agent under consideration, such as dose, the timing, and protocols used in humans. Of note, a handful of agents have even more robust effects and can actually reverse T1D in the NOD mouse. These very drugs are, in general, the ones that have shown greatest promise in humans, but durable clinical remissions have remained elusive. In addition, certain drugs, such as monoclonal antibodies, cannot be evaluated in animal models. Thus, investigators must also draw on clinical experiences in other settings, such as transplantation or other autoimmune conditions, to find other potential agents that could be applied to T1D.

What To Target?

Since T1D results from T-cell–mediated destruction of β-cells, the goal has been to identify therapies that target T-cells (see Figure 3.1 and chapter 2). Therapeutics may be subdivided into several broad categories based on their intended targets, including: *1) antigen-based therapies*, such as insulin or glutamate

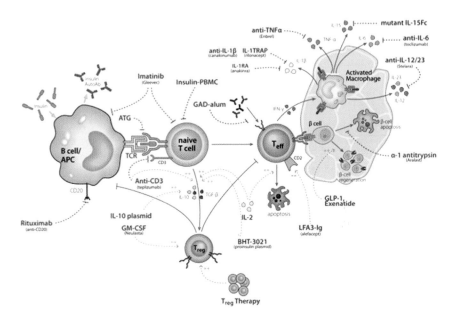

Figure 3.1 Overview of the current understanding of pathogenesis of T1D pathogenesis, highlighting a number of key pathways that are being targeted by current therapeutics. Source: Matthews JB, Staeva TP, Bernstein PL, Peakman M, Von Herrath M: ITN-JDRF Type 1 Diabetes Combination Therapy Assessment Group: Developing combination immunotherapies for type 1 diabetes: recommendations from the ITN–JDRF Type 1 Diabetes Combination Therapy Assessment Group. *Clin Exp Immunol* 160:176–184, 2010. Reprinted with permission from the publisher.

decarboxylase (GAD); *2) anti-inflammatory agents*, including docosahexaenoic acid (DHA), nicotinamide, α-1-anti-trypsin, and interleukin 1-blockade; and *3) immunosuppressants or immunomodulators*, such as anti-CD3 monoclonal antibody (mAb) and CTLA4 Ig. Preferably, the therapy would be tolerizing, meaning that it could be given for a brief period of time and withdrawn and have fundamentally changed the immune system so that continuous therapy is not needed. In addition to blocking the immune destruction, one would ideally *4) enhance β-cell repair and regeneration*. Specific growth factors for β-cells have proven elusive, although there have been suggestions that islet neogenesis-associated peptide and GLP-1 agonists and DPP-IV inhibitors may have salutary effects.

II. PREVENTION

In order to prevent disease, one must have an effective means to determine risk for T1D. As noted in chapter 2, a combination of immunologic, genetic, and metabolic indices can be used to assess risk. Prevention efforts can be broadly divided into those that serve as a means for *primary prevention* (those with underlying genetic risk but before the onset of autoimmunity) and *secondary prevention* (after autoimmunity has been detected but before the onset of clinical disease).

PRIMARY PREVENTION

The goal at this stage is to distinguish higher-risk subjects from the general population, and offer a therapy that will prevent progression to autoimmune destruction, and frank T1D. The challenge posed by studies at this level is that one has less predictive power in identifying individuals who will eventually develop diabetes, and thus one must conduct larger trials. Further, if diabetes occurs, the progression often happens over a long time period, sometimes 5–10 years or more, thereby necessitating longer trials. Individuals recruited for primary prevention trials are now targeted early in life, in some cases during pregnancy or in the newborn period, and are from families with an index case of T1D or with high-risk HLA haplotypes associated with T1D, or both. Because of the protracted timeline needed to follow such individuals to T1D onset, investigators may utilize a surrogate end point, such as the development of one or more β-cell autoantibodies, rather than T1D development. Nonetheless, the benefit of early intervention is that a less intense approach may prevent disease, as opposed to more aggressive interventions undoubtedly necessary to interdict autoimmune destruction later in the disease process. Given the nature of primary prevention studies, with large subject numbers, requisite long-term follow-up, and attendant expense, such studies are rarely undertaken. Fully powered studies are usually not initiated until a pilot study demonstrates safety and tolerability, feasibility and perhaps a hint of efficacy.

Trial to Reduce IDDM in the Genetically at Risk (TRIGR)

Animal studies and epidemiological evidence suggests that lack of breast-feeding, shorter breast-feeding duration, or early exposure to cow's milk may increase risk for β-cell autoimmunity. Postulated mechanisms include reduced gut inflammation, enhanced permeability to autoantigens, changes in regulatory T-cells (Tregs) in the lymphoid tissue lining the gut, modified gut microflora, or some combination thereof. A Finnish pilot study of infants with a high-risk HLA haplotype and a first-degree relative with T1D showed that weaning to a highly hydrolyzed formula was associated with ~50% risk reduction in development of 1 or more β-cell autoantibodies, as compared to those randomized to conventional cow's milk formula.[4]

TRIGR is a fully powered study that will definitively address this question.[5] This trial is an ongoing primary intervention study that is now fully enrolled. It is designed to determine if supplementation of breast-feeding with a highly hydrolyzed milk formula (Nutramigen) and, in the first 6–8 months of life, avoidance of foods containing bovine protein will decrease the cumulative incidence of islet-related autoantibodies, as opposed to those who are supplemented with usual cow's milk formula. The targeted population is newborns with a first-degree relative with T1D and a high-risk HLA haplotype. They will be followed until 10 years of age. The primary end point is T1D development. Secondary end points are diabetes associated islet antibodies (NCT00179777). If effective, this approach could then be tested in the general population, and could be adapted on a wider scale as a public health measure to lower T1D risk. The beauty of such an approach is that, if effective, it confers absolutely no risk, would be easy to implement, and a simple intervention early in life could have a huge impact on the general population.

Nutritional Intervention Program (NIP)

TrialNet conducted the Nutritional Intervention Program (NIP), evaluating if docosahexaenoic acid (DHA) (NCT00333554) in genetically at-risk newborns could prevent islet autoimmunity. The study was based on epidemiological evidence that a diet rich in omega-3 fatty acid and vitamin D lowers autoimmunity risk. Secular trends indicate that, over time, less DHA is being consumed. This randomized, placebo-controlled pilot study enrolled pregnant mothers and infants. The eligible subjects were required to have a first-degree relative with T1D and a high-risk HLA haplotype. Infants were supplemented with DHA until 36 months of age. Analysis of results and long-term follow-up are ongoing.

BABYDIET

The BABYDIET group conducted a pilot study to determine the effects of gluten avoidance on autoimmunity in infants of first-degree relatives with T1D (NCT01115621).[6] This study was based on both encouraging data from mouse models as well as human epidemiological studies linking age of gluten exposure with islet autoimmunity development. Delaying gluten exposure to 12 months of age did not reduce islet autoimmunity, but the study was not powered for efficacy, and compliance was problematic with this open-label study design.

Vitamin D

Interest also lies in vitamin D supplementation as a primary intervention. Aside from its effects on calcium and bone metabolism, vitamin D mediates many aspects of the immune response. Animal studies and epidemiological findings, particularly in pregnant women and infants deficient in vitamin D, support its role in ameliorating autoimmunity.[7] A case-controlled study aimed at early intervention found that in pregnant women the odds of T1D were more than twofold higher for the offspring of women with the lowest levels of 25-hydroxy-vitamin D versus those with levels above the upper quartile.[8] Clinical trials with vitamin D supplementation in recent onset T1D have not demonstrated efficacy. However, vitamin D may need to be administered earlier in the disease process, or the therapeutic dose for inducing a change in the immune response may need to be significantly higher than that for calcium and bone effects, or both. Further studies are underway in animal models with novel analogs that may have immunomodulatory effects without the effects on calcium and bone. While a randomized intervention trial is needed, these data suggest that enhancing maternal 25-hydroxy-vitamin D during pregnancy may be beneficial.

SECONDARY PREVENTION

Secondary prevention trials attempt to prevent progression to diabetes in those with evidence of autoimmunity, but without T1D. As noted in chapter 2, those with a single autoantibody are very unlikely to progress to T1D, whereas those with a greater number of autoantibodies, and higher titers, have progressively increased risk, starting from a 25–50% risk of developing T1D in the next 5 years.[9,10] Those who also exhibit altered glucose metabolism (e.g., low first-phase insulin secretion on an intravenous glucose tolerance test [IVGTT] or abnormalities on an oral glucose tolerance test [OGTT]) are at highest risk, >50%, for developing T1D in the ensuing 5 years. From the OGTT results, the DPT-1 study group and Trial-Net have defined an at-risk population with dysglycemia, referring to any one of the following: impaired fasting glucose or impaired 120-min glucose, as defined by American Diabetes Association criteria, or an intervening glucose on a 2-h OGTT >200 mg/dl. In general, secondary prevention trials are not as long or as large as primary prevention studies. However, they still require a significant effort by a well-funded network to screen, enroll, and follow enough subjects over a sufficient time period to evaluate the agent.

Given that these are prevention trials, investigators search for therapies that offer promise but do not pose significant risk for subjects. Such risks could include adverse side effects or toxicities, or possibly accelerating disease progression. The trials to date have primarily utilized antigen based or anti-inflammatory approaches, rather than immunosuppressive therapies. The Diabetes Prevention Trial-1, European Nicotinamide Diabetes Intervention Trial, and Finnish intranasal insulin prevention trial discussed in detail below represent signature efforts for T1D secondary prevention.[9,11-13]

Antigen-Based Therapies

Diabetes prevention trial–type 1 (DPT-1). Insulin is one of the primary antigens initially recognized by the immune system in T1D. NOD mice and early human pilot studies have suggested that exogenous insulin may alter disease course. DPT-1 was a randomized, controlled, nonblinded North American effort to determine if insulin exposure could prevent or delay T1D onset.[9,11] The study was notable for establishing a collaborative network throughout North America to efficiently screen a large number of subjects and for identifying an algorithm that identified an intermediate and high-risk cohort.

The DPT-1 study group screened ~100,000 first-degree relatives for the presence of β-cell autoantibodies. The antibody-positive subjects were subdivided into two arms: a high-risk group (>50% chance of developing T1D in the next 5 years), who were islet cell autoantibody (ICA) positive with abnormal β-cell function (e.g., low first-phase insulin secretion on IVGTT or dysglycemia on an OGTT); and an intermediate-risk group (25–50% risk of developing T1D in 5 years), with ICA and insulin autoantibodies present.

In a randomized, controlled, nonblinded trial, subjects in the high-risk group received parenteral insulin, with low-dose daily subcutaneous ultralente insulin and 4 days of intravenous insulin annually.[9] The therapy was safe but not effective in preventing progression to T1D. Possible reasons for study failure include the late stage at which the therapy was offered, and the dosing scheme (limited by hypoglycemia risk at higher insulin doses).

Subjects in the intermediate-risk group participated in a randomized, double-blinded, placebo-controlled trial with oral insulin.[11] The primary analysis showed that oral insulin did not delay progression to T1D. However, in a secondary post-hoc analysis, subjects with higher baseline insulin autoantibody titers appeared to have a statistically significant delay in the onset of T1D, by ~4.5 years with an IAA titer ≥80 nU/ml, and a 10-year delay with an IAA titer >300 nU/ml. Furthermore, the hazard rate for diabetes progression increased after cessation of therapy and approximated the rate in the placebo group, further suggesting that therapy was efficacious but that ongoing therapy may be needed.[14] A follow-up confirmatory study with oral insulin is ongoing in Trial-Net (NCT00419562). As a further extension of these efforts, the JDRF-funded POINT trial (Primary Oral/Intranasal INsulin Trial) is a randomized, placebo-controlled, multicentered, dose-finding study that will evaluate the optimal oral insulin dose in a primary intervention study, rather than as a secondary effort as described within TrialNet.[15] The hypothesis is that an even earlier exposure to antigen, prior to the initiation of autoimmunity, will have even greater efficacy in T1D prevention.

Type 1 Diabetes Prediction and Prevention Study (DIPP). DIPP was a randomized, double-blinded, placebo-controlled study evaluating the efficacy of intranasal insulin in children from the general population with high-risk genotypes and ≥2 autoantibodies (NCT00223613).[13] As in DPT-1, >100,000 children were screened, eventually identifying 264 at-risk individuals. In those with HLA susceptibility to T1D, intranasal insulin administered soon after detection of autoantibodies did not prevent or delay T1D.[13] The findings may be due to inadequate antigen dose, the method for antigen presentation, or the stage at which it was introduced.

Australian investigators have also evaluated intranasal insulin effects, initially in new-onset T1D adults. They found that it did not retard loss of residual β-cell function but noted that the treatment may induce tolerance, at least to exogenous insulin.[16] They have since launched a phase II prevention trial in first-degree relatives with ≥2 autoantibodies, Intranasal Insulin Trial II (INIT II) (NCT00336674).

Anti-Inflammatory Agents

European Nicotinamide Diabetes Intervention Trial (ENDIT). Like DPT-1, ENDIT represented a concerted European effort to screen over 30,000 individuals to identify first-degree relatives with autoantibodies and normal β-cell function.[12] Investigators enrolled subjects in a randomized, double-blinded, placebo-controlled trial. Rather than an antigen-based approach, the trial evaluated nicotinamide, which has demonstrated efficacy in T1D animal models and in smaller pilot studies. Nicotinamide presumably acts as a scavenger of free radicals and is postulated to prevent β-cell destruction.[17] Nicotinamide had a favorable safety profile but failed to document an effect, possibly due to insufficient doses, its use at a later stage in autoimmune destruction, or its inability to effectively block autoimmunity.

Immunosuppressants

Anti-CD3: Teplizumab. TrialNet has recently launched a study utilizing an immunosuppressant, teplizumab, a mAb directed against the CD3 portion of the T-cell receptor, for the highest-risk members of the prevention group, with ≥2 autoantibodies and dysglycemia (see Preservation section). This approach has shown early initial success in new-onset T1D trials. Subjects in this risk category are considered to be one step upstream from T1D, and the hypothesis is that earlier intervention may result in even greater efficacy than seen with this agent in new-onset T1D (NCT01030861).

Future Considerations

In the preceding decades, investigators have clearly delineated algorithms to identify populations at risk for T1D. Much of this work has centered on first-degree relatives, yet the majority of new-onset T1D cases occurs in families without a positive family history. At some point investigators will need to shift the focus to the general population. Initial screening to identify high-risk genotypes, as done by the Finnish study group in the intranasal insulin prevention trial, is a means to identify this higher-risk population, although more diverse populations like the U.S. may require additional modifications for race and ethnicity.[13,18]

There is a high hurdle for conducting T1D prevention trials. Earlier interventions may have the greatest chance to prevent T1D development. However, predicting disease requires conducting larger trials over longer time periods. Therefore, it is critical to ascertain, prior to study initiation, that the time and expense are warranted. Toward that end, one would expect to see preclinical studies and pilot studies that indicate convincing rationale in both safety and feasibility, although as noted from past trials, there is no guarantee of success.

The next iteration may require a different tack, with smaller trials utilizing surrogate measures as an end point rather than using T1D onset. The benefits include reducing trial size and time required to evaluate a particular therapy. These measures may be tailored to a particular therapy, such as an immunologic change that is predicted to lower disease risk. Studies have defined a risk score from DPT-1 data incorporating body mass index (BMI), age, fasting, and stimulated C-peptide from 2-h OGTT that may also be useful in evaluating incremental change before progression to overt T1D.[19,20] Further analysis from the TrialNet natural history study may define possible intermediate end points that could be employed for early prevention trials, reducing sample size and trial time (Krischer, *Diabetologia*, under review). Two-year changes in A1C and C-peptide from baseline, along with progression to abnormal OGTT and dysglycemia all appear to be promising. Changes in autoantibody status (such as number of antibodies, the particular antibody profile present, and titer) may also be helpful in marking progression along the continuum toward T1D. Surrogate measures that reflect other changes in immunological status, such as changes in T-cells, have proven elusive to date.

The other notable feature of prevention trials is that they have employed a single arm vs. comparison to a placebo or control group. Future studies may benefit from multiple arms, testing a range of doses for a particular agent, or evaluating a variety of other agents while all utilizing a single control group. The studies may benefit from incorporation of an adaptive or factorial trial design.

New Approaches for T1D Prevention

Those therapies that have proven safe and effective in new-onset T1D are obvious and logical considerations for use just upstream for those at high risk for developing T1D, such as the anti-CD3 mAb. For these reasons, CTLA4 Ig (Abatacept) is also being considered for use in a prevention trial. However, those agents that have not proven effective in new-onset T1D may still be worth considering for use earlier in the autoimmune process, as has been the case with oral insulin. Furthermore, not all therapeutics to be considered for diabetes prevention need to be necessarily evaluated first in new-onset T1D, although use in those with recent-onset or established diabetes may help determine if there are any unique safety or tolerability issues in this particular disease.

Antigen-based therapies will continue to be carefully considered for prevention trials. The challenge with antigen-based therapies lies in optimizing the administration route, dosing frequency, and adjuvant use; selecting the best antigen(s); and determining the best intervention time in the disease process. In evaluating insulin, for example, parenteral, oral, and intranasal, exposure has been utilized, and consideration has been given not only to the whole processed molecule, but also to proinsulin, B-chain, and peptide fragments that are considered to be of greatest relevance in the autoimmune response. Some of the groundwork has been laid in new onset trials. For example, insulin B-chain in incomplete Freund's adjuvant (IFA) and administered intramuscularly may induce a regulatory T-cell population (NCT00057499).[21] The safety and efficacy of a proinsulin DNA vaccine in T1D, with an intramuscular injection of a plasmid carrying proinsulin (NCT00453375), has been evaluated. Finally, investigators have identified peptide fragments from the insulin molecule that activate autoreactive, cytotoxic T-cells.[22] A cocktail of such peptides may be utilized in a future prevention trial. Other antigens, such as GAD and Hsp60 (Diapep277) may also have efficacy in T1D prevention (see preservation section).

Aside from antigen, various other approaches are being considered. These include anti-inflammatory drugs. Even though IL-1 blockade was not effective in new-onset T1D (see Preservation section), use earlier in the course of the autoimmune process may prove effective. There is also interest in non-steroidal anti-inflammatories and further assessment of omega-3 fatty acids, possibly in combination with vitamin D. Nonspecific immunostimulants, such as OM85 and BCG, could also prove effective. Emerging evidence links the intestinal microbiome with mucosal immunity and T1D risk. Probiotics, helminthes (such as trichuris suis ova), and even lactobacillus modified to over-express IL-10 may alter T1D risk.[23] As noted with antigen-based therapies, optimizing dose, frequency, and timing of administration in the disease course will be necessary for success. It may be that a combination of drugs working by different mechanisms is necessary to accomplish the task. Investigators will continue to closely monitor advances in related autoimmune diseases and transplantation, in search of therapies that warrant assessment in T1D prevention.

III. PRESERVATION

Preservation trials focus on halting further pancreatic β-cell destruction after T1D diagnosis. At the time of diagnosis, it has been estimated that 15–40% of β-cell function remains. However, this remnant can serve one well while it lasts, as evidenced by better overall glycemic control during this remission or honeymoon phase, with lower A1Cs, less glycemic variability, and less hypoglycemia risk. For several decades, investigators have attempted to define a safe and effective means to preserve β-cell function following diagnosis. However, intervening late in the process poses the challenge of daring to be aggressive enough to arrest further destruction while finding an intervention that is safe and tolerable. In those with long-standing disease, such therapy could be used in conjunction with a β-cell replacement strategy: even if replacement islets are generated from host stem cells, one must control the chronic autoimmune response to enable long-term cell survival. Over the past few decades, numerous agents have been evaluated with varying levels of success, with many efforts conducted with smaller number of subjects and often lacking a contemporaneous control group. A subset of these efforts is reviewed herein, with a focus on the well-powered randomized, placebo-controlled studies.

Antigen-Based Therapies

Antigen-based therapies have yielded disappointing results in new-onset T1D patients. Given its known role as a primary antigen in the NOD mouse and in humans, it is not surprising that various forms of insulin as an antigen-based therapy have been attempted in new-onset T1D studies. While some have shown early promise after disease onset, no large, placebo-controlled study has shown efficacy to date (reviewed in Prevention section). Animal studies and pilot human clinical studies with glutamate decarboxylase (GAD) were promising, but subsequent phase II and III trials have shown no effect.[24,25] As with the insulin antigen experience, there may be numerous reasons for the negative findings to date and opportunities to optimize responses. These include *1)* antigen use earlier in the course of disease (as a preventive measure), *2)* use of specific peptides vs. whole molecules, *3)* an alternate dose or frequency of antigen administration, *4)* an alternate route of administration, or *5)* use of an alternate adjuvant to improve efficacy.

Diapep277, an epitope of heat shock protein 60, is another antigen that may be involved in autoimmune responses against the β-cell, though it does not appear to be one of the primary initial targets. Phase II trials showed mixed results with statistically significant preservation of -1-cell function in adults but not in children, and there was no change in A1C and insulin requirements.[26] Results from a recently completed randomized, double-blind, phase III trial for adults with new-onset T1D reached the primary outcome, showing modest improvement in glucagon stimulated C-peptide at 24 months for the treated group, with improvement in some secondary measures of metabolic control (A1C, insulin use, hypoglycemia frequency), yet there was no difference in stimulated C-peptide on MMTT between the two groups (NCT01103284).[27] A follow-up phase III trial will soon be underway to confirm these findings. None of the Diapep277 trials has raised any safety concerns.

Anti-Inflammatory Agents

β-Cell destruction may result from inflammation as well as autoimmunity, and thus another approach to preserving β-cell function is through use of anti-inflammatory agents. Recent focus has centered on responses generated by the innate immune system, and IL-1 has been implicated as a primary proinflammatory cytokine and mediator of β-cell destruction. A TrialNet-sponsored phase II new-onset T1D clinical trial with the IL-1β receptor antagonist canakinumab failed to demonstrate efficacy in the initial analysis of the primary end point at 1 year (NCT00947427) (Moran, submitted manuscript).[28] Similarly, a phase II/III study with the IL-1 receptor antagonist anakinra also failed to reach the primary end point (NCT00711503) (Mandrup-Poulsen, TR, submitted manuscript). As with other therapies, it may be that dosing earlier in the course of autoimmune destruction is needed and may have efficacy in T1D prevention. In addition, IL-1 blockade in combination with an immunomodulatory drug such as anti-CD3 may offer synergy and prove effective in new-onset T1D. This combination has proven highly effective in NOD mice with new-onset T1D.[29]

Another anti-inflammatory approach of interest is utilizing α-1 anti-trypsin. Once again, this approach appeared promising in the NOD mouse. An ITN-funded, initial lead-in, dose-finding study has been conducted for adults and children with recent-onset T1D, and plans are underway for a phase II, placebo-controlled, randomized, new-onset T1D trial to follow (NCT01183468). Encouraging results have also been noted in independent smaller phase 1 trials conducted by P. Gottlieb et al., and by Y. Lebenthal et al. in Israel.

Immunosuppressants

Cyclosporine. Immunosuppression is capable of halting β-cell destruction, as demonstrated by a series of early studies with cyclosporine.[30,31] This drug is a general immunosuppressant that has been used widely in transplantation and suppresses humoral immunity but is even more effective against T-cell–dependent mechanisms. In the 1980s and 1990s, a series of clinical trials demonstrated clinical efficacy in new-onset T1D, but important limitations were noted. Not all treated subjects responded, and for those who did, continuous therapy was required. Furthermore, cyclosporine may be hepato- and nephrotoxic, and continuous immunosuppression may confer risk for infection and possibly cancer. Thus, while cyclosporine established proof of principle, it has not become a viable standard therapy for preserving β-cell function. Following these studies, further trials with immunosuppression were relatively quiescent as investigators sought novel, more targeted therapies, especially those not requiring continuous use.

Anti-CD3 monoclonal antibodies. One novel approach has been to block activation of potentially autoreactive T-cells (see chapter 2), which occurs following interaction between T-cells and antigen-presenting cells (APCs), via the T-cell receptor and costimulatory receptors at the immunologic synapse with antigen peptide/major histocompatability complex (MHC) and costimulatory molecules from APCs (Figure 3.1). Investigators have utilized a mAb that targets the CD3-ε subunit of the T-cell receptor, thereby altering the primary signaling between T-cell and APC. This approach exhibited remarkable findings in the NOD mouse, where a short-term course of antibody induced lasting remission in mice with new-onset diabetes. Investigators have since modified the parent OKT3 antibody in two ways to make a better-tolerated product for humans. These products are teplizumab (hOKT3γ1 (Ala-Ala)) and otelixizumab (ChA-glyCD3).

In an initial phase I/II trial, it was noted that a single 14-day course of teplizumab administered within 2 months of diagnosis preserved β-cell function in treated subjects out to 1 year, as opposed to ~50% decline for those in the open-label control group.[32] However, beyond 12 months the effect appeared to wane, although there was a statistically significant difference between treated and control subjects at 24 months, with long-term follow-up demonstrating persisting effects even at 5 years.[33,34] Related findings were seen with otelixizumab, in which a single 8-day course preserved β-cell function.[35] More extensive long-term follow-up confirmed β-cell preservation up to 4 years after the treatment was received.[36] Side effects from teplizumab have generally been mild, consisting of a flu-like reaction and skin rash in ~50%, with a much smaller percentage having a more marked cytokine release syndrome that necessitates early drug termination; somewhat greater side effects have been noted with otelixizumab, including transient Epstein-Barr viral reactivation in some subjects.

These initial observations have galvanized the field, and spawned a series of downstream trials with these drugs, and related approaches. The phase II AbATE trial evaluated the efficacy of a second course of teplizumab given 12 months after the initial dose (Herold, manuscript submitted, *Lancet* 2012). The trial achieved the primary outcome at 24 months, with loss of C-peptide delayed by 15.9 months, on average, in treated versus control subjects. In the post-hoc analysis, the treated subjects could be divided into two discrete groups: 45% of the treated subjects were considered responders, showing virtually no change in C-peptide by 24 months, whereas the remaining 55% were nonresponders, and were not distinguishable from controls, with progressive C-peptide loss of more than 40% at 24 months. One would ideally hope to determine why the drug works in some people but not others, and have a means to predict those more likely to respond. Analysis to date suggests that, at baseline, responders exhibited reduced frequencies of peripheral Th1-like T-cells as well as lower A1C levels and exogenous insulin use. Responders are also less likely to develop antidrug antibodies.

The Protégé trial was a similar industry-sponsored phase III placebo-controlled trial to evaluate the efficacy of teplizumab administered at baseline and 6 months to subjects with recent onset T1D.[2] The trial did not reach statistical significance for the composite end point (A1C <6.5% and exogenous insulin use <0.50 units/kg/day). However, the trial did achieve similar effects in preserving β-cell function to that observed in the aforementioned AbATE study: those enrolled earlier in their disease course, at younger ages, and treated in North America all appeared to have more favorable outcomes. The Protégé trial also evaluated dosing with several treatment arms, and the original full 14-day course of teplizumab was shown to be more effective than lower drug doses. Based on these promising findings in new-onset subjects, TrialNet launched a prevention trial with teplizumab (as mentioned in the Prevention section) (NCT01030861).

The phase III DEFEND trial evaluated the related anti-CD3 mAb, otelixizumab, electing to use a significantly lower dose to minimize side effects. There were no significant safety concerns, but the study failed to meet its primary efficacy end point of preserving C-peptide at 12 months in new-onset T1D subjects (www.gsk.com).[37]

Anti-thymocyte Globulin (ATG). Based upon the successful anti-CD3 mAb approach, investigators have postulated that a polyclonal antibody approach against T-cells may have even greater efficacy. In the NOD mouse, ATG is one of the few drugs that can induce a lasting remission for animals with recent-onset disease.[38] Although ATG is an effective T-cell depleting agent, that effect alone would not account for its lasting effects in T1D, as T-cells repopulate quickly via a mechanism called homeostatic proliferation. ATG may also foster induction of regulatory T-cells, and animal models suggest that G-CSF may enhance this effect. Several smaller clinical pilot studies with ATG alone have suggested that this approach may be effective.[39–41] The most successful approach to date in any of the new-onset T1D trials has come from combination therapy conducted in Brazil, with an aggressive attempt at immunological "re-booting" using an autologous nonmyeloablative hematopoietic stem cell transplant procedure.[41] Subjects were initially pretreated with cyclophosphamide and then G-CSF to mobilize a hematopoietic stem cell population. The emerging CD34+ bone marrow precursors were harvested and stored. The subjects were allowed to recover and then returned for an immune ablative conditioning regimen with ATG and cyclophosphamide. They received an infusion of their previously harvested cells and were then observed over time. Twenty of 23 subjects were able to discontinue insulin, 12 for a mean of 31 months. Some have remained off insulin with euglycemia for over 4 years. Side effects included infusion reactions, reports of azospermia, and opportunistic infection. Small follow-up studies (again open label, without a control group) have been conducted in China and Poland with this protocol, validating these findings.[42,43]

While this trial yielded impressive metabolic effects, many investigators remain concerned that the associated risks do not justify this approach for more widespread therapy. Investigators are now deconstructing the cocktail of ATG, G-CSF, and cyclophosphamide used in the Brazil study, with phase II recent-onset T1D trials evaluating ATG alone (NCT01106157), G-CSF alone (NCT00662519), and ATG plus GCSF (NCT01106157) to determine if an equally efficacious but safer approach is attainable.

Costimulatory Blockade

CTLA4 Ig (abatacept). Following on the heels of the anti-CD3 mAb successes, investigators have pursued trials with other drugs that provide co-stimulatory blockage of the interactions between APCs and T-cells, targeting secondary pathways. A phase II, double-blinded, randomized, placebo-controlled trial with CTLA4 Ig (abatacept) in new-onset T1D showed a 9.6-month delay in β-cell decline in the treated versus control group, although therapy was provided continuously over a 24-month period (NCT00505375).[44] Follow-up out to 3 years, with 1 year of observation off therapy, showed that β-cell function did not deteriorate at an accelerated rate in the treated group, with C-peptide decline in the treated group parallel to that of the control group and a statistically significant difference remaining between the two (Orban et al, *Lancet*, submitted 2012). It remains unclear why the treatment effect did not persist beyond the initial 9.6-month period. A T1D-prevention trial is being planned with abatacept, as earlier intervention may prove even more effective, and overall there was a favorable safety and tolerability profile in those with recent onset T1D (see Prevention section).

LFA-3 Ig (alefacept). Another approach with costimulatory blockade is an ongoing ITN-sponsored phase II new-onset T1D trial with alefacept (LFA-3 Ig, Amevive). This drug binds CD2, which is expressed on the T-cell surface, and blocks interactions with the costimulatory molecule LFA-3 on APCs and thereby interferes with activation and depletes autoreactive memory T-cells. This approach has proven quite effective and well tolerated in psoriasis patients, and may have long-term tolerizing effects when therapy is withdrawn (NCT00965458). The study has completed enrollment, and results are expected soon.

Role of Regulatory T-cells

In moving these studies from bedside back to bench, investigators have attempted to define what has been altered in the immune system that accounts for the success to date in these efforts. From immunological mechanistic assays of clinical samples, and from further evaluation in animal models with these agents, a leading thought now is that these therapies are not only functioning as depleting agents or in some direct way blunting T effector cells responses but in some cases may in turn foster the development of a novel population of T-cells regulatory T-cells (Tregs), that serve to keep autoreactive T-cells in check. Tregs constitute a small percentage of CD4+ T-cells and are identified by their constitutive expression of CD25 (the α chain of the IL-2 receptor) and the transcription factor FoxP3. One critical factor in Treg development is the cytokine IL-2, and thus one could consider exogenous IL-2 to directly augment this cell population. The complexity that has emerged however is that the dose of IL-2 is critical in how the immune system is affected, with higher-dose IL-2 serving as a nonspecific activator of multiple immune cell subsets, including T-cells and Natural Killer (NK) cells, while low-dose IL-2 selectively augments Tregs.[45]

IL-2 and rapamycin. One initial attempt to directly target this pathway has been an ITN-sponsored phase I trial with IL-2 (proleukin) plus rapamycin (sirolimus) (NCT00525889).[46] The latter drug was added as a means to keep autoreactive T-cells in check while Tregs expanded. Tregs did indeed expand, but NK cells and eosinophils did as well. Investigators terminated the trial early when they noted a transient decline in β-cell function. It may have been related to the dosing and timing of rapamycin or IL-2, or both, but the exact cause is unclear. β-cell function subsequently stabilized, and of interest from the mechanistic studies was a persistent change in IL-2 signaling in Tregs at 12 months. It may be that such an approach will be feasible with optimal dosing of rapamycin and a lower dose of IL-2. Studies with lower-dose IL-2 alone have proven effective in graft vs. host disease and hepatitis-C–related vasculitis.[47,48] A phase I/II, placebo-controlled trial is being conducted with low-dose IL-2 in T1D, investigating the relationship between low-dose IL-2 and Treg induction, and effects on β-cell function (Klatzmann, NCT01353833). Investigators are also considering alternate means to more selectively amplify Tregs via this axis. For example, there may be mutated forms of IL-2 that selectively bind to the receptor on target Tregs but not on other cell types, and thus do not confer the same risk for expansion of other cell types.

Therapeutic approaches with Tregs. As a means to bypass all the potential issues noted above, one could consider direct therapy with Tregs. Proof of principle has once again come from studies in the NOD mouse, where purified and ex vivo expanded Tregs given to mice with recent-onset T1D reverses the disease. Bluestone and colleagues subsequently developed a procedure for purifying and expanding a polyclonal Treg population for clinical use, and are conducting a phase I dose-escalation trial with autologous expanded Tregs (NCT01210664).[49] Safety and possible efficacy in a phase I study of children with new-onset T1D based on this same expansion protocol has been reported.[50] An open-label phase I trial in T1D subjects using umbilical cord blood (UCB), potentially another source of Tregs, has been conducted.[51] The study showed that autologous UCB infusion was safe and did induce changes in Treg frequency, but the therapy failed to preserve C-peptide (NCT00305344).[5] Follow-up studies using UCB coupled with vitamin D and omega-3 fatty acids are ongoing (NCT00873925). As with the drug trials, the challenge for these studies is to determine a safe and effective dose of cells. Rather than using polyclonal Tregs, investigators ultimately hope to develop more targeted clinical therapy with antigen-specific Tregs.

Additional Therapeutic Considerations

Other cellular therapies. Aside from augmenting Tregs, one can consider changing APCs. Toward this end, Giannoukakis et al. modified autologous monocyte-derived dendritic cells, treating the cells ex vivo with antisense phosphorothioate–modified oligonucleotides targeting costimulatory molecules.[52] They hypothesize that these modified APCs will have immunosuppressive properties via impaired T-cell costimulation. In a phase I T1D trial, they have shown that treatment with these modified autologous dendritic cells is safe and well tolerated and may upregulate the frequency of potentially beneficial β-cells (NCT00445913).[52] A larger phase II study is needed to further assess this approach.

An alternate approach to modifying T-cell activation has been noted in a phase I study in multiple sclerosis. Investigators are utilizing antigen coupled to peripheral blood leukocytes via ethylene carbodimide as a modified APC in an attempt to induce tolerance.[53] Such an approach may also be adapted as a T1D therapy. It is notable that a variety of different antigens can be coupled to a single cell, as peptides of interest are further defined in T1D. This approach may be one means to present antigens for tolerance induction. Mesenchymal stem cell infusions are also being evaluated in new-onset T1D, with the goal that they may differentiate into β-cells in vivo, modulate the immune response, or both (NCT00690066).

Augmentation of β-cell mass. The approaches mentioned to date address means to abrogate autoimmune destruction of β-cells. However, therapies to enhance β-cell repair, regeneration, or neogenesis may also be an important synergistic approach. Animal models suggest that glucagon-like peptide-1 (GLP-1) agonists and dipeptidyl peptidase-4 (DPP-IV) inhibitors have salutary effects. An ongoing new-onset T1D clinical trial with sitagliptin (DPP-IV inhibitor) and lansoprozole (GLP-1R agonist) (NCT01155284) will test this hypothesis. Other studies with related agents are also being considered for prevention and new-onset trials. Growth factors that have been evaluated in animal models and considered for clinical trials include insulin-like growth factor-1 (IGF-1) and islet neogenesis–associated peptide. Ultimately, one may consider β-cell replacement in those with new-onset T1D, particularly as more robust cells become available from stem cell–based approaches (see chapter 4). If the means become available to develop such cells from the affected individual, one would presume that immunotherapy would still be needed in the face of an ongoing autoimmune response, and thus the new-onset trials mentioned above will become quite important in informing the best choice of therapy to preserve such cells. Encapsulation could obviate the need for such immunotherapy, although there is ongoing concern about the integrity and function of such devices to date.

Rituximab. Despite the dogma that T1D is a T-cell–mediated disease, evidence from animal models suggests that β-cells, but not autoantibodies themselves, are involved in β-cell destruction. The hypothesis is that β-cells act as APCs, communicating with T-cells, and altering their behavior. To further explore this in a clinical trial, investigators conducted a phase II trial with an anti-CD20 mAb (rituximab) (NCT00279305).[54] They found that a single course of therapy resulted in a statistically significant difference in β-cell function at 1 year in the treatment vs. the placebo group. C-peptide was preserved in the treated group for 8.2 months, but thereafter the rate of decline in C-peptide was parallel between the drug-treatment and placebo groups. Adverse events included infusion reactions, depletion of β-cells (as expected) with low recovery over 1 year, and persisting lower IgM levels. These findings provide novel insights into the complexities of the autoimmune process in T1D, and highlight the potential role of other cell types in this process. Future studies could include repeated dosing with this or related anti-β-cell therapies in new-onset T1D, as has been used in other autoimmune disorders such as rheumatoid arthritis, although concern lies in risk from infectious diseases following chronic β-cell depletion. This approach is also under consideration for T1D prevention.

Metabolic control. Outside of the realm of immunology, one approach to preserve β-cell function is intensive glycemic control. In the DCCT, it was noted that improved metabolic control seemed to preserve β-cell function.[55,56] Another study, of an intensive 2-week inpatient treatment shortly after diagnosis, with continuous intravenous insulin regulated by a Biostator, resulted in better β-cell function at 1 year, compared to conventional controls.[57] One common observation from the aforementioned successful new-onset trials is a transient stabilization in β-cell function, for a variable period of time, followed by an inexorable decline in β-cell function that seems to parallel the control group, prompting speculation that there may be interplay between metabolic control, inflammation, and immune responses. TrialNet and DirecNet are collaborating to critically evaluate this concept: a randomized trial is evaluating subjects who receive intensive metabolic control, first with an in-hospital 5-day program utilizing a hybrid closed loop consisting of a continuous glucose sensor coupled with an insulin pump to optimize metabolic control. The algorithm uses every-minute glucose sensor readings to determine minute-by-minute pump insulin doses based on the present glucose, glucose rate of change, and pending insulin action. The subjects are followed at an outpatient program with openloop sensor and pump. Subjects are compared to those in the control group, who pursue usual diabetes care through their regular provider (NCT00891995).

PRESERVATION TRIALS: FUTURE CONSIDERATIONS

Next Steps for β-cell Preservation Studies

The trials conducted to date have laid important groundwork for the next generation of studies. Each of these past studies had compelling preclinical or related clinical rationale, yet there is ongoing concern about what most consider lukewarm results to date. No single agent or trial has safely and effectively restored β-cell function for an extended period of time without the need for exogenous insulin therapy in the vast majority of participants. Based on these findings, where should the field go from here?

The last few decades have taught us that the immunological defects of T1D are complex and not completely understood: elucidation of the underlying pathophysiology may guide more rational trials. Insights will continue to be gained from T1D animal models such as the NOD mouse, but, at best, these models will have limitations; an inbred mouse strain with a T1D-like disease process only crudely approximates the complexities of the human clinical condition. Identifying other T1D animal models, aside from the NOD, may prove helpful. Humanizing the mouse immune system, in which the mouse immune system is essentially replaced with human components, may help recapitulate the human derangements of the immune system in a mouse model.

There may be no substitute for trying to gain further information directly from humans. Ideally, one would utilize clinical samples. However, very real limitations are posed by the inability to gain direct access to the pancreas and pancreatic lymph nodes, and instead relying on peripheral blood samples, where the autoreactive T-cell repertoire may be present at very low numbers. T-cell assays, such as the tetramer assay, make it possible to detect autoreactive T-cells present at very low frequency. Means to visualize β-cell mass and function in vivo are currently in development and will be a major advancement for clinical trials. Finally, much may be learned from the Network for Pancreatic Organ Donation (nPOD), an organized network collecting and archiving pancreata and other tissues from recently deceased individuals with T1D for further study (www.jdrfnpod.org).[58]

Next Generation Study Design

Most trials in new-onset T1D patients have been conducted with a single agent, and often with a placebo control group. In addition to the drugs currently available, the number of potential agents in the pipeline continues to steadily expand (see Table 3.1). If we conduct business as usual with intermediate-sized phase II clinical trials with a single agent compared to placebo, then we face very inefficient means to evaluate and identify the most promising candidates and may never reach a definitive answer. In addition, we may need to revisit the primary end point utilized for most studies to date. Current practice uses the change in β-cell function over time, which often requires close observation over a 12- to 24-month period and is an indirect measure of the inciting autoimmune response. Thus, study design may need to be refocused on testing a series of agents, utilizing a common control group; where possible, study design may adopt surrogate immune markers that will allow a faster readout of promising agents that should be further evaluated.[59] If appropriate surrogate measures can be identified, an adaptive design may achieve this. Study size, study power, and effect size will also need to be addressed. For drugs with greater risk, one may want to demand a higher effect size, in order to consider the attendant risk acceptable. For a drug with no or minimal risk, one may be willing to accept a much smaller effect size. Greatest interest will be placed in those drugs that appear to have a tolerizing effect.

Furthermore, many now feel that the most successful approaches will require targeting more than one pathway in order to interdict this complex process of autoimmune destruction, much as has been necessary with organ transplantation and cancer therapy.[60,61] Targeting multiple pathways with two (or more) drugs poses considerable hurdles, including the following considerations:

- What is the best combination?
- What is the ideal dose and length of therapy for each component of the cocktail?
- What is the ideal timing for each agent relative to the others to be utilized?
- Could there be additive or synergistic toxicities that could result from the combination, such as an infectious disease risk from immunosuppression?
- For trial design, should there be arms to evaluate each therapy alone and then the combination, vs. a placebo, or is combination vs. placebo adequate?
- Will industry be willing to partner with investigators and other companies to evaluate combination therapies, or might they remain risk averse and avoid such trials in order to limit any potential for uncovering new toxicities with an emerging therapy?
- Will the investigators be able to work with the FDA to settle the associated regulatory and ethical concerns that such combination therapies will pose for T1D, in which evolving clinical therapies continue to improve over time?

Table 3.1 T1D Prevention and Preservation Studies (Partial Listing): Completed, Underway, or Under Active Consideration*

Primary Prevention	Intervention
TIGR	Bovine protein (cow's milk) or hydrolyzed casein formula
NIP	Docosahexanoic acid capsules vs. placebo
BabyDiet	Routine vs. delayed introduction of gluten
Vitamin D supplementation	Vitamin D supplementation
POINT	Oral insulin
Secondary Prevention	**Intervention**
DPT	Parenteral insulin (high-risk group)
	Oral insulin (intermediate-risk group)
DIPP	Intranasal insulin
INIT II	Nicotinamide
ENDIT	
Anti-CD3 mAb	Teplizumab
CTLA4 Ig (abatacept)	Abatacept
Helminthes	Trichuris suis ovae

Preservation

GAD
Hsp60 (Diapep277)
IL1β receptor blockade (canakinumab)
IL1 receptor antagonist (anakinra)
α-1-antitrypsin
Cyclosporine
Anti-CD3 (teplizumab, otelixizumab)
ATG
GCSF
ATG + GCSF
ATG + GCSF + cyclophosphamide
CTLA4 Ig (abatacept)
LFA-3 Ig (alefacept)
IL-2 + rapamycin
Autologous Tregs
UCB + vitamin D + Ω-3 fatty acids
Modified APCs
Sitagliptin +lansoprozole
CD20 (rituximab)
Intensive metabolic control
MMF/DZB

*Please refer to the text for a detailed explanation of listed acronyms.

These are clearly formidable hurdles to anticipate and overcome, and yet some combination trials have already been completed, such as the unsuccessful attempt with mycophenolate mofetil plus daclizumab (NCT00100178), the trial in Brazil with ATG, GCSF, and Cyclophosphamide, and the ongoing trial with sitagliptin plus lansoprozole (NCT01155284).[41,62,63] Furthermore, one should bear in mind that some single agents such as monoclonal antibodies are quite precise and focused in their target, whereas other monotherapies are more multifaceted, targeting multiple sites or multiple cell types, such as ATG, which cross-reacts with multiple cell surface T-cell antigens. Another example is a tyrosine kinase inhibitor, imatinib, which will soon be evaluated in a phase II new-onset T1D trial. This drug targets multiple tyrosine kinases, in a variety of cell types, but this broader targeting may be necessary to quell the autoimmune response in T1D.

There is ongoing discussion about the ideal drug combination for such a new-onset T1D trial. General guidelines have been suggested in an ITN-JDRF assessment group, including:

■ Initially assessing combination therapies in preclinical models
■ Limiting initial combination studies to two drugs at first
■ Giving priority toward drugs that have already shown some level of efficacy and safety in T1D trials as a monotherapy and to FDA-approved drugs
■ Selecting drugs that operate via independent and complementary mechanisms
■ Paying attention to safety, with sequential rather than simultaneous use of the drugs, if possible[60]

One cocktail now being explored further is with anti-CD3 mAb plus IL-1 β blockade (canakinumab). Data is available for each drug alone in new-onset T1D trials, and there is a larger safety experience from which to draw. Preclinical studies are promising with this combination, and the drugs have complementary effects, targeting both innate and adaptive immunity. Another natural combination under consideration is coupling anti-CD3 mAb to antigen-based–therapy in order to extend the benefits of initial immune modulation, and it appears promising in animal models. Drugs that may enhance β-cell repair or regeneration, such as GLP-1 agonists or DPP-IV inhibitors, may also serve well in combination with an immunomodulatory agent. As the list of completed clinical trials with a single agent in new-onset T1D grows, many promising potential combinations will no doubt continue to emerge.

Eligibility Criteria

New-onset studies have typically targeted subjects shortly after diagnosis, and indeed studies such as the cyclosporine trials and the recent Protégé trial with teplizumab suggest that those who enrolled earlier had better responses. However, several investigators are exploring that assumption further, to determine if there is a broader window than may have been previously appreciated in which interventions may be helpful. As metabolic control has improved and as investigators have evaluated subjects at various times from diagnosis, a substantial portion retain clinically significant amounts of stimulated C-peptide (i.e., above the 0.2

pmol/ml threshold established in the DCCT). A phase II trial with teplizumab for subjects 4–12 months from diagnosis noted a trend toward β-cell preservation 1 year later, though the effects do not appear as robust as those noted for newer onset subjects (NCT00378508).[64] Several early trials, in phase I or phase I/II, are now enrolling T1D subjects up to 2 years out from diagnosis. These are studies in which there is a focus on safety, with an attempt to get an early assessment of efficacy (NCT01106157, NCT01210664). If this window for possible therapy can be broadened from the usual study window of less than 3 months from diagnosis, then investigators will be able to enroll clinical trials more rapidly. As they are approved, there may ultimately be a broader target population for effective therapies.

As noted above, there is an ongoing challenge of how to best transition clinical trials into younger age-groups. Drugs are primarily studied in adult patients, to gain initial experience to prove safety and possibly efficacy, before exposing children to a potentially harmful drug. This approach poses several possible constraints from a clinical trials perspective. First, the disease process itself may be somewhat different in an older population than in children: the rate of β-cell decline following T1D diagnosis is faster in those aged <21 years,[65] and findings from several recent trials indicate that younger children may be more likely to respond to therapies than older participants (Herold, Lancet 2012, submitted).[2,54]

Standardize Approach to Trials and Reporting of Trials Outcomes

Ultimately, investigators will need to compare results from different agents from various clinical trials and determine which agents should be pursued further in larger phase III studies alone or in combination with other drugs. As has been suggested by others, in order to advance the field, it will be extremely helpful if key aspects of the study design and data analysis are conducted in similar fashion.[66,67] To a large extent, TrialNet and the Immune Tolerance Network have adopted very similar approaches, and many others are now doing so as well. There have been extensive past discussions about the choice of primary outcome to document preservation of endogenous β-cell function, and many agree with stimulated C-peptide, such as obtained with a mixed-meal tolerance test.[67] Some studies have utilized or are considering a composite end point, such as A1C and exogenous insulin use that may reflect endogenous insulin secretion.[2] A group of common secondary metabolic measures may also be helpful to include in all trials, such as exogenous insulin use, severe hypoglycemia, and A1C. For presentation of results, some common reported analysis will be helpful, such as for mixed-meal tolerance test providing 2- and 4-h C-peptide area under the curve as well as peak C-peptide; a shared definition of responder vs. nonresponder; similar approach on handling missing tests in the analysis (imputation or not); and how to handle results that are at the lower limit of detection (zero versus input one half the lower limit of detection).

IV. CONCLUSION

Current clinical therapy for T1D is suboptimal: the majority of patients are not able to consistently meet necessary glycemic targets to avoid long-term complications. Investigators now have the means to screen and identify those at risk for T1D, and a series of primary and secondary prevention trials offer promise for blocking progression to overt disease. For those with recent-onset T1D, several immunomodulatory agents have been found to delay β-cell destruction, and a series of intriguing trials are underway or are being planned. Ultimately, combination therapy, using complementary and synergistic agents, may be necessary to interdict the autoimmune process. New strategies are needed to more efficiently evaluate the emerging pipeline of therapies for both T1D prevention and β-cell preservation.

REFERENCES

1. Palmer JP, Fleming GA, Greenbaum CJ, Herold KC, Jansa LD, Kolb H, Lachin JM, Polonsky KS, Pozzilli P, Skyler JS, Steffes MW: C-peptide is the appropriate outcome measure for type 1 diabetes clinical trials to preserve beta-cell function: report of an ADA workshop, 21–22 October 2001. *Diabetes* 53:250–264, 2004 [Erratum in: *Diabetes* 53:1934, 2004]
2. Sherry N, Hagopian W, Ludvigsson J, Jain SM, Wahlen J, Ferry RJ, Bode B, Aronoff S, Holland C, Carlin D, King KL, Wilder RL, Pillemer S, Bonvini E, Johnson S, Stein KE, Koenig S, Herold KC:, Daifotis AG for the Protégé Trial Investigators: Teplizumab for treatment of type 1 diabetes (Protégé study): 1-year results from a randomised, placebo-controlled trial. *Lancet* 378:487–497, 2011
3. Shoda LK, Young DL, Ramanujan S, Whiting CC, Atkinson MA, Bluestone JA, Eisenbarth GS, Mathis D, Rossini AA, Campbell SE, Kahn R, Kreuwel HT: A comprehensive review of interventions in the NOD mouse and implications for translation. *Immunity* 23:115–126, 2005
4. Knip M, Virtanen SM, Seppä K, Ilonen J, Savilahti E, Vaarala O, Reunanen A, Teramo K, Hämäläinen AM, Paronen J, Dosch HM, Hakulienen T, Åkerblom HK: for the Finnish TRIGR Study Group: Dietary intervention in infancy and later signs of beta-cell autoimmunity. *N Engl J Med* 363:1900–1908, 2010
5. TRIGR Study Group: Study design of the Trial to Reduce IDDM in the Genetically at Risk (TRIGR). *Pediatr Diabetes* 8:117–137, 2007
6. Hummel S, Pfluger M, Hummel M, Bonifacio E, Ziegler AG: Primary dietary intervention study to reduce the risk of islet autoimmunity in children at increased risk for type 1 diabetes: the BABYDIET study. *Diabetes Care* 34:1301–1305, 2011
7. Hyppönen E, Läärä E, Reunanen A, Järvelin MR, Virtanen SM: Intake of vitamin D and risk of type 1 diabetes: a birth-cohort study. *Lancet* 358:1500–1503, 2001
8. Sorensen IM, Joner G, Jenum PA, Eskild A, Torjesen PA, Stene LC: Maternal serum levels of 25-Hydroxy-vitamin D during pregnancy and risk of type 1 diabetes in the offspring. *Diabetes* 61:175 –178, 2012
9. Diabetes Prevention Trial (DPT)—Type 1 Diabetes Study Group: Effects of insulin in relatives of patients with type 1 diabetes mellitus. *N Engl J Med* 346:1685–1691, 2002
10. Sosenko JM, Palmer JP, Greenbaum CJ, Mahon J, Cowie C, Krischer JP, Chase HP, White NH, Buckingham B, Herold KC, Cuthbertson D, Skyler JS, and the Diabetes Prevention Trial—Type 1 Study Group (DPT-1):

Patterns of metabolic progression to type 1 diabetes in the Diabetes Prevention Trial—Type 1. *Diabetes Care* 29:643–649, 2006

11. Skyler JS, Krischer JP, Wolfsdorf J, Cowie C, Palmer JP, Greenbaum C, Cuthbertson D, Rafkin-Mervis LE, Chase HP, Leschek E: Effects of oral insulin in relatives of patients with type 1 diabetes: the Diabetes Prevention Trial—Type 1. *Diabetes Care* 28:1068–1076, 2005

12. Gale EA, Bingley PJ, Emmett CL, Collier T: European Nicotinamide Diabetes Intervention Trial (ENDIT): European Nicotinamide Diabetes Intervention Trial (ENDIT): a randomized controlled trial of intervention before the onset of type 1 diabetes. *Lancet* 363:925–931, 2004

13. Näntö-Salonen K, Kupila A, Simell S, Siljander H, Salonsaari T, Hekkala A, Korhonen S, Erkkola R, Sipilä JI, Haavisto L, Siltala M, Tuominen J, Hakalax J, Hyöty H, Ilonen J, Veijola R, Simell T, Knip M, Simell O: Nasal insulin to prevent type 1 diabetes in children with HLA genotypes and autoantibodies conferring increased risk of disease: a double-blind, randomised controlled trial. *Lancet* 372:1746–1755, 2008. Epub 22 September 2008

14. Vehik K, Cuthbertson D, Ruhlig H, Schatz DA, Peakman M, Krischer JP: DPT-1 and TrialNet Study Groups: Long-term outcome of individuals treated with oral insulin: Diabetes Prevention Trial—Type 1 (DPT-1) oral insulin trial. *Diabetes Care* 34:1585–1590, 2011

15. Achenbach P, Barker J, Bonifacio E: Pre-POINT Study Group: Modulating the natural history of type 1 diabetes in children at high genetic risk by mucosal insulin immunization. *Curr Diab Rep* 8:87–93, 2008

16. Fourlanos S, Perry C, Gellert SA, Martinuzzi E, Mallone R, Butler J, Colman PG, Harrison LC: Evidence that nasal insulin induces immune tolerance to insulin in adults with autoimmune diabetes. *Diabetes* 60:1237–1245, 2011. Epub 9 February 2011

17. Kolb H, Burkart V: Nicotinamide in type 1 diabetes. Mechanism of action revisited. *Diabetes Care* 22 (Suppl. 2):B16–B20, 1999

18. Hsu WC, Boyko EJ, Fujimoto WY, Kanaya A, Karmally W, Karter A, King GL, Look M, Maskarinec G, Misra R, Tavake-Pasi F, Arakaki R: Pathophysiologic differences among Asians, native Hawaiians, and other Pacific Islanders and treatment implications. *Diabetes Care* 35:1189–1198, 2012

19. Sosenko JM, Krischer JP, Palmer JP, Mahon J, Cowie C, Greenbaum CJ, Cuthbertson D, Lachin JM, Skyler JS: Diabetes Prevention Trial-Type 1 Study Group. A risk score for type 1 diabetes derived from autoantibody-positive participants in the diabetes prevention trial-type 1. *Diabetes Care* 31:528–533, 2008. Epub 13 November 2007

20. Xu P, Beam CA, Cuthbertson D, Sosenko JM, Skyler JS, Krischer JP: DPT-1 Study Group: Prognostic accuracy of immunologic and metabolic markers for type 1 diabetes in a high-risk population: receiver operating characteristic analysis. *Diabetes Care.* 28 August 2012 [Epub ahead of print]

21. Orban T, Farkas K, Jalahej H, Kis J, Treszl A, Falk B, Reijonen H, Wolfsdorf J, Ricker A, Matthews JB, Tchao N, Sayre P, Bianchine P: Autoantigen-specific regulatory T cells induced in patients with type 1 diabetes mellitus by insulin B-chain immunotherapy. *J Autoimmun* 34:408–415, 2010

22. Unger WW, Velthuis J, Abreu JR, Laban S, Quinten E, Kester MG, Reker-Hadrup S, Bakker AH, Duinkerken G, Mulder A, Franken KL, Hilbrands

R, Keymeulen B, Peakman M, Ossendorp F, Drijfhout JW, Schumacher TN, Roep BO: Discovery of low-affinity preproinsulin epitopes and detection of autoreactive CD8 T-cells using combinatorial MHC multimers. *J Autoimmun* 37:151–159, 2011. Epub 1 June 2011

23. Takiishi T, Korf H, Van Belle TL, Robert S, Grieco FA, Caluwaerts S, Galleri L, Spagnuolo I, Steidler L, Van Huynegem K, Demetter P, Wasserfall C, Atkinson MA, Dotta F, Rottiers P, Gysemans C, Mathieu C: Reversal of autoimmune diabetes by restoration of antigen-specific tolerance using genetically modified Lactococcus lactis in mice. *J Clin Invest* 122:1717–1725, 2012. doi: 10.1172/JCI60530. Epub 9 April 2012

24. Wherrett DK, Bundy B, Becker DJ, DiMeglio LA, Gitelman SE, Goland R, Gottlieb PA, Greenbaum CJ, Herold KC, Marks JB, Monzavi R, Moran A, Orban T, Palmer JP, Raskin P, Rodriguez H, Schatz D, Wilson DM, Krischer JP, Skyler JS: Type 1 Diabetes TrialNet GAD Study Group: Antigen-based therapy with glutamic acid decarboxylase (GAD) vaccine in patients with recent-onset type 1 diabetes: a randomised double-blind trial. *Lancet* 378:319–327, 2011. Epub 27 June 2011

25. Ludvigsson J, Krisky D, Casas R, Battelino T, Castaño L, Greening J, Kordonouri O, Otonkoski O, Pozzilli P, Robert JJ, Veeze HJ, Palmer J: GAD65 antigen therapy in recently diagnosed type 1 diabetes mellitus. *N Engl J Med* 366:433–442, 2012

26. Tuccinardi D, Fioriti E, Manfrini S, D'Amico E, Pozzilli P: DiaPep277 peptide therapy in the context of other immune intervention trials in type 1 diabetes. *Expert Opin Biol Ther* 11:1233–1240, 2011. Epub 13 July 2011

27. Raz I: Oral presentation at the European Association for the Study of Diabetes, abstract 145, Berlin, Germany, 4 October 2012

28. Moran A: Canakinumab, and anti-IL-1 monocolonal antibody in recent-onset type 1 diabetes. 72nd Scientific Sessions, ADA, Philadelphia, PA, USA, 8–12 June, Oral Presentation.

29. Ablamunits V, Henegariu O, Hansen JB, Opare-Addo L, Preston-Hurlburt P, Santamaria P, Mandrup-Poulsen T, Herold KC: Synergistic reversal of type 1 diabetes in NOD mice with anti-CD3 and interleukin-1 blockade: evidence of improved immune regulation. *Diabetes* 61:145–154, 2012. Epub 31 October 2011

30. Bougneres PF, Carel JC, Castano L, Boitard C, Gardin JP, Landais P, Hors J, Mihatsch MJ, Paillard M, Chaussain JL, et al.: Factors associated with early remission of type I diabetes in children treated with cyclosporine. *N Engl J Med* 318:663–670, 1988

31. Stiller CR, Dupré J, Gent M, Jenner MR, Keown PA, Laupacis A, Martell R, Rodger NW, von Graffenried B, Wolfe BM: Effects of cyclosporine immunosuppression in insulin-dependent diabetes mellitus of recent onset. *Science* 223:1362–1367, 1984

32. Herold KC, Hagopian W, Auger JA, Poumian-Ruiz E, Taylor L, Donaldson D, Gitelman SE, Harlan DM, Xu D, Zivin RA, Bluestone JA: Anti-CD3 monoclonal antibody in new-onset type 1 diabetes mellitus. *N Engl J Med* 346:1692–1698, 2002

33. Herold KC, Gitelman SE, Masharani U, Hagopian W, Bisikirska B, Donaldson D, Rother K, Diamond B, Harlan DM, Bluestone JA: A single course

of anti-CD3 monoclonal antibody hOKT3gamma1(Ala-Ala) results in improvement in C-peptide responses and clinical parameters for at least 2 years after onset of type 1 diabetes. *Diabetes* 54:1763–1769, 2005

34. Herold KC, Gitelman S, Greenbaum C, Puck J, Hagopiang W, Gottliebh P, Sayrej P, Bianchinei P, Wong E, Seyfert-Margolis V, Bourcier K, Bluestone JA: Immune Tolerance Network ITN007AI Study Group: Treatment of patients with new onset type 1 diabetes with a single course of anti-CD3 mAb teplizumab preserves insulin production for up to 5 years. *Clin Immunol* 132:166–173, 2009

35. Keymeulen B, Vandemeulebroucke E, Ziegler AG, Mathieu C, Kaufman L, Hale G, Gorus F, Goldman M, Walter M, Candon S, Schandene L, Crenier L, De Block C, Seigneurin JM, De Pauw P, Pierard D, Weets I, Rebello P, Bird P, Berrie E, Frewin M, Waldmann H, Bach JF, Pipeleers D, Chatenoud L: Insulin needs after CD3-antibody therapy in new-onset type 1 diabetes. *N Engl J Med* 352:2598–2608, 2005

36. Keymeulen B, Walter M, Mathieu C, Kaufman L, Gorus F, Hilbrands R, Vandemeulebroucke E, Van de Velde U, Crenier L, De Block C, Candon S, Waldmann H, Ziegler AG, Chatenoud L, Pipeleers D: Four-year metabolic outcome of a randomised controlled CD3-antibody trial in recent-onset type 1 diabetic patients depends on their age and baseline residual beta cell mass. *Diabetologia* 53:614–23, 2010. Epub 14 January 2010

37. GlaxoSmithKline: Press Release Archive: Friday 11 March 2011. Available at http://www.gsk.com/media/pressreleases/2011/2011_pressrelease_10039.htm

38. Parker MJ, Xue S, Alexander JJ, Wasserfall CH, Campbell-Thompson ML, Battaglia M, Gregori S, Mathews CE, Song S, Troutt M, Eisenbeis S, Williams J, Schatz DA, Haller MJ, Atkinson MA: Immune depletion with cellular mobilization imparts immunoregulation and reverses autoimmune diabetes in nonobese diabetic mice. *Diabetes* 58:2277–2284, 2009. Epub 23 July 2009

39. Eisenbarth GS, Srikanta S, Jackson R, Rabinowe S, Dolinar R, Aoki T, Morris MA: Anti-thymocyte globulin and prednisone immunotherapy of recent onset type 1 diabetes mellitus. *Diabetes Res* 2:271–276, 1985

40. Saudek F, Havrdova T, Boucek P, Karasova L, Novota P, Skibova J: Polyclonal anti-T-cell therapy for type 1 diabetes mellitus of recent onset. *Rev Diabet Stud* 1:80–88, 2004. Epub 10 August 2004

41. Couri CE, Oliveira MC, Stracieri AB, Moraes DA, Pieroni F, Barros GM, Madeira MI, Malmegrim KC, Foss-Freitas MC, Simões BP, Martinez EZ, Foss MC, Burt RK, Voltarelli JC: C-peptide levels and insulin independence following autologous nonmyeloablative hematopoietic stem cell transplantation in newly diagnosed type 1 diabetes mellitus. *JAMA* 301:1573–1579, 2009

42. Li L, Shen S, Ouyang J, Hu Y, Hu L, Cui W, Zhang N, Zhuge YZ, Chen B, Xu J, Zhu D: Autologous hematopoietic stem cell transplantation modulates immunocompetent cells and improves β-cell function in Chinese patients with new onset of type 1 diabetes. *J Clin Endocrinol Metab* 97:1729–1736, 2012. Epub 14 March 2012

43. Snarski E, Milczarczyk A, Torosian T, Paluszewska M, Urbanowska E, Król M, Boguradzki P, Jedynasty K, Franek E, Wiktor-Jedrzejczak W:

Independence of exogenous insulin following immunoablation and stem cell reconstitution in newly diagnosed diabetes type I. *Bone Marrow Transpl* 46:562–566, 2011. Epub 28 June 2010

44. Orban T, Bundy B, Becker DJ, DiMeglio LA, Gitelman SE, Goland R, Gottlieb PA, Greenbaum CJ, Marks JB, Monzavi R, Moran A, Raskin P, Rodriguez H, Russell WE, Schatz D, Wherrett D, Wilson DM, Krischer J, Skyler JS: Type 1 Diabetes TrialNet Abatacept Study Group: Co-stimulation modulation with abatacept in patients with recent-onset type 1 diabetes: a randomised, double-blind, placebo-controlled trial. *Lancet* 378:412–419, 2011. Epub 28 June 2011

45. Rosenberg SA, Lotze MT: Cancer immunotherapy using interleukin-2 and interleukin-2-activated lymphocytes. *Annu Rev Immunol* 4:681–709, 1986

46. Long SA, Rieck M, Sanda S, Bollyky JB, Samuels PL, Goland R, Ahmann A, Rabinovitch A, Aggarwal S, Phippard D, Turka LA, Ehlers MR, Bianchine PJ, Boyle KD, Adah SA, Bluestone JA, Buckner JH, Greenbaum CJ: for Diabetes TrialNet and the Immune Tolerance Network: Rapamycin/IL-2 combination therapy in patients with type 1 diabetes augments Tregs yet transiently impairs β-cell function. *Diabetes* 61:2340–2348, 2012. Epub 20 June 2012

47. Koreth J, Matsuoka K, Kim HT, McDonough SM, Bindra B, Alyea EP 3rd, Armand P, Cutler C, Ho VT, Treister NS, Bienfang DC, Prasad S, Tzachanis D, Joyce RM, Avigan DE, Antin JH, Ritz J, Soiffer RJ: Interleukin-2 and regulatory T cells in graft-versus-host disease. *N Engl J Med* 365:2055–2066, 2011

48. Saadoun D, Rosenzwajg M, Joly F, Six A, Carrat F, Thibault V, Sene D, Cacoub P, Klatzmann D: Regulatory T-cell responses to low-dose Interleukin-2 in HCV-induced vasculitis. *N Engl J Med* 365:2067–2077, 2011

49. Putnam AL, Brusko TM, Lee MR, Liu W, Szot GL, Ghosh T, Atkinson MA, Bluestone JA: Expansion of human regulatory T-cells from patients with type 1 diabetes. *Diabetes* 58:652–662, 2009

50. Marek-Trzonkowska N, Mysliwiec M, Dobyszuk A, Grabowska M, Techmanska I, Juscinska J, Wujtewicz MA, Witkowski P, Mlynarski W, Balcerska A, Mysliwska J, Trzonkowski P: Administration of CD4+CD25highCD127- regulatory T cells preserves β-cell function in type 1 diabetes in children. *Diabetes Care* 35:1817–1820, 2012. Epub 20 June 2012

51. Haller MJ, Wasserfall CH, Hulme MA, Cintron M, Brusko TM, McGrail KM, Sumrall TM, Wingard JR, Theriaque DW, Shuster JJ, Atkinson MA, Schatz DA: Autologous umbilical cord blood transfusion in young children with type 1 diabetes fails to preserve C-peptide. *Diabetes Care* 34:2567–2569, 2011. Epub 19 October 2011

52. Giannoukakis N, Phillips B, Finegold D, Harnaha J, Trucco M. Phase I (safety) study of autologous tolerogenic dendritic cells in type 1 diabetic patients. *Diabetes Care* 34:2026–2032, 2011. Epub 16 June 2011

53. Turley DM, Miller SD: Prospects for antigen-specific tolerance based therapies for the treatment of multiple sclerosis. *Results Probl Cell Differ* 51:217–235, 2010

54. Pescovitz MD, Greenbaum CJ, Krause-Steinrauf H, Becker DJ, Gitelman SE, Goland R, Gottlieb PA, Marks JB, McGee PF, Moran AM, Raskin R,

Rodriguez H, Schatz DA, Wherrett D, Wilson DM, Lachin JM, Skyler JS: for the Type 1 Diabetes TrialNet Anti-CD20 Study Group: Rituximab, B-lymphocyte depletion, and preservation of beta-cell function. *N Engl J Med* 361:2143–2152, 2009

55. Diabetes Control and Complications Trial Research Group: The effect of intensive treatment of diabetes on the development and progression of long-term complications in insulin-dependent diabetes mellitus. *N Engl J Med* 329:977–986, 1993

56. Diabetes Control and Complications Trial Research Group: Effect of intensive therapy on residual beta-cell function in patients with type 1 diabetes in the diabetes control and complications trial. A randomized, controlled trial. *Ann Intern Med* 128:517–523, 1998

57. Shah SC, Malone JI, Simpson NE: A randomized trial of intensive insulin therapy in newly diagnosed insulin-dependent diabetes mellitus. *N Engl J Med* 320:550–554, 1989

58. Network for Pancreatic Organ Donors with Diabetes website. Available at http://www.jdrfnpod.org.

59. Roep BO, Peakman M: Surrogate end points in the design of immunotherapy trials: emerging lessons from type 1 diabetes. *Nat Rev Immunol* 10:145–152, 2010

60. Matthews JB, Staeva TP, Bernstein PL, Peakman M, Von Herrath M: ITN-JDRF Type 1 Diabetes Combination Therapy Assessment Group: Developing combination immunotherapies for type 1 diabetes: recommendations from the ITN–JDRF Type 1 Diabetes Combination Therapy Assessment Group. *Clin Exp Immunol* 160:176–184, 2010

61. Skyler JS, Ricordi C: Stopping type 1 diabetes: attempts to prevent or cure type 1 diabetes in man. *Diabetes* 60:1–8, 2011

62. Voltarelli JC, Couri CE, Stracieri AB, Oliveira MC, Moraes DA, Pieroni F, Coutinho M, Malmegrim KC, Foss-Freitas MC, Simões BP, Foss MC, Squiers E, Burt RK: Autologous nonmyeloablative hematopoietic stem cell transplantation in newly diagnosed type 1 diabetes mellitus. *JAMA* 297:1568–1576, 2007

63. Gottlieb PA, Quinlan S, Krause-Steinrauf H, Greenbaum CJ, Wilson DM, Rodriguez H, Schatz DA, Moran AM, Lachin JM, Skyler JS: Type 1 Diabetes TrialNet MMF/DZB Study Group: Failure to preserve beta-cell function with mycophenolate mofetil and daclizumab combined therapy in patients with new onset type 1 diabetes. *Diabetes Care* 33:826–832, 2010. Epub 12 January 2010

64. Herold KC, Gitelman SE, Willi SM, Gottlieb PA, Waldron-Lynch F, Devine L, Sherr J, Rosenthal SM, Adi S, Jalaludin MY, Michels AW, Dziura J, Bluestone JA: Teplizumab treatment may improve C-peptide responses in participants with type 1 diabetes after the new-onset period: a randomised controlled trial. *Diabetologia*. 2012 Oct 21. [Epub ahead of print]

65. Greenbaum CJ, Beam CA, Boulware D, Gitelman SE, Gottlieb PA, Herold KC, Lachin JM, McGee P, Palmer JP, Pescovitz MD, Krause-Steinrauf H, Skyler JS, Sosenko JM: Type 1 Diabetes TrialNet Study Group. Fall in C-peptide during first 2 years from diagnosis: evidence of at least two distinct phases from composite Type 1 Diabetes TrialNet data. *Diabetes* 61(8):2066–2073, 2012. Epub 2012 June 11

66. Greenbaum CJ, Harrison LC: Immunology of Diabetes Society: Guidelines for intervention trials in subjects with newly diagnosed type 1 diabetes. *Diabetes* 52:1059–1065, 2003. Erratum in *Diabetes* 52:2643, 2003
67. Palmer JP, Fleming GA, Greenbaum CJ, Herold KC, Jansa LD, Kolb H, Lachin JM, Polonsky KS, Pozzilli P, Skyler JS, Steffes MW: C-peptide is the appropriate outcome measure for type 1 diabetes clinical trials to preserve beta-cell function: report of an ADA workshop, 21-22 October 2001. *Diabetes* 53:250–264, 2004

4

β-Cell Replacement Therapy

Andrew M. Posselt, MD, PhD, FACS, and Peter Stock, MD, PhD

INTRODUCTION

The goal of curing type 1 diabetes (T1D) is best achieved with β-cell replacement therapy because this allows physiologic blood glucose control. Currently, the only way to restore normal blood glucose levels in individuals with T1D without the associated risk of hypoglycemia is to replace the patient's islets of Langerhans, which normally produce insulin but have been destroyed by an autoimmune reaction. This replacement can be achieved by either the transplantation of a whole pancreas or by the injection of islets of Langerhans, which are isolated from donor pancreata.[1] Solid organ pancreas transplantation, particularly when performed in conjunction with a renal transplant in the uremic patient with diabetes, has become an increasingly successful procedure.[2-4] Unfortunately, the procedure continues to carry significant perioperative morbidity and requires potent, long-term immunosuppression, and this has limited the target population to individuals who are <50 years old and who do not have significant cardiovascular disease.[5,6]

Pancreatic islet transplantation represents a minimally invasive alternative to vascularized whole organ transplantation. It offers a safer means of restoring euglycemia and insulin independence early in the course of diabetes, thereby preventing acute complications such as hypoglycemia, and long-term complications such as diabetic nephropathy, retinopathy, and neuropathy.[7] The avoidance of the surgical complications associated with pancreas transplantation also significantly increases the safety and applicability of islet transplantation early in the course of diabetes. Unfortunately, multiple donors usually are required to isolate sufficient islets to achieve insulin independence, and islet function appears to wane over time.[8-10] As with pancreas transplantation, lifelong aggressive immunosuppression is necessary to protect islets from the alloimmune and autoimmune responses of the host. Thus, the acceptability of clinical islet transplantation will in part depend on the development of less toxic immunosuppressive protocols and on the identification of alternative sources for donor islets, such as xenogeneic grafts and islets developed from stem cell progenitors. This chapter examines the history and current state of each β-cell replacement option and provides a rational approach to the treatment of patients with T1D.

WHOLE ORGAN PANCREAS TRANSPLANTATION

The first successful pancreas transplant was performed at the University of Minnesota in 1966.[11] For a number of years after this achievement, the applicability of the whole organ pancreas transplantation was hampered by both technical and immunologic factors. Pancreas grafts were frequently lost to thrombosis, rejection,

DOI: 10.2337/9781580404785ch04

61

bleeding, and anastomotic leaks at the donor duodenum.[12] Over the past several years, however, advances in operative technique, perioperative management, and monitoring have resulted in significant improvements in graft and patient survival. In discussing outcomes, we will refer to graft survival and loss.[3,5,13] *Graft survival* refers to the success of the graft and takes into account all possible causes of graft loss. *Graft loss* is a term that specifies the cause of graft failure (e.g., rejection, thrombosis, etc.).

Advances in immunosuppression have been an important component of the improved outcomes. New agents have allowed adequate suppression of the immune system without the chronic use of steroids, which are known to be toxic to β-cells.[14] For example, lymphocyte-depleting antibodies, such as antithymocyte globulin are now routinely used for induction therapy as well as for the treatment of acute episodes of cellular rejection.[15] The introduction of sirolimus, an mTor inhibitor that has little nephrotoxicity, has improved renal allograft survival in patients with simultaneous pancreas and kidney (SPK) transplants by permitting reduction of tacrolimus dosing. With these new agents, rejection rates for SPK transplants have dropped from 80% to <20% in the past 10 years.[16] The most recent national data for recipients of SPK transplants demonstrate a one-year and a five-year pancreatic graft survival of 87% and 72%, respectively (SRTR Annual Report, 2007).

Pancreas transplants alone (PTA) and pancreas after kidney (PAK) transplants traditionally have been less successful compared with SPK.[13,15,17] Immunologic and technical factors play a role in this discrepancy. Because these patients do not suffer from the uremia associated with renal failure, their platelet function is not impaired, which places them at higher risk for thrombosis in the low-flow vessels of the pancreas. Treatment of these patients with heparin and dipyridamole in the perioperative period has decreased graft thrombosis rates; however, this has also increased bleeding risk significantly. In the past, PTA and PAK patients have experienced more graft loss because of rejection as compared with SPK recipients. In 1998, the University of Minnesota reported that one- and three-year rates of graft loss because of rejection were 2% and 6% for SPK transplants, 12% and 19% for PAK transplants, and 22% and 43% for PTA, respectively.[5,18] Since then, improvements in monitoring (such as with protocol graft biopsies) and immuno-suppression have resulted in pancreas graft survival rates of 85% and 52% at one year and five years, respectively, in patients receiving a pancreas only (PTA; SRTR Annual Report, 2007), results that are approaching those achieved in SPK.

Although pancreas transplantation can achieve long-term insulin-independence in >80% of patients and stabilizes some of the diabetes-associated complications such as retinopathy and neuropathy, it has significant limitations. First, the number of pancreata that are suitable for transplantation is quite low. Of the ~8,000 deceased donors in the U.S. annually, only ~1,400 (16%) are potentially suitable for whole organ transplantation.[19] Second, because of the accelerated course of cardiovascular disease among patients with T1D, many patients who could benefit from the normal insulin physiology conferred by a pancreas transplant are poor candidates for this complex operation due to their underlying cardiovascular disease and resultant increased risk of perioperative complications.[6,20] This perioperative cardiac risk coupled with the surgical complications that some patients experience have led researchers to look for other methods to restore β-cell function in patients with diabetes. In the U.S., as with other organs, pancreas transplants are covered by insurance.

PANCREATIC ISLET TRANSPLANTATION

The pancreas is an organ with numerous functions, yet the function relevant to transplantation is its endocrine function in controlling blood glucose. Soon after the first successful whole organ pancreas transplant, researchers began to develop methods of transplanting isolated pancreatic islets rather than the entire organ. In theory, such a transplant would restore β-cell function, while not requiring a physiologically stressful operation, and would eliminate the complications that can result from the nonendocrine portions of the gland (Fig. 4.1). In 1972, transplantation of isolated islets succeeded in treating hyperglycemia in a rat model of diabetes.[21] Shortly afterward in 1974, islet transplantation was attempted in a patient with diabetes, although only brief, partial function was observed (Fig. 4.2).[22] These early achievements raised hope that long-term insulin independence using islet transplantation was imminent; however, the ensuing decades failed to see the realization of the tremendous potential for islet cell transplants in achieving this goal. In 1999, the international registry at Giessen reported that of the 405 islet cell allotransplants performed, <10% were able to achieve and sustain insulin independence for >6 months.[23]

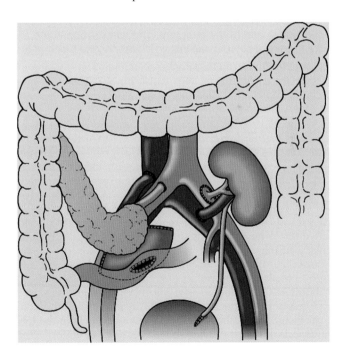

Figure 4.1 Simultaneous pancreas-kidney transplantation with enteric drainage of the pancreatic exocrine secretions into the ileum. The vessels of the pancreas and kidney are connected to the right and left iliac vessels of the recipient, respectively. Source: John D. Pirsch, Jon S. Odorico, and Hans W. Sollinger. Reprinted with permission from the publisher.

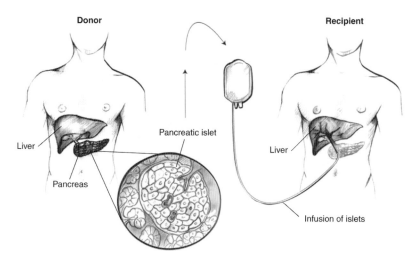

Figure 4.2 Human pancreatic islet manufacture and transplantation. Islets are isolated from a deceased donor pancreas using a multi-step process and infused directly into the portal vein of the recipient. The islets lodge in the small portal venules and eventually begin to make insulin in response to blood glucose levels.

Source: National Institute of Diabetes and Digestive and Kidney Diseases: *Pancreatic Islet Transplantation*. NIH publ. no. 07-4693. Bethesda, MD, National Diabetes Information Clearinghouse, 2007.

Interestingly, patients who underwent islet autotransplants for indications other than diabetes had far better clinical outcomes than those who underwent islet allotransplants. In a series reported by the University of Minnesota, patients undergoing total or completion pancreatectomy for chronic pancreatitis with subsequent islet transplantation derived from their own tissue achieved insulin independence rates of >70%.[24] One such patient was able to sustain insulin independence for >13 years without the need for immunosuppression.[25,26] This was proof that islet transplantation could achieve long-lasting insulin independence. It also identified the immune response as an important barrier to clinical success in islet allotransplantion.

Multiple aspects of the islet transplant process were thought to contribute to the poor clinical outcomes observed in islet allotransplants; nonetheless, despite the general dysphoria surrounding islet allotransplantation, the groups at the University of Giessen and at the University of Alberta in Edmonton continued to work on the problem. This resulted in encouraging advances in the technical and immunologic aspects of islet transplantation.[26,27] Studies of donor factors revealed that better islet yields could be obtained from patients with higher BMIs, and the importance of short cold ischemia times (<8 h) for pancreata destined for islet isolation was also evident.[28,29] Ironically, the characteristics that make pancreata suitable for islet isolation (older donor, high BMI) also make them less desirable for whole organ transplantation, thus avoiding competition for organs and increasing overall organ utilization.

Improvements in the islet isolation process also had dramatic effects on islet yields and rates of insulin independence. The isolation process is extremely complex, and many of the steps are difficult to control (Fig. 4.3). Most important among these is the initial digestion of the exocrine tissue by enzymes that release the islets from the organ without destroying them. Historically, the purity and the activity of these enzymes were not well quantitated or standardized, and this resulted in inconsistent yields and highly variable results. Over the past few years, commercially available collagenase cocktails and neutral protease enzymes have become available, and although some variation still exists between lots, islet isolation centers are gaining more experience with these reagents and are able to achieve more consistent results.[30,31] Other aspects of the islet isolation process, such as the separation, purification, and culture of the islets have been refined.[32] These technical advancements have improved the islet yields obtained from each donor pancreas and have helped achieve insulin independence in up to 50% of patients after transplantation of islets from a single donor.[33,34]

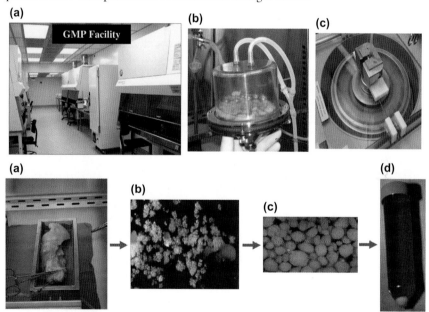

Figure 4.3 Steps in the islet manufacturing process. Top row: (a) Islets are isolated in a Good Manufacturing Practice (GMP) facility using stringent protocols. (b) Enzymatic digestion in a temperature-controlled chamber is the first step in the isolation process. (c) Islets are separated from exocrine tissue using gradient centrifugation.

Bottom row: Appearance of the islet product at various stages of the manufacturing process. (a) Donor pancreas at the beginning of digestion. (b) Islets (stained red) with contaminating exocrine tissue. (c) The purified islet product. (d) Settled islet product in culture medium. The islets comprise the light colored pellet at the bottom of the tube.

The importance of the immune response in islet cell transplants was made evident by the vastly improved outcomes in patients undergoing autotransplantation versus allotransplantation. In addition to the allogeneic immune response, patients with T1D also have an autoimmune destruction of their native β-cells as the etiology of their disease. This autoimmune response needs to be suppressed if the transplanted β-cells are to survive. In 2000, the group at the University of Alberta reported consistent insulin independence using a strategy that is now known as the Edmonton protocol.[27] This protocol consisted of infusing at least 8,000–9,000 islet equivalents (IEQs) per kilogram of body weight (this usually required two to three separate infusions). A normal-size pancreas has an estimated ~1 million islets. It is thought that stable independence needs ~8,000–9,000 IEQs (essentially islets), so a 70-kg person needs ~600,000–700,000 islets, which represents an extremely good yield from a single pancreas.[35] However, although more is better, islet number is not the only factor.

The Edmonton protocol also included an immunosuppressive regimen that avoided steroids and minimized calcineurin inhibitors, both toxic to β-cells. An antibody against the interleukin-2 receptor (daclizumab) was used for induction

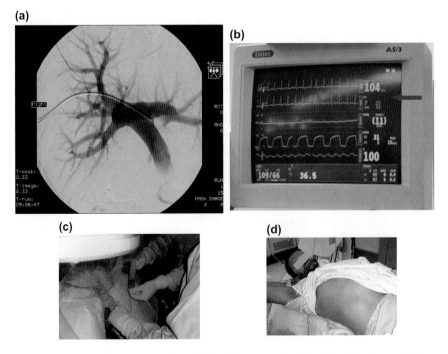

Figure 4.4 Islet transplantation. (a) Angiogram showing the infusion catheter within the main portal vein. (b) Monitoring of recipient vital signs, including portal pressure (arrow). (c) Infusion of the islets under fluoroscopic guidance. (d) Patient in the recovery room showing the small puncture site.

therapy, and sirolimus and low-dose tacrolimus were used for long-term immunosuppression. Using these techniques, researchers were able to achieve insulin independence in seven patients.[27,36]

These results set off a new wave of interest in islet cell transplantation, and multiple other centers in the U.S. and worldwide began to perform islet transplants (Fig. 4.4).[37] A 2007 report from the Collaborative Islet Transplant Registry showed that 28 centers in the U.S. were currently or had been active in islet transplantation and that 783 patients had received this treatment. In addition, ~65% of patients were able to achieve insulin independence, and 24% were still free of the need for insulin at three years time.[38] This improvement in results has continued. The most recent report from the Collaborative Islet Transplant Registry (CITR; 2011) showed insulin independence rates of ~45% at three years.[39]

Hypoglycemia Unawareness

Hypoglycemic unawareness in islet transplant recipients decreased from 60% pretransplant to 4% at three years post-transplant, even in patients who returned to insulin use. One possible explanation for this result is that nearly 80% of patients did retain some graft function, as defined by the presence of C-peptide at three years, which helped control glucose regulation, even if exogenous insulin use was resumed.[40,41] More recently, the National Institutes of Health (NIH) have supported an ongoing, multicenter trial of clinical islet transplantation that is designed to serve as a stepping stone for standardization of islet isolation and transplantation, and to provide data that can be used to support efforts to make islet transplantation a U.S. Food and Drug Administration (FDA)–approved procedure (see http://www.citisletstudy.org).

Adverse Events

Adverse events were noted that related to infusion of the islets into the portal vein, such as elevation in liver enzymes, bleeding, and portal vein thrombosis, but these were well tolerated.[42,43] More serious consequences included the development of neoplasms that were likely related to immunosuppression, a death from viral meningitis, and development of antidonor alloantibodies when immunosuppressive drugs were discontinued. Such sensitization was concerning because it could place patients at increased risk for rejection in the future and also limit the pool of acceptable donors for future islets or kidneys.[44,45]

PATIENT SELECTION FOR PANCREAS VERSUS PANCREATIC ISLET TRANSPLANTATION

Although solid organ pancreas transplantation has been the gold standard for the achievement of long-term insulin independence, recent advances in islet transplantation have made cellular transplants an increasingly attractive alternative for β-cell replacement. In fact, some studies using more aggressive immunosuppression with lymphodepletion as induction therapy have demonstrated five-year insulin independence rates in greater than 50% of islet recipients. These results are now approximating those seen with PTA.

At this point, islet transplants remain in the domain of experimental trials and rarely are covered by insurance. Islet transplants after kidney transplants are covered by Medicare, and if they are part of an NIH-sponsored trial, islet transplants alone are also covered by Medicare. At this time, other insurance companies do not cover islet transplants. Islet transplantation, however, likely will become an FDA-approved procedure in the near future. By the time it is approved, the algorithm by which β-cell replacement therapy is offered to a given patient will change. Until this change, any patient with T1D who is a candidate for pancreas transplantation (SPK, PAK, or PTA) and has a cardiovascular system that can tolerate whole organ pancreas transplantation should be offered that procedure. For patients with advanced cardiovascular disease or patients who do not wish to or cannot undergo an open surgical procedure, islet transplantation can be offered but only as part of an experimental trial (see citisletstudy.org, niddk.nih. gov, and clinicaltrials.gov). Until islet transplantations can be offered routinely as a covered service, the algorithm of who should be offered an islet versus pancreas transplant will depend on the state of the art of islet transplantation available at the time. Currently, patients who are highly sensitized or have high insulin requirements remain better candidates for solid organ pancreas transplants.

CONCLUSION

Pancreas transplantation is a safe and durable strategy to achieve insulin independence in patients with T1D. Long-term insulin independence can be achieved as well as stabilization of the devastating secondary complications of long-standing diabetes. Rigorous immune monitoring combined with aggressive immunosuppression have resulted in excellent outcomes, even in PTA recipients who remain at an increased risk for acute rejection. Nonetheless, the number of patients who can benefit from this procedure is limited by the surgical and cardiovascular stresses associated with solid organ pancreas transplantation. Although islet transplantation remains an experimental procedure, progress continues in long-term success utilizing aggressive immunosuppression protocols. Further improvements in islet isolation, immunosuppression, and new sources of β-cells derived from stem cells will move islet transplantation into the realm of FDA-approved procedures within the next few years. Upon approval, the number of options available for β-cell replacement will increase and potentially benefit more patients with T1D who currently are not candidates for β-cell replacement via whole organ pancreas transplantation. These would include patients who are too old or have significant medical comorbidities, such as heart disease, that would put them at higher risk for perioperative complications.

Significant advances in the technology of islet isolation, as well as improvements in the ability to protect transplanted islets from both the alloimmune and autoimmune responses, have led to major improvements in long-term rates of insulin independence. The logistics of isolating sufficient islets from a limited pool of donors remains a major limiting factor for widespread application as a treatment for diabetes. Potential solutions for new sources include xenogeneic tissue, embryonic stem cells (ES) differentiated into insulin-producing cells, and induced pluripotent stem cells (iPS) cells.[46,47]

Although clinical trials using porcine islets likely will move forward in the near future, success will require novel immunosuppressive strategies to overcome the potent xenogeneic response. In addition, concerns persist regarding the risk of transmitting infectious diseases from one species to another. Although iPS-derived β-cells have the promise of providing a source of human leukocyte antigen (HLA)–matched β-cells for the diabetic patient, this technology has not evolved as far as the ES-derived β-cell.[48]

The first clinical trials of ES-derived β-cells will likely be moving forward in the near future. Several teams have produced insulin-producing β-cells derived from human ES lines by culturing the cells with selected differentiation factors. These cells have been capable of reversing diabetes in immunodeficient mice. As these ES-derived β-cells move closer to clinical trials, they will still require protection from both the alloimmune and autoimmune responses, as they express HLA derived from the ES cell line.[49-51] Strategies that are being considered include the immunosuppressive regimens found to be effective in the human islet trials as well as use of an immunoisolation barrier.[52] The latter strategy also will provide a barrier for undifferentiated cells, which could develop from the pluripotent ES cell line. Current platforms and immunosuppressive strategies that are successful for islet allotransplantation will form the basis for the first clinical trials for ES-derived β-cells. The potential for an unlimited source of β-cells undeniably will have a profound impact on the treatment of T1D.

GAPS ACCORDING TO THE EDITORS

1. There is a need for the identification of additional sources of β-cells for replacement, either from donor organs, iPS cells, ES cells, or other options, with additional investigations aimed at improved isolation, purification, and differentiation processes.
2. There is a need for β-cell replacement approaches that limit or reduce exposure to toxic immunosuppressive therapies.
3. Although many of the issues related to optimizing islet replacement therapy remain within the realm of research, there is a need to ensure rapid insurance reimbursement for effective treatments, such as islet transplantation.

REFERENCES

1. Group TDCaCTR: The effect of intensive treatment of diabetes on the development and progression of long-term complications in insulin-dependent diabetes mellitus. The Diabetes Control and Complications Trial Research Group. *N Engl J Med* 329:977–986, 1993
2. Gruessner AC, Sutherland DE: Report for the international pancreas transplant registry, 2000. *Transplant Proc* 33:1643–1646, 2001
3. Sutherland DE, Gruessner RW, Gruessner AC: Pancreas transplantation for treatment of diabetes mellitus. *World J Surg* 25:487–496, 2001
4. Feng S, Barr M, Roberts J, Oberbauer R, Kaplan B: Developments in clinical islet, liver thoracic, kidney and pancreas transplantation in the last 5 years. *Am J Transplant* 6:1759–1767, 2006

5. Sutherland DE, Gruessner RW, Dunn DL, et al.: Lessons learned from more than 1,000 pancreas transplants at a single institution. *Ann Surg* 233:463–501, 2001
6. Gruessner RW, Sutherland DE, Gruessner AC: Mortality assessment for pancreas transplants. *Am J Transplant* 4:2018–2026, 2004
7. Fiorina P, Folli F, Zerbini G, et al.: Islet transplantation is associated with improvement of renal function among uremic patients with type I diabetes mellitus and kidney transplants. *J Am Soc Nephrol* 14:2150–2158, 2003
8. Shapiro AM, Ricordi C, Hering BJ, et al.: International trial of the Edmonton protocol for islet transplantation. *N Engl J Med* 355:1318–1330, 2006
9. Rother KI, Harlan DM: Challenges facing islet transplantation for the treatment of type 1 diabetes mellitus. J Clin Invest 114:877–883, 2004
10. Cravedi P, van der Meer IM, Cattaneo S, Ruggenenti P, Remuzzi G: Successes and disappointments with clinical islet transplantation. *Advances in Experimental Medicine and Biology* 654:749–769, 2010
11. Sutherland DE, Goetz FC, Chinn PL, et al.: Clinical pancreas and islet transplantation. Part 2: pancreas transplantation at the University of Minnesota. *Primary Care* 10:717–722, 1983
12. Sutherland DE, Moudry KC: Clinical pancreas and islet transplantation. *Transplant Proc* 19:113–120, 1987
13. Gruessner RW, Sutherland DE, Najarian JS, Dunn DL, Gruessner AC: Solitary pancreas transplantation for nonuremic patients with labile insulin-dependent diabetes mellitus. *Transplant* 64:1572–1577, 1997
14. Gruessner RW, Sutherland DE, Parr E, Humar A, Gruessner AC: A prospective, randomized, open-label study of steroid withdrawal in pancreas transplantation—a preliminary report with 6-month follow-up. *Transplant Proc* 33:1663–1664, 2001
15. Humar A, Ramcharan T, Kandaswamy R, et al.: Pancreas after kidney transplants. *Am J Surg* 182:155–161, 2001
16. Singh RP, Stratta RJ: Advances in immunosuppression for pancreas transplantation. *Curr Opin Organ Transplant* 13:79–84, 2008
17. Najarian JS, Gruessner AC, Drangsteveit MB, et al.: Insulin independence of more than 10 years after pancreas transplantation. *Transplant Proc* 30:1936–1937, 1998
18. Sutherland DE: Pancreas and pancreas-kidney transplantation. *Curr Opin Nephrol Hypertens* 7:317–325, 1998
19. Gruessner AC, Sutherland DE, Gruessner RW: Pancreas transplantation in the United States: a review. *Curr Opin Organ Transplant* 15:93–101, 2010
20. Nathan DM: Isolated pancreas transplantation for type 1 diabetes: a doctor's dilemma. *JAMA* 290:2861–2863, 2003
21. Ballinger WF, Lacy PE: Transplantation of intact pancreatic islets in rats. *Surgery* 72:175–186, 1972
22. Sutherland DE: Pancreas and islet transplantation. II. Clinical trials. *Diabetologia* 20:435–450, 1981
23. Bretzel RG, Brendel M, Eckhard M, et al.: Islet transplantation: present clinical situation and future aspects. *Experimental and Clinical Endocrinology & Diabetes* 109 (Suppl. 2):S384–S399, 2001

24. Blondet JJ, Carlson AM, Kobayashi T, et al.: The role of total pancreatectomy and islet autotransplantation for chronic pancreatitis. *Surg Clin North Am* 87:1477–1501, 2007
25. Sutherland DE, Radosevich DM, Bellin MD, et al.: Total pancreatectomy and islet autotransplantation for chronic pancreatitis. *J Am Coll Surg* 214:409–424, 2012; discussion 24-6
26. Bretzel RG: Current status and perspectives in clinical islet transplantation. *J Hepatobiliary Pancreat Surg* 7:370–373, 2000
27. Shapiro AM, Lakey JR, Ryan EA, et al.: Islet transplantation in seven patients with type 1 diabetes mellitus using a glucocorticoid-free immunosuppressive regimen. *New Engl J Med* 343:230–238, 2000
28. Tsujimura T, Kuroda Y, Kin T, et al.: Human islet transplantation from pancreases with prolonged cold ischemia using additional preservation by the two-layer (UW solution/perfluorochemical) cold-storage method. *Transplantation* 74:1687–1691, 2002
29. Lakey JR, Burridge PW, Shapiro AM: Technical aspects of islet preparation and transplantation. *Transplant Int* 16:613–632, 2003
30. Balamurugan AN, Breite AG, Anazawa T, et al.: Successful human islet isolation and transplantation indicating the importance of class 1 collagenase and collagen degradation activity assay. *Transplantation* 89:954–961
31. Anazawa T, Balamurugan AN, Bellin M, et al.: Human islet isolation for autologous transplantation: comparison of yield and function using SERVA/Nordmark versus Roche enzymes. *Am J Transplant* 9:2383–2391, 2009
32. Posselt AM, Szot GL, Frassetto LA, Masharani U, Stock PG: Clinical islet transplantation at the University of California, San Francisco. *Clin Transplant*, 235–243, 2010
33. Hering BJ, Kandaswamy R, Ansite JD, et al.: Single-donor, marginal-dose islet transplantation in patients with type 1 diabetes. *JAMA* 293:830–835, 2005
34. Posselt AM, Szot GL, Frassetto LA, et al.: Islet transplantation in type 1 diabetic patients using calcineurin inhibitor-free immunosuppressive protocols based on T-cell adhesion or costimulation blockade. *Transplantation* 90:1595–1601, 2010
35. Shapiro AM: State of the art of clinical islet transplantation and novel protocols of immunosuppression. *Current Diabetes Reports* 11:345–354, 2011
36. Ryan EA, Lakey JR, Rajotte RV, et al.: Clinical outcomes and insulin secretion after islet transplantation with the Edmonton protocol. *Diabetes* 50:710–719, 2001
37. Ricordi C, Inverardi L, Kenyon NS, et al.: Requirements for success in clinical islet transplantation. *Transplantation* 79:1298–1300, 2005
38. 2007 update on allogeneic islet transplantation from the Collaborative Islet Transplant Registry (CITR). *Cell Transplant* 18:753–767, 2009
39. Seventh annual data report, 2011. Available at http://www.citregistry.org/reports/reports.htm. Accessed 1 August 2012
40. Ryan EA, Paty BW, Senior PA, Bigam D, Alfadhli E, Kneteman NM, Lakey JRT, Shapiro AMJ: Five-year follow-up after clinical islet transplantation. *Diabetes* 54:2060–2069, 2005

41. Ryan EA, Shandro T, Green K, et al.: Assessment of the severity of hypoglycemia and glycemic lability in type 1 diabetic subjects undergoing islet transplantation. *Diabetes* 53:955–962, 2004

42. Kawahara T, Kin T, Kashkoush S, et al.: Portal vein thrombosis is a potentially preventable complication in clinical islet transplantation. *Am J Transplant* 11:2700–2707, 2011

43. Rafael E, Ryan EA, Paty BW, et al.: Changes in liver enzymes after clinical islet transplantation. *Transplantation* 76:1280–1284, 2003

44. Chhabra P, Brayman KL: Current status of immunomodulatory and cellular therapies in preclinical and clinical islet transplantation. *J Transplant*, 637–692, 2011

45. Naziruddin B, Wease S, Stablein D, et al.: HLA class I sensitization in islet transplant recipients: report from the Collaborative Islet Transplant Registry. *Cell Transplant* 21:901–908, 2012

46. Miszta-Lane H, Mirbolooki M, James Shapiro AM, Lakey JR: Stem cell sources for clinical islet transplantation in type 1 diabetes: embryonic and adult stem cells. *Med Hypoth* 67:909–913, 2006

47. Bretzel RG, Eckhard M, Brendel MD: Pancreatic islet and stem cell transplantation: new strategies in cell therapy of diabetes mellitus. *Panminerva Medica* 46:25–42, 2004

48. Casu A, Trucco M, Pietropaolo M: A look to the future: prediction, prevention, and cure including islet transplantation and stem cell therapy. *Pediatr Clin North Am* 52:1779–1804

49. Kandeel F, Smith CV, Todorov I, Mullen Y: Advances in islet cell biology: from stem cell differentiation to clinical transplantation: conference report. *Pancreas* 27:e63–78, 2003

50. Dominguez-Bendala J, Inverardi L, Ricordi C: Stem cell-derived islet cells for transplantation. *Curr Opin Organ Transplant*, 2010

51. Duprez IR, Johansson U, Nilsson B, Korsgren O, Magnusson PU: Preparatory studies of composite mesenchymal stem cell islets for application in intraportal islet transplantation. *Upsala J Med Sci* 116:8–17, 2011

52. Vaithilingam V, Tuch BE: Islet transplantation and encapsulation: an update on recent developments. *Rev Diabet Stud* 8:51–67, 2011

5

Initial Evaluation and Follow-up

Linda M. Siminerio, RN, PhD, CDE, Lori Laffel, MD, MPH, and Anne Peters, MD

CLINICAL ASSESSMENTS FOR INDIVIDUALS WITH TYPE 1 DIABETES: PEDIATRICS AND ADULTS

Our goal for this chapter is to clarify the care for a patient with type 1 diabetes (T1D) at any age. More than 80% of children with T1D are cared for by a diabetes specialist, as a part of a multidisciplinary pediatric team.[1] However, this is not necessarily true for adults, where many adult patients with T1D receive care from generalists without the expertise of adult-trained endocrinologists or diabetologists (some of whom are generalists with a particular focus on diabetes). Furthermore, adult providers predominantly see type 2 diabetes (T2D) patients so they may not be as well versed in the details and demands of intensive insulin therapy that is standard in the care of individuals with T1D.

As envisioned for this book, we discuss the care of patients of all ages with T1D. Much of this information derives from the 2012 American Diabetes Association (ADA) Clinical Practice Recommendations, but we have eliminated approaches that apply exclusively to T2D patients. We do not intend to reinvent the standards of care per se, so we utilize the current recommendations as annually published by the ADA along with updated approaches from the literature and expert consensus, when gaps in the published literature exist. In this chapter, we will not discuss topics covered in other chapters, such as setting treatment targets (chapter 6) and monitoring (chapter 9). We want providers to know that patients with T1D *are not* the same as patients with T2D; thus, we describe the specific approaches for patients with T1D across the life span.

INTRODUCTION

All patients with T1D require close evaluation and follow-up. There are common elements for initial assessment and follow-up care, although one must always recognize that unique circumstances and personal needs support the individualization of treatment recommendations and care delivery. Assessment and care delivery vary across the life span: for infants and young children, parents and other adult caregivers provide the management and become the focus of the care delivery. As diabetes care progresses through childhood, adolescence, and into emerging adulthood, there is a gradual transfer and, hopefully, acceptance of self-management responsibilities. This necessitates a change in the focus of care delivery to the patient along with provision of different yet ongoing support. The transition into middle adulthood heralds autonomous decision making and treatment shifts almost exclusively to the patient. Finally, in the older, geriatric population, care delivery may again shift back to caregivers who once again play an increasingly critical role in a patient's diabetes management.

At each developmental and life stage, a defined infrastructure for care should exist, with a specific focus on the safe and effective use of insulin; on matching the diabetes treatment program to fit the patient's unique psychosocial needs; and on ongoing screening, prevention, and treatment of comorbidities and complications. Of particular importance is the transition from the pediatric to the adult provider. As emphasized earlier, the level of care provided by a pediatric specialist team may be substantially different from that given by adult providers. Both pediatric and adult health care providers are responsible for facilitating this transition process, so that young adult patients receive quality, uninterrupted care.

Assessment

Assessment is the cornerstone of the care and educational process. The information gathered provides a sense of who patients are, their medical history, the results of physical exams, and their experiences and beliefs. These give insights into how they might best master diabetes knowledge and the self-management skills essential for optimal clinical, psychosocial, and long-term outcomes. It is critical that clinicians realize that assessment is an ongoing process. Information collected initially must be reviewed on a continual basis and updated throughout the course of diabetes care, especially as the patient enters different developmental stages. In this way, individual care and education plans with realistic and achievable goals can be developed that promote effective care and self-management aimed at achieving desired health and psychosocial outcomes.

Multiple studies indicate the importance of individualizing plans for care and education based on a thorough assessment. While a thorough medical evaluation is necessary, attention to patients' educational and psychosocial needs is also important. An education and psychosocial assessment needs to include specific information about lifestyle, cultural influences and beliefs, health beliefs and attitudes, diabetes knowledge, self-management skills and behaviors, readiness to learn, health literacy level, physical limitations, family and social support, and financial status.

People with T1D should receive medical care from a physician-coordinated multidisciplinary team. Such teams may include, but are not limited to, physicians with specialty training in endocrinology or diabetes, nurse practitioners, physician's assistants, nurses, dietitians, pharmacists, eye care specialists, and mental health professionals with expertise and a special interest in diabetes. For pediatric patients, child-life specialists can also be valuable members of the pediatric team to assist with reducing stress and providing comfort to pediatric patients while parents attend diabetes education and management appointments or when the patient's condition requires uncomfortable procedures such as phlebotomy, an initial insulin injection, insertion of a pump infusion set, or insertion of a continuous glucose sensor. As patients age, additional specialists such as cardiologists and nephrologists may be needed. It is essential in this collaborative and integrated team approach that individuals with diabetes assume an active role in their care.

The management plan should be formulated as a collaborative therapeutic alliance among the patient and family, the physician, and other members of the health care team. A variety of strategies and techniques should be used to provide adequate education and development of problem-solving skills in the various aspects of diabetes management. Implementation of the management plan requires that each aspect is understood and agreed to by the patient and the care providers and that the goals and treatment plan are reasonable and realistic. Plans should recognize diabetes self-management education (DSME) and ongoing diabetes support as integral components of care. In developing the plan, consideration should be given to the patient's age, school or work schedule and conditions, physical activity, eating patterns, social situation and cultural factors, and the presence of complications of diabetes or other medical conditions.

The information outlined below is designed to aid the clinician in the evaluation and treatment of the patient initially and over time during follow-up. In addition, both the initial evaluation and ongoing follow-up approaches clarify the unique needs of pediatric and adult patients. Children with diabetes are not just small adults. Their diabetes treatment program must reflect the particular needs of childhood growth and development, puberty, social and emotional changes, and the particular requirement for the involvement of adults in care delivery both at home and at school.

Approaches that are similar for pediatric and adult patients will be presented together, followed by sections that clarify the distinctions between the patient populations. The approaches are modeled after the current ADA recommendations for care, but are not meant to supplant those recommendations. They have been amended to focus on the needs of persons with T1D. When possible, approaches to care result from clinical trials; when such data do not exist, expert consensus provides the suggested approaches.

An overview of the clinical assessments and laboratory tests that should be performed routinely in individuals with T1D is presented in the Appendix: Components of Assessments. These can serve as a reference for the basic requirements for care. Although similar to care approaches for individuals with T2D, the focus for patients with T1D includes a greater concern for detecting coexistent autoimmune diseases and less on cardiovascular evaluation, particularly in younger individuals. Few data exist to support these clinical recommendations, which exist largely as expert opinion relying heavily on the recommendations made by the ADA Professional Practice Committee.

INITIAL EVALUATION

An initial evaluation may be performed at the time of presentation of hyperglycemia or when a patient begins care with a new provider. The key elements of the initial diabetes evaluation are listed in Table 5.1 (for details of classification, see chapter 1 and chapter 2, Natural History and Prediction of T1D).

After a focused history and physical examination are completed, a diabetes management plan should be formulated, involving other providers as indicated. The management plan should create a basis for ongoing care. Laboratory tests appropriate to the evaluation of each patient should be performed. At the end of

---

Table 5.1 Initial Evaluation of Patients with New-Onset or Established T1D

■ Diabetes classification to confirm T1D

■ Review of symptoms and signs at presentation and initial treatment (in- or outpatient)

■ Diabetes history including past hospitalizations and occurrence of acute complications

■ Family history

■ Current treatment approaches (for patients with established diabetes)

■ A review of symptoms of uncontrolled diabetes

■ Assessment of patient's (and family's, if pediatric) psychosocial and educational needs

■ Evaluation for diabetes complications (if applicable) and other autoimmune conditions

■ Establishment of a follow-up care plan

---

the initial visit each patient or caregiver should be capable of basic T1D management skills and should understand the plan for follow-up care.

Assessment through the Life Span

Infants and preschool children. Child, parent, and caregiver assessments are all necessary to provide optimal care of the child. In this age-group, parents are the primary care providers, so examination of metabolic, psychosocial, and developmental issues as well as general parenting concerns and family interactions is necessary. How parents learn has to do with their current emotional state as well as their specific learning abilities. Parents confronted with diabetes often exhibit enormous guilt, fears, and frustration because of the diagnosis or because of prior stresses in their own upbringing and family situations. Exploring these areas and identifying support systems are important.

School-age children. As children grow and move toward more independence, assessing the school-age child's self-care competencies is crucial. Attending school forces the child with diabetes to begin assuming self-care tasks, such as recognizing hypoglycemia and making healthy meal choices. Identifying the available resources in the school and community is important in supporting the school-aged child's self-care and providing a safe environment. This developmental stage is also the time when children are building relationships with peers. Understanding the school-aged child's relationships with peers is particularly important in understanding the child's psychosocial needs.

Adolescents. Adolescents with diabetes are notorious for maladjustment to the rigors of diabetes care. Adolescence is associated with major hormonal and body changes, many competing academic and athletic demands, and psychosocial stresses and challenges. Diabetes, peer pressures, and all of the changes associated with adolescence place tremendous demands on the adolescent and family. A comprehensive assessment needs to address themes relevant to this age-group: driving, dating, sex, smoking, alcohol, drugs, eating disorders, and career choices. Identifying the need for counseling services may be necessary.

Young adults. An assessment in young adults spans a variety of relevant life changes. Accepting responsibility for living well with diabetes comes to bear as young adults move away from their families, start jobs, purchase their own diabetes supplies, and engage in long-lasting relationships. Independent living, buying and preparing foods, managing finances, and dealing with insurance and health care costs directly affect their diabetes self-management. Young adults may require medical and psychosocial adjustment assistance in managing early diabetes complications and with the accompanying feelings of depression, guilt, anger, and fear. These areas need to be considered in helping young adults plan for ongoing medical care and promoting their relationships with the diabetes health care team.

Adults. Adults with diabetes face unique challenges that need to be examined. Diabetes may significantly affect decisions related to marriage and relationships with friends and family. When an adult with diabetes decides to marry or partner, the spouse or significant other needs to be educated about diabetes and about the spousal or partner role in diabetes care. Diabetes may affect a couple's decision about whether and when to have children. Diabetes may affect an individual's choice of employment. Jobs that involve significant physical activity or unpredictable hours can affect diabetes control; certain occupations such as commercial airline pilot or interstate truck driver may not accept individuals with T1D (although in many cases, restrictions are removed for those who are well controlled). The health care team can help identify workplace challenges in an effort to construct a diabetes care plan to accommodate a job that involves irregular hours. The cost of diabetes care may be an issue, especially when finances are limited. The health care team must be aware of an individual's special needs and goals, assess them regularly, and develop care plans to meet them.

Older adults. The older adult who has lived with T1D for many years may be facing changes that come with aging that require ongoing assessment. Older adults have an increased incidence of comorbid illnesses, surgeries, and chronic complications. These factors often require further modifications in meal-planning and nutrition goals, the physical activity plan, and strategies for coping with stress. The physiological changes of aging (e.g., loss of sensation; declines in visual, auditory, and olfactory acuity; cognition impairment; and memory loss) may require adapted teaching methods and equipment (e.g., large print teaching materials; a syringe magnifier). In addition, physical limitations such as osteoarthritis, which limit degree of activity and ability to perform activities of daily living, may directly or indirectly affect diabetes management capabilities.

Multiple medications may require intervention by family and home health care aides to assure adherence to the prescribed regimen and accuracy in administration. Older adults may be making management decisions based on outdated or inaccurate information that needs updating. Identifying sources of information is important. Assessing family or support systems for the older adult cannot be stressed enough. Social support is an important predictor of physical and psychological health. Numerous studies have found that patients with good metabolic control and quality of life report having family support. Including such a support person in the assessment process is desirable.

INITIAL TREATMENT FOR PEDIATRIC PATIENTS

Although exact numbers are unknown, more than half of all patients with T1D appear to be diagnosed during childhood. In pediatric patients, the SEARCH for Diabetes in Youth Study has reported that 30% of youth with T1D present at diagnosis with diabetic ketoacidosis (DKA) while almost 40% of those aged <5 years present with DKA.[2,3] Initial evaluation occurs in the acute care hospital setting for almost all (>90%) patients who present with DKA, with the remaining minority managed in the emergency room setting. Further, 40% of patients diagnosed with hyperglycemia without DKA are managed in the hospital setting.[2] This amounts to 50% of pediatric patients newly diagnosed with T1D being managed initially in the hospital setting. Outpatient management has been shown to reduce costs and has not been associated with poorer glycemic control nor need for future hospitalizations.[4-6] In fact, there is greater opportunity for a quicker return to usual school and family activities with outpatient management. Outpatient management requires staff availability to provide initial education and management, relative ease for families to travel to and from the diabetes center, and absence of metabolic decompensation and DKA. Many centers will also hospitalize very young patients aged <2 years, independent of metabolic status at diagnosis.

Independent of location of initial evaluation and treatment, there is a need for patient and family education, implementation of individualized intensive insulin therapy, and ongoing close case management with frequent telephone contact between the diabetes team and the family for a few weeks following the diagnosis. (Approaches to insulin management are detailed in chapter 12, Insulin.)

Initiation of insulin therapy in pediatric patients depends on presence or absence of DKA and the pubertal status of the patient. (DKA management is reviewed in chapter 15.) DKA is associated with greater insulin needs due to the insulin resistance that accompanies ketosis and the presence of more severe β-cell failure in those youth who present with DKA. In addition, insulin needs are greater during puberty due to the recognized insulin resistance associated with pubertal growth and development.[7] Estimates of initial insulin dosing in youth according to weight appear in Table 5.2.

Table 5.2 Subcutaneous Insulin Administration at Diagnosis of T1D in Youth

	No DKA	DKA
Prepubertal	0.25–0.5 U/kg/day	0.75–1 U/kg/day
Pubertal	0.5–0.75	1–1.25
Postpubertal	0.25–0.5	0.75–1

INITIAL TREATMENT FOR ADULTS

Adult patients can vary greatly at presentation, from a more acute picture, with DKA and marked hyperglycemia, to a more gradual course such as is often seen in LADA. Although the natural history of LADA is not well characterized, in many adults it appears to be a slower onset of autoimmune T1D, where individuals are treated as though they have T2D before they are diagnosed with T1D. Regardless of the initial course of the diabetes, all patients will end up on insulin. For those presenting acutely as well as those presently more indolently, starting insulin is the mainstay of therapy.

Chapter 12 discusses insulin use in the management of T1D. In general, the starting dose is similar to that seen in postpubertal children, at 0.25–0.5 units/ kg/day. However, this can have significant variability. Higher initial doses often need to be reduced as glucotoxicity is reduced and residual β-cell function returns following normalization of glycemia. For most, basal insulin should be given initially (or as soon as the diagnosis of autoimmune T1D is made) with small doses of prandial insulin. These mealtime doses may be much smaller than in patients with longer duration of disease, often on the order of 1 unit per 25–30 g of carbohydrates. Dosing can be titrated upward as indicated by blood glucose levels, but initial instruction in basal-bolus insulin therapy and carbohydrate counting seems appropriate for most individuals.

ONGOING MANAGEMENT: PEDIATRICS AND ADULTS

For most individuals with T1D, ongoing management should involve quarterly follow-up to assess glycemic control and evaluate ongoing needs and concerns. For the pediatric patient with T1D, these quarterly visits are particularly important as the needs of children frequently change. Continued growth and pubertal development, expected and unexpected schedule alterations as the school year progresses, and changes in activity levels (as the school year ends and summer begins) require constant adjustments. Initially, ongoing management for the pediatric patient and family requires a focus on parental involvement in diabetes management tasks for the child. Family involvement is a fundamental component of diabetes management throughout childhood and into adolescence. Health care providers who care for children and adolescents must attend to the behavioral, emotional, and psychosocial factors that may interfere with implementation of the child's diabetes treatment program, and then they must work with the child and family to problem solve and modify treatment goals as needed.

Since a substantial proportion of a child's waking hours are spent in school, close communication and ongoing cooperation with school or day care personnel are important components of optimal diabetes management, safety, and maximal academic performance for youth with T1D. (Details are provided in chapter 18.II.)

Eventually, a gradual shift from parental to self-care management needs to occur, so that the older teen and emerging young adult can be fully independent in diabetes self-management tasks (see Table 5.3).

Although adults are not necessarily changing in the same physical ways as children, there are often many life changes that can impact diabetes, such as going to college and graduate school, moving, getting married, having children, changing

Table 5.3 Major Developmental Issues and Their Effect on Diabetes in Children and Adolescents

Developmental Stages (Ages)	Normal Developmental Tasks	T1D Management Priorities	Family Issues in T1D Management
Infancy (0–12 months)	Developing a trusting relationship or bonding with primary caregiver(s)	Preventing and treating hypoglycemia Avoiding extreme fluctuations in BG levels	Coping with stress Sharing the burden of care to avoid parent burnout
Toddler (13–26 months)	Developing a sense of mastery and autonomy	Preventing hypoglycemia Avoiding extreme fluctuations in BG levels due to irregular food intake	Establishing a schedule Managing the picky eater Limit setting and coping with toddler's lack of cooperation with regimen Sharing the burden of care
Preschooler and early elementary school (3–7 years)	Developing initiative in activities and confidence in self	Preventing hypoglycemia Coping with unpredictable appetite & activity Positively reinforcing cooperation with regimen Trusting other caregivers with diabetes management	Reassuring child that diabetes is no one's fault Educating other caregivers about diabetes management
Older elementary school age (8–11 years)	Developing skills in athletic, cognitive, artistic, social areas Consolidating self-esteem with respect to the peer group	Making diabetes regimen flexible to allow for participation in school or peer activities Child learning short- and long-term benefits of optimal control	Maintaining parental involvement in insulin and BGM tasks while allowing for independent self-care for special occasions Continuing to educate school and other caregivers

Continued

Table 5.3 Major Developmental Issues and Their Effect
on Diabetes in Children and Adolescents (Continued)

Early adolescence (12–15 years)	Managing body changes Developing a strong sense of self-identity	Increasing insulin requirements during puberty Diabetes management and BG control becoming more difficult Weight and body image concerns	Renegotiating parent and teen's roles in diabetes management to be acceptable to both Learning coping skills to enhance ability to self-manage Preventing and intervening with diabetes-related family conflict Monitoring for signs of depression, eating disorders, risky behaviors
Later adolescence (16–19 years)	Establishing a sense of identity after high school (decisions about location, social issues, work, education)	Beginning and ongoing discussion of transition to a new diabetes team (discussion may begin in earlier adolescent years) Integrating diabetes into new lifestyle	Supporting the transition to independence Learning coping skills to enhance ability to self-manage Preventing and intervening with diabetes-related family conflict Monitoring for signs of depression, eating disorders, risky behaviors

jobs, caring for an aging parent, developing nondiabetes-related diseases, and possibly developing diabetes-related complications. Therefore, adults with T1D need ongoing assessment of glycemic control and their diabetes treatment plan. Adults may have changes in physical activity goals, from sustaining injuries, joining a gym, or training for a marathon. Thus, frequent contact allows for diabetes management changes that can be customized for the patients' current life situations.

Screening

Ongoing management of the individual with T1D also involves screening for common comorbidities like thyroid autoimmunity and celiac disease, microvascular complications involving the eyes and kidneys, and risk of macrovascular disease, with attention to weight, blood pressure, and lipid levels. Further, there is a need to screen for behavioral issues like treatment nonadherence, disordered eating behaviors, and psychosocial distress including symptoms of depression, anxiety, fear of hypoglycemia, or diabetes burnout. These topics are covered in chapters 8 and 14. Details regarding microvascular and macrovascular complications appear in chapter 16. Routine ongoing screening and management of complications and comorbidities follow.

SCREENING AND MANAGEMENT OF COMORBIDITIES AND COMPLICATIONS

Retinopathy

Diabetic retinopathy is extremely unusual under the age of 10 years or within the first 5 years following the T1D diagnosis. Thus, screening for diabetic retinopathy usually begins after the age of 10 years and after T1D has been diagnosed for 3–5 years. However, children and teens with diabetes need ongoing routine eye exams with respect to assessment of visual acuity and need for refractive corrections, especially upon entry into grade school and during the pubertal years, when need for corrective lens may arise. Similarly, adults need routine screening for ocular and retinal disorders, including cataracts, glaucoma, and macular degeneration. Additionally, refraction needs may change with age. Treatments for eye problems will not be discussed.

Recommendations: Pediatrics

- Children with T1D should have an initial dilated and comprehensive eye examination by an ophthalmologist or optometrist once the child is ≥10 years of age and has had diabetes for 3–5 years.
- Subsequent examinations should be repeated annually by an ophthalmologist or optometrist. Less frequent exams (every 2–3 years) may be considered following one or more normal eye exams. Examinations will be required more frequently if retinopathy is present or progressing.

Recommendations: Adults

- Adults with T1D should have an initial dilated and comprehensive eye examination by an ophthalmologist or optometrist within 5 years after the onset of diabetes.
- Subsequent examinations should be repeated annually by an ophthalmologist or optometrist. Less frequent exams (every 2–3 years) may be considered following one or more normal eye exams. Examinations will be required more frequently if retinopathy is progressing.
- Women with T1D who are planning pregnancy or who have become pregnant should have a comprehensive eye examination and be counseled on the risk of development or progression of diabetic retinopathy. Eye examination should occur in the first trimester with close follow-up throughout pregnancy and for 1 year postpartum.

Nephropathy

The first evidence of diabetic nephropathy is the appearance of elevated urinary albumin excretion, termed microalbuminuria. It is extremely unusual to find elevations in urinary albumin excretion related to diabetes in youth under the age of 10 years. If albuminuria is identified in pediatric patients, it is important to consider orthostatic proteinuria as the etiology. This can be assessed by collecting a first morning urine sample for microalbumin determination, which is then compared with a midday urine sample. If the first morning void is normal and the midday sample has an elevation, one can be assured that the benign condition of orthostatic proteinuria is likely present.

Risk factors for microalbuminuria in both pediatric and adult patients include poor glycemic control, smoking, and a positive family history of hypertension or diabetic nephropathy. The treatment goal is to reduce the risk or slow the progression of nephropathy, optimize glucose, and control blood pressure. Neither ACE inhibitors nor ARBs have been shown to prevent microalbuminuria in normotensive patients with T1D.

Recommendations: Pediatrics
Screening:

- Begin annual screening for microalbuminuria, with a random spot urine sample for albumin-to-creatinine (ACR) ratio, once the child is 10 years of age and has had diabetes for 5 years.

Treatment:

- Begin treatment with an ACE inhibitor, titrated to normalization of albumin excretion, when persistent elevations in ACR are confirmed in an additional specimen or in two out of three specimen from different days. It is important to recognize that intermittent elevations in urinary albumin excretion are common in pediatric patients. Regression of microalbuminuria is as common as progression, independent of treatment with ACE inhibitors.

Recommendations: Adults
Screening:

- Perform an annual test to assess urine albumin excretion in patients with T1D with diabetes duration of ≥5 years.
- Measure serum creatinine at least annually in all adults with diabetes regardless of the degree of urine albumin excretion. The serum creatinine should be used to estimate GFR and stage the level of chronic kidney disease (CKD) if present.

Treatment:

- In the treatment of the nonpregnant patient with micro- or macroalbuminuria, either ACE inhibitors or ARBs should be used.
- If one class is not tolerated, the other should be substituted.
- Reduction of protein intake to 0.8–1.0 g $\times$ kg body wt^{-1} $\times$ day^{-1} in individuals with diabetes and the earlier stages of CKD and to 0.8 g $\times$ kg body wt^{-1} $\times$ day^{-1} in the later stages of CKD may improve measures of renal function (urine albumin excretion rate, GFR) and is recommended.
- When ACE inhibitors, ARBs, or diuretics are used, monitor serum creatinine and potassium levels for the development of increased creatinine and hyperkalemia.

- Continued monitoring of urine albumin excretion to assess both response to therapy and progression of disease is reasonable.
- When eGFR <60 ml.min/1.73 m^2, evaluate and manage potential complications of CKD.
- Consider referral to a physician experienced in the care of kidney disease for uncertainty about the etiology of kidney disease, difficult management issues, or advanced kidney disease.

Neuropathy

The two broad categories of neuropathies include focal (e.g., carpal tunnel syndrome, nerve palsies) and generalized neuropathies (e.g., sensorimotor polyneuropathy and autonomic neuropathies—vomiting, diarrhea, abnormal heart rates).

Recommendations: Pediatrics. Because diabetic neuropathy is so rare in children, there are limited prospective studies and screening information. Diabetic neuropathies occur in children, but because most are asymptomatic, detection and screening are difficult and more detailed assessments remain within the realm of ongoing clinical research.[8]
Screening:

- Assess peripheral and autonomic neuropathy by history and physical examination in patients from age 11 years with 2 or more years diabetes duration (ISPAD recommendation).[9]
- Take history: questions regarding numbness, persistent pain, or paresthesias.
- Perform sensorimotor nerve tests: physical exam of ankle reflexes, vibration, light touch, 10-gram monofilament, and possibly thermal sensation.
- Consider performing autonomic nerve tests: heart rate response to deep breathing and after rising from lying down, pupillary responses to light and dark.

Recommendations: Adults

- All patients should be screened for distal symmetric polyneuropathy (DPN) starting 5 years after the diagnosis of T1D and at least annually thereafter, using simple clinical tests.
Screening:

- Testing includes an annual comprehensive foot examination to identify risk factors predictive of ulcers and amputations. The foot examination should include inspection, assessment of foot pulses, and testing for loss of protective sensation (10-g monofilament plus testing any one of: vibration using 128-Hz tuning fork, pinprick sensation, ankle reflexes, or vibration perception threshold).
- Provide general foot self-care education to all patients with diabetes but this should be tailored to the age and risk factors present in the patient.

- Refer patients who smoke, have loss of protective sensation, have structural abnormalities, or have history of prior lower-extremity complications to foot care specialists for ongoing preventive care and lifelong surveillance.
- In older patients with signs and symptoms of peripheral arterial disease (PAD), an ankle-brachial index (ABI) should be measured. If positive (see Chapter 16.I), considered as an ankle-to-brachial systolic pressure ratio outside of 0.9–1.2, refer the patient for vascular assessment.

Hypertension

Elevations in blood pressure in patients with T1D are relatively common, especially in the current era when one out of three youth is either overweight or obese and over half the adults with T1D are either overweight or obese. Blood pressure elevations in pediatric patients are based upon the child's age, sex, and height and are defined as prehypertension (or high normal) when values are ≥90th percentile and <95th percentile and defined as hypertension when values are ≥95th percentile. Normal blood pressure levels for age, sex, and height and appropriate methods for determinations are available online (www.nhlbi.nih.gov/health/prof/heart/hbp/hbp_ped.pdf).

It is important to use a proper cuff size for blood pressure measurements in all patients (pediatric and adult) and to access electronic or paper tables to classify pediatric patients correctly as normotensive, prehypertensive, or hypertensive. The individual should be seated and relaxed. Values need to be confirmed on three separate occasions prior to diagnosis of hypertension and implementation of any treatments.

Recommendations: Pediatrics
Screening:

- Blood pressures should be obtained at each quarterly visit.
- For the pediatric patient, the school nurse can often be asked to obtain blood pressure measurements between visits as a means to confirm previously identified elevations.

Treatment:

- Initial treatment of high-normal blood pressure (systolic or diastolic blood pressure consistently >90th percentile for age, sex, and height) begins with lifestyle intervention focused on diet and exercise, aimed at weight control and increased physical activity, if appropriate. If target blood pressure is not reached within 3–6 months, pharmacologic treatment should be considered.
- Pharmacologic treatment of hypertension (systolic or diastolic blood pressure consistently >95th percentile for age, sex, and height or consistently >130/80 mmHg, if the 95th percentile exceeds that value) should be considered when the diagnosis is confirmed.
- ACE inhibitors should be used for the initial treatment of hypertension, following appropriate reproductive counseling due to potential teratogenic effects of ACE inhibitors (or ARBS).

■ The goal of treatment is a blood pressure consistently <130/80 or <90th percentile for age, sex, and height, whichever is lower.

Recommendations: Adults

■ Blood pressure should be measured at every routine diabetes visit. Based on studies done in individuals with T2D, patients found to have systolic blood pressure ≥130 mmHg or diastolic blood pressure ≥80 mmHg should have blood pressure confirmed on a separate day. Repeat systolic blood pressure ≥130 mmHg or diastolic blood pressure ≥80 mmHg confirms a diagnosis of hypertension.
■ Adults may perform blood pressure monitoring at home. Any values at or above 130/80 mmHg are considered elevated.

Treatment:

■ Patients with a systolic blood pressure of 130–139 mmHg or a diastolic blood pressure of 80–89 mmHg may be given lifestyle therapy alone for a maximum of 3 months and then, if targets are not achieved, be treated with addition of pharmacological agents.
■ Pharmacologic therapy for patients with T1D and hypertension should be with a regimen that includes either an ACE inhibitor or an ARB. If one class is not tolerated, the other should be substituted.
■ Do not use ACE-I/ARBs in women contemplating pregnancy (or who are not using contraception).
■ Patients with more severe hypertension (systolic blood pressure ≥140 or diastolic blood pressure ≥90 mmHg) at diagnosis or follow-up should receive pharmacologic therapy in addition to lifestyle therapy.
■ If ACE inhibitors, ARBs, or diuretics are used, kidney function and serum potassium levels should be monitored.
■ In pregnant patients with diabetes and chronic hypertension, blood pressure target goals of 110–129/65–79 mmHg are suggested in the interests of long-term maternal health and minimizing impaired fetal growth. ACE inhibitors and ARBs are contraindicated during pregnancy (see chapter 17, Pregnancy).

Dyslipidemia

Elevations in lipid levels are also common in pediatric patients with T1D, especially in association with uncontrolled diabetes.[10] Youth with A1C levels <7.5% have lipid levels similar to youth without T1D. However, achieving such optimal glycemic control in pediatric patients with T1D is challenging. Therefore, screening for lipid abnormalities remains important. Usually, lipid screening can occur at the time of routine diabetes appointments, when fasting has not occurred, because total and LDL cholesterol levels are generally independent of prandial state. However, if there are concerns about triglyceride abnormalities in pediatric patients, fasting samples are required. Adults also commonly have lipid abnormalities (see chapter 16.I, Macrovascular Complications), and annual screening is recommended.

Recommendations: Pediatrics

■ If there is a family history of hypercholesterolemia or of premature cardiovascular disease (CVD) before the age of 55 years, or if family history is unknown, obtain lipid profiles on children >2 years of age soon after diagnosis once glucose control has been achieved. If family history is not concerning, then lipid screening can begin at puberty (≥10 years) although one would likely want to confirm normal lipid levels with a single lipid screen during childhood. For children diagnosed with diabetes at or after puberty, obtain lipid profiles soon after diagnosis once glucose control has been established.

■ For both younger and older pediatric patients, if lipids are abnormal, annual monitoring is appropriate. If LDL cholesterol values are within the accepted risk levels (<100 mg/dl [2.6 mmol/l]), a lipid profile repeated every 5 years is reasonable.

Treatment:

■ Initial therapy generally consists of optimization of glucose control and medical nutrition therapy (MNT) using a Step 2 American Heart Association (AHA) diet aimed at decreasing the amount of saturated fat in the diet. The Step 2 AHA diet limits saturated fat to 7% of total calories and dietary cholesterol to 200 mg per day.

■ After the age of 10 years, pharmacologic treatment with a statin is recommended for patients who, after MNT and lifestyle changes, have persistent elevations in LDL-C >160 mg/dl or LDL-C >130 mg/dl and one or more CVD risk factors.

■ The goal of therapy is an LDL-C value <100 mg/dl (2.6 mmol/l).

There are no long-term safety data or cardiovascular outcome data of efficacy related to statin therapy in children. However, short-term data are reassuring with respect to safety and provide some information related to the efficacy of lowering LDL-C upon endothelial function and regression of carotid intimal thickening.[11-13] For postpubertal girls, issues of pregnancy prevention are important since statins are Category X in pregnancy. (See chapter 17.I for more information.)

Recommendations: Adults
Screening:

■ In most adult patients, measure fasting lipid profile at least annually. In adults with low-risk lipid values (LDL-C <100 mg/dl, HDL-C >50 mg/dl, and triglycerides <150 mg/dl), lipid assessments may be repeated every 2 years.

■ If fasting is not possible in a patient with T1D, measure a direct LDL cholesterol level.

Treatment recommendations and goals:

■ Lifestyle modification should focus on the reduction of saturated fat, trans fat, and cholesterol intake; increase of omega-3 fatty acids, viscous fiber, and plant stanols/sterols; and weight loss (if indicated). Increased physical activity should be recommended to improve the lipid profile in patients with diabetes.

- Statin therapy should be added to lifestyle therapy, regardless of baseline lipid levels, for patients with T1D:
  - ❏ with overt CVD
  - ❏ without CVD who are over the age of 40 and have one or more other CVD risk factors
- For lower risk patients than the above (e.g., without overt CVD, age ≤40 years with no CVD risk factors or with high HDL cholesterol levels), statin therapy should be considered on a case-by-case basis.
- Women of child-bearing age should not be treated with statin therapy if contemplating pregnancy or sexually active, or both, without use of contraception.
- In individuals without overt CVD, the primary goal is an LDL-C <100 mg/dl although in younger, low-risk patients the threshold for starting statin therapy may be increased. This should be evaluated on an individual basis.
- In individuals with overt CVD, a lower LDL-C goal of <70 mg/dl is recommended.
- Triglycerides levels <150 mg/dl (1.7 mmol/l) and HDL-C >40 mg/dl (1.0 mmol/l) in men and >50 mg/dl (1.3 mmol/l) in women are desirable. However, LDL-C-targeted statin therapy remains the preferred strategy.
- If targets are not reached on maximally tolerated doses of statins, combination therapy using statins and other lipid-lowering agents may be considered to achieve lipid targets. Combination therapy has not been evaluated in outcome studies for either CVD outcomes or safety in individuals with T1D. Data on individuals with T2D have not shown benefit with the addition of a fibric acid derivative or niacin.
- Statin therapy is contraindicated in pregnancy.

CVD and Antiplatelet Agents

Antiplatelet agents are important for patients at high risk for CVD or with known CVD. Data do not specifically exist for patients with T1D, however. Consider aspirin therapy (75–162 mg/day) as a primary prevention strategy in those with T1D at increased cardiovascular risk (10-year risk >10%).

Screening:

- In asymptomatic patients with T1D, routine screening for CAD is not recommended, as it does not improve outcomes as long as CVD risk factors are treated.
- Anecdotally, in some individuals with T1D where it is not clear if they need treatment for indeterminate lipid values, a coronary calcium scan can be useful in determining if atherosclerotic plaque is present.

Treatment:

- Aspirin should not be recommended for CVD prevention for adults with diabetes at low CVD risk (10-year CVD risk <5%), since the potential adverse effects from bleeding likely offset the potential benefits.
- In patients with a history of CVD, use aspirin therapy (75–162 mg/day) as a secondary prevention strategy.

■ In patients with known CVD, consider ACE inhibitor therapy, aspirin, and statin therapy (if not contraindicated) to reduce the risk of cardiovascular events.

■ In patients with a prior myocardial infarction, β-blocker therapy should be considered but the risks vs. benefits of these agents in terms of masking symptoms of hypoglycemia should be addressed. If used, they should be continued for at least 2 years after the event.

ASSESSMENT OF COMORBID CONDITIONS

Metabolic Syndrome or Obesity

Individuals with T1D may also develop the metabolic syndrome, with hypertension, dyslipidemia, and central obesity. This confers an increased risk for CVD and is discussed in chapter 16.I on macrovascular complications. Overall obesity rates are similar or slightly higher in people with T1D compared to the general population and should be addressed similarly with the caveat that caloric restriction can lead to hypoglycemia and needs to be monitored by a health care professional to assist with appropriate insulin adjustments.

Recommendations: Pediatrics and adults

■ Encourage weight loss (if overweight or obese) and physical activity.
■ Treat lipid disorders to achieve lipid targets described in ADA guidelines. Most will need statin therapy, especially if >40 years of age.
■ Treat blood pressure to <130/80 mmHg as discussed above.
■ Aspirin therapy recommendations should be followed based on ADA guidelines.
■ Assess for and treat obesity-related comorbidities such as sleep apnea and fatty liver.

Smoking Cessation
Recommendations: Pediatrics and adults

■ Advise all patients not to smoke.
■ Include smoking cessation counseling and other forms of treatment as a routine component of diabetes care.

Celiac Disease

Celiac disease is a common immune-mediated disease of the small intestine that occurs in genetically susceptible individuals upon repeated exposure to the gliadin moiety of gluten, which is found in wheat, rye, barley, and possibly oats. The disease is linked to the human leukocyte antigen (HLA)-DQ2 and HLA-DQ8 haplotypes. The immune-mediated damage to the mucosa of the small intestine destroys the absorptive surfaces of the villi, leading to malabsorption. Estimates vary but up to 10% of children with T1D may have celiac disease.[14,15] General symptoms of celiac disease include diarrhea, weight loss or poor weight gain, growth failure, abdominal pain, fatigue, irritability, nutritional deficiencies, and other gastrointestinal problems. Symptoms specific to patients with diabetes include unpredictable blood glucose levels with unexplained hypo- or hyperglycemia due to disordered absorption of food, often leading to poor glycemic control.

Recommendations: Pediatrics
Screening:

- Following glucose stabilization after the diagnosis of T1D, screen children and adolescents with T1D for celiac disease by serologic measurements of tissue transglutaminase, antiendomysial, or deamidated gliadin IgA antibodies; documentation of normal total serum IgA levels is needed. In patients with IgA deficiency, measurement of IgG to tissue transglutaminase, antiendomysial, or deamidated gliadin is recommended.
- Following an initial negative screening test, retesting should occur whenever clinical concerns of celiac disease arise or possibly every 2 years in the absence of symptoms or signs.
- Testing should be performed in youth with growth failure, failure to gain weight, weight loss, diarrhea, flatulence, abdominal pain, signs of malabsorption, or frequent unexplained hypo- or hyperglycemia.
- Refer to a gastroenterologist for evaluation and possible endoscopy and small bowel biopsy for confirmation of celiac disease in asymptomatic children with positive antibodies.
- Children with biopsy- or serology-confirmed celiac disease should receive a gluten-free diet with families undergoing comprehensive consultation with a dietitian experienced in managing both diabetes and celiac disease.

Recently published guidelines by the European Society for Pediatric Gastroenterology, Hepatology, and Nutrition recommend that endoscopy and small bowel biopsy can be avoided in pediatric patients with high titer antibodies (>10 times the upper limit of normal).[16] These patients may still benefit from referral to a pediatric gastroenterologist to review with parents and older pediatric patients options of performing additional lab studies (serology, genetics) to make the diagnosis of celiac disease without biopsy. Positive serology should always be rechecked in case of lab errors with false positives resulting from mislabeling of blood samples or assay errors. With serology confirmation, celiac can be confirmed without biopsy and a gluten-free diet begun. The new recommendations include checking HLA haplotypes to reaffirm the celiac diagnosis.

Recommendations: Adults
Although more common in children, celiac disease may also develop in adults with T1D. It is not known, however, how often this occurs. In adult patients with T1D who exhibit possible symptoms of celiac disease (see above), the same evaluation that is performed in children should occur.
Screening:

- Consider screening adults with T1D for celiac disease by measuring tissue transglutaminase, antiendomysial, or deamidated gliadin, with documentation of normal total serum IgA levels, soon after the diagnosis of diabetes.

- Testing should be considered in adults with weight loss, diarrhea, flatulence, abdominal pain, or signs of malabsorption, or with frequent unexplained hypoglycemia or deterioration in glycemic control.
- Consider referral to a gastroenterologist for evaluation with endoscopy and biopsy for confirmation of celiac disease in asymptomatic adults with positive antibodies.
- Adults with biopsy-confirmed celiac disease should be placed on a gluten-free diet and have consultation with a dietitian experienced in managing both diabetes and celiac disease.

Hypothyroidism

Thyroid autoimmunity is the most common comorbid autoimmune disease in individuals with T1D, with a reported prevalence of at least 17–30%.[17] Autoimmune thyroid disease can result in normal thyroid function, hypothyroidism, or hyperthyroidism. In children, untreated hypothyroidism can negatively impact growth and development and lead to unpredictable hypoglycemia. On the other hand, untreated hyperthyroidism may increase the rate of insulin metabolism, leading to hyperglycemia and uncontrolled diabetes. Individuals with T1D should be screened for autoimmune thyroid disease at disease onset with measurement of thyroid autoantibodies and TSH to assess thyroid dysfunction. Confirmed biochemical or clinical hypothyroidism or hyperthyroidism should be treated and followed with ongoing laboratory monitoring at routine diabetes follow-up visits.

Recommendations: Pediatrics and adults

- In children, screen for thyroid peroxidase and thyroglobulin antibodies shortly after diagnosis of T1D. No such recommendation exists for adults with new-onset T1D so the decision to draw thyroid antibodies should be made on an individual basis.
- Measure TSH concentrations soon after diagnosis of T1D, once glycemic control has been established. If normal, consider rechecking every 1–2 years, or if the patient develops any symptoms of abnormal thyroid dysfunction, thyromegaly, an abnormal growth rate (in children), or uncontrolled diabetes for unknown reasons.

Polyglandular Autoimmune Failure

- Rarely individuals with T1D develop other endocrinopathies. These include adrenal insufficiency, primary hypogonadism, diabetes insipidus, and vitiligo.
- Testing should be performed based on symptoms or clinical findings, or both.

Osteoporosis

T1D is associated with osteoporosis. Age-matched hip fracture risk is significantly increased in T1D (summary relative risk [RR] 6.3) in both sexes.[18]

Recommendations: Adults

- Assess fracture history and risk factors in older patients with diabetes with bone mineral density (BMD) testing if appropriate for the patient's age and gender.
- For at-risk patients, it is reasonable to consider standard primary or secondary prevention strategies (reduce risk factors for falls; ensure adequate calcium and vitamin D intake; avoid use of medications that lower BMD, such as glucocorticoids) and to consider pharmacotherapy based on current osteoporosis treatment guidelines.

SPECIAL CIRCUMSTANCES

Diabetes and Driving

Epidemiologic and simulator data suggest that people with insulin-treated diabetes have a small increase in risk of motor vehicle accidents, primarily due to hypoglycemia and decreased awareness of hypoglycemia. This increase (RR 1.12–1.19) is much smaller than the risks associated with teenage male drivers (RR 42), driving at night (RR 142), driving on rural roads compared to urban roads (RR 9.2), and obstructive sleep apnea (RR 2.4), all of which are accepted for unrestricted licensure.

The ADA position statement, Diabetes and Driving, recommends against blanket restrictions based on the diagnosis of diabetes and urges individual assessment by a health care professional knowledgeable in diabetes if restrictions on licensure are being considered.[19] Patients should be evaluated for decreased awareness of hypoglycemia, episodes of hypoglycemia while driving, or severe hypoglycemia. Patients with retinopathy or peripheral neuropathy require assessment to determine if those complications interfere with operation of a motor vehicle. Health care professionals should be cognizant of the potential risk of driving with diabetes and counsel their patients about detecting and avoiding hypoglycemia while driving. Following treatment of hypoglycemia, cognitive recovery likely varies among persons and needs to be reviewed individually with patients.

Recommendation: Pediatrics and adults

- Individuals with T1D should measure their blood glucose level before driving and every hour during prolonged drives and treat with 15 g of carbohydrate if blood glucose is <70 mg/dl.
- Driving should not begin or resume until BG is consistently >70 mg/dl.
- Clinicians treating patients with T1D who drive should discuss strategies and guidelines for safe driving when initially evaluating a patient and periodically thereafter as indicated. This is especially true for youth who are obtaining a learner's permit and license for the first time.
- Rapid-acting carbohydrate should be available in the car at all times to treat hypoglycemia.

Sick Day Rules: Pediatrics and Adults

Intercurrent illnesses occur frequently and are exceptionally common in pediatric patients, with youth experiencing up to 7–10 acute illnesses each year. Any illness or surgical procedure places substantial stress upon the body and initiates a counterregulatory hormone response, which in turn can lead to hyperglycemia and ketosis. Illness prevention is important, when possible, for example, by provision of annual flu shots and routine immunizations. Simple procedures, like good hand washing and not sharing drinks between friends, can help to reduce risk of intercurrent illness. Regardless, acute illnesses remain common and thus patients and families with T1D should be taught sick day rules as part of routine care and reminded about sick day management on an annual basis. Problems with insulin pump infusion sets can masquerade as an acute illness with onset of hyperglycemia, ketosis, and nausea and vomiting. At such times, insulin should be given by injection and the pump set changed. Unfortunately, sick day management is often taught when patients are well, so the fundamental principles of sick day management frequently are forgotten (see Table 5.4). There are a number of detailed reviews of sick day management and insulin dose recommendations that can help avoid progression of ketosis to DKA.[20,21]

CONCLUSION

All individuals with T1D need a comprehensive initial evaluation with routine follow-up. The key elements of this care are presented in this chapter, although as with all medical care, the treatment needs to be individualized. A multidisciplinary team to facilitate care and follow-up is beneficial, although for each patient, the emphasis may differ and will change over time. Regardless, having consistent, accessible care is vital to the continued health and well-being of people with T1D.

Table 5.4 Sick Day Management

- NEVER OMIT INSULIN. Continue to give usual insulin dose, although the dose may need to be changed (more insulin at times of hyperglycemia and less insulin at times of hypoglycemia).

- Provide supplemental insulin by injection (and not by pump in case of infusion site problem) based upon the blood glucose and ketone levels and the recommendations of the diabetes health care team (usually with additional rapid- or short-acting insulin every 2–4 h at doses of 10–20% of the total daily dose).

- Prevent dehydration by giving extra fluids (sugar-free fluids at times of hyperglycemia and sugar-containing fluids at times of hypoglycemia).

- Check blood glucose levels every 2–4 h.

- Check blood or urine ketones every 2–4 h during intercurrent illness or if blood glucose exceeds 250 mg/dl on two consecutive checks.

- Treat intercurrent illness (e.g., strep throat).

- Call the diabetes health care team for support in adjusting insulin dose and food.

The currently available ADA Standards of Care provide an excellent framework for the basic treatment necessary for all individuals with diabetes, and some of those recommendations are presented here. However, in other areas of concern, the treatment of the person with T1D is different, with unique challenges and solutions. Thus, we discuss these distinct areas in this chapter, in the hope that it will bring more awareness in managing the unique needs of people with T1D so that they receive the comprehensive but individualized care they deserve.

APPENDIX: COMPONENTS OF ASSESSMENT

For examples of educational assessment questions, refer to Table 7.3.

Table 5.A1 Medical History

- Age and characteristics of onset of diabetes (e.g., DKA, asymptomatic laboratory finding)
- Eating patterns, physical activity habits, nutritional status, and weight history
- Whether or not patient wears medical alert identification
- Diabetes education history; health literacy assessment
- Review of previous insulin treatment regimens and response to therapy (A1C records); treatment preferences; and prior difficulty with therapies
- Current treatment of diabetes, including medications and medication adherence, meal plan, physical activity patterns, and readiness for behavior change
- Use of insulin, insulin pumps, carbohydrate ratios, corrections; knowledge of sick day rules, ketone testing, pump troubleshooting (if applicable)
- Results of glucose monitoring including SMBG and CGM and patient's use of data
- DKA frequency, severity, and cause
- Hypoglycemic episodes
  - ❑ Hypoglycemia awareness
  - ❑ Any severe hypoglycemia: frequency and cause
  - ❑ Whether or not patient has glucagon available and someone to administer it
- History of diabetes-related complications
  - ❑ Microvascular: retinopathy, nephropathy, neuropathy (sensory, including history of foot lesions; autonomic, including sexual dysfunction and gastroparesis)
  - ❑ Macrovascular: CHD, cerebrovascular disease, PAD
  - ❑ Other: psychosocial problems, dental disease
- History of pregnancy and any diabetes-related complications; desire for future pregnancies
- Contraception (if female, of childbearing age)
- Smoking
- ETOH (alcohol) use, abuse, and impact on blood glucose levels
- Illicit drug use
- Driving

Table 5.A2 Clinical Evaluation: Children and Adolescents*

	Initial	Annual	Quarterly Follow-Up
Height	X	X	X
Weight	X	X[†]	X[†]
BMI percentile	X	X	X
BP	X	X	X
General PE	X	X	
Thyroid exam	X	X	X
Injection/infusion sites	X (if already on insulin)	X	X
Comprehensive foot exam[‡]	If needed based on age	Beginning with older teens with diabetes since childhood	
Visual foot exam		X	If needed based on high-risk characteristics
Retinal exam by eye care specialist	X[§]	In some cases may be done every 2–3 years, see ADA standards of care	
Depression screen	X	X	
Hypoglycemia assessment	X	X	X
Diabetes self-management skills	X	X	X
Physical activity assessment	X	X	X
Assess clinically relevant issues (e.g., ETOH, drugs, tobacco, use of contraception, driving)	X	As needed for teens	As needed for teens
Nutritional knowledge	X	X	As needed
Query for evidence of other autoimmune disease	X	As needed	As needed

*Assumes that patient has a health care provider to manage the nondiabetes-related health assessments and to perform annual evaluations.

†Patient may opt out of measurement if psychologically distressing.

‡Foot inspection should be done at each visit and self foot exams taught if high risk characteristics present. Comprehensive foot exam: inspection, palpation of dorsalis pedis and posterior tibial pulses, presence or absence of patellar and Achilles reflexes, determination of proprioception, vibration, and monofilament sensation.

§Within 5 years after diagnosis.

Table 5.A3 Laboratory Assessments: Children and Adolescents

	Initial	Annual	Follow-Up
A1C	X	X	Every 3 months
Cr/eGFR	X	X	
Lipid panel *If triglycerides elevated in a non-fasting specimen, measure a direct LDL cholesterol level.	Once glycemia is stable	X	As needed based on treatment
TSH	X	X Frequency of testing varies, based on clinical symptoms, presence of antibodies, and/or if on treatment.	As needed based on treatment
Antithyroid Abs	X Frequency of testing is unknown. Test if symptoms are present or for periodic screening.	Repeat as indicated by exam	
Celiac Ab panel	X Frequency of testing is unknown. Test if symptoms are present or for periodic screening.	Every other year	
Urine A/C ratio	Starting 5 years after diagnosis	X	As needed based on treatment
Autoantibodies: AntiGAD/IA2/ IAA/ ZnT8	X May be needed in new-onset patients to establish diagnosis		
C-peptide levels	X Occasionally needed to establish T1D in patient on insulin or to verify T1D for insurance purposes—always measure a simultaneous blood glucose level.		

Table 5.A4 Clinical Evaluation: Adults*

	Initial	Annual	Follow-Up
Height	X		
Weight	X	X[†]	X[†]
BMI	X	X	
BP	X	X	X
General PE	X		
Thyroid exam	X	If indicated	
Injection/infusion sites	X	X	X
Comprehensive foot exam[‡]	Exam defined below	X	
Visual foot exam			As needed—at each visit, if high-risk foot
Retinal exam by eye care specialist[§]	Starting 5 years after diagnosis; earlier if visual symptoms and/or true date of diagnosis is unknown	In some individuals screening may be done less often than annually, see ADA standards of care	
Depression screen	X	X	
Hypoglycemia assessment	X	X	X
Diabetes self-management skills	X	X	X
Physical activity assessment	X	X	X
Assess clinically relevant issues (e.g., ETOH, drugs, tobacco, use of contraception, driving)	X	As needed	As needed
Nutritional knowledge	X	X	As needed
Query for evidence of other autoimmune disease	X	As needed based on clinical scenario	As needed based on clinical scenario

*Assumes that patient has a health care provider to manage the nondiabetes-related health assessments and to perform annual evaluations.

[†]Patient may opt out of measurement if psychologically distressing.

[‡]Foot inspection should be done at each visit and self foot exams taught if high-risk characteristics present. Comprehensive foot exam: inspection, palpation of dorsalis pedis and posterior tibial pulses, determination of presence or absence of patellar and Achilles reflexes, determination of proprioception, vibration, and monofilament sensation.

[§]In some instances may not need to be done yearly.

Table 5.A5 Laboratory Assessments: Adults

	Initial	Annual	Follow-Up
A1C	X	X	Every 3 months
Cr/eGFR	X	X	
Fasting lipid panel*	X	X	As needed based on treatment
TSH	X	X[†]	As needed based on treatment
Antithyroid Abs	X[‡]		
Celiac Ab panel	X[‡]		
Urine A/C ratio	X	X	
Anti-GAD Abs	X[§]		
C-peptide levels	X[¶]		

*If patient unable to undertake a fasting test due to hypoglycemia, measure a direct LDL cholesterol level.

[†]Frequency of testing varies based on clinical symptoms, presence of antibodies, or if on treatment.

[‡]Frequency of testing unknown; test if symptoms or for periodic screening.

[§]May be needed in new-onset patients to establish diagnosis.

[¶]Occasionally needed to establish T1D in patient on insulin or to verify T1D for insurance purposes—always measure a simultaneous blood glucose level.

Table 5.A6 Referrals

- Eye care professional for annual dilated eye exam
- Family planning for women of reproductive age
- Registered dietitian for MNT
- Educator for diabetes self-management
- Exercise physiologist for advanced management of physical activity and elite athletics
- Dentist for comprehensive periodontal examination
- Mental health professional if needed
- Cardiologist if heart disease
- Nephrologist if renal insufficiency or refractory hypertension
- Physical therapist if needed for balance or strength issues
- Cognitive testing if indicated for elderly patients

REFERENCES

1. Petitti DB, Klingensmith GJ, Bell RA, Andrews JS, Dabelea D, Imperatore G, Marcovina S, Pihoker C, Standiford D, Waitzfelder B, Mayer-Davis E; SEARCH for Diabetes in Youth Study Group: Glycemic control in youth with diabetes: the SEARCH for Diabetes in Youth Study. *J Pediatr* 155:668–672. e1–e3, 2009. Epub 29 Jul 2009
2. Rewers A, Klingensmith G, Davis C, Petitti DB, Pihoker C, Rodriguez B, Schwartz ID, Imperatore G, Williams D, Dolan LM, Dabelea D: Presence of diabetic ketoacidosis at diagnosis of diabetes mellitus in youth: the Search for Diabetes in Youth Study. *Pediatrics* 121:e1258–e1266, 2008
3. Quinn M, Fleischman A, Rosner B, Nigrin DJ, Wolfsdorf JI: Characteristics at diagnosis of type 1 diabetes in children younger than 6 years. *J Pediatr* 148:366–371, 2006
4. Chase HP, Crews KR, Garg S, Crews MJ, Cruickshanks KJ, Klingensmith G, Gay E, Hamman RF: Outpatient management vs in-hospital management of children with new-onset diabetes. *Clin Pediatr (Phila)* 31:450–456, 1992
5. Kostraba JN, Gay EC, Rewers M, Chase HP, Klingensmith GJ, Hamman RF: Increasing trend of outpatient management of children with newly diagnosed IDDM. Colorado IDDM Registry, 1978-1988. *Diabetes Care* 15:95–100, 1992
6. Rewers A, Chase P, Bothner J, Hamman RF, Klingensmith G: Medical Care Patterns at the onset of type 1 diabetes in Colorado children, 1978-2001. *Diabetes* 52 (Suppl. 1):A62, 2003
7. Amiel SA, Sherwin RS, Simonson DC, Lauritano AA, Tamborlane WV: Impaired insulin action in puberty. A contributing factor to poor glycemic control in adolescents with diabetes. *N Engl J Med* 315:215–219, 1986
8. Blankenburg M, Kraemer N, Hirschfeld G, Krumova EK, Maier C, Hechler T, Aksu F, Magerl W, Reinehr T, Wiesel T, Zernikow B: Childhood diabetic neuropathy: functional impairment and non-invasive screening assessment. *Diabet Med* 16 Apr 2012. doi: 10.1111/j.1464-5491.2012.03685.x. [Epub ahead of print]
9. International Society for Pediatric and Adolescent Diabetes, International Diabetes Federation. *Global IDF/ISPAD Guideline for Diabetes in Childhood and Adolescence*. Brussels, Belgium, International Diabetes Federation, 2011
10. Guy J, Ogden L, Wadwa RP, Hamman RF, Mayer-Davis EJ, Liese AD, D'Agostino R Jr, Marcovina S, Dabelea D: Lipid and lipoprotein profiles in youth with and without type 1 diabetes: the SEARCH for Diabetes in Youth case-control study. *Diabetes Care* 32:416–420, 2009. Epub 17 Dec 2008
11. McCrindle BW, Ose L, Marais AD: Efficacy and safety of atorvastatin in children and adolescents with familial hypercholesterolemia or severe hyperlipidemia: a multicenter, randomized, placebo-controlled trial. *J Pediatr* 143:74–80, 2003
12. de Jongh S, Lilien MR, op't Roodt J, Stroes ES, Bakker HD, Kastelein JJ: Early statin therapy restores endothelial function in children with familial hypercholesterolemia. *J Am Coll Cardiol* 40:2117–2121, 2002

13. Wiegman A, Hutten BA, de Groot E, Rodenburg J, Bakker HD, Büller HR, Sijbrands EJ, Kastelein JJ: Efficacy and safety of statin therapy in children with familial hypercholesterolemia: a randomized controlled trial. *JAMA* 292:331–337, 2004
14. Holmes GK: Screening for coeliac disease in type 1 diabetes. *Arch Dis Child* 87:495–498, 2002
15. Rewers M, Liu E, Simmons J, Redondo MJ, Hoffenberg EJ: Celiac disease associated with type 1 diabetes mellitus. *Endocrinol Metab Clin North Am* 33:197–214, xi, 2004
16. Husby S, Koletzko S, Korponay-Szabó IR, Mearin ML, Phillips A, Shamir R, Troncone R, Giersiepen K, Branski D, Catassi C, Lelgeman M, Mäki M, Ribes-Koninckx C, Ventura A, Zimmer KP; ESPGHAN Working Group on Coeliac Disease Diagnosis; ESPGHAN Gastroenterology Committee; European Society for Pediatric Gastroenterology, Hepatology, and Nutrition: European Society for Pediatric Gastroenterology, Hepatology, and Nutrition guidelines for the diagnosis of coeliac disease. *J Pediatr Gastroenterol Nutr* 54:136–160, 2012
17. Roldán MB, Alonso M, Barrio R: Thyroid autoimmunity in children and adolescents with Type 1 diabetes mellitus. *Diabetes Nutr Metab* 12:27–31, 1999
18. Janghorbani M, Van Dam RM, Willett WC, Hu FB: Systematic review of type 1 and type 2 diabetes mellitus and risk of fracture. *Am J Epidemiol* 166:495–505, 2007. Epub 16 Jun 2007
19. American Diabetes Association, Lorber D, Anderson J, Arent S, Cox DJ, Frier BM, Greene MA, Griffin JW Jr, Gross G, Hathaway K, Hirsch I, Kohrman DB, Marrero DG, Songer TJ, Yatvin AL: Diabetes and driving. *Diabetes Care* 35 (Suppl. 1):S81–S86, 2012
20. Bismuth E, Laffel L: Can we prevent diabetic ketoacidosis in children? *Pediatr Diabetes* 8 (Suppl. 6):24–33, 2007
21. Brink S, Laffel L, Likitmaskul S, Liu L, Maguire AM, Olsen B, Silink M, Hanas R: Sick day management in children and adolescents with diabetes. *Pediatr Diabetes* 10 (Suppl. 12):146–153, 2009

6

Setting Treatment Targets

Nora Alghothani, MD, and Kathleen Dungan, MD, MPH

INTRODUCTION

The Diabetes Control and Complications Trial (DCCT)[1] was a landmark medical study conducted by the National Institute of Diabetes and Digestive and Kidney Diseases (NIDDK). It was the largest clinical trial focusing exclusively on patients with type 1 diabetes (T1D) and significantly changed T1D management principles. In particular, it established targets (glucose, A1C, and frequency of blood glucose testing) and their impact on long-term complications.

The United Kingdom Prospective Diabetes Study (UKPDS) studied patients with type 2 diabetes (T2D) and helped inform standards for blood pressure and glycemic control.[2] In the UKPDS, blood glucose control reduced the risk of microvascular complications, although the effect was not as pronounced as in the DCCT, and blood pressure control was clearly important. As a result of the two studies, there was a paradigm shift in the way clinicians managed patients with T1D and T2D.

In this chapter, our goals are to provide an overview of the current targets, specifically discussing the Diabetes Control and Complications Trial, present differences for those with T1D versus T2D, review relevant targets for children and adults with T1D, and conclude with recommendations for future clinical research. We hope to emphasize that targets for individuals with T1D are fundamentally different from those with T2D, particularly with respect to glucose management. We will discuss pediatrics first and then will proceed to adults.

T1D VERSUS T2D

Guidelines for glucose targets are available for diabetes in general and will be discussed later in this chapter. However, glucose targets for patients with T1D deserve separate consideration from those with T2D because T1D differs significantly from T2D in many regards:

- Pathophysiology
- Demographics
- Prevalence of nonglycemic risk factors in complications
- Disease course
- Risk for hypoglycemia
- Disease management
- Role of glycemic control
- Labile glycemic control

The pathophysiology of the two diseases differ on a basic pathophysiologic level such that T1D is marked by insulinopenia while T2D is characterized by obesity, hyperinsulinemia, insulin resistance, and relative insulinopenia. The age of onset is typically much younger in patients with T1D, and with modern treatment, the duration of disease spans many decades, necessitating management that must be adapted to individual needs over an entire lifetime. Other than hyperglycemia, patients with T1D are less likely to have other risk factors (e.g., hypertension, dyslipidemia, and obesity) for microvascular and macrovascular complications.

In addition, the disease course differs markedly. In T2D, complications such as kidney disease[3] and cardiovascular disease (CVD) [4,5] are often well established at the time of diagnosis of diabetes, potentially hampering the individual effect of glycemic control. In contrast, the development of complications in T1D follows a more scripted course, developing several years after the diagnosis. Therefore, it is postulated that glycemic control may be a more important relative predictor of complications in patients with T1D compared to T2D, as suggested in a large registry study.[6] These observations do not mean that management of other risk factors for microvascular and macrovascular complications, such as hypertension and hyperlipidemia, should be overlooked in patients with T1D but simply that the approach may be framed in a way that is specific to the needs of patients with T1D.

The risk of hypoglycemia and hypoglycemia unawareness differs,[7] potentially raising the stakes for intensive glycemic control. Management of T1D typically involves more complex insulin regimens and more frequent glycemic monitoring, yielding more circumstances for which glycemic targets are needed and utilized. While hemoglobin A1C (A1C) alone (without glucose monitoring) could be used to manage some patients with T2D, it cannot typically be used to implement changes in therapy in T1D. T1D is associated with more labile blood glucose levels,[8,9] for which targets reflecting measures of glycemia other than A1C must be considered.

PEDIATRICS

Targets for glucose, blood pressure, and lipids are informed by data from adult diabetes patients and smaller studies of pediatric patients. However, since young children in particular are not included in these studies, the effects of interventions are not always clear. Where available, recommendations from professional organizations in addition to that of the ADA are summarized. In some cases, relaxed targets are recommended according to age group, but in general, targets are individualized in a particular patient according to the balance of risks and benefits. Further data are necessary.

Glucose

It is important to note that young children were not included in the DCCT and therefore the long-term effects of the intervention in this age group are not known. Cognitive and behavioral problems associated with hypoglycemia have traditionally created more concern in children than in adults. Adult brain volume is not reached until age 7–10 years.[10] In a cohort study that enrolled 117 youths age 5–16 years and 58 nondiabetic sibling controls, verbal[11] intelligence was reduced with exposure to hyperglycemia, not hypoglycemia. However, performance on spatial intelligence and delayed recall tests were reduced with repeated severe hypoglycemia (marked by seizure, loss of consciousness, or the need for assistance in treatment), particularly when it occurred before age 5 years.[11] In preschool-age children with T1D, hyperglycemia was associated with lower cognitive ability, slower fine motor speed, and lower receptive language scores, but hypoglycemia was not.[12] In a meta-analysis of 2,144 children, hypoglycemic seizures were associated overall with negligible or inconsistent effects on cognition.[13] However the study could not rule out potential synergistic effects in children with early onset disease or poor overall glycemic control. In a 12-year follow-up of patients who were diagnosed at an average age of 8 years, severe hypoglycemia was associated with lower verbal IQ and thalamic volume on MRI.[14] Another small but long-term (16-year follow-up) study demonstrated decreased problem solving, verbal function, and psychomotor efficiency among young adults who experienced severe hypoglycemia before age 10 years.[15] These risks need to be interpreted in light of additional, perhaps clearer, adverse effects of hyperglycemia[16,17] or insulin deficiency[18] on cognitive function.

Glucose targets (see Table 6.1).[19–20] There is limited scientific evidence for age-specific glucose targets. Pediatric health care providers must individualize blood glucose targets for each child, walking the tightrope of near-term hypoglycemia risks and long-term hyperglycemic complications. In young children, higher targets are recommended, but only with some reservation. This is due to the clear risks of hyperglycemia long-term, and the concerning observation that early poor metabolic control is a predictor of continued poor control, an observation that has been termed *metabolic tracking*.[21,22] Targets for older children, particularly adolescents, with T1D should be similar to that of adults, provided that it can be done safely (Table 6.1).

Blood Pressure (See Table 6.2)

With hypertension present in up to 16% of children[23] with T1D and predictive of future microalbuminuria, blood pressure should be closely monitored and controlled. In children, blood pressure targets are based on age-, sex-, and height-specific percentiles. The American Diabetes Association (ADA)[19] and International Society Pediatric and Adolescent Diabetes (ISPAD) both recommend a target blood pressure of <90th percentile by age, sex, and height (Table 6.2).[24] Blood pressure values that fall between the 90th and 95th percentile are classified as prehypertension. Children with blood pressure readings persistently above the 95th percentile for age, sex, and height, despite lifestyle modification and weight loss (if indicated), should be started on pharmacologic therapy based on recommendations for children without diabetes. ACE inhibitors have been safe and effective in children ages 6–16 years of age in short-term studies[25,26] and

Table 6.1 Children and Adolescents

	A1C (%)	Premeal Glucose (mg/dl)	Postmeal Glucose (mg/dl)	Nocturnal (mg/dl)
ADA[19]				
<6	<8.5	100–180	—	110–200
6–12	<8.0	90–180	—	100–180
13–18	<7.5	90–130	—	90–150
NICE[20]	<7.5	72–144	<180	—
Australia[21]				
Older children	<7.5	72–126	90–180	90–144
Infants/young children	—	90–180	108–180	—
Canada[22]				
<6	<8.5	108–216	—	—
6–12	<8.0	72–180	—	—
13–18	≤7.0	72–126	90–180	—
ISPAD[23,24]*	<7.5	90–145	90–180	80–162

* Targets listed are those considered optimal. Additional cutoffs whereby additional action is either suggested or mandatory are also published.

are to be initiated in those with persistent hypertension with a treatment goal of blood pressure <130/80 or <90th percentile, whichever is lower.

Microalbuminuria. Based on its effectiveness in adults, ACE inhibitors are also indicated for children with persistent microalbuminuria. Angiotensin receptor blockers (ARBs) have had similar clinical benefits but have not been studied in children with hypertension and diabetes. Despite the long-term renal protective effect of ACE inhibitors seen in adults, their use in children without hypertension remains of concern given the potential adverse effects after decades of exposure. According to the ADA guidelines, annual screening for microalbuminuria should start once a child is 10 years old and has had diabetes for 5 years.[19] The National

Table 6.2 Blood Pressure Targets in Children

Blood Pressure	Category	Recommendations
<90% age, sex, height	Normal	None
90–95%	Prehypertension	Lifestyle + weight loss
>95%	Hypertension	Lifestyle + weight loss; consider ACEi

Institutes of Health and Clinical Excellence (NICE) guidelines suggest measuring blood pressure and microalbumin annually starting at 12 years of age,[20] while the Canadian Clinical practice guidelines recommend screening all children with T1D for hypertension at least twice annually.[22]

Lipids (See Table 6.3)

Atherosclerosis starts during childhood,[27] and children with T1D who have poor glycemic control develop long-term diabetic complications sooner. As per ADA guidelines, lipid screening should be targeted at those >10 years old unless there is a family history of a cardiovascular (CV) event prior to 55 years of age.[19] If so, then a fasting lipid profile should be obtained soon after diagnosis. If LDLc is abnormal or >100 mg/dl, repeat annually, otherwise, it may be repeated in five years. Short-term trials have shown statin therapy to be effective and safe in children over 10 years of age,[28,29] who despite optimized glucose control and compliance with a Step 2 AHA diet[30], have LDLc levels >160 mg/dl or >130 mg/dl with one or more CV risk factors. The treatment goal is an LDLc <100 mg/dl (Table 6.3).[19, 31–33] No randomized trials have determined the long-term safety or CV efficacy of statin therapy in children with T1D.

ADULTS

Glucose

Current trends. In the National Health and Nutrition Examination Survey (NHANES), the proportion of patients with diabetes with an A1C <7% has improved over time but still accounts for only 56% of patients.[34] However, NHANES data do not distinguish between T1D and T2D, and only 16% of subjects received insulin therapy only. Therefore, it is possible that a smaller proportion of patients with T1D attain effective glycemic control.

Table 6.3 Lipid Targets in Children

Lipid Panel	Recommendation
No family history	>10 years of age
Positive family history (CVD <55 years)	Baseline lipid panel after diagnosis
LDLc	
≤100 mg/dl	Screen every 5 years
>100 mg/dl	Annual screening
>10 years of age & 130 mg/dl & >1 CVD risk factor	Consider statin treatment
>10 years of age & >160 mg/dl	Consider statin treatment

The Type 1 Diabetes Exchange cohort of 7,477 U.S. adults had a mean A1C of 8.7, 8.2, 7.7, and 7.4% in subjects of age 18–20, 21–25, 26–64, and >65 years respectively.[31] Lower A1C was associated with older age, non-Hispanic white race, higher income, higher education, marriage, and private insurance, and greater use of insulin pumps, sensors, and self-monitoring of blood glucose.

In a Swedish national registry of over 13,000 patients with T1D, the frequency of obtaining an A1C <7% increased only slightly from 17.4% in 1997 to 21.2% in 2004 and the mean A1C decreased from 8.2 to 8.0%.[32] In a large German and Austrian database of over 30,000 children and adolescents, mean A1C improved over time from 8.7 to 8.1% and the rate of severe hypoglycemia declined (RR 0.917, 95% CI 0.885–0.950) from 1995 to 2009.[33] The decline in hypoglycemia was not completely attributable to insulin modality such as the introduction of continuous subcutaneous insulin infusions. However, it may be possible that a combination of new technologies may be able to lower A1C without increasing the risk of hypoglycemia. In the DCCT, the initiation of intensive insulin therapy resulted in an A1C reduction that was accompanied by an increase in severe hypoglycemia. However, after the introduction of rapid-acting analogs (lispro) there was an additional reduction in A1C without further increase in frequency of hypoglycemia.[35] In the Pittsburgh Epidemiology of Diabetes Complications (EDC) Study, A1C fell only about 0.5% in 1995, approximately in concert with publication of findings from the DCCT, and after 30 years of follow-up, only 17% achieved an A1C <7%.[36] Clearly, more needs to be done to ensure that targets are reached.

Association with complications: A1C. Since the DCCT did not randomize subjects to multiple A1C targets, the appropriate target for A1C is based upon epidemiologic analysis of data from the DCCT. The DCCT randomly assigned 1,441 patients to conventional (one to two injections of insulin per day with a goal of freedom from severe hyperglycemia or hypoglycemia symptoms) or intensive treatment (at least three injections per day with the goal of attaining near normoglycemia) arms.[37] Over the 6.5 years of the study, there was a reduction in the risk of nephropathy, retinopathy, and neuropathy in the intensive arm. Mean A1C during the study was the dominant predictor of the development of microvascular complications,[38] and although the risk was nonlinear, there was no threshold below which further reduction in risk was identified.[39] In addition, the risk of microvascular complications was dependent upon the duration of diabetes, emphasizing the relevance of glycemic control at the lower end of the A1C spectrum early in the disease course in order to improve long-term complications.

Long-term epidemiologic follow-up of the DCCT, known as the Epidemiology of Diabetes Interventions and Complications (EDIC) Study, demonstrated persistent beneficial effects of the intensive therapy that were explained mostly by A1C levels during the randomized portion of the trial.[40,41,42] In the EDIC cohort, emergent reduction in CV events was observed in the intensively treated group, again explained by A1C reduction during the intervention phase of the trial.[43] Thus a clear legacy effect exists for multiple complications.

In the Pittsburgh EDC Study, A1C was not a predictor of long-term risk of CVD in patients with T1D.[44] This finding differs from the EDIC and may be at least in part due to greater A1C reduction in the DCCT, which enrolled patients earlier in the disease course, or due to renal disease.[45] However, the EDC did confirm the findings of the relationship between A1C and microvascular complications.[46]

The EURODIAB study was another prospective observational cohort of patients with T1D. In EURODIAB, there was an increased risk of progression of microalbuminuria in a stepwise relationship with A1C.[47] In fact, no threshold for complications was apparent, such that each percentage increase in A1C above 5.5% was associated with increased risk, although only levels >6.5% were significantly different. Similar findings were observed for retinopathy.[48] There was an association of A1C with CV events only in men.[49]

Data from another large national prospective observational study confirmed the strong association between A1C and microvascular complications, with no apparent threshold below which complications are avoided.[50]

Association with complications: Hypoglycemia. Hypoglycemia may be defined in a variety of ways in the literature, but is most concerning when it results in neurologic sequelae such as seizure, or loss of consciousness or requires the assistance of someone other than the patient for treatment. Such events are typically considered to be severe. Severe hypoglycemia is often the only presentation of hypoglycemia that is reported in the literature. Intensive insulin therapy in the DCCT was associated with a threefold increase in severe hypoglycemia,[51] and as the A1C falls, the hypoglycemia risk increases exponentially.[1] Severe hypoglycemia was not associated with the development of microvascular complications[52] or decline in cognitive function in the overall cohort[16] or in the youngest cohort age 13–19 years[17] after 18 years in the study. However, severe hypoglycemia should be minimized as the acute effects are not inconsequential.[53,54]

Association with complications: Glucose variability. In an earlier DCCT publication, there was a difference in outcomes not explained by A1C between the two groups. This was originally attributed to glycemic excursions that might be more prevalent in the less intensive group.[55] However, the same data were reanalyzed, and this finding was attributed to an artifact of the Poisson model as well as to inadequate adjustment for baseline variables.[42] In addition, variability of the relationship between mean glucose and A1C may be significant, further supporting the need for A1C to be supplemented by self-monitored blood glucose readings.[56] In fact, total glucose exposure (A1C and diabetes duration) only explained 11% of the total variation in retinopathy risk overall, after adjustment for treatment group in the DCCT.

Post-hoc analysis of seven-point glucose profiles (self-monitored blood glucose obtained before and after meals and at bedtime) did not demonstrate a relationship between complications and various measures of glycemic variability, except for a weak association between mean amplitude of glycemic excursion (MAGE) and retinopathy.[57,58] Unfortunately, seven-point profiles are limited for capturing glycemic variability, and this question remains incompletely answered.

There is stronger evidence for the use of glycemic variability measures to identify patients at risk of severe hypoglycemia. Lower mean glucose and higher glucose variability (measured as standard deviation [SD]) further contributed to the risk of severe hypoglycemia after controlling for A1C.[59] For example, each 18 mg/dl increase in SD was associated with a 1.09-fold increase in risk of severe hypoglycemia, and the association strengthened for subsequent events. SD, but not mean glucose, predicted overnight hypoglycemia. The authors suggested that optimizing glycemic variability rather than bedtime glucose might be a better way of minimizing nocturnal hypoglycemia. A similar relationship between fasting glucose variability and nocturnal hypoglycemia was reported elsewhere.[60]

Of more recent interest are observations that long-term glycemic variability, assessed with intrapersonal SD of A1C, has been associated with renal disease and CVD, even after adjusting for mean A1C and other known risk factors.[61]

GUIDELINES

Current guidelines for glycemic control from select organizations worldwide are shown in Table 6.4.[19-22,62] Due to the special nature of T1D, only those guidelines that are intended for T1D or that specify self-monitored blood glucose targets are included. In general, guidelines reflect glucose targets established by the DCCT. However, all guidelines recommend that targets be individualized based upon life expectancy and risk for severe hypoglycemia. Conversely, most guidelines allow lower targets for those in which it can be achieved safely, but as noted above, most patients with T1D have difficulty reaching current targets.

Interpretation of Guidelines

A1C (see Table 6.4). The current guidelines for A1C reflect the balance between the continuous benefits achieved by lowering A1C with the increased risk of hypoglycemia as A1C declines (Table 6.4).[19-22,63] As the A1C falls, the hypoglycemia risk increases exponentially.[1] However, since many people with T1D live beyond the duration of time captured in the DCCT, even a small increase in A1C will likely have cumulative adverse effects over time. Based upon evidence from the DCCT, an A1C <7% still appears reasonable for most. However, in select patients for whom it can be done safely, a lower target should be considered. Indeed, as technologies such as continuous glucose monitoring and closed-loop insulin pumps evolve, lower glucose targets may be achievable without increasing the risk of severe hypoglycemia. Such interventions, if successfully established, would warrant a reappraisal of the target A1C.

Glucose (see Table 6.4). Because most patients with T1D are treated with complex insulin regimens, actual insulin titration relies more upon frequent self-monitored or continuous glucose profiles than it does on A1C. Targets by various organizations generally reflect those used by the DCCT (Table 6.4).[19-22,63] Post-meal targets should be considered, particularly in those patients not meeting A1C targets. Although some normative data exist for continuous glucose monitoring, there are no long-term outcomes studies to warrant the reestablishment of separate targets.[64]

Table 6.4 Glucose Targets in Adults

	A1C (%)	Premeal Glucose (mg/dl)	Postmeal Glucose (mg/dl)	Nocturnal (mg/dl)
ADA[19]	<7.0	70–130	<180	<140
AACE[63]	<6.5	<110	<140	—
NICE[20]	<7.5	72–126	<162	—
Australia[21]	<7.0	See DCCT	See DCCT	See DCCT
Canada[22]	<7.0	72–126	90–180 (UL 126 if A1C target not met)	—
DCCT[1]	<6.1%	70–121	90–180	>65

Glycemic Variability. A measure of glycemic variability, such as SD, should be considered to guide interventions aimed at preventing severe hypoglycemia, since such episodes are preceded by periods of increased glycemic variability.[65,66] This is of particular relevance in patients with prior episodes of severe hypoglycemia or with hypoglycemia unawareness. There are currently few data to support the use of one measure over another. However, SD is readily available from downloaded reports of many insulin pumps and glucose meters. Since SD is directly proportional to mean glucose (MG), it must be reported as a percentage of mean glucose, known as the coefficient of variation (%CV). One simple approach proposes that the optimal MG/SD value should be <3, whereas a value >2 is proposed as poor.[63] Further data are needed to determine whether these cutoffs are the best predictors of outcomes such as severe hypoglycemia. CGM data show that the cutoff for the interquartile range for %CV among patients with diabetes is 33.5–40.6%.[67] Glycemic variability should be assessed using continuous glucose monitoring or frequent glucose measurements (minimum of every 4 h) for optimal use.[68]

Alternative markers. Where there are known conditions that affect the accuracy of A1C or where A1C and self-monitored blood glucoses are discrepant, alternative markers of glycemia, such as fructosamine, glycoalbumin, or 1,5-anhydroglucitol, could be considered.[19] While there are insufficient data to warrant the establishment of a specific target level for alternative markers of glycemia, these markers can be used to track patients over time.[69] These markers have not been studied adequately as predictors of long-term complications and it is unclear whether interventions utilizing these markers will improve outcomes over time.

Special Considerations

Severe hypoglycemia. Higher targets are reasonable in patients with severe hypoglycemia or hypoglycemia unawareness in order to restore hypoglycemia sensitivity.[70] In these cases, a higher target A1C may be reasonable, but relaxed blood glucose targets, particularly for fasting glucose, are more important. For example, instead of a premeal target of 70–130 mg/dl, the premeal target would be 90–180 mg/dl. Ultimately, the degree of relaxation of glucose targets is that which eliminates hypoglycemia without causing severe hyperglycemia or ketoacidosis. Relaxation of glycemic targets for only a short period of time may restore hypoglycemia awareness, which may allow for resumption of somewhat tighter targets.

Limited life expectancy/cognitive limitations. We advise higher targets for patients with limited life expectancy and patients with cognitive limitations in which tighter glucose targets are not considered feasible or safe. These targets must be individualized for each patient and their circumstances.

Pregnancy (see Table 6.5). Targets for pregnancy are mainly derived from large randomized controlled trials of women with gestational diabetes (Table 6.5).[19,22,71–72] However, some data from T1D are available. In pregnancy, women with T1D maintained with meal glucose <95 mg/dl in the second and third trimesters minimize the risk of fetal macrosomia.[73] A CGM study determined that early-onset large-for-gestational-age is associated with hyperglycemia in all three trimesters.[74] In another cohort study of 289 patients with T1D, A1C <7% was present in 84% but macrosomia still occurred in nearly half of pregnancies.[75] A1C was a significant predictor but only explained 5% of the variance in macrosomia. This is believed to be due to a greater importance of postprandial hyperglycemia.[76,77,78] In addition, suboptimal glycemic control (A1C >8.0% early pregnancy, >6.1% at 26 weeks, or >7.0% at 34 weeks) was associated with increased risk of preeclampsia.[79] A randomized controlled trial demonstrated that postprandial glucose targeting reduced this risk.[72] Finally, suboptimal first trimester median blood glucose >120 mg/dl[80] and A1C >7%[81] were associated with increased risk of congenital malformations and abortions. Both ACOG75 and ADA[9] have published guidelines for specific glucose targets as well as other countries.[22,76–78] Most guidelines recommend fasting glucose in the <100 mg/dl range and postprandial glucose <140 mg/dl as well as an A1C as close to 6.0% as possible during pregnancy, if it can be done without severe hypoglycemia. (See chapter 17.)

Hospitalized patients (see Table 6.6). There are no guidelines that specifically address glucose targets for patients with T1D in the hospital. Most of these recommendations are based upon extrapolation from randomized controlled trials of predominantly patients with stress hyperglycemia or T2D (Table 6.6).[82]

The current American Diabetes Association/American Association of Clinical Endocrinology hospital guidelines recommend a target glucose of 140–180 mg/dl in the ICU for most patients, with targets of 110–140 possible for selected patients if it can be safely attained. In non-ICU settings, recommendations are for fasting glucose <140 mg/dl and random glucose <180 mg/dl until further data are available.[83] The Endocrine Society published recommendations for meal-specific targets for non–critical care settings, including a fasting glucose <140 mg/dl and postprandial target of <180 mg/dl,[84] while the American College of Physicians allowed a higher range of 140–200 mg/dl.[85] These targets are generally higher than that advocated for most outpatients

Table 6.5 Glucose Targets in Pregnancy

	A1C (%)	Premeal Glucose (mg/dl)	Postmeal Glucose (mg/dl)	Nocturnal (mg/dl)
ADA[19]	<6.0	60–99	100–129 peak postprandial	—
ACOG[75]	<6.0	Fasting: 95 Premeal: 100	1 h: <140 2 h: <120	60
NICE[76]	Not recommended in second and third trimester	63–106	1 h: <140	—
Canada[22]	—	68–94	1 h: 99–139 2 h: 90–119	>65
Australia[77]	"within the normal range"	72–99	1 h: <144 2 h: <126	
IDF[78]	<6.0	60–120		

with diabetes. The recommendations are based largely upon the NICE-SUGAR study (both T1D and T2D patients), which showed that tight glycemic control (target glucose 80–110 mg/dl) compared to standard care (target glucose 140–180 mg/dl) resulted in higher frequency of severe hypoglycemia and mortality in the intensively treated group [86] However, NICE-SUGAR did not address whether glycemic control targeting a more modest glucose range (110–140 mg/dl) is better. As a result, the guidelines suggest that an intermediate target glucose range between 110–140 mg/dl may be reasonable in certain populations (for example, postcardiac surgery) and institutions and patients where it can be done safely. In children, higher targets may be advised in the hospital.[87] Improvements in technology, such as more precise methods of glucose monitoring and computerized (or even closed-loop) intravenous infusion algorithms are ultimately needed to determine whether achievement of normoglycemia is beneficial.[87,88]

Table 6.6 Glucose Targets during Hospitalization

	Premeal Glucose (mg/dl)	Random Glucose (mg/dl)
ADA/AACE[89]		140–180
Endocrine Society[90]	<140	<180
ACP[91]		140–200

Blood Pressure

Current trends. In the DCCT, 44% of patients developed incident hypertension during the 15-year follow-up, for which hyperglycemia was a major risk factor of CV events.[89] Thus, hypertension is felt to be a consequence rather than a cause of nephropathy. However, patients were excluded from the DCCT if they had hypertension (defined as >140/90 mmHg) at entry. In the EDC and EURO-DIAB studies, the prevalence of treatment for hypertension was 7–10% (mean diabetes duration 14–19 years).[48] In a large Swedish study of patients with T1D there was a slow improvement in blood pressure and cholesterol over time, but only 61% of patients achieved a mean blood pressure <130/80 mmHg.[37] Other studies demonstrate that hypertension is suboptimally managed in patients with T1D, although this has improved over time.[90,91]

Association with complications. Diabetes significantly increases the prevalence of CVD, with T1D conferring an independent risk factor for premature morbidity and mortality related to its duration, control, and association with traditional CV risk factors including hypertension and hyperlipidemia.[48,92]

Blood pressure management was not a salient feature of the DCCT. In the UKPDS (which enrolled patients with T2D), a 10 mmHg increase in systolic blood pressure was associated with an 11% rise in myocardial infarction, a 13% rise in microvascular disease, and a 15% rise in diabetes-related mortality.[93] Numerous other large trials, including the HOT trial, HOPE, LIFE, and ALLHAT studies have also shown significant improvement in CV outcomes and slowed progression of microvascular complications when aggressive blood pressure targets are achieved, albeit largely in individuals with T2D.[94,95,96,97] Achievement of *tighter control* to <130 mmHg systolic that was examined in 6,400 patients with diabetes and CVD in the International Verapamil/Trandolapril Study (INVEST) did not reveal further improvement of CV outcomes compared with the usual 130–140 mmHg, but patients were not randomized to different targets.[98] Nor was randomization to tighter blood pressure control (systolic <120 mmHg) found to be beneficial on the primary outcome in patients with T2D in the ACCORD study, although there was a statistically significant reduction in strokes, a secondary outcome.[99]

Guidelines. On the basis of these findings, although not specifically conducted for T1D, ADA guidelines recommend a blood pressure target of <130/80.[19] The NICE guidelines recommend intervention at 135/85 mmHg unless the individual has an abnormal albumin excretion rate or at least two of the metabolic syndrome features, in which case it should be initiated at 130/80 mmHg.[20]

Interpretation of guidelines. Individuals should have routine blood pressure checks at diabetes visits.[19] According to the ADA, those with systolic blood pressure >130 mmHg and diastolic blood pressure >80 mmHg, despite lifestyle interventions for a maximum of 3 months, should be started on a pharmacologic agent blocking the renin angiotensin system.[19] Although a systolic blood pressure of >140 mmHg clearly results in worse outcomes, further evidence is needed to support targeting a systolic blood pressure significantly <130 mmHg in T1D. Some variation may be appropriate based on individual response and tolerance to therapy as well as specific characteristics.

Special circumstances: Nephropathy. In patients who develop diabetic nephropathy characterized by persistent proteinuria, optimization of blood pressure can slow the progression of renal damage. The blood pressure targets are the same for individuals with T1D with or without nephropathy per ADA,[19] AACE,[63] NICE,[20] and Canadian[22] guidelines. The Australian guidelines, however, conclude a blood pressure target <125/75 mmHg in the presence of 1 g daily or more of proteinuria.[21] In addition to controlling blood pressure, ACE inhibitor therapy has decreased albuminuria and prevented worsening nephropathy while ARBs have reduced proteinuria. These renal-protective effects were demonstrated in a study of 698 microalbuminuric patients without hypertension.[100] Those receiving ACE inhibitors had a reduction in progression to macroalbuminuria and an increase in regression to nonalbuminuria.[101]

Special circumstances: Pregnancy. In pregnant women with T1D, hypertension is more commonly associated with preeclampsia and complicates the pregnancy 40–45% of the time.[102] Hypertension may result in very adverse outcomes, and thus the blood pressure target throughout the pregnancy is lower, at 110–129/65–79 mmHg, to protect maternal health and fetal growth.[76] ACE inhibitors and ARBs are contraindicated during pregnancy given associated risk of increased congenital malformations. Instead, calcium channel blockers, β blockers, hydralazine, and methyldopa should be used to achieve blood pressure target goal.[103] (Also see chapter 17.)

Low Density Lipoprotein Cholesterol

Current trends. While T2D most commonly presents with hypertriglyceridemia, low HDLc, and increased LDLc,[104] in T1D, lipid and lipoprotein concentrations may be normal but present with impaired function and increased atherogenicity due to oxidation and glycation of lipoproteins.[105,106,107] In a large Swedish national registry study, only 48% of patients receiving lipid lowering agents achieved the goal LDLc of <100 mg/dl.[37] Suboptimal control has also been reported in the U.S., with only 5.5% meeting targets, particularly children.[48]

Association with complications. Dyslipidemia is highly prevalent in people with diabetes, further increasing the risk of microvascular complications as seen in DCCT/EDIC[108] along with CVD and associated mortality. Overall, in T1D evidence indicates an effect of statin on lipids consistent with the general population. The Heart Protection Study (HPS) is one of a few studies that examined the effect of a statin in patients with T1D, and nearly 600 patients were included. The HPS found a CV risk reduction similar to that of patients with T2D.[109] This study supported the reduction of baseline LDLc level by about 30–40% as an alternative therapeutic goal. A large meta-analysis of statin trials demonstrated similar CV risk reduction in patients with T1D (1,566 patients) compared to patients with T2D and patients without diabetes.[110]

Guidelines. According to the ADA and the National Cholesterol Education Program's Adult Treatment Panel III, the primary goal for individuals without overt CVD is an LDL <100 mg/dl and <70 mg/dl with overt CVD or more than two major CV risk factors.[19,111] However, statins should be started in individuals over the age of 40 years or with CV risk factors or overt disease, regardless of baseline lipid levels.[19] The Adult Treatment Panel III guidelines were last updated in 2002 and an updated version is expected to be released soon.[112] The target HDLc is >40 mg/dl for men and >50 mg/dl for women, while that for triglycerides is <150 mg/dl.[19]

Interpretation of guidelines. To screen adult patients for dyslipidemia, a fasting lipid profile should be checked at least annually, and then repeated every 1–2 years. To achieve target goals for lipid measures, aggressive lifestyle and medical management of dyslipidemia is necessary.

SPECIAL CIRCUMSTANCES

Pregnancy

Statins are contraindicated during pregnancy (category X) and should be stopped prior to conception.[113] Thus, adequate patient education and family planning counseling are necessary for women with T1D of childbearing age.

Other Lipid Targets

Additional measures of atherogenic lipid lipoproteins have been explored. The TC/HDLc ratio (or non-HDL cholesterol) has been proposed as a specific index of CV risk and a secondary goal of therapy to <4.0 (for the ratio) or 30 mg/dl above the LDLc target for non-HDLc) is suggested.[19,114] The use of apo B to predict CVD events with target of <80 mg/dl in patients with CVD and <90 mg/dl in those without has been recommended by some,[115] but inadequate supporting evidence exists.

Other Metabolic Variables

Intensive glycemic control was associated with greater weight gain and risk of metabolic syndrome compared to the standard group in the DCCT.[116] However, the benefits of glycemic control appear to mitigate any observed increase in risk of complications. In contrast, insulin resistance at baseline (assessed with estimated glucose disposal rate) but not metabolic syndrome or insulin dose predicted the onset of both microvascular and macrovascular complications. In another study within the DCCT, waist circumference was associated with increased risk of incident microalbuminuria but not decline in creatinine clearance.[117] However, those patients in the intensive group who did not gain weight still experienced a survival benefit and lower risk of complications compared to those who gained weight.[118]

In EURODIAB, waist-to-hip ratio and triglycerides (as markers of insulin resistance) were independent predictors of incident retinopathy.[119] Furthermore, waist-to-hip ratio and triglycerides were nearly as strong as albumin excretion rate for predicting microalbuminuria.[120] Increased weight was a predictor of progression from microalbuminuria to macroalbuminuria.[51]

As noted above, dyslipidemia commonly associated with metabolic syndrome or T2D may be observed in patients with T1D. If low HDLc results in a persistently elevated ratio, niacin therapy may be added to statin. Niacin combined with statin was associated with >13% absolute risk reduction for CV outcomes in the HATS nondiabetic cohort.[121] However, CV risk reduction was not confirmed in a large prospective study of patients with T2D who were already receiving statin therapy, and there was suggestion of increased risk of stroke.[122] Fibrate therapy is recommended for individuals with significantly elevated triglyceride levels although it revealed no reduction in CV outcomes in a large trial of T2D patients unless there was dyslipidemia present at baseline.[19,123] Outside of lowering triglycerides to prevent pancreatitis, further research is needed to determine the optimal role of managing dyslipidemia beyond statin therapy in patients with T1D.

FUTURE CLINICAL RESEARCH: FILLING THE GAPS

There are many unanswered questions surrounding optimal targets for risk factors of microvascular and macrovascular complications. The following is a list of more urgent questions.

Pediatrics

Glucose

■ Effects of severe hypoglycemia on cognitive function in children with T1D stratified by age in order to more closely establish any threshold effect

Blood pressure

■ Optimal blood pressure targets and long-term safety and efficacy of blockade of the renin-angiotensin system

LDLc

■ Optimal targets and long-term safety and efficacy of statins

Adults

Glucose

■ Updated risk of complications and hypoglycemia risk at various A1C strata and duration of diabetes
■ Assessment of the long-term risk of complications using continuous glucose monitoring data, including glucose area under the curve, time spent in hyperglycemic and hypoglycemic ranges, and measures of glycemic variability

■ Robust longitudinal assessment of the prevalence of severe hypoglycemia in relationship to newer technologies, such as insulin analogues, continuous subcutaneous insulin infusion, and continuous glucose monitoring

■ Optimal targets for avoidance of hypoglycemia in hypoglycemia-associated autonomic failure

■ Utility and comparison of measures of glycemic variability for preventing severe hypoglycemia

■ Utility of alternative markers of glycemia for predicting long-term complications

Blood pressure

■ Further characterization of the relative role of blood pressure in the development of microvascular and macrovascular complications

■ Optimal target blood pressure in patients by duration of diabetes (with separate attention to essential hypertension and that presumably mediated by early nephropathy)

■ Optimal blood pressure targets in nephropathy

LDLc

■ Optimal LDLc level for CV prevention in patients with T1D by age and duration of diabetes

■ Prospective studies further characterizing the role of lipids in the development of microvascular complications

■ Longitudinal studies assessing and comparing the association between various components of the lipid profile, including lipoprotein analysis on risk of CVD in patients with T1D

■ Investigation of any additive benefit of managing dyslipidemia associated with metabolic syndrome

CONCLUSION

It is clear that the optimal targets for T2D cannot always be extrapolated to patients with T1D, since the pathophysiology, disease course, and management differ so markedly. In patients with T1D, it is likely that glycemic control is even more important than for T2D, although other factors such as blood pressure and lipids play a key role. Targets should include A1C, but A1C alone has little utility for making specific adjustments in glucose-lowering therapy. Instead targets should include goals for glucose in a variety of circumstances, such as fasting, premeal and postmeal, and possibly for glycemic variability. In general, targets must be individualized to fit the specific circumstances of the patient, taking into account the risks and benefits of the intervention, particularly in the case of glucose targets. Newer technologies may allow tighter targets over time without increasing the risk of hypoglycemia. Therefore, targets should be frequently reevaluated among individuals and among the population as a whole.

REFERENCES

1. Diabetes Control and Complications Trial Research Group: The effect of intensive treatment of diabetes on the development and progression of long-term in insulin-dependent diabetes mellitus. *N Engl J Med* 329:977–986, 1993
2. Stratton IM, Adler AI, Neil HA, Matthews DR, Manley SE, Cull CA, Hadden D, Turner RC, Holman RR: Association of glycaemia with macrovascular and microvascular complications of type 2 diabetes (UKPDS 35): prospective observational study. *BMJ* 321:405– 1412, 2000
3. Fox CS, Larson MG, Leip EP, Meigs JB, Wilson PW, Levy D: Glycemic status and development of kidney disease: the Framingham Heart Study. *Diabetes Care* 28:2436–2440, 2005
4. Selvin E, Steffes MW, Zhu H, Matsushita K, Wagenknecht L, Pankow J, Coresh J, Brancati FL: Glycated hemoglobin, diabetes, and cardiovascular risk in nondiabetic adults. *N Engl J Med* 362:800–811, 2010
5. Taubert G, Winkelmann BR, Schleiffer T, März W, Winkler R, Gök R, Klein B, Schneider S, Boehm BO: Prevalence, predictors, and consequences of unrecognized diabetes mellitus in 3266 patients scheduled for coronary angiography. *Am Heart J* 145:285–291, 2003
6. Juutilainen A, Lehto S, Rönnemaa T, Pyörälä K, Laakso M: Similarity of the impact of type 1 and type 2 diabetes on cardiovascular mortality in middle-aged subjects. *Diabetes Care* 31:714–719, 2008
7. Donnelly LA, Morris AD, Frier BM, Ellis JD, Donnan PT, Durrant R, Band MM, Reekie G, Leese GP: DARTS/MEMO Collaboration: Frequency and predictors of hypoglycaemia in type 1 and insulin-treated type 2 diabetes: a population-based study. *Diabet Med* 22:749–755, 2005
8. Kuenen JC, Borg R, Kuik DJ, Zheng H, Schoenfeld D, Diamant M, Nathan DM, Heine RJ: ADAG Study Group: Does glucose variability influence the relationship between mean plasma glucose and HbA1c levels in type 1 and type 2 diabetic patients? *Diabetes Care* 34:1843–1847, 2011
9. Greven WL, Beulens JW, Biesma DH, Faiz S, de Valk HW: Glycemic variability in inadequately controlled type 1 diabetes and type 2 diabetes on intensive insulin therapy: a cross-sectional, observational study. *Diabetes Technol Ther* 12:695–699, 2010
10. Lawrie SM, Whalley H, Kestelman JN, Abukmeil SS, Byrne M, Hodges A, Rimmington JE, Best JJ, Owens DG, Johnstone EC: Magnetic resonance imaging of brain in people at high risk of developing schizophrenia. *Lancet* 353:30–33, 1999
11. Perantie DC, Lim A, Wu J, Weaver P, Warren SL, Sadler M, White NH, Hershey T: Effects of prior hypoglycemia and hyperglycemia on cognition in children with type 1 diabetes mellitus. *Pediatr Diabetes* 9:87–95, 2008
12. Patiño-Fernández AM, Delamater AM, Applegate EB, Brady E, Eidson M, Nemery R, Gonzalez-Mendoza L, Richton S: Neurocognitive functioning in preschool-age children with type 1 diabetes mellitus. *Pediatr Diabetes* 11:424–430, 2010
13. Gaudieri PA, Chen R, Greer TF, Holmes CS: Cognitive function in children with type 1 diabetes: a meta-analysis. *Diabetes Care* 31(9):1892–1897, 2008

14. Northam EA, Rankins D, Lin A, Wellard RM, Pell GS, Finch SJ, Werther GA, Cameron FJ: Central nervous system function in youth with type 1 diabetes 12 years after disease onset. *Diabetes Care* 32:445–450, 2009
15. Asvold BO, Sand T, Hestad K, Bjørgaas MR: Cognitive function in type 1 diabetic adults with early exposure to severe hypoglycemia: a 16-year follow-up study. *Diabetes Care* 33:1945–1947, 2010
16. Jacobson AM, Musen G, Ryan CM, Silvers N, Cleary P, Waberski B, Burwood A, Weinger K, Bayless M, Dahms W, Harth J: Diabetes Control and Complications Trial/Epidemiology of Diabetes Interventions and Complications Study Research Group: Long-term effect of diabetes and its treatment on cognitive function. *N Engl J Med* 356:1842–1852, 2007
17. Musen G, Jacobson AM, Ryan CM, Cleary PA, Waberski BH, Weinger K, Dahms W, Bayless M, Silvers N, Harth J, White N: Diabetes Control and Complications Trial/Epidemiology of Diabetes Interventions and Complications Research Group: Impact of diabetes and its treatment on cognitive function among adolescents who participated in the Diabetes Control and Complications Trial. *Diabetes Care* 31:1933–1938, 2008
18. Sima AAF: Encephalopathies: the emerging diabetic complications. *Acta Diabetol* 47:279–293, 2010
19. American Diabetes Association: Standards of medical care in diabetes: 2012. *Diabetes Care* 35 (Suppl. 1):S11–S63, 2012
20. Rewers M, Pihoker C, Donaghue K, Hanas R, Swift P, Klingensmith GJ: Assessment and monitoring of glycemic control in children and adolescents with diabetes. *Pediatr Diabetes* 10 (Suppl. 12):71–81, 2009
21. Chemtob CM, Hochhauser CJ, Shemesh E, Schmeidler J, Rapaport R: Does poor early metabolic control predict subsequent poor control in young children with type 1 diabetes: an exploratory study. *J Diabetes* 3:153–157, 2011
22. Shalitin S, Phillip M: Which factors predict glycemic control in children diagnosed with type 1 diabetes before 6.5 years of age? *Acta Diabetol* 49:355–362, 2012 [Epub ahead of print]
23. Eppens MC, Craig ME, Cusumano J, Hing S, Chan AK, Howard NJ, Silink M, Donaghue KC: Prevalence of diabetes complications in adolescents with type 2 compared with type 1 diabetes. *Diabetes Care* 29:1300–1306, 2006
24. Hanas R, Donaghue KC, Klingensmith G, Swift PG: ISPAD clinical practice consensus guidelines 2009 compendium. *Pediatr Diabetes* 10 Suppl 12: 1–2, 2009
25. Soffer B, Zhang Z, Miller K, Vogt BA, Shahinfar S: A double-blind, placebo-controlled, dose-response study of the effectiveness and safety of lisinopril for children with hypertension. *Am J Hyperten* 16:795–800, 2003
26. Wells T, Frame V, Soffer B, Shaw W, Zhang Z, Herrera P, Shahinfar S: Enalapril Pediatric Hypertension Collaborative study group: A double-blind, placebo-controlled, dose-response study of the effectiveness and safety of enalapril for children with hypertension. *J Clin Pharma* 42: 870–880, 2002
27. Järvisalo MJ, Raitakari M, Toikka JO, Putto-Laurila A, Rontu R, Laine S, Lehtimäki T, Rönnemaa T, Viikari J, Raitakari OT: Endothelial dysfunction and increased arterial intima-media thickness in children with type 1 diabetes. *Circulation* 109:1750–1755, 2004

28. De Jongh S, Ose L, Szamosi T, Gagné C, Lambert M, Scott R, Perron P, Dobbelaere D, Saborio M, Tuohy MB, Stepanavage M, Sapre A, Gumbiner B, Mercuri M, van Trotsenburg AS, Bakker HD, Kastelein JJ: Simvastatin in Children Study Group: Efficacy and safety of stain therapy in children with familial hypercholesterolemia: a randomized, double-blind, placebo-controlled trial with simvastatin. *Circulation* 106:2231–2237, 2002
29. Wiegman A, Hutten BA, de Groot E, Rodenburg J, Bakker HD, Büller HR, Sijbrands EJ, Kastelein JJ: Efficacy and safety of statin therapy in children with familial hypercholesterolemia: a randomized controlled trial. *JAMA* 292:331–337, 2004
30. Dietary Intervention Study in Children (DISC): Writing Group for the DISC Collaborative Research Group: Efficacy and safety of lowering dietary intake of fat and cholesterol in children with elevated low-density lipoprotein cholesterol. *JAMA* 273:1429–1435, 1995
31. Beck RW, Tamborlane WV, Bergenstal RM, Miller KM, Dubose SN, Hall CA, for the T1D Exchange Clinic Network. *J Clin Endocrinol Metab* 20 September 2012. [Epub ahead of print] PMID: 22996145
32. Eeg-Olofsson K, Cederholm J, Nilsson PM, Gudbjörnsdóttir S, Eliasson B: Steering Committee of the Swedish National Diabetes Register: Glycemic and risk factor control in type 1 diabetes: results from 13,612 patients in a national diabetes register. *Diabetes Care* 30:496–502, 2007
33. Rosenbauer J, Dost A, Karges B, Hungele A, Stahl A, Bächle C, Gerstl EM, Kastendieck C, Hofer SE, Holl RW: DPV Initiative and the German BMBF Competence Network Diabetes Mellitus: Improved metabolic control in children and adolescents with type 1 diabetes: a trend analysis using prospective multicenter data from Germany and Austria. *Diabetes Care* 35:80–86, 2012
34. Hoerger TJ, Segel JE, Gregg EW, Saaddine JB: Is glycemic control improving in U.S. adults? *Diabetes Care* 31:81–86, 2008
35. Chase HP, Lockspeiser T, Peery B, Shepherd M, MacKenzie T, Anderson J, Garg SK: The impact of the diabetes control and complications trial and humalog insulin on glycohemoglobin levels and severe hypoglycemia in type 1 diabetes. *Diabetes Care* 24:430–434, 2001
36. Nathan DM, Zinman B, Cleary PA, Backlund JY, Genuth S, Miller R, Orchard TJ: Diabetes Control and Complications Trial/Epidemiology of Diabetes Interventions and Complications (DCCT/EDIC) Research Group: Modern-day clinical course of type 1 diabetes mellitus after 30 years' duration: the diabetes control and complications trial/epidemiology of diabetes interventions and complications and Pittsburgh epidemiology of diabetes complications experience (1983-2005). *Arch Intern Med* 169:1307–1316, 2009
37. Writing Team for the Diabetes Control and Complications Trial/Epidemiology of Diabetes Interventions and Complications Research Group: Effect of intensive therapy on the microvascular complications of type 1 diabetes mellitus. *JAMA* 287:2563–2569, 2002
38. Lachin JM, Genuth S, Nathan DM, Zinman B, Rutledge BN: DCCT/EDIC Research Group: Effect of glycemic exposure on the risk of microvascular

complications in the diabetes control and complications trial—revisited. *Diabetes* 57:995–1001, 2008

39. Diabetes Control and Complications Trial Research Group: The absence of a glycemic threshold for the development of long-term complications: the perspective of the Diabetes Control and Complications Trial. *Diabetes* 45:1289–1298, 1996

40. White NH, Sun W, Cleary PA, Tamborlane WV, Danis RP, Hainsworth DP, Davis MD: DCCT-EDIC Research Group: Effect of prior intensive therapy in type 1 diabetes on 10-year progression of retinopathy in the DCCT/EDIC: comparison of adults and adolescents. *Diabetes* 59:1244–1253, 2010

41. Albers JW, Herman WH, Pop-Busui R, Feldman EL, Martin CL, Cleary PA, Waberski BH, Lachin JM: Diabetes Control and Complications Trial/Epidemiology of Diabetes Interventions and Complications Research Group: Effect of prior intensive insulin treatment during the Diabetes Control and Complications Trial (DCCT) on peripheral neuropathy in type 1 diabetes during the Epidemiology of Diabetes Interventions and Complications (EDIC) Study. *Diabetes Care* 33:1090–1096, 2010

42. Writing Team for the Diabetes Control and Complications Trial/Epidemiology of Diabetes Interventions and Complications Research Group: Sustained effect of intensive treatment of type 1 diabetes mellitus on development and progression of diabetic nephropathy: the Epidemiology of Diabetes Interventions and Complications (EDIC) Study. *JAMA* 290:2159–2167, 2003

43. Nathan DM, Cleary PA, Backlund JY, Genuth SM, Lachin JM, Orchard TJ, Raskin P, Zinman B: Diabetes Control and Complications Trial/Epidemiology of Diabetes Interventions and Complications (DCCT/EDIC) Study Research Group: Intensive diabetes treatment and cardiovascular disease in patients with type 1 diabetes. *N Engl J Med* 353:2643–2653, 2005

44. Zgibor JC, Ruppert K, Orchard TJ, Soedamah-Muthu SS, Fuller J, Chaturvedi N, Roberts MS: Development of a coronary heart disease risk prediction model for type 1 diabetes: the Pittsburgh CHD in type 1 diabetes risk model. *Diabetes Res Clin Pract* 88:314–321, 2010

45. Prince CT, Becker DJ, Costacou T, Miller RG, Orchard TJ: Changes in glycaemic control and risk of coronary artery disease in type 1 diabetes mellitus: findings from the Pittsburgh Epidemiology of Diabetes Complications Study (EDC). *Diabetologia* 50:2280–2288, 2007

46. Vergouwe Y, Soedamah-Muthu SS, Zgibor J, Chaturvedi N, Forsblom C, Snell-Bergeon JK, Maahs DM, Groop PH, Rewers M, Orchard TJ, Fuller JH, Moons KG: Progression to microalbuminuria in type 1 diabetes: development and validation of a prediction rule. *Diabetologia* 53:254–262, 2010

47. Giorgino F, Laviola L, Cavallo Perin P, Solnica B, Fuller J, Chaturvedi N: Factors associated with progression to macroalbuminuria in microalbuminuric type 1 diabetic patients: the EURODIAB Prospective Complications Study. *Diabetologia* 47:1020–1028, 2004

48. Rottiers R, Veglio M, Fuller JH: EURODIAB Prospective Complications Study Group: Risk factors for progression to proliferative diabetic retinopathy in the EURODIAB Prospective Complications Study. *Diabetologia* 44:2203–2209, 2001

49. Soedamah-Muthu SS, Chaturvedi N, Toeller M, Ferriss B, Reboldi P, Michel G, Manes C, Fuller JH: EURODIAB Prospective Complications Study Group: Risk factors for coronary heart disease in type 1 diabetic patients in Europe: the EURODIAB Prospective Complications Study. *Diabetes Care* 27:530–537, 2004

50. Hammes HP, Kerner W, Hofer S, Kordonouri O, Raile K, Holl RW: DPV-Wiss Study Group: Diabetes retinopathy in type 1 diabetes—a contemporary analysis of 8,784 patients. *Diabetologia* 43:1977–1984, 2011

51. Diabetes Control and Complications Trial Research Group: Adverse events and their association with treatment regimens in the diabetes control and complications trial. *Diabetes Care* 18:1415–1427, 1995

52. Kilpatrick ES, Rigby AS, Atkin SL, Frier BM: Does severe hypoglycaemia influence microvascular complications in type 1 diabetes? An analysis of the diabetes control and complications trial database. *Diabet Med* doi: 10.1111/j.1464-5491.2012.03612.x, 2012. [Epub ahead of print]

53. Cox D, Clarke W, Gonder-Frederick L, Kovatchev B: Driving mishaps and hypoglycaemia: risk and prevention. *Int J Clin Pract (Suppl.)*38–42, 2001

54. Gonder-Frederick LA, Zrebiec JF, Bauchowitz AU, Ritterband LM, Magee JC, Cox DJ, Clarke WL: Cognitive function is disrupted by both hypo- and hyperglycemia in school-aged children with type 1 diabetes: a field study. *Diabetes Care* 32:1001–1006, 2009

55. Diabetes Control and Complications Trial Research Group: The relationship of glycemic exposure (HbA1c) to the risk of development and progression of retinopathy in the diabetes control and complications trial. *Diabetes* 44:968–983, 1995

56. Kilpatrick ES, Rigby AS, Atkin SL: Variability in the relationship between mean plasma glucose and HbA1c: implications for the assessment of glycemic control. *Clin Chem* 53:897–901, 2007

57. Kilpatrick ES, Rigby AS, Atkin SL: The effect of glucose variability on the risk of microvascular complications in type 1 diabetes. *Diabetes Care* 29:1486–1490, 2006

58. Service FJ, O'Brien PC: The relation of glycaemia to the risk of development and progression of retinopathy in the diabetic control and complications trial. *Diabetologia* 44:1215–1220, 2001

59. Kilpatrick ES, Rigby AS, Goode K, Atkin SL: Relating mean blood glucose and glucose variability to the risk of multiple episodes of hypoglycaemia in type 1 diabetes. *Diabetologia* 50:2553–2561, 2007

60. Niskanen L, Virkamäki A, Hansen JB, Saukkonen T: Fasting plasma glucose variability as a marker of nocturnal hypoglycemia in diabetes: evidence from the PREDICTIVE Study. *Diabetes Res Clin Pract* 86:e15–e18, 2009

61. Wadén J, Forsblom C, Thorn LM, Gordin D, Saraheimo M, Groop PH: Finnish Diabetic Nephropathy Study Group: A1C variability predicts incident cardiovascular events, microalbuminuria, and overt diabetic nephropathy in patients with type 1 diabetes. *Diabetes* 58:2649–2655, 2009

62. Handelsman Y, JI, Blonde L, Grunberger G, Bloomgarden ZT, Bray GA, Dagogo-Jack S, Davidson JA, Einhorn D, Ganda O, Garber AJ, Hirsch IB, Horton ES, Ismail-Beigi F, Jellinger PS, Jones KL, Jovanovič L, Lebovitz H, Levy P, Moghissi ES, Orzeck EA, Vinik AI, Wyne KL: AACE Task Force

for Developing Diabetes Comprehensive Care Plan: American Association of Clinical Endocrinologists medical guidelines for clinical practice for developing a diabetes mellitus comprehensive care plan. *Endocr Pract* 17 (Suppl. 2):1–53, 2011

63. Hirsch IB: Glycemic variability: it's not just about A1C anymore! *Diabetes Technol Ther* 7:780–783, 2005

64. Hill NR, Oliver NS, Choudhary P, Levy JC, Hindmarsh P, Matthews DR: Normal reference range for mean tissue glucose and glycemic variability derived from continuous glucose monitoring for subjects without diabetes in different ethnic groups. *Diabetes Technol Ther* 13:921–928, 2011

65. Breton M, Clarke W, Farhy L, Kovatchev B: A model of self-treatment behavior, glucose variability, and hypoglycemia-associated autonomic failure in type 1 diabetes. *J Diabetes Sci Technol* 3:331–337, 2007

66. Kovatchev BP, Cox DJ, Farhy LS, Straume M, Gonder-Frederick L, Clarke WL: Episodes of severe hypoglycemia in type 1 diabetes are preceded and followed within 48 hours by measurable disturbances in blood glucose. *J Clin Endocrinol Metab* 85:4287–4292, 2000

67. Rodbard D: Clinical interpretation of indices of quality of glycemic control and glycemic variability. *Postgrad Med* 123:107–118, 2011

68. Baghurst PA, Rodbard D, Cameron FJ: The minimum frequency of glucose measurements from which glycemic variation can be consistently assessed. *J Diabetes Sci Technol* 4:1382–1385, 2010

69. Foo JP, Mantzoros CS: The quest for the perfect biomarker of long-term glycemia: new studies, new trials and tribulations. *Metabolism* 60:1651–1654, 2011

70. Dagogo-Jack S, Rattarasarn C, Cryer PE: Reversal of hypoglycemia unawareness, but not defective glucose counterregulation, in IDDM. *Diabetes* 43:1426–1434, 1994

71. ACOG Committee on Practice Bulletins. ACOG Practice Bulletin. Clinical Management Guidelines for Obstetrician-Gynecologists. Number 60, March 2005. Pregestational diabetes mellitus. *Obstet Gynecol* 105:675, 2005

72. International Diabetes Federation Clinical Guidelines Taskforce. Chapter 17: Pregnancy in *Global Guideline for Type 2 Diabetes.* 2005. International Diabetes Federation, Brussels. Available at http://www.idf.org/webdata/docs/GGT2D%2017%20Pregnancy.pdf. Accessed 20 March 2012

73. Mello G, Parretti E, Mecacci F, La Torre P, Cioni R, Cianciulli D, Scarselli G: What degree of maternal metabolic control in women with type 1 diabetes is associated with normal body size and proportions in full-term infants? *Diabetes Care* 23:1494, 2000

74. Kerssen A, de Valk HW, Visser GH: Increased second trimester maternal glucose levels are related to extremely large-for-gestational-age infants in women with type 1 diabetes. *Diabetes Care* 30:1069–1074, 2007

75. Evers IM, De Balk HW, Mol BWJ, ter Braak EW, Visser GH: Macrosomia despite good glycaemic control in type I diabetic pregnancy: results of a nationwide study in the Netherlands. *Diabetologia* 45:1484–1489, 2002

76. Jovanovic-Peterson L, Peterson CM, Reed GF, Metzger BE, Mills JL, Knopp RH, Aarons JH: Maternal postprandial glucose levels and infant birth weight: the Diabetes in Early Pregnancy Study. National Institute

of Child Health and Human Development: Diabetes in Early Pregnancy Study. *Am J Obstet Gynecol* 164:103–111, 1991

77. Combs CA, Gunderson E, Kitzmiller JL, Gavin LA, Main EK: Relationship of fetal macrosomia to maternal postprandial glucose control during pregnancy. *Diabetes Care* 15:1251–1257, 1992

78. Manderson JG, Patterson CC, Hadden DR, Traub AI, Ennis C, McCance DR: Preprandial versus postprandial blood glucose monitoring in type 1 diabetic pregnancy: a randomized controlled clinical trial. *Am J Obstet Gynecol* 189:507–512, 2003

79. Holmes VA, Young IS, Patterson CC, Pearson DW, Walker JD, Maresh MJ, McCance DR: Diabetes and Pre-eclampsia Intervention Trial Study Group: Optimal glycemic control, pre-eclampsia, and gestational hypertension in women with type 1 diabetes in the diabetes and pre-eclampsia intervention trial. *Diabetes Care* 34:1683, 2011

80. Rosenn B, Miodovnik M, Combs CA, Khoury J, Siddiqi TA: Glycemic thresholds for spontaneous abortion and congenital malformations in insulin-dependent diabetes mellitus. *Obstet Gynecol* 84:515–520, 1994

81. Nielsen GL, Møller M, Sørensen HT: HbA1c in early diabetic pregnancy and pregnancy outcomes: a Danish population-based cohort study of 573 pregnancies in women with type 1 diabetes. *Diabetes Care* 29:2612–2616, 2006

82. Tridgell DM, Tridgell AH, Hirsch IB: Inpatient management of adults and children with type 1 diabetes. *Endocrinol Metab Clin N Am* 39:595–608, 2010

83. Moghissi ES, Korytkowski MT, DiNardo M, Einhorn D, Hellman R, Hirsch IB, Inzucchi SE, Ismail-Beigi F, Kirkman MS, Umpierrez GE: American Association of Clinical Endocrinologists, American Diabetes Association: American Association of Clinical Endocrinologists and American Diabetes Association consensus statement on inpatient glycemic control. *Diabetes Care.* 32:1119–1131, 2009

84. Umpierrez GE, Hellman R, Korytkowski MT, Kosiborod M, Maynard GA, Montori VM, Seley JJ, Van den Berghe G: Management of hyperglycemia in hospitalized patients in non-critical care setting: an endocrine society clinical practice guideline. *J Clin Endocrinol Metab* 97:16–38, 2012

85. Qaseem A, Humphrey LL, Chou R, Snow V, Shekelle P: Clinical Guidelines Committee of the American College of Physicians: Use of intensive insulin therapy for the management of glycemic control in hospitalized patients: a clinical practice guideline from the American College of Physicians. *Ann Intern Med* 154:260–267, 2011

86. Finfer S, Chittock DR, Su SY, Blair D, Foster D, Dhingra V, Bellomo R, Cook D, Dodek P, Henderson WR, Hébert PC, Heritier S, Heyland DK, McArthur C, McDonald E, Mitchell I, Myburgh JA, Norton R, Potter J, Robinson BG, Ronco JJ: NICE-SUGAR Study Investigators: Intensive versus conventional glucose control in critically ill patients. *N Engl J Med* 360:1283–1297, 2009

87. Fort A, Narsinghani U, Bowyer F: Evaluating the safety and efficacy of Glucommander, a computer-based insulin infusion method, in management of diabetic ketoacidosis in children, and comparing its clinical performance with manually titrated insulin infusion. *J Pediatr Endocrinol Metab* 22:119–125, 2009

88. Hirsch IB: Intravenous bolus insulin delivery: implications for closed-loop control and hospital care. *Diabetes Technol Ther* 14:6–7, 2012

89. de Boer IH, Kestenbaum B, Rue TC, Steffes MW, Cleary PA, Molitch ME, Lachin JM, Weiss NS, Brunzell JD: Diabetes Control and Complications Trial (DCCT)/Epidemiology of Diabetes Interventions and Complications (EDIC) Study Research Group: Insulin therapy, hyperglycemia, and hypertension in type 1 diabetes mellitus. *Arch Intern Med* 168:1867–1873, 2008

90. Soedamah-Muthu SS, Colhoun HM, Abrahamian H, Chan NN, Mangili R, Reboldi GP, Fuller JH: the EURODIAB Prospective Complications Study Group: Trends in hypertension management in type 1 diabetes across Europe, 1989/1990–1997/1999. *Diabetologia* 45:1362–1371, 2002

91. Zgibor JC, Orchard TJ: Has control of hyperlipidemia and hypertension in patients with type 1 diabetes improved over time? *Diabetes* 50:1049, 2001

92. Laing SP, Swerdlow AJ, Slater SD, Botha JL, Burden AC, Waugh NR, Smith AW, Hill RD, Bingley PJ, Patterson CC, Qiao Z, Keen H: British Diabetic Association Cohort Study, II: Cause-specific mortality in patients with insulin-treated diabetes mellitus. *Diabet Med* 16:466–471, 1999

93. Adler AI, Stratton IM, Neil HA, Yudkin JS, Matthews DR, Cull CA, Wright AD, Turner RC, Holman RR: Association of systolic blood pressure with macrovascular and microvascular complications of type 2 diabetes (UKPDS 36): prospective observational study. *BMJ* 321:412–419, 2000

94. Hansson L, Zanchetti A, Carruthers SG, Dahlöf B, Elmfeldt D, Julius S, Ménard J, Rahn KH, Wedel H, Westerling S: Effects of intensive blood-pressure lowering and low dose aspirin in patients with hypertension: principal results of the Hypertension Optimal Treatment (HOT) randomized trial, HOT Study Group. *Lancet* 351:1755–1762, 1998

95. Heart Outcomes Prevention Evaluation Study Investigators: Effects of ramipril on cardiovascular and microvascular outcomes in people with diabetes mellitus: results of the HOPE study and MICRO-Hope substudy. *Lancet* 355:253–259, 2000

96. Dahlöf B, Devereux RB, Kjeldsen SE, Julius S, Beevers G, de Faire U, Fyhrquist F, Ibsen H, Kristiansson K, Lederballe-Pedersen O, Lindholm LH, Nieminen MS, Omvik P, Oparil S, Wedel H: LIFE Study Group: Cardiovascular morbidity and mortality in the Losartan Intervention for Endpoint reduction in hypertension study (LIFE): a randomized trial against atenolol. *Lancet* 359:995–1003, 2002

97. Whelton PK, Barzilay J, Cushman WC, Davis BR, Iiamathi E, Kostis JB, Leenen FH, Louis GT, Margolis KL, Mathis DE, Moloo J, Nwachuku C, Panebianco D, Parish DC, Pressel S, Simmons DL, Thadani U: ALLHAT collaborative Research Group: Clinical outcomes in antihypertensive treatment of type 2 diabetes, impaired fasting glucose concentration, and normoglycemia: antihypertensive and lipid-lowering treatment to prevent heart attack trail (ALLHAT). *Arch Intern Med* 165:1401–1409, 2005

98. Cooper-DeHoff RM, Gong Y, Handberg EM, Bavry AA, Denardo SJ, Bakris GL, Pepine CJ: Tight blood pressure control and cardiovascular outcomes among hypertensive patients with diabetes and coronary artery disease. *JAMA* 304:61–68, 2010

99. Cushman WC, Evans GW, Byington RP, Goff DC Jr, Grimm RH Jr, Cutler JA, Simons-Morton DG, Basile JN, Corson MA, Probstfield JL, Katz L, Peterson KA, Friedewald WT, Buse JB, Bigger JT, Gerstein HC, Ismail-Beigi F, ACCORD Study Group: Effects of intensive blood-pressure control in type 2 diabetes mellitus. *N Engl J Med* 362:1575–1585, 2010
100. ACEI Trialist Group (ACE Inhibitors in Diabetic Nephropathy Trialist Group): Should all patients with type 1 diabetes mellitus and microalbuminuria receive angiotensin-converting enzyme inhibitors? A meta-analysis of individual patient data. *Ann Intern Med* 134:370–379, 2001
101. Strippoli GF, Craig M, Deeks JJ, Schena FP, Craig JC: Effects of angiotensin converting enzyme inhibitors and angiotensin II receptor antagonists on mortality and renal outcomes in diabetic nephropathy: systematic review. *BMJ* 329:828, 2004
102. Cundy T, Slee F, Gamble G, Neale L: Hypertensive disorders of pregnancy in women with type 1 and type 2 diabetes. *Diabet Med* 19:482–489, 2002
103. Chobanian AV, Bakris GL, Black HR, Cushman WC, Green LA, Izzo JL Jr, Jones DW, Materson BJ, Oparil S, Wright JT Jr, Roccella EJ: Joint National Committee on Prevention, Detection, Evaluation, and Treatment of High Blood Pressure, National Heart, Lung, and Blood Institute, National High Blood Pressure Education Program Coordinating Committee: Seventh report of the Joint National Committee on Prevention, Detection, Evaluation, and treatment of high blood pressure. *Hypertension* 42:1206–1252, 2003
104. Watts GF, Karpe F: Triglycerides and atherogenic dyslipidaemia: extending treatment beyond statins in the high-risk cardiovascular patient. *Heart* 97:350–356, 2011
105. Kara C, Cetinkaya S, Sezgin N, Kinik ST: The effects of metabolic control on oxidized low-density lipoprotein antibodies in children and adolescents with type 1 diabetes mellitus. *Pediatr Diabetes* 9:17–22, 2008
106. Lopes-Virella MF, Baker NL, Hunt KJ, Lachin J, Nathan D, Virella G: DCCT/EDIC Research Group: Oxidized LDL immune complexes and coronary artery calcification in type 1 diabetes. *Atherosclerosis* 214:462–467, 2011
107. Lopes-Virella MF, Hunt KJ, Baker NL, Lachin J, Nathan DM, Virella G: Diabetes Control and Complications Trial/Epidemiology of Diabetes Interventions and Complications Research Group: Levels of oxidized LDL and advanced glycation end products-modified LDL in circulating immune complexes are strongly associated with increased levels of carotid intima-media thickness and its progression in type 1 diabetes. *Diabetes* 60:582–589, 2011
108. Jenkins AJ, Lyons TJ, Zheng D, Otvos JD, Lackland DT, McGee D, Garvey WT, Klein RL: Diabetes Control and Complications Trial/Epidemiology of Diabetes Interventions and Complications (DCCT/EDIC) Research Group: Lipoproteins in the DCCT/EDIC cohort: associations with diabetic nephropathy. *Kidney Internat* 64:817–828, 2003
109. Collins R, Armitage J, Parish S, Sleigh P, Peto R: Heart Protection Study Collaborative Group: MRC/BHF Heart Protection Study of cholesterol-lowering with simvastatin in 5963 people with diabetes: a randomized placebo-controlled trial. *Lancet* 361:2005–2016, 2003

110. Kearney PM, Blackwell L, Collins R, Keech A, Simes J, Peto R, Armitage J, Baigent C, Cholesterol Treatment Trialists' (CTT) Collaborators: Efficacy of cholesterol-lowering therapy in 18,686 people with diabetes in 14 randomised trials of statins: a meta-analysis. *Lancet* 371:117–125, 2008

111. National Cholesterol Education Program (NCEP) Expert Panel on Detection, Evaluation, and Treatment of High Blood Cholesterol in Adults (Adult Treatment Panel III): Third report of the National Cholesterol Education Program (NCEP) Expert Panel on Detection, Evaluation, and Treatment of High Blood Cholesterol in Adults (Adult Treatment Panel III) final report. *Circulation* 106:3143–3421, 2002

112. Available at http://www.nhlbi.nih.gov/guidelines/cholesterol/atp4/index .htm. Accessed 8 October 2012

113. Kitzmiller JL, Block JM, Brown FM, Catalano PM, Conway DL, Coustan DR, Gunderson EP, Herman WH, Hoffman LD, Inturrisi M, Jovanovic LB, Kjos SI, Knopp RH, Montoro MN, Ogata ES, Paramsothy P, Reader DM, Rosenn BM, Thomas AM, Kirkman MS: Managing preexisting diabetes for pregnancy: summary of evidence and consensus recommendations of care. *Diabetes Care* 31:1060–1079, 2008

114. Fodor JG, Frohlich JJ, Genest JJ Jr, McPherson PR: Working Group on Hypercholesterolemia and Other Dyslipidemias: Recommendations for the management of dyslipidemia and the prevention of cardiovascular disease: summary of the 2003 update. *CMAJ* 169:921–924, 2003

115. Brunzell JD, Davidson M, Furberg CD, Goldberg RB, Howard BV, Stein JH, Witztum JL, American Diabetes Association, American College of Cardiology Foundation: Lipoprotein management in patients with cardiometabolic risk: consensus statement from the American Diabetes Association and the American College of Cardiology Foundation. *Diabetes Care* 31:811–822, 2008

116. Kilpatrick ES, Rigby AS, Atkin SL: Insulin resistance, the metabolic syndrome, and complication risk in type 1 diabetes: "double diabetes" in the Diabetes Control and Complications Trial. *Diabetes Care* 30:707–712, 2007

117. de Boer IH, Sibley SD, Kestenbaum B, Sampson JN, Young B, Cleary PA, Steffes MW, Weiss NS, Brunzell JD: Diabetes Control and Complications Trial/Epidemiology of Diabetes Interventions and Complications Study Research Group: Central obesity, incident microalbuminuria, and change in creatinine clearance in the epidemiology of diabetes interventions and complications study. *J Am Soc Nephrol* 18:235–243, 2007

118. Palmer AJ, Roze S, Valentine WJ, Minshall ME, Lammert M, Nicklasson L, Spinas GA: Deleterious effects of increased body weight associated with intensive insulin therapy for type 1 diabetes: increased blood pressure and worsened lipid profile partially negate improvements in life expectancy. *Curr Med Res Opin* 20 (Suppl. 1):S67-S73, 2004

119. Chaturvedi N, Sjoelie AK, Porta M, Aldington SJ, Fuller JH, Songini M, Kohner EM: Markers of insulin resistance are strong risk factors for retinopathy incidence in type 1 diabetes. *Diabetes Care* 24:284–289, 2001

120. Chaturvedi N, Bandinelli S, Mangili R, Penno G, Rottiers RE, Fuller JH: Microalbuminuria in type 1 diabetes: rates, risk factors and glycemic threshold. *Kidney Int* 60:219–227, 2001

121. Brown BG, Zhao XQ, Chait A, Fisher LD, Cheung MC, Morse JS, Dowdy AA, Marino EK, Bolson EL, Alaupovic P, Frohlich J, Albers JJ: Simvastatin and niacin, antioxidant vitamins, or the combination for the prevention of coronary disease. *N Engl J Med* 345:1583–1592, 2001
122. AIM-HIGH Investigators: Niacin in patients with low HDL cholesterol levels receiving intensive statin therapy. *N Engl J Med* 365:2255–2267, 2011
123. Keech A, Simes RJ, Barter P, Best J, Scott R, Taskinen MR, Forder P, Pillai A, Davis T, Glasziou P, Drury P, Kesäniemi YA, Sullivan D, Hunt D, Colman P, d'Emden M, Whiting M, Ehnholm C, Laakso M: FIELD Study Investigators: Effects of long-term fenofibrate therapy on cardiovascular events in 9795 people with type 2 diabetes mellitus (the FIELD Study): randomized controlled trial. *Lancet* 366:1849–1861, 2005

7

Diabetes Self-Management Education

Martha M. Funnell, MS, RN, CDE, and Linda M. Siminerio, RN, PhD, CDE

INTRODUCTION

Type 1 diabetes (T1D) is largely a self-managed disease with as much as 99% of the daily care provided by the person who has it or, in the case of a child, the family. Diabetes self-management education (DSME) has long been thought of as a cornerstone of quality diabetes care. However, in recent years DSME has evolved from simply providing information to providing patients with the knowledge, skills, and abilities identified as necessary to effectively assume the daily self-management responsibilities for their own care.

EVIDENCE FOR DSME IN T1D

In spite of the significant self-management demands of T1D, there is very little information about how to best provide effective DSME and diabetes self-management support (DSMS) for this population, as recommended by the National Standards for Diabetes Self-Management Education and Support.[1] The majority of studies and meta-analyses about the effectiveness of DSME have been conducted among adults with type 2 diabetes (T2D).[2-8] Studies of DSME in T1D have largely been focused on assisting patients to intensify insulin therapy.

A review by Loveman and colleagues identified four studies of DSME in T1D as part of treatment intensification that resulted in improved metabolic control and fewer complications; however, only one of these, Terent et al., was a true test of an educational intervention.[9-13] All of these interventions were designed to educate participants about the metabolic processes and the relationship between eating, exercise, insulin doses, and blood glucose levels. The goal was to help participants self-adjust insulin doses based on variations in eating, activity, and glucose values. While the Diabetes Control and Complications Trial (DCCT) included education as a component of the intervention, the education provided was not predetermined or consistent across sites and was given primarily to assist individuals achieve the established A1C targets.[14]

More recently, based on 25 years of study, the Dose Adjustment for Normal Eating (DAFNE) program in the United Kingdom has reported clinically and statistically significant improvements in glycemic control without increased severe hypoglycemia, as well as improvements in quality of life and treatment satisfaction.[15] The DAFNE program is based on the earlier work by Muhlhauser

DOI: 10.2337/9781580404785ch07

et al., which used the Assal model of therapeutic education, which incorporates the physical, psychological, and behavioral aspects of care.[11,16] Within DAFNE, participants are taught to match their insulin doses to their food intake on a meal-by-meal basis. This program has been widely implemented elsewhere in Europe, Australia, and New Zealand.[17,18] A follow-up study of the DAFNE model implemented in routine clinical practice showed reduced A1C, reduced severe hypoglycemia, and improved well-being with reduced psychological distress.[19]

STANDARDS OF DSME AND T1D

The Standards of Medical Care in Diabetes recommend that people with diabetes receive DSME at the time of diagnosis and as needed thereafter.[20] The National Standards for DSME define diabetes self-management education as the on going process of facilitating the knowledge, skill, and ability necessary for diabetes self-care.[1] They further state that the process needs to incorporate the needs, goals, and life experiences of the person with diabetes and be guided by the evidence and standards of care. The overall objectives of DSME are to support informed decision making, self-care behaviors, problem solving, active collaboration with the health care team and to improve clinical outcomes, health status, and quality of life.[1] Based on the current evidence, the DSME Standards recommend that the education should emphasize practical, problem-solving skills, collaborative care, psychosocial issues, behavior change, and strategies to sustain self-management efforts.[1,21] The educational process begins with an assessment. Specific content areas that need to be assessed are identified in the DSME Standards (Table 7.1). Because most community-based group DSME programs are designed for people with T2D, DSME is usually provided individually for those with either newly diagnosed or long-standing T1D.

Children vs. Adults

It is important to acknowledge that the education and management of T1D in infants, toddlers, young children (≤6 years), youths, and adolescents differ vastly from that of adults. With infants and toddlers, parents or caregivers exclusively manage diabetes care. As the child develops, a gradual transition occurs with the youth performing more self-care. Over time, the youth still requires parental supervision, but less hands-on management. In adolescence, the patient performs most, if not all, of the daily care. As they age, individuals, once again, may need supervision and support. In this chapter, we will address best practices for DSME, initially focusing on children and then on the adult population.

PEDIATRICS

Introduction

Children and adolescents with T1D have unique care and educational requirements that need to be considered. Limited ability to provide self-care and growth and developmental issues are some of the distinct challenges associated with

Table 7.1 DSME Content Areas[1]

Describing the *diabetes disease process* and *treatment options*

Incorporating *nutritional management* into lifestyle

Incorporating *physical activity* into lifestyle

Using *medication(s)* safely and for maximum therapeutic effectiveness

Monitoring blood glucose and other parameters and interpreting and using the results for self-management decision making

Preventing, detecting, and treating *acute complications*

Preventing, detecting, and treating *chronic complications*

Developing personalized strategies to address psychosocial issues and concerns

Developing personalized strategies to promote health and behavior change

children and T1D. Therefore, we strongly recommend that an experienced, multidisciplinary team (diabetes educators, pediatric diabetologists, nurses, dietitians, and social workers or psychologists), with a strong understanding of childhood diabetes and the complexities in this young cohort, provide this comprehensive diabetes care and education.

Assessment

Since diabetes education and support set the stage for self-management and long-term health, it is important that the child's and family's educational needs be assessed routinely. A careful assessment that includes attention to learning styles and diabetes management needs, like schedules, activity, and eating habits, is an important first step. When performing an assessment, distress needs to be considered in both the child and parent. Attention to the child's psychosocial needs may be identified through social cues and interactions. Questions regarding friendships, school attendance, and participation in activities can provide insights into a child's acceptance of T1D. Parental distress and guilt also need to be considered when providing DSME to the family.[22] Children and parents should receive the emotional support needed to cope and not be bombarded with unrealistic expectations from a well-meaning diabetes treatment team. Children and parents should be encouraged to proceed with education and self-management at their own pace.

DSME

The initial diagnosis usually overwhelms children and their families. Therefore, delivering education must be balanced with empathy and support. Families need time to grieve the loss of a healthy child, to adjust, and to heal. While ongoing DSME may be provided at various time points and settings, the hospital setting can provide a safe place to begin. Historically, DSME was always provided at the time of hospitalization with initiation of insulin therapy. Now, unless the child presents in diabetic ketoacidosis (DKA), is metabolically unstable, or social circumstances are prohibitive, DSME is being provided in an outpatient setting in many pediatric diabetes centers.[23] For children, we recommend that DSME be provided at diagnosis. A comprehensive day-treatment program staffed by a multidisciplinary diabetes team is an effective alternative for those not hospitalized. Table 7.2 identifies specific content areas that are important at each stage of life.

Strategies for DSME. Since there is limited evidence about specific interventions and learning theories applied to pediatric DSME, it is important to tailor education to the age and developmental stage of the child and to include their parents (caregivers). For children, teaching strategies should focus on their maturity level and developmental stage.[24]

Providing education for the child with diabetes requires age-appropriate teaching methods and tools. Children are other directed, have had few life experiences, are subject centered, and have a delayed application of learning. Creative, innovative methods are needed to engage the child in the educational process. For example, picture drawing, role playing, stories, diabetes camps, computer programs, and support groups are effective diabetes education interventions.[24] Social media (e.g., Facebook and Twitter), open doors to educational venues and self-management support.

Psychosocial Stages of Development

Erik Erikson identified psychosocial life stages,[25] which can serve as a guide for specific themes that need to be addressed in DSME as the child moves through these developmental stages. Although the specific ages vary, the stages defined by Erikson are:

Infancy: Birth to 18 months: Trust vs. mistrust. This stage of infancy is referred to as the *oral sensory stage* (as anyone who watches a baby put everything in her mouth will appreciate) where the major emphasis is on the parent's positive and loving care for the child, with a big emphasis on visual contact and touch. Parents of babies with diabetes have an additional burden in communicating a sense of trust while doing necessary injections and blood glucose pricks. Parents have enormous guilt and performing the requisite testing can be difficult.[22,26]

At this earliest stage, the parent or caregiver is the only person who is able to manage diabetes care. Key issues during this stage include the child's inadequate verbal and cognitive abilities to convey hypoglycemic symptoms, difficulties of administering small insulin doses, and erratic eating and activities. Two important aspects of care that need to be discussed during education are *1)* sharing treatment responsibilities between parents/family members, and *2)* preventing and treating hypoglycemia.

Early childhood: 18 months to 3 years: Autonomy vs. shame. During this stage, the child has the opportunity to build self-esteem and autonomy as they gain more control over their bodies and acquire new skills, learning right from wrong. One of the skills during the terrible twos is the ability to use the powerful

Table 7.2 DSME Content Based on Life Stages (Children)

For the very young child, education will be directed to the adult caregivers. Adult learning theories and principles can be applied to the caregiver. When providing education to the adult caregiver, attention to specific content is necessary based on the child's developmental stage.

Infancy (Birth to 18 months)

Period of trust versus mistrust

Providing warmth and comfort measures after invasive procedures is important

Feeding and sleeping or nap routines

Vigilance for hypoglycemia

Need to support parents

Play age (3–5 years)

Reassurance that body is intact, use of band-aids, kisses after procedures

Identification of hypoglycemic signs & symptoms (temper tantrums & nightmares common)

Include child in choosing injection and finger prick sites

Positive reinforcement for cooperation

Begin process for teaching child awareness of hypoglycemia

School age (6–12 years)

Integrate child into educational experience

Determine skill level

Identify self-care skills

Determine roles and responsibilities

Who or when to tell peers and school staff

Adolescence (12–18 years)

Personal meaning of diabetes

Determine roles and responsibilities in care

Social situations and dating

Who or when to tell about diabetes

Driving

Sex and preconception counseling

Alcohol and drugs

College and career planning

6566669666666444444444

word "NO!" For parents of toddlers with diabetes, autonomy and terrible two behaviors can cause confusion when children are refusing food and injections or having a temper tantrum that can be masking hypoglycemia.

Toddlers are unable to understand why cooperating with an intrusive, painful procedure is required, causing blood glucose checks and insulin injections to become battlegrounds between the resisting toddler and the weary parent. Parents need to be told that providing comfort, warmth, and positive feedback to the very young child can help promote assurance and trust. Performing these invasive tasks can be a difficult assignment for parents and caregivers. Caregivers need to know that taking a well-deserved break from time to time and sharing the management tasks is important.[26]

Play age: 3 to 5 years: initiative vs. guilt. Although parents still are the primary contact and recipients of diabetes education during this period, the child experiences a desire to imitate adults and takes initiative in creating play situations. The preschooler begins to use the universal word for exploring the world: "WHY?" Conveying an abstract concept like diabetes, and the need for the associated care tasks, to a preschooler can be challenging. Play offers a unique opportunity to convey educational messages. Encouraging the youngster to inject a doll or stuffed animal can be very therapeutic.[26]

Children may begin to use cause-effect thinking. A young child may blame himself for having the disease or see the injections and restrictions as punishments. The child needs to be reassured that diabetes is not their fault, and caregivers should avoid using punitive language when referring to necessary diabetes management tasks. For example, avoid castigatory communications like "You better not eat the extra cookie or you'll need another shot." In addition, engaging the child in simple motor and cognitive skills enables the child to share in minor diabetes care tasks, such as choosing snacks and picking and cleaning an injection site.

Going to day care, nursery school, or kindergarten may represent the first time for separation and the social consequences of diabetes, including the need to educate others who will be responsible for care.[27]

School age: 6 to 12 years: industry vs. inferiority. During this stage, often called *latency*, the youngster is capable of learning, creating, and accomplishing numerous new skills and gaining new knowledge, thus developing a sense of industry. This is a very social stage of development. If the school-aged child experiences feelings of inadequacy and inferiority among peers, problems in terms of competence and self-esteem can appear. He may also wonder why he (and not someone else) has diabetes.

As the world expands for the child, the most significant relationship is with the school and community. Parents are no longer the complete authorities they once were, although they are still important. Engaging school-aged children in diabetes education is critically important as they begin to explore the world outside the care of their parents.

The goal for elementary school children is to engage them in diabetes care in a positive, empowering manner and not to impart premature or unrealistic expectations.[26] Parents and school staff remain the primary caregivers, with children playing a more active role (doing their own monitoring and injections, but with adult supervision as needed). It is important to emphasize parent-child teamwork.

Health care providers should begin to direct more education toward the child and begin to involve the child in the decision-making process.

As children begin to socialize and seek peer approval, adult caregivers need to foster a strong, positive self-image. Children with diabetes should be encouraged to participate in regular activities. The child's life should not adapt to diabetes; rather, diabetes management should accommodate the child's life.

Adolescence: 12 to 18 years: identity vs. role confusion. Adolescence is a stage at which the teen is neither a child nor an adult. Life becomes more complicated for the teen in an attempt to find identity, struggle with social interactions, and grapple with moral issues. The most significant relationships can be with peer groups. Adolescents with diabetes are notorious for having problems adjusting to the rigors of diabetes self-care. Major hormonal and body changes, psychosocial stresses, and challenges accompany the transition to adulthood. Peer pressures increase and teenagers naturally experiment with societal and personal issues and limits. Teen support groups, teen-only weekends, and camp programs can promote appropriate experimentation, education, and self-growth.

Early adolescence (12–15 years old) is characterized by changes in puberty, cognitive development, family dynamics, school experiences, and social networks. The tumultuous teenage years are compounded by challenges imposed by diabetes. Pubertal hormones increase insulin resistance and may wreak havoc on blood glucose levels. Teenagers become aware that their diabetes makes them different and may hide or ignore their diabetes from their peer groups. It is during this time that parents should begin to transfer responsibility for diabetes management to the adolescent. Both care providers and parents have been known to overestimate the adolescent's ability to manage their disease,[28] and it has been recommended that parents and teens begin shifting roles by sharing responsibilities.[29] Because of the social and psychological issues, parents and health care providers need to assess the teen's self-care abilities and the level of supervision required. To help the teen assume independence it is important to allow her to make decisions about her own care. Setting small goals and rewarding positive self-care behaviors are useful approaches in transitioning responsibility for care. Camps and weekend retreats with other youth with diabetes may provide the education, self-care, and support opportunities that are needed.[26]

Later adolescence (16–18 years old) is a stage when physical growth and development are usually complete and conflicts tend to decrease. Insulin requirements stabilize. However, families and health care providers must address the recurring issues of independence, responsibility, and teenage issues (drugs, alcohol, sexual intimacy, driving, etc.). Teenage girls should receive preconception and pregnancy counseling.[30]

Specific Pediatric Issues

Self-monitoring of blood glucose (SMBG) and insulin delivery. When training the child and parents on SMBG and injections, careful consideration should be made in regards to the children's developmental stage and psychosocial needs. For example, the parents of a very young child may have enormous guilt when pricking their child at a time when bonding and developing a sense of trust is paramount.

For a school-aged child, performing SMBG and administering insulin can lead them to feeling different from peers. SMBG and injections hold special challenges for the teen with diabetes where testing is bothersome. Management tasks can serve as a platform for rebellious behavior and challenge adherence[31] (see chapter 12).

Medical nutrition therapy (MNT) diet. MNT requires special approaches that attend to the eating nuances of the various developmental stages. For example, parents of the picky or belligerent toddler will need strategies to encourage the child to eat enough after insulin has been given, or alternatively inject insulin after a meal is consumed. Packing lunches for the school-aged child may be a necessity when school lunches don't meet the child's diabetes needs. Providing MNT for the growing adolescent may require weight management, snacking, and fast food choice strategies[31] (see chapter 10, Nutrition).

Exercise. Children with T1D should be encouraged to participate in physical activity. Education needs to focus on fitting activities into the diabetes regimen. With the benefits of exercise comes the risk of blood glucose swings. Education regarding monitoring, food intake, and hypoglycemia recognition are key[31] (refer to chapter 11).

Hypoglycemia management. Educating the child and family on hypoglycemia is highly age dependent. For example, for the very young child who cannot identify and express symptoms of low blood glucose, constant vigilance is necessary. Educating all of the individuals in contact with the young child about early symptoms of hypoglycemia is paramount. For the older child and adolescent, making sure that the child is aware of symptoms and can identify appropriate treatment, whether at school or while driving is critical. Since hypoglycemia presents one of the greatest immediate risks in children with T1D, education needs to be provided to a very broad audience[31] (refer to chapter 14, Hypoglycemia).

Sick-day education. This requires attention to essential elements that include guidelines on fluid intake, monitoring, the need for continued insulin administration, and, most importantly, when and whom to call for help. Sick days almost always require connection to the health care team and, at the very least, families and caretakers need contact numbers[31] (refer to chapter 5, Initial Evaluation and Follow-Up, and chapter 18.II, Schools).

ADULTS

Introduction

The number of adults with T1D, both newly diagnosed and those who have had diabetes since childhood, is increasing, and it is estimated that 85% of people currently living with T1D in the U.S. are adults.[32] As summarized by Heisler and Resnicow, patients need:

- sufficient knowledge and skills
- internal (autonomous) motivation
- confidence in their abilities (self-efficacy)
- effective coping[33]

In addition, because of both the changes in treatment and life circumstances that occur across the lifespan, DSME and ongoing DSMS must be ongoing processes throughout the life of the person with T1D so that self-management can be sustained.

Although the data are mixed about declines in cognitive function among adults with T1D, mental slowing has been noted in some studies. Among older adults with T1D, speed of information processing has been shown to be significantly poorer than among similarly aged nondiabetic adults.[34,35] Cognitive function therefore needs to be included in the educational assessment. Questions that can be used as part of the assessment process are listed in Table 7.3. Based on the assessment, a *personal education plan* is then developed in collaboration with the patient. The content areas delineated by the DSME standards provide an outline for developing the curriculum, however it is important that the content be tailored to match each individual's needs and adapted as necessary.[1,21] Each of these content areas also needs to be adapted for initial education, a comprehensive review, or ongoing education.

DSME can occur at the time of diagnosis or during a first clinical or educational visit as an adult for patients diagnosed as children or teens. Although those transitioning to adult care may have been taking insulin for many years, their information may be outdated, they may not have been formally educated, or they may have acquired habits that interfere with getting the most from their efforts. Education for both groups needs to focus on emotional and psychosocial issues and concerns, insulin administration and management, self-monitoring of blood glucose, hypo- and hyperglycemia, and nutrition. Further education is based on the educational assessment and the collaboratively developed education plan.

T1D may appear to occur out of the blue during a time of life when those affected expect to be healthy. Adults with T1D are twice as likely to be depressed as those without diabetes, and rates are even higher among those with complications (see chapter 9).[36] Diabetes-related distress is also common, with reported rates as high as one-third of young adults with T1D.[37,38] Providing information about mental health resources or a referral is important for patients with depression or for whom the emotional response to diabetes interferes with their self-management efforts.

Even when clinical depression is not present, patients with long-standing T1D may experience strong feelings about their illness and diabetes-related distress at different times during their lives, particularly if complications occur.[37,39,40] Although diabetes-related distress is linked to poorer glycemic control and emotional responses to diabetes significantly influence self-management behaviors, these issues are rarely addressed.[41,42] Both initial and continuing DSME and DSMS therefore need to include an assessment of emotional concerns and strategies to assist patients to cope with diabetes-related distress, which includes both the ongoing emotional impact of living with a chronic illness that can result in multiple complications and premature death, and the everyday anger, fear, guilt, and frustration that often accompany self-management efforts. Beginning each DSME or clinical visit by asking patients to identify their greatest concern or what is hardest for them helps to provide a meaningful focus for the visit. It is also important to keep in mind that A1C may not truly reflect the patient's struggles and good control does not mean that patients are coping well.

Table 7.3 Examples of Educational Assessment Questions[78]

What language do you prefer to speak? To read?

What is your favorite way to learn (e.g., reading, discussion, videos, computers, Internet, group class, individual teaching)?

Where do you get most information about health and diabetes?

Do you have difficulty with your hearing or vision, such as reading regular-size print?

How far did you go in school?

Do you have any cultural or religious practices or beliefs that affect how you care for your health and diabetes?

Do you ever have difficulty paying for your diabetes supplies or medicines?

Do you have trouble remembering things?

Have you ever known other people with type 1 or type 2 diabetes? How did it affect them?

Do you have health problems that you manage other than diabetes? What helps you to manage them?

Have you ever lost weight or increased your physical activity? What helped you to make those changes? What got in your way?

About what areas of diabetes are you most interested in learning?

What are you currently doing to manage your diabetes at home?

How much flexibility do you need in managing your diabetes?

How much do you want to be involved in planning your care?

On a scale of 1–10 with 10 being the most important, how important is managing diabetes in your life?

On a scale of 1–10 with 10 being the most confident, how confident do you feel that you can manage your diabetes?

How much stress are you experiencing in your life?

Have you felt sad and blue most of the time for the past two weeks? Two months?

Do you often feel overwhelmed by caring for your diabetes?

What kind of support do you want and need from you family and friends to care for your diabetes?

What kind of support do you receive from your family and friends to care for your diabetes?

Who helps you the most to care for your diabetes?

What is your greatest concern about your diabetes?

What is the hardest thing for you in caring for your diabetes? What is the easiest?

What were your thoughts or feelings when you first learned that you had diabetes? What are your thoughts or feelings now?

What is your preferred way to get support for managing diabetes (support group, reading, online groups, blogs)?

How can I be most helpful to you?

Strategies for DSME

The evidence about effective strategies for providing DSME for adults with T1D is extremely limited. While there is no one best program or approach, the evidence supports incorporating insulin dose self-adjustment and meal-planning strategies designed for maximum flexibility.[15] In addition, based primarily on studies among adults with T2D, DSME that incorporates psychosocial and behavioral strategies such as goal setting and are culturally and age appropriate can improve outcomes.[43–49]

In light of the limited evidence about specific interventions, adult learning theory and tailoring DSME to the age and life stage of the participant can be used to guide the development and implementation of DSME interventions for adults.

Adult learning theory. The field of adult learning was pioneered by Malcom Knowles.[50,51] He identified the characteristics of adult learners as:

- Autonomous and self-directed
- Based on a foundation of life experiences and knowledge
- Goal oriented
- Relevancy oriented
- Practical
- Desirous of respect

Based on these principles, DSME designed for adults with T1D should:

- Involve the patient in the development of the learning plan, including teaching strategies and learning goals
- Be based on patient experiences that are relevant to diabetes self-management
- Be applicable to the patient's goals and objectives
- Provide content that is personally relevant and useful
- Acknowledge the expertise of patient about their own lives, values, and goals

Based on learning theory (ALT), the educator needs to move from a teacher role to a facilitator role in order to promote learning through self-discovery. It is important to keep in mind that adults generally want to know what they want to know when they want to know it. They are usually not interested in learning about diabetes for its own sake, so the DSME content needs to relate to their lives, concerns, and experiences. As an example, a question often asked by adults newly diagnosed with T1D is "Why did I get diabetes?" While it is common to respond with an explanation of diabetes pathophysiology, they are usually more interested in understanding why it happened to *them* on a personal level and how it will affect their daily lives and future.[52]

Rather than focusing on the mechanics of diabetes, asking patients to identify their greatest fear about this new diagnosis helps to establish a relationship based on mutual respect. It also provides information that is relevant to managing the disease and guides the discussion toward the reality of living with T1D and the importance of their role in self-management.

DSME and DSMS programs based on questions asked by patients have been shown to be effective in T2D and are more consistent with ALT than providing a lecture or leading a discussion on an educator-determined topic.[53–55] Providing written materials or referring to resources that are specific for adults with T1D rather than to more generic diabetes materials is also in keeping with ALT. An example of using ALT in the development of T1D educational resources are tool kits developed for both newly diagnosed adults and those with long-standing T1D (www.jdrf.org/adults). These tool kits were written by both people with diabetes and health professionals, and focus first on topics of concern for adults, rather than on pathophysiology.

Currently 77% of the U.S. population uses the Internet (see http://www.internetworldstats.com/am/us.htm), and 80% of Internet users look online for health information (http://www.marketingcharts.com/direct/8-in-10-web-users-look-for-online-health-data-16107/). While the largest group of Internet users is in the age range of 18–44 years, the largest growth in Internet use is among those in the age range of 70–75 years, with almost half of that group currently online (http://pewresearch.org/pubs/1093/generations-online). In addition, the development and use of smart phone applications for health is also expanding (www.mobilehealthnews.com). Therefore, creating Internet or other electronic methods for DSME and DSMS is a reasonable and promising approach for adults with T1D, however there are no reported research findings of these programs developed and tested specifically for adults with T1D to date.[56]

Psychosocial life stages. While most of the focus on self-management education is on the management aspects, focusing on the self is just as important. As identified by Erikson, the psychosocial life stages can be used as a guide for DSME and DSMS.[25] Although the specific ages vary, the stages and questions asked by adults as defined by Erikson are:

- Young adulthood, ages 19–40 years old: *intimacy vs. isolation*, when the primary focus is on relationships. The main question that needs to be answered is "Shall I share my life with someone?"
- Middle adulthood, ages 40–60 years old: *generativity vs. stagnation*, when the primary focus is on children and work. The main question that needs to be answered is "Will I produce something of real value?"
- Maturity, ages 65 years old to–death: *ego-integrity vs. despair*, when the primary focus is looking back on life. The main question that needs to be answered is "Have I lived a full life?"

Because of the impact of T1D on the lives of people who have it, DSME needs to include content that reflects each of these stages and questions. Table 7.4 identifies specific content areas that are important at each stage of adulthood. It is important to keep in mind that some issues go across the life stages (e.g., clarifying the differences between T1D and T2D, which is often perceived as a childhood illness; roles and responsibilities in diabetes care) and for more than one life stage (e.g., safety issues when living alone for young adult singles and older adults who are widowed). In addition, there is variation among individuals within each stage. For example, the needs of a 22-year-old single person are different from those of a 35-year-old juggling parenthood and a career, just as the needs of a newly retired and otherwise healthy 66-year-old are different from those of an 80-year-old with multiple chronic illnesses. Thus, just as the treatment plan and education about the management aspects needs to be personalized

Table 7.4 DSME Content Based on Life Stages (Adults)

Young Adults

Personal meaning of diabetes

Roles and responsibilities in care

Social situations and dating

Who or when to tell about diabetes

Genetic risks, conception and preconception

Travel

Choosing or pursuing a career

Workplace rights

Health or life insurance

Involving friends and significant others in diabetes care

Safety

Creating a support network

Establishing or maintaining independence

Middle Adults

Personal meaning of diabetes

Roles and responsibilities in care

Involving spouse or significant other in care

Obtaining a support network

Travel

Pursing a career

Workplace rights

Health or life insurance

Talking with children or other family members about diabetes

Balancing other responsibilities with diabetes care

Safety

Facing complications

Older Adults

Personal meaning of diabetes

Roles and responsibilities in care

Maintaining independence

Obtaining assistance with diabetes care tasks

Involving spouse or significant other in care

Travel

(continued)

Table 7.4 DSME Content Based on Life Stages (Adults) (Continued)

Talking with adult children or other family members about diabetes

Safety

Caring for diabetes along with other chronic illnesses or comorbidities

Obtaining health care when living in multiple locations

Community resources

Care of T1D in long-term or other care facilities

for each patient, so does the education and support needed to incorporate diabetes into one's life.

The average life span of the person with diabetes is increasing.[57] While the majority of patients in nursing home settings currently have T2D, the number of T1D patients can be expected to increase as this larger population ages.[58] There are currently no guidelines for providing diabetes care and education in nursing homes for T1D patients. However, DSME may need to be provided to the staff in long-term care settings, with a focus on the differences in T1D and T2D and the importance of insulin administration and frequent monitoring.

Effective Approaches to Support Diabetes Self-management

Traditional views of DSME were based on providing knowledge in order to help patients be compliant or adherent to the recommendations made by health care professionals.[59] However, current approaches to DSME recognize the right and responsibility of adults to make informed decisions and set self-selected behavioral goals based on their priorities, values, and lives. The purpose of providing DSME within that context is to help patients make informed decisions and evaluate the costs and benefits of those choices and to help patients become effective self-managers.

Self-determination theory is a theoretical framework that can be used to develop and implement DSME and DSMS for adults with T1D.[59] Self-determination theory states that an individual is more likely to be motivated (autonomy motivation) to develop the skills and capacity to self-regulate the behaviors needed to function effectively, if that individual views those behaviors as personally meaningful.[60] In the context of diabetes care, autonomy motivation refers to the extent to which patients feel they are initiating and valuing specific diabetes self-management behaviors.[61,62] Autonomy support refers to the behaviors that professionals explicitly use to enhance motivation and self-directed behavior change. Strategies that are consistent with autonomy support are conveying empathy through active listening and using an open-ended, collaborative communication style.[59]

DSME approaches based on self-determination theory are particularly relevant for adults with T1D, who are often using intensive regimens. While this offers the best hope for a healthier future, it also increases the complexity and demands for self-management and behavior change.

Two approaches to facilitate self-management that can be used as part of the DSME and DSMS process that are consistent with self-determination theory and autonomy support are patient empowerment and motivational interviewing.

Patient empowerment. Patient empowerment is defined as helping patients discover and develop the inherent capacity to be responsible for one's own life.[63] Since initially proposed in diabetes, there has been a growing evidence of its effectiveness and recognition that, although health professionals are experts on diabetes care, patients are the experts on their own lives.[53,55,64–67] The principles that form the basis for patient empowerment are listed in Table 7.5. It is best understood as a philosophy rather than a technique.[63,68]

The communication strategy used within the empowerment approach is Ask, Listen, Empathize (ALE) which is a nondirective communication style based on active and reflective listening.[69] With this approach, the health professional asks questions to elicit the patient's concerns and emotions and barriers to treatment or self-management; listens to the patient's responses without offering opinions, judgments, or advice; and then empathizes and encourages further reflection and discussion. The goal is to help patients understand the issue so that they can then develop their own solutions and gain confidence (self-efficacy) as they carry them out.[69]

Motivational interviewing. Motivational interviewing (MI) is a process used to help patients build motivation and confidence to make the behavioral changes necessary for effective diabetes self-management that has shown some success in diabetes.[33,70–72] MI is a system of communication that is nondirective, nonjudgmental and empathetic, and there is no attempt to motivate or persuade

Table 7.5 Fundamental Principles of Patient Empowerment[68]

1. Patients provide 98% of their own diabetes care.

2. The greatest impact on the patient's health and well-being is a result of their self-management decisions/actions during the routine conduct of their daily life.

3. Diabetes is so woven into the fabric of the patient's life that many, if not most, of the routines of daily living affect and are affected by diabetes and its self-management.

4. Because patients are in control of their daily self-management decisions, they are responsible for those decisions and the resulting consequences.

5. Patients cannot surrender the control or responsibility they have for their diabetes self-management no matter how much they wish to do so. Even if patients turn their self-management completely over to a health care professional, they can change their mind about that decision at any time. Thus, they remain in control at all times.

6. Health care professionals cannot control and therefore cannot be responsible for the self-care decisions of their patients.

7. Health care professionals are responsible for doing all they can to ensure their patients are making informed self-management decisions, i.e., informed by an adequate understanding of diabetes self-management and an awareness of the aspects of their personal lives that influence their self-management decisions.

patients. Instead, *health professionals assist patients to determine their own internal motivation through active and reflective listening.* It is best understood as a system or process rather than a technique.[73] Extensive training is generally required to use MI effectively.

Self-directed goal setting. One of the most powerful strategies that providers can use to support behavior change is to create behavioral goals and action plans in collaboration with patients.[47,74] In keeping with autonomy motivation, goals chosen by patients are more likely to be attained. However, most patients will need to be taught how to set meaningful, measurable, and realistic goals as part of DSME. Table 7.6 outlines a 5-step process for goal setting developed as part of the empowerment approach.

When setting goals, teach patients to think of these as experiments rather than as absolutes that will result in a success or a failure. Begin the next visit or DSME session by asking patients about their experiment and what they learned as a result to set the agenda for the rest of the visit and for future goal setting.[65,69]

DSMS

While DSME is essential for behavior change, it is generally not adequate for patients to maintain the number of behaviors needed for effective diabetes self-management throughout their lives. The DSME standards recommend that a personalized follow-up plan for ongoing DSMS be developed collaboratively with each participant. DSMS is defined as activities to assist the individual with diabetes to implement and sustain the ongoing behaviors needed to manage

Table 7.6 5-Step Behavioral Goal Setting[65]

1. Identify the problem

   What is the most difficult or frustrating part of caring for your diabetes at this time? What makes this difficult for you?

2. Determine feelings and their influence on behavior

   What are your thoughts about this issue? How are your feelings influencing your behavior?

3. Set a long-term goal

   What do you want? What do you need to do? What problems to you expect to encounter? What support do you have to overcome these problems? Are you willing or able to take action to address this problem?

4. Make a plan for a behavioral step

   What will you do this week to get started working toward your goal? How important is this to you? How confident do you feel that you can do this step?

5. Assess how the experiment worked

   How did it work? What did you learn? What might you do differently next time?

their illness.[1] DSMS can include behavioral, educational, psychosocial, or clinical support.

DSMS can be provided in multiple formats. Unfortunately, the number of support groups for adults with T1D is often limited. Some patients can obtain the support that they need online or through blogs with others who are similar in age and concerns. Use of trained peers to provide ongoing support has been effective for patients with T2D, but has not been tested in T1D.[75–77] Assessing the preferred method of support will help the educator provide information about available and reliable resources.

FUTURE CLINICAL RESEARCH/FILLING THE GAPS

Very little is known about how to effectively provide DSME for individuals with T1D. This is particularly true for adults with both newly diagnosed and long-standing T1D, where most DSME is based on research among T2D patients. As the need for DSME for individuals with T1D increases, greater emphasis on this population of patients is essential in order to provide the best possible information and support. Specifically, additional research is needed to better understand:

- How to provide DSME for newly diagnosed children, adolescents and their families
- How to provide DSME and DSMS for newly diagnosed adults with T1D and for the person diagnosed as a child who is now receiving care in the adult setting
- How to provide behavioral and psychosocial support for children and adults with T1D
- How to provide ongoing DSMS for children and adults with T1D
- What setting and who is best suited to provide DSME and DSMS for these populations
- How to best use electronic, social media, and other methods of DSME and DSMS for these populations
- How self-determination theory and approaches such as empowerment, goal setting, problem solving, and motivational interviewing are most effectively used when providing DSME and DSMS for children and adolescents with T1D

CONCLUSION

Effective DSME acknowledges the patient's (whether a child or parent or an adult) role as a collaborator, decision maker, and expert on his or her own life and provides ongoing self-management support. DSME can help relieve the burden of diabetes care on practices by helping patients become informed, active participants in their own care. Patients make multiple decisions each day that directly affect their outcomes. They experience the consequences of their daily choices and self-care efforts. The key to closing the gap between the promise and reality of diabetes care is through the development of collaborative relationships and patient-centered practices that support patients' self-management efforts.

REFERENCES

1. Haas L, Maryniuk M, Beck J, et al., 2012 Standards Revision Task Force: National standards for diabetes self-management education and support. *Diabetes Care*. In press
2. Norris SL, Engelgau MM, Naranyan KMV: Effectiveness of self-management training in type 2 diabetes: a systematic review of randomized controlled trails. *Diabetes Care* 24:561–587, 2001
3. Norris SL, Lau J, Smith SJ, Schmid CH, Engelgau MM: Self-management education for adults with type 2 diabetes. *Diabetes Care* 25:1159–1171, 2002
4. Duncan I, Birkmeyer C, Coughlin S, Li QE, Sherr D, Boren S: Assessing the value of diabetes education. *Diabetes Educ* 35:752–760, 2009
5. Duncan I, Ahmed T, Li Q(E), Stetson B, Ruggerio L, Burton K, Rosenthal D, Fitzner K: Assessing the value of the diabetes educator. *Diabetes Educ* 37:638–658, 2011
6. Gary TL, Genkinger JM, Guallar E, Peyrot M, Brancati FL: Meta-analysis of randomized educational and behavioral interventions in type 2 diabetes. *Diabetes Educ* 28:488–501, 2003
7. Renders CM, Valk GD, Griffin SJ, Wagner EH, Eijk Van JT, Assendelft WJ: Interventions to improve the management of diabetes in primary care, outpatient, and community settings: a systematic review. *Diabetes Care* 24:1821–1833, 2001
8. Deakin T, McShane CE, Cade JE, Williams RD: Review: group based training for self-management strategies in people with type 2 diabetes mellitus. *Cochrane Database Syst Rev* CD003417, 2005
9. Loveman E, Cave C, Green C, Royle P, Dunn N, Waugh N: The clinical and cost-effectiveness of patient education models for diabetes: a systematic review and economic evaluation. *Health Technol Assess* 7:iii, 1–190, 2003
10. Mühlhauser I, Bruckner I, Berger M, et al.: Evaluation of an intensified insulin treatment and teaching programme as routine management of type 1 (insulin-dependent) diabetes. The Bucharest–Düsseldorf Study. *Diabetologia* 30:681–690, 1987
11. Reichard P, Britz A, Cars I, Nilsson BY, Sobocinsky-Olsson B, Rosenqvist U: The Stockholm Diabetes Intervention Study (SDIS): 18 months' results. *Acta Med Scand* 224:115–122, 1988
12. Starostina EG, Antsiferov M, Galstyan GR, et al.: Effectiveness and cost–benefit analysis of intensive treatment and teaching programmes for type 1 (insulin-dependent) diabetes mellitus in Moscow: blood glucose versus urine glucose self-monitoring. *Diabetologia* 37:170–176, 1994
13. Terent A, Hagfall O, Cederholm U: The effect of education and self-monitoring of blood glucose on glycosylated hemoglobin in type I diabetes: a controlled 18-month trial in a representative population. *Acta Med Scand* 217:47–53, 1985
14. DCCT Research Group: The effect of intensive treatment of diabetes on the development and progression of long-term complications in insulin-dependent diabetes mellitus. *N Engl J Med* 329:977–986, 1993
15. DAFNE Study Group: Training in flexible, intensive insulin management to enable dietary freedom in people with type 1 diabetes: the dose adjustment for normal eating (DAFNE) randomised controlled trial. *BMJ* 325:746–749, 2002

16. Assal JP, Mühlhauser I, Pernet A, Gfeller R., Jörgens V, Berger M: Patient education as the basis for diabetes care in clinical practice and research. *Diabetologia* 28:602–613,1985
17. Pieber TR, Brunner GA, Schnedl WJ, Schattenberg S, Kaufmann P, Krejs GJ: Evaluation of a structured outpatient group education program for intensive insulin therapy. *Diabetes Care* 18:625–630, 1995
18. Plank J, Köhler G, Rakovac I, et al.: Long-term evaluation of a structured outpatient education programme for intensified insulin therapy in patients with type 1 diabetes: a 12 year follow-up. *Diabetologia* 47:1370–1375, 2004
19. Hopkins D, Lawrence I, Mansell P, et al.: Improved biomedical and psychological outcomes 1 year after structured education in flexible insulin therapy for people with type 1 diabetes: the U.K. DAFNE experience. *Diabetes Care* 35:1638–1642, 2012
20. American Diabetes Association: Standards of medical care in diabetes: 2012. *Diabetes Care* 35 (Suppl. 1):S11–S63, 2012
21. Glazier RH, Bajcar J, Kennie NR, Willson K: A systematic review of interventions to improve diabetes care in socially disadvantaged populations. *Diabetes Care* 26:1675–1688, 2006
22. Betschart J: Parents' understanding of and guilt over their children's blood glucose control. *Diabetes Educ* 13:398–401, 1987
23. Charron-Prochownik D, Maihle T, Siminerio L, Songer T: Outpatient vs. inpatient care of children newly diagnosed with IDDM. *Diabetes Care* 20:657–660, 1997
24. Siminerio L, Charron-Prochownik D, Banion C, Schreiner B. Comparing outpatient and inpatient diabetes education for newly diagnosed pediatric patients. *Diabetes Edu* 25:895–906, 1999
25. Erikson EH: *Identity and the Lifecycle.* New York, W.H. Norton, 1994
26. Siminerio L (Ed.), McLaughlin S, and Polonsky W (Contributing Ed.): *American Diabetes Association Diabetes Education Goals.* 3rd ed. Alexandria, VA American Diabetes Association, 2002.
27. Betschart-Roemer J: *American Diabetes Association Guide to Raising a Child with Diabetes.* 3rd ed. Alexandria, VA, American Diabetes Association, 2011
28. Wysocki T, Mcinhold P, Abrams K, et al.: Parental and professional estimates of self-care independence of children and adolescents with IDDM. *Diabetes Care* 15:40–52, 1992
29. Anderson BJ, Auslander WF, Jung KC, Miller JP, Santiago JV: Assessing family sharing of diabetes responsibilities. *J Pediatr* 4:477–492, 1990
30. Charron-Prochownik: Evidence-based clinical decision making: a framework to guide clinical practice (exemplar: preconception counseling). *Diabetes Spectrum* 20:69–70, 2007
31. Siminerio L, Betschart J. *Raising a Child with Diabetes.* 5th ed. Alexandria, VA, American Diabetes Association, 1995
32. JDRF: Type 1 diabetes, 2010. Prime Group for JDRF, Mar. 2011
33. Heisler M, Resnicow K: Helping patients make and sustain health changes: a brief introduction to motivational interviewing. *Clin Diabetes* 26:161–165, 2008
34. Brands AMA, Biessels G-J, De Haan EHF, Kappelle LJ, Kessels RPC: The effects of type 1 diabetes on cognitive performance: a meta-analysis. *Diabetes Care* 28:726–735, 2005

35. Brands AMA, Kessels RPC, Biessels G-J, et al.: Cognitive performance, psychological well-being, and brain magnetic resonance imaging in older patients with type 1 diabetes. *Diabetes* 55:1800–1806, 2006
36. Gendelman N, Snell-Bergeon JK, McFann K, et al.: Prevalence and correlates of depression in individuals with and without type 1 diabetes. *Diabetes Care* 32:575–579, 2009
37. Lloyd CE, Pambianco G, Orchard TJ: Does diabetes-related distress explain the presence of depressive symptoms and/or poor self-care in individuals with type 1 diabetes? *Diabetic Med* 27:234–237, 2010
38. Hislop AL, Fegan PG, Schlaeppi MJ, Duck M, Yeap BB: Prevalence and associations of psychological distress in young adults with type 1 diabetes. *Diabetic Medicine* 25:91–96, 2008
39. Polonsky, WH, Anderson, BJ, Lohrer, PA, et al.: Assessment of diabetes-related distress. *Diabetes Care* 18:754–760, 1995
40. Polonsky WH, Fisher L, Earles J, et al.: Assessing psychosocial distress in diabetes. *Diabetes Care* 28:626–631, 2005
41. Peyrot M, Rubin RR, Lauritzen T, Snoek FJ, Matthews DR, Skovlund SE: Psychosocial problems and barriers to improved diabetes management: results of the cross-national Diabetes Attitudes, Wishes and Needs study. *Diabetic Med* 22:1379–1385, 2005
42. Skovlund SE, Peyrot M, DAWN International Advisory Panel: Lifestyle and behavior: the diabetes attitudes, wishes and needs [DAWN] program: a new approach to improving outcomes of diabetes care. *Diabetes Spectrum* 18:136–142, 2005
43. Roter DL, Hall JA, Merisca R, Nordstrom B, Cretin D, Svarstad B: Effectiveness of interventions to improve patient compliance: a meta-analysis. *Med Care* 36:1138-1161, 1998
44. Barlow J, Wright C, Sheasby J, et al: Self-management approaches for people with chronic conditions: a review. *Patient Education and Counseling* 48:177–187, 2002
45. Skinner TC, Cradock S, Arundel F, Graham W: Lifestyle and behavior: four theories and a philosophy: self-management education for individuals newly diagnosed with type 2 diabetes. *Diabetes Spectrum* 16:75–80, 2003
46. Sarkisian CA, Brown AF, Norris CK, Wintz RL, Mangione CM: A systematic review of diabetes self-care interventions for older, African American or Latino adults. *Diabetes Educ* 28:467–479, 2003
47. Bodenheimer T, MacGregor K, Sharifi C: *Helping Patients Manage Their Chronic Conditions.* Oakland, CA, California Healthcare Foundation, 2005
48. Chodosh J, Morton SC, Mojica W, et al.: Meta-analysis: chronic disease self-management programs for older adults. *Ann Intern Med* 143:427–438, 2005
49. Winkely K, Landau S, Eisler I, Ismail K: Psychological interventions to improve glyceaemic control in patients with type 1 diabetes: systematic review and meta-analysis of randomized controlled trials. *Brit Med J* 333:65, 2006
50. Knowles M: *The Modern Practice of Adult Education, from Pedagogy to Andragogy.* Englewood Cliffs, NJ, Prentice Hall, 1980
51. Knowles M: *The Adult Learner: A Neglected Species.* 4 ed. Houston, TX, Gulf Publishing, 1990

52. Weiss MA, Funnell MM: In the beginning: setting the stage for effective diabetes care. *Clin Diabetes* 27:149–151, 2009
53. Anderson RM, Funnell MM, Nwankwo R, Gillard ML, Oh M, Fitzgerald JT: Evaluating a problem-based empowerment program for African Americans with diabetes: results of a randomized controlled trial. *Ethnicity and Disease* 15:671–678, 2005
54. Funnell MM, Nwankwo R, Gillard ML, Anderson RM, Tang TS: Implementing an empowerment-based diabetes self-management education program. *Diabetes Educ* 31:53–61, 2005
55. Tang TS, Funnell MM, Brown MB, Kurlander JE: Self-management support in "real-world" settings: an empowerment-based intervention. *Patient Educ Couns* 79:176–184, 2010
56. Piette JD: Interactive behavior change technology to support diabetes self-management. *Diabetes Care* 30:2425–2432, 2007
57. Secrest AM, Becker DJ, Kelsey SF, LaPorte RE, Orchard TJ: All-cause mortality trends in a large population-based cohort with long-standing childhood-onset type 1 diabetes: the Allegheny County type 1 diabetes registry. *Diabetes Care* 33:2573–2579, 2010
58. Resnick HE, Heineman J, Stone R, Shorr RI: Diabetes in Nursing Homes: United States 2004. *Diabetes Care* 31:287–288, 2008
59. Anderson B, Funnell MM: Theoretical and behavioral approaches to self-management of health. In *The Art and Science of Diabetes Self-Management Education*. 2nd ed. Mensing C, Ed. Chicago, American Association of Diabetes Educators, 2011, p. 71–94
60. Deci EL, Eghrari H, Patrick BC, Leone DR: Facilitating internalization: the self-determination theory perspective. *J Pers* 62:119–142, 1994
61. Williams GC, Grow VM, Freedman Z, Ryan RM, Deci EL: Motivational predictors of weight loss and weight loss maintenance. *J Pers Soc Psychol* 70:115–126, 1996
62. Williams GC, Ryan RM, Rodin GC, Grolnick WS, Deci EL: Autonomous regulation and long-term medication adherence in adult outpatients. *Health Psychol* 17:269–276, 1998
63. Funnell, MM, Anderson, RM, Arnold MS, et al.: Empowerment: an idea whose time has come in diabetes education. *Diabetes Educ* 17:37–41, 1991
64. Anderson RM, Funnell MM, Butler PM, Arnold MS, Feste CC. Patient empowerment: results of a randomized controlled trial. *Diabetes Care* 18:943–949, 1995
65. Funnell MM, Anderson RM: Empowerment and self-management education. *Clin Diabetes* 22:123–127, 2004a
66. Anderson RM, Funnell MM, Aikens JE, et al.: Evaluating the efficacy of an empowerment-based self-management consultant intervention: results of a two-year randomized controlled trial. *Ther Patient Educ* 1:3–11, 2009
67. Funnell MM, Anderson RM: Patient empowerment: a look back, a look ahead. *Diabetes Educ* 29:454–462, 2003
68. Anderson RM, Funnell MM: Patient empowerment: myths and misconceptions. *Patient Educ Couns* 79:277–282, 2010

69. Funnell MM, Anderson RM: Behavior change strategies. In *Medical Management of Type 2 Diabetes*. 5th ed. CF Burant, Ed. Alexandria, VA, American Diabetes Association, 2004b, 124–129
70. Rubak S, Sandboek A, Lauritzen T, Christensen B: Motivational interviewing: a systematic review and meta-analysis. *Brit J Gen Pract* 55:305–312, 2005
71. Ismail K, Maissi E, Thomas S, et al.: A randomised controlled trial of cognitive behaviour therapy and motivational interviewing for people with type 1 diabetes mellitus with persistent sub-optimal glycaemiccontrol: A Diabetes and Psychological Therapies (ADaPT) study. *Health Technol Assess* 14(22):1–101, 2010
72. Martins RK, McNeil DW: Review of motivational interviewing in promoting health behaviors. *Clin Psychol Rev* 29:283–293, 2009
73. Miller WR, Rollnick S: Ten things motivational interviewing is not. *Behav Cogn Psychoth* 37:129–140, 2009
74. Bodenheimer T, Davis C, Holman H: Helping patients adopt healthier behaviors. *Clin Diabetes* 25:66–70, 2007
75. Tang TD, Ayala GX, Cherrington A, Rana G: A review of volunteer-based peer support interventions in diabetes. *Diabetes Spectrum* 24:85–98, 2011
76. Heisler M, Vijan S, Makki F, Piette JD: Diabetes control with reciprocal peer support versus nurse care management. *Ann Intern Med* 153:507–515, 2010
77. Funnell, MM: Peer-based behavioural strategies to improve chronic disease self-management and clinical outcomes: evidence, logistics, evaluation considerations and needs for future research. *Fam Pract* 27 (Suppl. 1):17–22, 2010
78. Funnell MM, Mensing CR: Education in the management of diabetes. In *Textbook of Nursing Care for Diabetes*. 2nd ed. Childs BP, Cypress M, Spollett G, Eds. Alexandria, VA, American Diabetes Association, 2010

8

Psychosocial Issues in Type 1 Diabetes
I. Psychosocial Assessment

Barbara J. Anderson, PhD

INTRODUCTION

In this section, we will discuss the importance of psychosocial assessments and provide examples of diabetes-specific tools to help health care providers better support their patients in managing type 1 diabetes (T1D). We will focus only on practical diabetes-specific psychosocial assessments that are most useful for providers treating youth or adults with T1D. We will discuss when to refer to mental health specialists and how the diabetes provider may best partner with mental health professionals in managing the complex psychosocial issues associated with T1D.

This section will *not* provide an exhaustive discussion of all diabetes-specific psychosocial measures. Assessment of depression and eating disorders is covered in later sections of this chapter. In addition, our review will not include the following measures of the following diabetes-specific domains: diabetes knowledge, diabetes treatment adherence, or diabetes-related cognitive functions such as health literacy and health numeracy skills.

In the two major parts of this section, we will discuss diabetes-specific psychosocial assessments for children and then for adults. In both the pediatric and adult sections, we will include what the American Diabetes Association (ADA) as well as other major diabetes organizations state about the role of psychosocial assessment in T1D. The final part of each section will summarize the current state of psychosocial assessments in T1D and suggest future directions for clinical research in this area to move toward more widespread clinical psychosocial assessments of individuals with T1D. Before discussing formal pediatric and adult psychosocial assessment instruments, we will overview several important psychosocial dimensions that apply to both children and adults with T1D and that are important for providers to assess informally during dialogue with the patient and family.

Significant Psychosocial Issues of Children/Adolescents and Adults with T1D for Clinicians to Assess Informally

At diagnosis. The diagnosis of T1D is a period of crisis for most children, adults, and their families. Patients and family members face two complex and often conflicting tasks: *1)* to begin grieving the loss of health and a spontaneous lifestyle, and *2)* to begin to learn the complex new language and set of skills involved in

DOI: 10.2337/9781580404785ch08s1

managing T1D. The diagnosis of a serious chronic illness like T1D can trigger strong emotions as well as stir up existing emotional issues. Therefore, it is important to consider patients carefully at diagnosis with respect to the following:

- *Patient's developmental stage*: What are the normal developmental tasks for a person of this age?
- *Mental health history of patient and family members:* What current and past mental health diagnoses, especially depression, anxiety disorders, and learning problems have the patient or family members experienced? Has the patient recently (within the past 2 years) had mental health treatment?
- *Current life stresses that are potential psychosocial barriers to effective management of T1D:* Are patient or family currently experiencing financial problems; other health or mental health problems; health insurance or health care access problems; educational or learning problems; a recent move, change of schools or job; or stresses in job, marriage, or family relationships?
- *Emotional responses to diagnosis:* It is important for providers to understand that patients and family members normally experience a wide range of emotions at diagnosis and in the following 3–6 months. Some of these normal emotional responses at diagnosis are: sadness, anxiety, denial, guilt, and blame.

After diagnosis. It is important for the provider periodically to ask the person with diabetes about any sources of diabetes-related distress. There is mounting evidence that at all stages of life, patients and families living with diabetes experience diabetes-related distress that interferes with diabetes management and blood glucose control. Diabetes-related distress is the primary potentially modifiable variable that the provider can address with the patient. Diabetes-related distress in patients can include such feelings as:

- Feelings of deprivation regarding food and meals
- Feeling burned out by the constant effort needed to manage diabetes[1]

In parents and other family members, diabetes-related distress can include feelings such as:

- I feel upset when my child's diabetes management is off track.
- I feel upset when my child's blood sugars are out of range.[2]

There are several formal diabetes-related distress assessment instruments that will be discussed in the following pediatric and adult sections.

PSYCHOSOCIAL ASSESSMENT OF CHILDREN, ADOLESCENTS, AND YOUNG ADULTS

Introduction

It is important for providers to understand the age-appropriate developmental tasks for the child and the family's role in diabetes management at each developmental stage.

Table 8.I.1 Major Developmental Issues and Their Effect on Diabetes in Children and Adolescents[3]

Developmental Stage (approximate ages)	Normal Developmental Tasks	T1D Management Priorities	Family Issues in T1D Management
Infancy (0–12 months)	Developing a trusting relationship/ bonding with primary caregiver(s)	Preventing and treating hypoglycemia	Coping with stress
		Avoiding extreme fluctuations in blood glucose levels	Sharing the burden of care to avoid parent burnout
Toddler (13–36 months)	Developing a sense of mastery and autonomy	Preventing and treating hypoglycemia	Establishing a schedule
		Avoiding extreme fluctuations in blood glucose levels due to irregular food intake	Managing the picky eater Setting limits and coping with toddler's lack of cooperation with regimen Sharing the burden of care
Preschooler and early elementary school age (3–7 years)	Developing initiative in activities and confidence in self	Preventing and treating hypoglycemia	Reassuring child that diabetes is no one's fault
		Unpredictable appetite and activity	Educating other caregivers about diabetes management
		Positive reinforcement for cooperation with regimen	
		Trusting other caregivers with diabetes management	
Older elementary school age (8–11 years)	Developing skills in athletic, cognitive, artistic, social areas	Making diabetes regimen flexible to allow for participation in school/peer activities	Maintaining parental involvement in insulin and blood glucose monitoring tasks while allowing for independent self-care for special occasions

(Continued)

Table 8.I.1 Major Developmental Issues and Their Effect on Diabetes in Children and Adolescents[3] (Continued)

Developmental Stage (approximate ages)	Normal Developmental Tasks	T1D Management Priorities	Family Issues in T1D Management
	Consolidating self-esteem with respect to the peer group	Child learning short- and long-term benefits of optimal control	Continue to educate school and other caregivers
Early adolescence (12–15 years)	Managing body changes	Managing increased insulin requirements during puberty	Renegotiating parents' and teen's roles in diabetes management to be acceptable to both
	Developing a strong sense of self-identity	Diabetes management and blood glucose control become more difficult	Learning coping skills to enhance ability to self-manage
		Weight and body image concerns	Preventing and intervening with diabetes-related family conflict
			Monitoring for signs of depression, eating disorders, risky behaviors
Later adolescence (16–19 years)	Establishing a sense of identity after high school (decision about location, social issues, work, education)	Begin discussion of transition to a new diabetes team	Supporting the transition to independence
		Integrating diabetes into new lifestyle	Learning coping skills to enhance ability to self-manage
			Preventing and intervening with diabetes-related family conflict
			Monitoring for signs of depression, eating disorders, risky behaviors

Table 8.I.1 provides an overview of normal developmental tasks as well as diabetes priorities and challenges facing families across developmental stages. For infants and toddlers, the patient is the parent. As the child becomes school-aged, the parent continues as the primary manager of the child's diabetes, with the child taking on some roles in decision making such as which finger to poke for the blood glucose check or what mid-morning snack to have at school. In addition, the parent has to continually educate school personnel about diabetes management in order to keep the child safe at school. As the child enters puberty and adolescence the parents must learn to work with their teenager in managing diabetes. There is much empirical evidence that across adolescence, developmentally appropriate parental involvement in, and low family conflict around, diabetes management is critical for positive health outcomes.

Neither the child nor the parent must be blamed for elevated blood glucose level or a higher A1C at the clinic visit. It is imperative that the provider explore with the child and parent possible barriers to acceptable blood glucose control in the child's or family's life, at home or at school. This informal psychosocial assessment will give the provider clues as to any changes in the management plan that might make diabetes care fit more easily into the child's or family's daily schedule. Also, by engaging the family in this type of problem-solving conversation, the clinician will help to build a more collaborative relationship with the child and family.

Diabetes-Related Distress in Pediatric T1D

Diabetes-related distress is common in patients and their family members living with T1D. Importantly, diabetes-related distress is one barrier to optimal disease management that the clinician can identify and work with the patient and family to improve. Several recent diabetes-related distress measures have been validated for pediatric T1D populations. First, Weissberg-Benchell and colleagues developed and validated a measure of diabetes-specific emotional distress experienced by adolescents with T1D.[4] This survey was based on the widely used Problem Area in Diabetes (PAID) measure of diabetes-specific emotional distress in adults with T1D.[1] Weissberg-Benchell and colleagues established the feasibility, reliability, and validity of the Problem Areas in Diabetes–Teen version (PAID-T).[4] This 26-item survey "is brief and easy to administer as a routine screening tool at clinic visits to identify potential problem areas and sources of distress for adolescents. Responses could be quickly viewed by the clinician and discussed directly during the clinic appointment."[4] Second, Markowitz and colleagues at the Joslin Diabetes Center in Boston designed and validated a measure of perceived parental burden associated with caring for a child with diabetes in the current era of intensive insulin therapy.[2] The Problem Areas in Diabetes Survey–Parent Revised version (PAID-PR) is an 18-item parent-report survey with excellent psychometric characteristic. It requires only 5–10 min for the parent to complete, and thus it is feasible to use in a busy diabetes clinic.

STANDARDS OF CARE

National (ADA) and international (International Society for Pediatric and Adolescent Diabetes [ISPAD]) standards of care for children and adolescents with T1D have specific recommendations concerning psychosocial assessment of youth and families living with T1D.[3,5]

ADA recommendations state:

- Ideally, every child newly diagnosed with T1D should be evaluated by a diabetes care team (consisting of a pediatric endocrinologist, a nurse educator, a dietitian, and a mental health professional) qualified to provide up-to-date pediatric-specific education and support.
- It is important to assess both the risk factors and the strengths of the child and family at the time of diagnosis, with the hope of intervening before child and family behavior patterns become firmly established.
- With respect to the initial diabetes visit, a behavioral specialist should be part of the initial team education or referral as needed optimally for evaluation and counseling of a patient and family at diagnosis, then as indicated to enhance support and empowerment to maintain family involvement in diabetes care tasks and to identify and discuss ways to overcome barriers to successful diabetes management.... Depression screening annually for children 10 years of age and older, with referral as indicated.[3]

With respect to adjustment in adolescents with T1D, the ADA Standards of Care recommends:

- Psychiatric illness is a serious complication of diabetes and is often associated with poor metabolic control and adaptation. Thus, regular screening for psychiatric disorders in adolescents with diabetes is warranted.... Routine screening of psychosocial functioning, especially depression and family coping, should be performed. Youth with positive screening should be referred promptly for treatment.
- Adolescent risk behaviors [i.e., "tobacco and recreational drugs and unprotected sexual intercourse"] should be routinely assessed by the diabetes team and counseling provided.[3]

ISPAD Guidelines

The 2009 Consensus Guidelines of the International Society for Pediatric and Adolescent Diabetes provide recommendations concerning psychosocial assessment of children and families living with T1D.[6] The recommendations of this 2009 document build on guidelines by the ADA as well as pediatric diabetes organizations in Australia, Canada, and the United Kingdom. ISPAD recommendations concerning psychosocial assessment include:

- Assessment of developmental progress in all domains of quality of life (physical, intellectual, academic, emotional, and social development) should be conducted on a routine basis.
- Quality of life can be reliably measured with good clinical utility.
- Routine assessment should be made of developmental adjustment to and understanding of diabetes management.
- Identification of psychosocial adjustment problems, depression, eating disorders, and other psychiatric disorders should be conducted at planned intervals by mental health professionals.

- Assessment of general family functioning (conflict, cohesion, adaptability, parental psychopathology) and diabetes-related functioning (communication, parental involvement and support, roles and responsibilities for self-care behaviors) especially when there is evidence of cultural, language or family problems.[6]

REFERRAL TO MENTAL HEALTH SPECIALISTS

Pediatric providers need to understand the value of psychosocial assessments and the appropriate screening questions and know when to refer to mental health providers specializing in diabetes management. At each clinic visit, providers should discuss all aspects of developmental progress (i.e., physical, intellectual, academic, emotional, and social development). For example, if a child has continued or new issues with adherence, develops complications, has a disruptive home environment, or new onset academic difficulties, providers should probe further, with prompt referral to mental health professionals, if indicated. Sociodemographic factors such as single parenthood, lower income and ethnic minority status are associated with greater risk for poor diabetes control.[6]

TRANSITIONING INTO YOUNG ADULTHOOD

For many young adults with T1D, the transition from adolescence into young adulthood, a period of development called *emerging adulthood* including ages 18–30 years, may be very challenging.[7] The physiological and psychosocial changes often result in deterioration in adherence. First, the older adolescent is often moving into a different life stage, whether college or work, isolated from both a familiar environment and a supportive family structure. This newfound independence and environment may lead to poor decision making. Second, transition from a known pediatric care team to an unknown adult health care team potentially requires the patient to relearn diabetes management. This may overwhelm the young adult who is undergoing multiple transitions developmentally. Third, issues with health insurance can pose barriers to accessing health care and diabetes medications and supplies. Given the above factors, this vulnerable population is at high risk for loss to follow-up care and poor psychosocial and health outcomes.

The ADA recently published a position statement, "Diabetes Care for Emerging Adult: Recommendations for Transition from Pediatric to Adult Diabetes Care Systems."[8] With respect to psychosocial assessment, this document recommends:

- Recognizing that trajectories of depressive symptoms worsen and impact physical and psychosocial well-being as older teens transition into young adulthood, it is important to monitor and refer older adolescents and young adults with T1D or T2D to appropriate mental health resources.
- In summary, eating disorders and affective disorders are especially serious in emerging adults who have diabetes because insulin omission, depression, anxiety, and fear of hypoglycemia interfere with diabetes self-care

behavior during a time when these patients may have fallen between the cracks of the pediatric and adult health care systems. … Clinicians who care for emerging adults with T1D need to evaluate the mental as well as the physical health history of their new patients and foster access to mental health providers for consultation and collaborative care for the diagnosis and treatment of eating disorders, depression, anxiety and fear of hypoglycemia.[8]

This statement highlights the types of diabetes-related distress that can be experienced by emerging adults with T1D:

Psychosocial challenges are common during emerging adulthood, occur more often in those with diabetes compared to those without diabetes, and occur more commonly during emerging adulthood than during other stages of life. Living with diabetes often brings with it a broad range of diabetes-related distresses. Diabetes-specific stressors that occur frequently and interfere with effective self-care include not having clear and concrete goals for diabetes care; feeling discouraged and overwhelmed with the diabetes regimen; uncomfortable interactions concerning diabetes with family, friends, or coworkers who do not have diabetes; feelings of guilt or anxiety about getting off track with diabetes self-care; and worrying about the future and the possibility of serious complications.[8]

RECOMMENDED CHANGES TO GUIDELINES

All pediatric diabetes care guidelines recommend psychosocial screening at the time of diabetes diagnosis. However, to date, only one published study reports on a psychosocial screening program at the diagnosis of T1D in youth.[9] Schwartz and colleagues implemented one of the first psychosocial screening protocols for children and adolescents newly diagnosed with T1D, in order to identify patients and families at risk for maladjustment or nonadherence to the diabetes regimen.[9] They integrated psychosocial screening into routine care at initial diagnosis. This screening protocol identified families at risk for nonadherence and lack of follow-up care within the first year following diagnosis.

In a controlled study, a pediatric diabetes team in the Netherlands demonstrated the positive effects of on going psychosocial assessment with adolescents with T1D. They performed an annual assessment of health-related quality of life of adolescents with T1D at diabetes outpatient visits with immediate feedback to physicians, so that the adolescent's quality of life could be discussed with the teen at the office visit. This was acceptable to teens and resulted in improved psychosocial well-being.[10] However, these investigators also demonstrated that when the routine annual assessment of quality of life was terminated, and physician-adolescent conversations about quality of life ceased, the improvements in psychosocial well-being were not sustained.[11]

The studies reviewed above indicate:

■ That psychosocial screening at diagnosis of T1D can identify families at risk for nonadherence and lack of follow-up care

■ That ongoing assessment and discussion of health-related quality of life between providers and adolescents with T1D during regular outpatient diabetes visits can improve psychosocial well-being

In a comprehensive review of psychological screening in youth with T1D, Cameron and colleagues conclude that "sequential use of validated functional health and behavioral questionnaires can be used in a step-wise fashion to screen for children and families exhibiting latent or overt behavioral difficulties."[12] Current guidelines all recommend risk-factor screening at diagnosis; however, we suggest that the standards of care should more strongly emphasize the benefits of routine monitoring and discussing of health-related quality of life between diabetes clinicians and their adolescent patients.

FUTURE CLINICAL RESEARCH/FILLING THE GAPS

There are two obvious gaps in the pediatric psychosocial assessment literature. The first concerns older adolescents transitioning to young adulthood. Currently there is no empirical evidence focused on psychosocial screening of older adolescents who are transitioning to adult care and more independent living. However, there is compelling evidence that psychosocial and mental health problems in childhood and adolescence persist into early adulthood and predict poor diabetes control and the early onset of diabetes-related complications.[13–15] Given this documented high vulnerability of older adolescents with T1D transitioning to young adulthood, psychosocial screening, and intervention prior to this transition would likely assure a more successful transition to adult care and more optimal glycemic and mental health outcomes.

A second gap in the pediatric literature is the scarcity of efficacy research on psychosocial screening of youth and their parents at the time of diagnosis of T1D. All international standards of care for youth with T1D recommend psychosocial screening of youth and families at diagnosis, therefore priority should be given to research documenting the efficacy of screening at diagnosis.

Filling the Gaps

Before psychosocial assessments of patients and families are widely adopted in pediatric clinical settings, research is needed that documents that these screenings are acceptable to youth and their parents. For youth, parents, and providers, psychosocial screening must also be easily integrated into routine care without adding excessive cost or time to clinical care. Furthermore, in order for psychosocial assessment to be reimbursed, we need cost-effectiveness research that establishes that psychosocial screening and appropriate intervention result in optimal psychosocial and glycemic outcomes as well as health care savings.

In addition to informal assessment during clinician-patient conversations of developmental functioning, risk factors and diabetes-related distress, providers may want to use formal, diabetes-specific assessments. Table 8.I.2 presents a list of some well-validated diabetes-specific psychosocial assessment instruments that may be of use in clinical care.

Table 8.I.2 Diabetes-Specific Psychosocial Assessment Instruments Appropriate for T1D Youth and Their Families

Construct Being Measured	Diabetes-Specific Measures
Social support	Diabetes Social Support Questionnaire–Friends version[16]
Family functioning	Diabetes Family Conflict Scale–Revised (DFC)[17]
	Diabetes Family Responsibility Questionnaire (DFRQ)[18]
	Diabetes Social Support Questionnaire–Family version[19]
	Diabetes Family Behavior Checklist (DFBC)[20]
	Diabetes Family Behavior Scale (DFBS)[21]
Diabetes quality of life and well-being	Pediatric Quality of Life Type 1 Diabetes Module (Peds QL 3.0 type 1 diabetes)[22]
	Diabetes Quality of Life for Youth (DQOL-Y)[23]
Diabetes self-efficacy	Self-efficacy in Diabetes (SED)[24]
	Self-efficacy for diabetes self-management[25]
Diabetes-related distress	Problem Areas in Diabetes–Teen version (PAID-T)[3]
	Problem Areas in Diabetes–Parent Revised version (PAID-PR)[2]
Eating disorders	Diabetes Eating Problem Survey (DEPS)[26]
Anxiety	Fear of Hypoglycemia Scale for Parents and Adolescents[27]

PSYCHOSOCIAL ASSESSMENT OF ADULTS WITH T1D

Introduction

For adults with T1D, the American Diabetes Association's Standards of Medical Care in Diabetes: 2012 recommends that "Diabetes Self-Management Education (DSME) should address psychosocial issues, since emotional well-being is associated with positive outcomes. Better outcomes were reported for DSME interventions that addressed psychosocial issues and incorporated behavioral strategies."[28]

Screening

Studies document that for adults with T1D, high quality of life and minimal depressive symptoms are critical for optimal glycemic outcomes.[29] Assessing depression should be routine for adults newly diagnosed with T1D, and annual screening for depressive symptoms and for quality of life should be the standard care, similar to the recommended annual screenings for eyes and feet.

Psychosocial screening should begin at diagnosis and be an ongoing part of the individual's diabetes management. "Individuals should be screened for psychosocial problems such as depression and diabetes-related distress, anxiety, eating disorders, and cognitive impairment when self-management is poor."[28] It should include, but is not limited to, attitudes about the illness, expectations for medical management and outcomes, affect/mood, general and diabetes-related quality of life, resources (financial, social, and emotional), and psychiatric history.

Diabetes-Related Distress in Adults with T1D

As discussed in the pediatric section above, diabetes-related distress is common in patients and their family members living with T1D. Diabetes-related distress is one barrier to optimal disease management that the clinician can identify and work with the patient to try to improve. Two diabetes-related distress measures have been validated for adults with T1D: the PAID Survey and the Diabetes Distress Scale (DDS).[1,30,31] We will discuss PAID and include a copy of this survey in Table 8.I.3, as PAID is the instrument with the longest use and most empirical support in 2012.

Because PAID is a brief survey, requiring only about 5 min for the adult with T1D to complete, it is feasible for the provider to ask the patient to complete PAID immediately before the medical visit. Based on patient responses, the provider can ask about those items that the patient marked as a "somewhat serious problem" or as a "serious problem." If a patient checked more than one item as a "serious problem," the provider can ask the patient, "What would s/he like to focus on in today's visit?" Then, using open-ended questions, the provider can learn about some of the real barriers to optimal self-management with which the patient is struggling.

Table 8.I.3 Items from the PAID Scale

Worrying about the future and the possibility of serious complications

Feeling guilty or anxious when you get off track with your diabetes management

Feeling scared when you think about having/living with diabetes

Feeling discouraged with your diabetes regimen

Feeling depressed when you think about having/living with diabetes

Feeling constantly concerned about food and eating

Feeling "burned out" by the constant effort to manage diabetes

Feeling angry when you think about having/living with diabetes

Coping with complications of diabetes

Feeling that diabetes is taking up too much mental and physical energy

Worrying about reactions

Not knowing if the mood or feelings you are experiencing are related to your blood glucose

Feeling overwhelmed by your diabetes regimen

Feeling alone with diabetes

Feelings of deprivation regarding food and meals

Not "accepting" diabetes

Not having clear and concrete goals for your diabetes care

Uncomfortable interactions around diabetes with family/friends

Feeling that friends/family are not supportive of diabetes management efforts

Feeling unsatisfied with your diabetes physician

n = 451. Items are listed in descending order of reported severity.[1]

In an informal psychosocial assessment, open-ended questions help patients feel secure and unhurried. For example:

■ Ask patients to share any stressful events or situations.
■ Explore if patients have adequate social and family support.
■ Ask about the patient's mood, anxiety, and sense of well-being.
■ For those at risk for eating disorders: inquire about skipped insulin doses, excessive dieting, binge eating, or induced emesis.

The use of open-ended questions helps patients to feel heard and unhurried and thus strengthens the patient-provider relationship. A strong patient–provider relationship helps to foster regular clinic visits and to facilitate early detection of complex psychosocial factors. It enables a patient to willingly disclose concerns and accept treatment options, if the need arises.[32]

Standards of Care

In Standards of Medical Care in Diabetes: 2012, the ADA made the following recommendations concerning psychosocial screening:

■ Effective self-management and quality of life are the key outcomes of diabetes self-management education and should be measured and monitored as part of care.
■ It is reasonable to include assessment of the patient's psychological and social situation as an ongoing part of the medical management of diabetes.
■ Psychosocial screening and follow-up may include, but is not limited to, attitudes about the illness, expectations for medical management and outcomes, affect/mood, general and diabetes-related quality of life, resources (financial, social, and emotional), and psychiatric history.
■ Consider screening for psychosocial problems such as depression and diabetes-related distress, anxiety, eating disorders, and cognitive impairment when self-management is poor.[28]

Referral to Mental Health Specialist

Providers of diabetes medical care should try to identify a mental health specialist in their local area (psychologist, psychiatrist, and clinical social worker) who is experienced in working with adults with T1D. The mental health provider must be familiar with the daily and complex burden of diabetes management for adults and their families living with T1D. The provider should consider the following patients for referral to a mental health specialist:

■ Two or more episodes of severe hypoglycemia or diabetic ketoacidosis without obvious causes in 1 year
■ No response to efforts to negotiate and implement a treatment plan
■ Comorbid psychiatric disorders that complicate diabetes management
■ Serious family dysfunction that is a barrier to improving diabetes management
■ Suspicion of depression or chronic diabetes-related distress

Table 8.I.4 Diabetes-Specific Psychosocial Assessment Tools

Psychosocial Construct Being Measured	Diabetes-Specific Assessment Tools
Social support	None identified
Marital relationships	None identified
Family functioning	Diabetes Family Behavior Checklist-II[34]
Quality of life and well-being	Diabetes Quality of Life[35]
Stress	Problem Areas in Diabetes (PAID)[1]
	Diabetes Distress Scale (DDS)[33]
Self-efficacy and empowerment	Diabetes Self-Efficacy Scale[36]
	Diabetes Empowerment Scale: a measure of Psychosocial Self-efficacy (DES)[37]
	Diabetes Empowerment Scale-Short Form (DES-SF)[38]
Locus of control	Diabetes Locus of Control (DLC)[39]
	Perceived Control of Diabetes Scales[40]
Anxiety and fear of hypoglycemia	Fear of Hypoglycemia Scale[41]

FUTURE CLINICAL RESEARCH/FILLING THE GAPS

There are numerous gaps in literature concerning psychosocial assessment of T1D adults. First and most fundamentally, we need research documenting the efficacy of psychosocial assessments for improved glycemic and mental health outcomes in adults with T1D. A second gap concerns the identification of adult patients who are suffering from diabetes-related distress.[33] A third gap is the lack of systematic screening for psychological disorders, especially depression and other mood disorders.[29] A fourth gap concerns the lack of research to demonstrate that psychosocial screening can be integrated into routine clinical practice without burdening busy clinicians. A fifth gap pertains to research that demonstrates that psychosocial assessments are cost effective in terms of health outcomes. Table 8.I.4 provides a listing of some psychosocial assessment instruments that may be of use in clinical practice.

Filling the Gaps

Multisite research projects consistently using the same core battery of psychosocial assessments would substantiate the evidence base for the benefits of psychosocial assessments. Funding opportunities that prioritize psychosocial assessments would encourage research in this area. Finally, once the evidence base is established for the efficacy and cost effectiveness of psychosocial assessments for improving diabetes outcomes, then national and international guidelines for the care of adults with T1D must make stronger and specific recommendations for psychosocial assessments in adult T1D patients.

In addition to assessing the adult patient with T1D by informal dialogue about diabetes-related distress and barriers to care the provider may want to carry out more formal psychosocial assessment.

CONCLUSION

There is consensus that psychosocial screening for youth and adults with T1D is necessary to optimize adherence behavior and glycemic control, yet there has been little research on the integration of psychosocial assessment into routine diabetes clinical care. In order to facilitate more widespread implementation of psychosocial assessments as part of routine pediatric and adult diabetes care, research is needed to document that assessments can be feasibly and effectively integrated into routine clinical practice without excess cost and time burdens. Future research is needed to document who can most effectively provide these assessments. More studies are needed to indicate that psychosocial screenings are acceptable to patients and their parents and to adults with T1D. Finally, future research is needed to demonstrate that psychosocial problems, once identified, can be effectively managed or treated and that this process is cost effective.

REFERENCES

1. Polonsky WH, Anderson BA, Lohrer PA Welch GW, Jacobson AM: Assessment of diabetes-related emotional distress. *Diabetes Care* 18:754–760, 1995
2. Markowitz JT, Volkening LK, Butler DA, Antisdel-Lomaglio JE, Anderson BJ, Laffel LM: Reexamining a measure of diabetes-related burden in parents of young people with type 1 diabetes: the Problem Areas in Diabetes Survey-Parent Revised version (PAID-PR). *Diabet Med* 28:1–5, 2011
3. Silverstein J, Klingensmith G, Copeland K, Plotnick L, Kaufman F, Laffel L, Deeb L, Grey M, Anderson B, Holzmeister LA, Clark N: Care of children and adolescents with type 1 diabetes: a statement of the American Diabetes Association. *Diabetes Care* 28:186–212, 2005
4. Weissberg-Benchell J, Antisdel-Lomoglio J: Diabetes-specific emotional distress among adolescents: feasibility, reliability and validity of the Problem Areas in Diabetes–Teen version. *Pediatric Diabetes* 12:341–344, 2011
5. Delamater AM: Psychological care of children and adolescents with diabetes: ISPAD Clinical Practice Consensus Guidelines 2009 Compendium. *Pediatr Diabetes* 10 (Suppl. 12):175–184, 2009
6. ISPAD Clinical Practice Consensus Guidelines 2009 Compendium. *Pediatr Diabetes* 10 (Suppl. 12), 2009
7. Arnett JJ: *Emerging Adulthood: The Winding Road from the Later Teens through the Twenties.* New York, Oxford University Press, 2004
8. Peters A, Laffel L: ADA Transitions Working Group: Diabetes care for emerging adults: recommendations for transition from pediatric to adult diabetes care systems. *Diabetes Care* 34: 2477–2485, 2011
9. Schwartz DD, Cline VD, Axelrad ME, Anderson BJ: Feasibility, acceptability, and predictive validity of a psychosocial screening program for children

and youth newly diagnosed with type 1 diabetes. *Diabetes Care* 34:326–331, 2011

10. de Wit M, Delemarre-van de Waal HA, Bokma JA, Haasnoot K, Houdijk MC, Gemke RJ, Snoek FJ: Monitoring and discussing health-related quality of life in adolescents with type 1 diabetes improve psychosocial well-being: a randomized controlled trial. *Diabetes Care* 31:1521–1526, 2008

11. de Wit M, Delemarre-van de Waal HA, Bokma JA, Haasnoot K, Houdijk MC, Gemke RJ, Snoek FJ: Follow-up results on monitoring and discussing health-related quality of life in adolescent diabetes care: benefits do not sustain in routine practice. *Pediatr Diabetes* 11:175–181, 2010

12. Cameron FJ, Northam EA, Ambler GR, Daneman D: Routine psychological screening in youth with type 1 diabetes and their parents: a notion whose time has come? *Diabetes Care* 30:2716–2724, 2007

13. Kovacs M, Mukerje P, Iyengar S, Drash A: Psychiatric disorder and metabolic control among youths with IDDM: a longitudinal study. *Diabetes Care* 19:318–323, 1996

14. Bryden KS, Dunger DB , Mayou RA, Peveler RC, Neil HA: Poor prognosis of young adults with type 1 diabetes: a longitudinal study. *Diabetes Care* 26:1052–1057, 2003

15. Northam EA, Matthews LK, Anderson PJ, Cameron FJ, Werther GA: Psychiatric morbidity and health outcomes in type 1 diabetes: perspectives from a prospective longitudinal study. *Diabet Med* 22:152–157, 2005

16. Bearman KJ, La Greca AM: Assessing friend support of adolescents' diabetes care: the Diabetes Social Support Questionnaire: Friends Version. *J Ped Psychol* 27:417–428, 2002

17. Hood KK, Butler DA, Anderson BJ, Laffel LMB: Updated and revised Diabetes Family Conflict Scale. *Diabetes Care* 30:1764–1769, 2007

18. Anderson BJ, Auslander WF, Jung KC, Miller JP, Santiago JV: Assessing family sharing of diabetes responsibilities. *J Pediatr Psychol* 15:477–492, 1990

19. La Greca AM, Bearman MS: The Diabetes Social Support Questionnaire—Family version: Evaluating adolescents' diabetes-specific support from family members. *J Pediatr Psychol* 27:665–676, 2002

20. Schafer LC, McCaul KD, Glasgow RE: Supportive and nonsupportive family behaviors: relationships to adherence and metabolic control in persons with type 1 diabetes. *Diabetes Care* 9:170–185, 1986

21. McKelvey J, Waller DA, North AJ, Marks JF, Schreiner B, Travis LB, Murphy J: Reliability and validity of the Diabetes Family Behavior Scale (DFBS). *Diabetes Educ* 19:125–132, 1993

22. Varni JW, Burwinkle TM, Jacobs JR, Gottschalk M, Kaufman F, Jones KL: The Peds QL in type 1 and type 2 diabetes. *Diabetes Care* 26: 631–637, 2003

23. Ingersoll GM, Marrero DG: A modified quality-of-life measures for youths. *Diabetes Educ* 17:114–118, 1991

24. Grossman HY, Brink S, Hauser ST: Self-efficacy in adolescent girls and boys with insulin-dependent diabetes mellitus. *Diabetes Care* 10:324–329, 1987

25. Iannotti RM, Schneider S, Nansel TR, Haynie D, Plotnick LP, Clark LM, Sobel DO, Simons-Morton B: Self-efficacy, outcome expectations, and

diabetes self-management in adolescents with type 1 diabetes. *J Dev Behav Pediatr* 27:98–105, 2006

26. Markowitz JT, Butler DA, Volkening LK, Antisdel JE, Anderson BJ, Laffel LM: Brief screening tool for disordered eating in diabetes: internal consistency and external validity in a contemporary sample of pediatric patients with type 1 diabetes. *Diabetes Care* 33:495–500, 2010

27. Gonder-Frederick LA, Fisher CD, Ritterband LM, Cox DJ, Hou L, Das-Gupta AA, Clarke WL: Predictors of fear of hypoglycemia in adolescents with type 1 diabetes and their parents. *Pediatr Diabetes* 7:215–222, 2006

28. American Diabetes Association: Standards of medical care in diabetes: 2012. *Diabetes Care* 35 (Suppl. 1):S11–S63, 2012

29. Peyrot M, Rubin RR: Behavioral and psychosocial interventions in diabetes: a conceptual review. *Diabetes Care* 30:2433–2440, 2007

30. Fisher L, Glasgow RE, Mullan JT, Skaff MM, Polonksy WH: Development of a brief diabetes distress screening instrument. *Ann Fam Med* 6:246–252, 2008

31. Fisher L, Hessler DM, Polonsky WH, Mullan J: When is diabetes distress clinically meaningful: establishing cut points for the Diabetes Distress Scale. *Diabetes Care* 35:259–264. 2012

32. Anderson BJ, Mansfield AK:Psychological issues in the treatment of diabetes. In Beaser R, and Staff of Joslin Diabetes Center. *Joslin's Diabetes Deskbook.* 2nd ed. Boston, Joslin Diabetes Center, 2007, p. 641–661

33. Polonsky WH, Fisher L, Earles J, Dudl RJ, Lees J, Mullan J, Jackson RA: Assessing psychosocial distress in diabetes: development of the Diabetes Distress Scale. *Diabetes Care* 28:626–631, 2005

34. Glasgow RE, Toobert DJ: Social environment and regimen adherence among type 2 diabetic patients. *Diabetes Care* 11:377–386, 1988

35. Jacobson AM and the DCCT Research Group: The diabetes quality of life measure. In *Handbook of Psychology and Diabetes.* Bradley C, Ed. Chur, Switzerland, Harwood Academic Publishers, 1994, p. 65–87

36. Skaff M, Mullan J, Fisher L, Chesla C: A contextual model of control beliefs, behavior, and health: Latino and European Americans with type 2 diabetes. *Psychol Health* 18:295–312, 2003

37. Anderson RM, Funnell MM, Fitzgerald JT, Marrero DC: The Diabetes Empowerment Scale: a measure of psychosocial self-efficacy. *Diabetes Care* 23: 739–743, 2000

38. Anderson RM, Fitzgerald JT, Gruppen LD, Funnell MM, Oh MS: The Diabetes Empowerment Scale-Short Form (DES-SF). *Diabetes Care* 26:1641–1642, 2003

39. Peyrot M, Rubin RR: Structure and correlates of diabetes-specific locus of control. *Diabetes Care* 17:994–1001, 1994

40. Bradley C, Brewin CR, Gamsu DS, Moses JKL: Development of scales to measure perceived control of diabetes mellitus and diabetes-related health beliefs. *Diabet Med* 1:213–218, 1984

41. Cox D, Irvine A, Gonder-Frederick L, Nowacek G, Butterfield J: Fear of hypoglycemia: quantification, validation, and utilization. *Diabetes Care* 10:617–621, 1987

II. Depression

Jeffrey S. Gonzalez, PhD

INTRODUCTION

In this section, we provide a brief overview of the evidence regarding the importance of depression in type 1 diabetes (T1D) by reviewing data regarding prevalence, associated adverse diabetes outcomes, and potential mechanisms that may explain the link between depression and T1D outcomes. This will serve as a background for a more focused discussion of important methodological issues relating to assessment of depression in patients with T1D. We conclude the section with clinical practice recommendations and areas for future clinical research.

PREVALENCE

Pediatrics and Young Adults

Several studies conducted in youth with T1D suggest a prevalence rate of depression that is approximately twice that found in youth without diabetes.[1-3] However, a recently published meta-analysis of depression in youth with T1D suggests that these differences, though significant, may be smaller overall and are often amplified by inadequate comparison group equivalence. The magnitude of this difference also appears to be smaller in more recently published data, perhaps suggesting a link between newer treatment approaches and improved well-being.[4] Data suggest that young adults may be at particularly high risk for experiencing significant psychological distress and depressive symptoms. For example, approximately one-third of consecutively screened young adult Australian patients (ages 18–28 years old) reported significant psychological distress and nearly one-quarter reported severe levels of depressive symptom severity.[5] In adolescents with diabetes, including 18–20 year olds, 15–33% report depressive symptoms, while 23–35% of emerging adults (18–28 years of age) with diabetes report such symptoms.[5,6]

Adults

A widely cited meta-analysis of the literature on the prevalence of depression in adults with diabetes (including T1D and T2D) concluded that individuals with diabetes were twice as likely as those without diabetes to be depressed.[7] However, the number of studies (n = 9) focusing on T1D was much smaller than the number that included either type 2 diabetes (T2D) or mixed samples (n = 33) and only three of these were controlled comparisons. An updated systematic literature

DOI: 10.2337/9781580404785ch08s2

review on depression in adults with T1D included five additional studies that were published since the earlier meta-analysis but failed to reach a stronger conclusion; the authors determined that there was insufficient evidence to conclude that depression is more prevalent in adults with T1D than in well-matched control groups.[8] Both reviews noted that prevalence rates were much higher in adults with T1D as compared to those without diabetes when self-report measures were used than when depression was evaluated with the gold standard assessment, a structured diagnostic interview. This is an important point that we will return to below, as it suggests that the prevalence of psychiatric presentations of clinical depression may be less elevated in individuals living with diabetes than nonpsychiatric emotional distress.

A more recent examination of depression in adults with and without T1D that used age- and sex-matched controls found that individuals living with T1D were 3.5 times more likely to self-report clinically significant elevations in depressive symptoms, 2.5 times more likely to have a history of depression, and nearly twice as likely to be on antidepressants than nondiabetic controls. T1D patients with diabetic complications were significantly more likely to report depressive symptoms than those without, indicating the possible role of health and functional impairments in explaining increased risk of depression in diabetes.[9] Thus, although there is some variation across studies, it appears that adults with T1D are significantly more likely to experience depression, particularly self-reported symptoms that may not qualify for a diagnosis of clinical depression.

ADVERSE OUTCOMES

In understanding the relationship between T1D and depression, it is important to be aware of likely bidirectional influences. T1D may contribute to the development of depressive symptoms; however, the converse is also true: depressive symptoms can significantly impact diabetes self-management and increase risk of poor treatment outcomes. The relentless demands of blood glucose monitoring, insulin adjustments and dosing, maintaining health visits, managing complications, along with juggling life's ordinary demands often strain individuals and lead to significant emotional distress. Emotional distress can, in turn, further impact patients' ability to cope with stressors and self-manage diabetes, resulting in a negative cycle that may be difficult for patients to reverse.

Although questions of directionality and causality remain unresolved, meta-analyses have shown that depression is consistently associated with increased risk of hyperglycemia, diabetes complications, and poorer adherence to diabetes self-management and treatment across both T1D and T2D.[10-12] Although the literature in aggregate does not suggest differences in these relationships between T1D and T2D, individual studies have suggested a stronger relationship between depression and glycemic control in T1D.[13,14] Some of the best longitudinal data available on the relationship between depression and diabetes complications has been conducted in individuals with T1D; these data suggest depressive symptoms are an important risk factor for diabetes complications. For example, African American patients with T1D who reported elevations on a self-report measure of depressive symptoms were nearly 2.5 times more likely to show progression of

diabetic retinopathy and over 3 times more likely to show progression to proliferative diabetic retinopathy based on detailed ophthalmologic exams and retinal
photographs over 6 years of follow-up than those with low depression scores.
These relationships persisted after controlling for baseline glycemic control, diabetes duration, and presence of hypertension.[15] In a related study from the same
cohort, depression scores also predicted increased risk for the development of
proteinuria after controlling for physiological risk factors.[16] Thus, there is strong
and consistent evidence to suggest that depression is an important risk factor for
poor health outcomes in T1D. However, evidence regarding the causal nature
and potential mechanisms for this relationship is inconclusive.

POTENTIAL MECHANISMS

The mechanisms that link depression and worse outcomes in T1D are poorly
understood but likely to be multifactorial. Direct biological effects of psychological distress on glucose metabolism are plausible but may be modest, at least in
regards to acute stress.[17,18] Evidence suggests that variability in daily stress level
may have a closer relationship to glycemic control than average stress over time,
independent of self-management behaviors.[19] The consistent association between
depression and problems with diabetes self-care and treatment adherence suggests that behavioral pathways may be important in explaining the link between
depression and worse diabetes outcomes.[12]

Although meta-analysis of the literature on depression and diabetes self-
management did not reveal significant differences between T1D and T2D, the
relationship was found to be significantly stronger in children and adolescents
than adults, though it was significant for both groups.[12] Thus, to the extent that
impaired self-management explains the link between depression and adverse outcomes in T1D, this pathway may be particularly important for younger patients.
Although two studies have failed to demonstrate a mediating role for self-management in the relationship between depression and glycemic control in T1D,
the use of self-reported composite measures of diet, exercise, and glucose testing
may have resulted in a less precise measure of important aspects of self-management (e.g., adherence to insulin regimen) that are causally related to glycemic
control.[19,20]

In contrast, one study of adolescents with T1D focused on frequency of blood
glucose monitoring, assessed by electronically downloaded data from glucom-
eters and self-report data adjusted for inflation biases, as a mediating pathway
between depression and glycemic control. This study did find significant evidence
for mediation, which suggested that 38% of the relationship between depression
and A1C was explained by self-monitoring frequency.[21] A subsequent study demonstrated that the link between depression and less frequent glucose monitoring
is enduring: baseline depression scores from adolescents with T1D predicted less
frequent monitoring over one year of follow-up.[22] Thus, although few studies
are available, there is better evidence for a mediating role of impaired T1D self-
management in adolescents than for adults.

While it may seem uncontroversial to expect that depression may cause poorer
outcomes in patients with T1D through associated impairments in self-management

and adherence to treatment, it should be noted that the causal nature of the link between depression and diabetes outcomes has not been clearly supported by studies using designs that can adequately evaluate change in these factors over time. A number of longitudinal studies have failed to find relationships between changes in depression and changes in glycemic control in either T1D or T2D.[23] Furthermore, intervention studies have failed to clearly demonstrate that reducing depression severity per se results in either improved self-management or treatment adherence or better glycemic control.[24,25]

It is possible that depression is not a causal risk factor but rather represents a confounding between problems with self-management or failing health and the assessment of depression. Depression and emotional distress may arise as a result of increasing health burden and functional impairments and therefore predict poor health outcomes in epidemiological studies without necessarily having a causal influence on these outcomes. Therefore, it seems that the best-supported conclusion regarding treatment of depression in diabetes is that it may be necessary but not sufficient to improve health-related outcomes. However, even if we conservatively assume that the data reviewed above on depression and adverse diabetes outcomes are not causal, it is clear that depression, poor self-management, and worse diabetes treatment outcomes are interrelated and co-occurring problems. Assessment and treatment approaches that comprehensively address these factors are likely to have a greater impact than approaches that target these issues in isolation.

ASSESSMENT OF DEPRESSION

Standards of Care

Although it is clear that living with the burden of T1D and its complex management can contribute to significant emotional distress for many individuals, it is important for providers to avoid complacency and take active steps to recognize and appropriately address distress in their patients. Data consistently demonstrate under recognition of depression in patients with diabetes by their health care providers. For example, in a mixed sample of T1D and T2D patients, diabetes nurses recorded the presence of an emotional problem in patient files for only 20% of patients who screened positive for significant depression. Nurses were no more likely to document such problems in patients who screened positive for depression than for those who did not.[26] This under recognition of depression by health care providers is consistent with the wider literature on the recognition of depression in primary care and in various other chronic illness populations. Given the increased prevalence of depression in T1D and problems with under recognition and under treatment, a number of investigators have called for routine depression screening to be implemented in both adults and in youth with diabetes. The current (2012) recommendations of the ADA for management of diabetes encourage health care providers to screen for depression, especially when self-management is poor, but the evidence base for these recommendations is based on poorly controlled or uncontrolled studies and clinical experience or expert consensus.

It has yet to be empirically demonstrated that routine screening for depression can improve outcomes in diabetes care. One recent study showed very high levels of acceptability for routine psychosocial screening among newly diagnosed T1D patients (96.8% accepted offered screening) and demonstrated that the procedures were feasible for clinical practice.[27] However, the impact of screening on access to treatment and improved outcomes remains understudied. Results from a mixed sample of adults with either T1D or T2D suggest that screening, diagnostic evaluation, and referrals for treatment have minimal impact on depression or diabetes outcomes.[28]

While the results of Pouwer and colleagues demonstrate a reasonably high level of patient acceptability of a thorough evaluation for the presence of a mood disorder (84% of those who screened positive on a self-report measure agreed to participate in a clinical interview to conclusively evaluate depression), they also reveal the problems inherent with such an approach. Specifically, a greater proportion of patients with a positive screen for depression were false-positives (54%) than true positives (33%), with the remainder qualifying for psychiatric diagnoses other than mood disorders.[28] This is consistent with findings from a comprehensive review showing acceptable sensitivity and specificity of screening measures for depression in diabetes but quite high false-positive rates; positive predictive values ranged from 26–53% across reviewed instruments. In contrast, negative predictive values were quite high in all reviewed studies (>90%).[29] Thus, providers may be relatively confident about negative screening results but positive screening results will need to be followed by further evaluation.

The problem of false positives goes beyond misallocated resources and time and points to a current lack of empirically supported intervention approaches for those patients who may be experiencing emotional distress that is significant but that would not meet criteria for a psychiatric diagnosis. Treatments that may be effective for clinical depression may not be appropriate to address subclinical symptoms. For example, the wider depression treatment literature strongly suggests that treatment with antidepressants is unlikely to be more effective than placebo for patients experiencing subclinical or mild presentations of depression.[30,31] Thus, a comprehensive approach to the full range of emotional distress, from subclinical symptoms of depression to full psychiatric presentations, is needed. Many patients experiencing symptoms of depression that do not meet criteria for a diagnosis could be effectively supported as part of comprehensive diabetes care, while patients with more severe presentations may benefit from referrals to mental health specialty care.[32] Such systems of care are likely to be most effective when they take advantage of key opportunities to screen for depression (see Table 8.II.1) and when they match screened patients to appropriate interventions.

Based on a Systematic Review, Are There Changes that Should Be Made?

Emotional distress, even at levels of severity below the threshold of a psychiatric diagnosis, should be recognized among health care providers as a common risk factor associated with poorer self-management and treatment outcomes in individuals with T1D. For example, meta-analysis of the literature on depression and diabetes self-management failed to find any indication of weaker relationships

Table 8.II.1 Key Opportunities to Screen for Depression

Diagnosis

End of honeymoon period

Intensified treatment

Hospitalizations

New complications

Pregnancy

Change in resources (financial, social, emotional)

Insurance changes

Problems with glucose control, quality of life, adherence

in studies that used self-report measures of depressive symptoms in comparison to those that used structured clinical interviews or other means of diagnosing clinical depression.[12] Furthermore, many studies linking depression and risk of complications in patients with diabetes use self-report scales that are more likely to reflect subclinical emotional distress than a psychiatric disorder.[15,16,33] In fact, evidence suggests that subclinical emotional distress, particularly diabetes-related distress (i.e., significant negative emotional reactions to the threat of complications, self-management demands, unresponsive providers, or unsupportive interpersonal relationships), is quite common and may be more closely related to problems with self-management and diabetes control.[32] Qualitative work shows that even when structured clinical interviews are used to evaluate symptoms of depression, adults with T1D often explain these symptoms as stemming from the burden of managing diabetes.[34] Therefore, it is important that clinicians evaluate symptoms of depression and the context for these symptoms (e.g., diabetes related vs. related to other life stressors) when assessing patients, as the severity of (subclinical vs. psychiatric) and context for these symptoms will inform the selection of the most appropriate treatments.

Screening should be considered a potentially useful tool but all measures designed to detect the presence of clinical depression have a problem with a high rate of false positives. A recent critical review of these instruments could not recommend any one instrument as superior.[29] Screening per se is unlikely to improve outcomes unless it is integrated within a system that can also provide effective treatment and care. Because of the heterogeneity of issues that may result in positive screening results (e.g., subclinical depressive symptoms, major depressive disorder, diabetes-related distress), further evaluation will be necessary for those patients who screen positive. The current state of the science suggests that the best approach would be for all diabetes care teams to have competence in evaluating and differentiating among these issues.[29,32] Given the prevalence of emotional distress in individuals living with diabetes, all team members should have training and be comfortable with empathic listening, sensitive verbal inquiry, and the use of reflective comments in working with their patients. Treatment of diabetes-related distress may be best delivered as part of comprehensive diabetes care while referrals to mental health specialists, who may not be part of the care team in many settings, may be indicated for more severe presentations of depression.[32]

When clinical depression is identified through the use of diagnostic interviews, psychotherapy and antidepressants are empirically supported treatments. However, interventions for clinical depression that target depression in isolation from the context of the challenges of living with diabetes are unlikely to result in improved self-management or glycemic control. Thus, even when mental health specialty care is needed, this should be supplemented by more intensive support for self-management and treatment adherence. While some mental health specialists have the training to work with diabetes patients on these issues, most do not. Therefore, it is important for diabetes care providers to work collaboratively with mental health providers in order to maximize treatment benefits for these patients. This coordination of care can be difficult to accomplish in a fragmented health care system. Developing successful and sustainable models of comprehensive diabetes care remains an important area for further research.

Where Are the Gaps in Clinical Research?

Although research clearly demonstrates that depression is important in the treatment of diabetes, there has been lack of clarity in our conceptualization of depression and the measures implemented in studies often have serious limitations. Because most studies use self-report measures that were not designed for diagnostic purposes and that can be influenced by diabetes-related distress, there is still considerable confusion about how best to conceptualize depression in diabetes. Important questions remain unanswered. For example, is depression a comorbid illness linked with diabetes through biological pathways, or is what we often call depression in most epidemiological studies often not an illness at all but rather a reflection of the distress associated with struggling with illness self-management, family and interpersonal conflict, or other difficult life stressors? Further research is necessary to clarify these issues in ways that will inform the best models of care delivery. Because most intervention studies have focused on treatments that were developed to treat psychiatric presentations of depression, we have less available evidence regarding how best to approach subclinical depression symptoms and diabetes-related distress. However, alternative models of care may hold promise. For example, relatively short-term structured group sessions using strategies from cognitive behavioral therapy have been effective in improving depression symptom severity, glycemic control, well-being, perceived stress, and diabetes-related distress in adults with T1D who were selected for treatment based on poor glycemic control.[35] Peer-led interventions have shown promise in improving diabetes-related distress and glycemic control in adults with T2D.[36] Whether lower-cost models of care such as group-based interventions and peer-delivered approaches can be successfully implemented in clinical practice to address emotional distress and depression in individuals with diabetes deserves further investigation.

How Do We Fill the Gaps?

Although insights have been gained by depression treatment studies in individuals with diabetes, the largest studies have focused on antidepressants as an important component of treatment. However, accruing evidence suggests that antidepressants may be no more effective than placebo for subclinical or mild cases of clinical depression.[30, 31] The evidence is also mixed, at best, for their ability to impact glycemic control outcomes.[25] Furthermore, antidepressants also cause significant side effects for many patients. Finally, although it is too early to draw clear conclusions, there is evidence that antidepressant use may be associated with risk for the development of T2D, even when potential confounds are statistically controlled, perhaps suggesting an accumulation of negative effects on glycemic control over time.[37,38] Although important challenges exist in translating psychotherapy- and behavioral intervention–based interventions to clinical practice settings, these approaches hold promise and may be most adaptable to responding to the variety of presentations of depression and emotional distress that are experienced by children, adolescents and adults with T1D. Translational research that addresses the challenges of sustainably implementing these approaches in practice settings could make an important impact on the ability of care providers to more effectively and comprehensively address the problem of depression in their patients.

CONCLUSION

Based on the available evidence, clinicians should be attuned to the emotional distress that is often part of the experience of diabetes for many patients. Depression, although not necessarily indicative of a psychiatric illness, appears to be more common in individuals living with T1D than in those who are not struggling with the burden of a chronic illness. This is true across the developmental lifespan and particularly in young adults. When depression is present, it is often associated with poorer diabetes self-management and, either as a result or through other as yet poorly understood biological pathways, is often a harbinger of risk for poor health outcomes. Thus, it is important for providers to recognize that addressing depression and other forms of emotional distress is an important part of delivering comprehensive diabetes care. While accurate identification of depression and the differentiation between subclinical and psychiatric presentations is an important first step, we must recognize that screening alone is not sufficient. Successful models of care delivery must differentiate between the varied presentations of emotional distress and link these to appropriate treatments. Many of these interventions are best delivered by the diabetes care team, particularly when symptoms of depression or distress appear to be related to the burden of living with diabetes and its intensive self-management demands. Other more severe presentations may require more intensive mental health specialist care, whether delivered by a specialist member of the diabetes care team or via referral. In both cases, an integrative approach that optimizes the management of depression along with the management of diabetes is likely to be most effective. The available literature strongly suggests that such integrative approaches are needed and have the best promise for improving both depression and diabetes health outcomes.

REFERENCES

1. Kovacs M, Obrosky DS, Goldston D, Drash A: Major depressive disorder in youths with IDDM. A controlled prospective study of course and outcome. *Diabetes Care* 20:45–51, 1997
2. Grey M, Whittemore R, Tamborlane W: Depression in type 1 diabetes in children: natural history and correlates. *J Psychosom Res* 53:907–911, 2002
3. Hood KK, Huestis S, Maher A, Butler D, Volkening L, Laffel LMB: Depressive symptoms in children and adolescents with type 1 diabetes: associations with diabetes-specific characteristics. *Diabetes Care* 29:1389–1391, 2006
4. Reynolds KA, Helgeson VS: Children with diabetes compared to peers: depressed? Distressed? *Ann Behav Med* 42:29–41, 2011
5. Hislop AL, Fegan G, Schlaeppi MJ, Duck M, Yeap BB: Prevalence and associations of psychological distress in young adults with type 1 diabetes. *Diabet Med* 25:91–96, 2008
6. Lawrence JM, Standiford DA, Loots B, Klingensmith GJ, Williams DE, Ruggiero A, Liese AD, Bell RA, Waitzfelder BE, McKeown RE: Prevalence and correlates of depressed mood among youth with diabetes: the SEARCH for Diabetes in Youth Study. *Pediatrics* 117:1348–1358, 2006
7. Anderson R, Freedland K, Clouse R, Lustman P: The prevalence of comorbid depression in adults with diabetes: a meta-analysis. *Diabetes Care* 24:1069–1078, 2001
8. Barnard KD, Skinner TC, Peveler R: The prevalence of co-morbid depression in adults with type 1 diabetes: systematic literature review. *Diabetic Med* 23:445–448, 2006
9. Gendelman N, Snell-Bergeon JK, McFann K, Kinney G, Wadwa RP, Bishop F, Rewers M, Maahs DM: Prevalence and correlates of depression in individuals with and without type 1 diabetes. *Diabetes Care* 32:575–579, 2009
10. Lustman PJ, Anderson RJ, Freedland KE, de Groot M, Carney RM, Clouse RE: Depression and poor glycemic control. *Diabetes Care* 23:934–942, 2000
11. de Groot M, Anderson R, Freedland KE, Clouse RE, Lustman PJ: Association of depression and diabetes complications: a meta-analysis. *Psychosomatic Med* 63:619–630, 2001
12. Gonzalez J, Peyrot M, McCarl L, Collins E, Serpa L, Mimiaga M, Safren S: Depression and diabetes treatment nonadherence: a meta-analysis. *Diabetes Care* 31:2398–2403, 2008
13. de Groot M, Jacobson AM, Samson JA, Welch G: Glycemic control and major depression in patients with type 1 and type 2 diabetes mellitus. *J Psychosom Res* 46:425–435, 1999
14. Van Tilburg MAL, McCaskill CC, Lane JD, Edwards CL, Bethel A, Feinglos MN, Surwit RS: Depressed mood is a factor in glycemic control in type 1 diabetes. *Psychosom Med* 63:551–555, 2001
15. Roy MS, Roy A, Affouf M: Depression is a risk factor for poor glycemic control and retinopathy in African-Americans with type 1 diabetes. *Psychosom Med* 69:537–542, 2007
16. Roy MS, Affouf M, Roy A: Six-year incidence of proteinuria in type 1 diabetic African Americans. *Diabetes Care* 30:1807–1812, 2007
17. Wiesle P, Schmid C, Kerwer O, Nigg-Koch C, Klaghofer R, Seifert B, Spinas GA, Schwegler K: Acute psychological stress affects glucose concentrations

in patients with type 1 diabetes following food intake but not in the fasting state. *Diabetes Care* 28:1910–1915, 2005

18. Wiesle P, Krayenbuhl PA, Kerwer O, Seifert B, Schmid C: Maintenance of glucose control in patients with type 1 diabetes during acute mental stress by riding high-speed roller coasters. *Diabetes Care* 30:1599–1601, 2007

19. Aikens JE, Wallander JL, Bell DSH, Cole JA: Daily stress variability, learned resourcefulness, regimen adherence, and metabolic control in type I diabetes mellitus: evaluation of a path model. *J Consult Clin Psychol* 60:113–118, 1992

20. Lustman PJ, Clouse RE, Ciechanowski PS, Hirsch IB, Freedland KE: Depression-related hyperglycemia in type 1 diabetes: a mediational approach. *Psychosom Med* 67:195–199, 2005

21. McGrady ME, Laffel L, Drotar D, Repaske D, Hood KK: Depressive symptoms and glycemic control in adolescents with type 1 diabetes: mediational role of blood glucose monitoring. *Diabetes Care* 32:804–806, 2009

22. Hilliard ME, Herzer M, Dolan LM, Hood KK: Psychological screening in adolescents with type 1 diabetes predicts outcomes one year later. *Diabetes Res Clin Pr* 94:39–44, 2011

23. Georgiades A, Zucker N, Friedman KE, Mosunic CJ, Applegate K, Lane JD, Feinglos MN, Surwit RS: Changes in depressive symptoms and glycemic control in diabetes mellitus. *Psychosom Med* 69:235–241, 2007

24. Lin EHB, Katon W, Rutter C, Simon GE, Ludman EJ, Von Korff M, Young B, Oliver M, Ciechanowski PC, Kinder L, Walker E: Effects of enhanced depression treatment on diabetes self-care. *Ann Fam Med* 4:46–53, 2006

25. Markowitz S, Gonzalez JS, Wilkinson JL, Safren SA: Treating depression in diabetes: emerging findings. *Psychosomatics* 52:1–18, 2011

26. Pouwer F, Beekman AT, Lubach C, Snoek FJ: Nurses' recognition and registration of depression, anxiety and diabetes-specific emotional problems in outpatients with diabetes mellitus. *Patient Educ Couns* 60:235–240, 2006

27. Schwartz DD, Depp Cline V, Axelrad ME, Anderson BJ: Feasibility, acceptability and predictive validity of a psychosocial screening program for children and youth newly diagnosed with type 1 diabetes. *Diabetes Care* 34:326–331, 2011

28. Pouwer F, Tack CJ, Geelhoed-Duijvestijn PHLM, Bazelmans E, Beekman AT, Heine RJ, Snoek FJ: Limited effect of screening for depression with written feedback in outpatients with diabetes mellitus: a randomized controlled trial. *Diabetologia* 54:741–748, 2011

29. Roy T, Lloyd CE, Pouwer F, Holt RIG, Sartorius N: Screening tools used for measuring depression among people with type 1 and type 2 diabetes: a systematic review. *Diabetic Medicine* 29:164–175, 2012

30. Kirsch I, Deacon BJ, Huedo-Medina TB, Scoboria A, Moore TJ, Johnson BT: Initial severity and antidepressant benefits: a meta-analysis of data submitted to the food and drug administration. *PLOS Med* 5:e45, 2008

31. Fournier JC, DeRubeis RJ, Hollon SD, Dimidjian S, Amsterdam JD, Shelton RC, Fawcett J: Antidepressant drug effects and depression severity: a patient-level meta-analysis. *JAMA* 303:47–53, 2010

32. Gonzalez JS, Fisher L, Polonsky WH: Depression in diabetes: have we been missing something important? *Diabetes Care* 34:236–239, 2011

33. Coyne JC: Self-reported distress: analog or ersatz depression? *Psychol Bull* 116:29–45, 1994
34. Tanenbaum ML, Gonzalez JS: The influence of diabetes on a clinician-rated assessment of depression in adults with type 1 diabetes. *Diabetes Educator* 2012 [published online before print 19 July]
35. Amsberg S, Anderbro T, Wredling R, Lisspers J, Lins PE, Adamson U, Johansson UB: A cognitive behavior therapy-based intervention among poorly controlled type 1 diabetes patients: a randomized controlled trial. *Patient Educ Couns* 77:72–80, 2009
36. Lorig K, Ritter PL, Villa F, Piette JD: Spanish diabetes self-management with and without automated telephone reinforcement: two randomized trials. *Diabetes Care* 31:408–414, 2008
37. Rubin RR, Ma Y, Marrero DG, Peyrot M, Barrett-Connor EL, Kahn SE, Haffner SM, Price DW, Knowler WC: Diabetes Prevention Program Research Group: Elevated depression symptoms, antidepressant medicine use, and risk of developing diabetes during the Diabetes Prevention Program. *Diabetes Care* 31:420–426, 2008
38. Rubin RR, Ma Y, Peyrot M, Marrero DG, Price DW, Barrett-Connor E, Knowler WC: Diabetes Prevention Program Research Group: Antidepressant medicine use and risk of developing diabetes during the Diabetes Prevention Program and Diabetes Prevention Program outcomes study. *Diabetes Care* 33:2549–2551, 2010

III. Eating Disorders

Ann E. Goebel-Fabbri, PhD

INTRODUCTION

Disturbed eating behavior, usually mild in severity, is common among adolescent girls and young women in the general population. However, those with type 1 diabetes (T1D) are more likely to exhibit two or more disturbed eating behaviors than their peers without diabetes.[1] Such behaviors may include dieting for weight loss, binge eating, or calorie purging through self-induced vomiting, laxative or diuretic use, excessive exercise, or insulin restriction, in the case of T1D.[2] Women with diabetes also have access to a unique calorie purging behavior—namely intentional insulin restriction, strategically induced hyperglycemia, and the loss of calories through glycosuria. Dehydration and the loss of lean body tissue will result from prolonged hyperglycemia. As many as 31% of women with T1D report intentional insulin restriction with rates of this disturbed eating behavior peaking in late adolescence and early adulthood (40% of women between ages of 15 and 30 years).[3] Evidence suggests women with T1D are 2.4 times more at risk for developing an eating disorder and 1.9 times more at risk for developing subthreshold eating disorders than women without diabetes and that these behaviors persist, become more common, and increase in severity over time.[1,4,5]

It remains unclear why girls and women with T1D have increased rates of eating disorder behaviors; however, T1D is strongly associated with a number of the risk factors that are known to be eating disorder risk factors in women without diabetes. As mentioned in the previous section, people with diabetes have twice the risk of clinically significant depression than those without diabetes.[6] Women and girls with T1D are also heavier on average than their peers without diabetes. For example, one study reported that by the age of 18 years, females with T1D were an average of 14 pounds heavier than matched controls.[7] Treatment itself may increase the risk of weight gain.

The Diabetes Control and Complications Trial (DCCT), established that maintaining near normal blood glucose ranges—through dietary management, exercise, and multiple daily blood glucose checks and insulin doses—improves long-term health outcomes in diabetes.[8] However, in the first year of the DCCT, the research team also found that intensive diabetes management conveyed a significantly increased risk of weight gain (an average of 6 pounds more in the intensive treatment cohort than in the standard treatment cohort), and long-term follow-up indicated that this weight was difficult to lose.[9,10] Women with T1D expressed particular concern about intensive insulin management causing weight gain.[11] However, it is important to note that the DCCT was conducted when very different treatment options were available. Today, intensive insulin

 DOI: 10.2337/9781580404785ch08s3

therapy most commonly involves basal/bolus insulin delivered by syringe, pen, or an insulin pump; these methods are better able to mimic physiological insulin secretion and in this way may lower the risk of weight gain associated with older treatment options.

Apart from weight gain, other aspects of current diabetes treatment may also increase the risk for developing disturbed eating behaviors. The attention to food portions and weight may parallel the rigid thinking about food and body image found in women with eating disorders who do *not* have diabetes.[12] Studies found disturbed eating behaviors to be strongly predicted by higher body mass index (BMI), higher weight and shape concerns, and depressed mood. By contrast, absence of depression, lower BMI, and positive feelings about appearance emerged as potential protective factors.[2,13–15] These findings support a model of disordered eating and T1D previously proposed by Goebel-Fabbri and colleagues.[16] In order to examine these issues further, Young-Hyman and colleagues are currently conducting a prospective study of the factors that might be predictive of disordered eating behaviors. Thus far, level of depression at diabetes diagnosis, premorbid body size dissatisfaction, and premorbid calorie restricting and purging behaviors appear to be associated with eating disorder risk in this cohort of youth with T1D.[17] This study holds promise for identifying some possible risk factors that could then be incorporated into routine screening in diabetes practice.

Women with T1D and eating disorders are in poorer glycemic control with A1C's approximately 2 or more percentage points higher than similarly aged women without eating disorders; they also have higher rates of hospital and emergency room visits, higher rates of neuropathy and retinopathy, and more negative attitudes toward diabetes than women who do not report insulin restriction.[3,18,19] Even subthreshold disturbed eating behaviors are strongly associated with significant medical and psychological consequences in the context of diabetes.[20] In fact, endorsing insulin restriction alone was recently shown to increase mortality risk threefold over an 11-year follow-up period.[21]

Less is known about boys and men with eating disorders, whether or not they have diabetes. Very few studies have included boys with T1D when investigating disordered eating behaviors. When compared to healthy controls, Svensson et al. found no eating disorders in either cohort but found that the males with T1D were significantly larger than their peers and had higher scores on the Drive for Thinness subscale of the Eating Disorder Inventory.[22] Indeed, larger body size appears to be a risk factor for developing disordered eating. Bryden and colleagues reported that as weight increased in both males and females with T1D, disordered eating behaviors increased.[19] Because there is such a paucity of research on males with T1D and disordered eating, the focus of the remainder of this section will be on girls and women.

ASSESSMENT OF DISTURBED EATING BEHAVIORS

Olmsted argues for early and routine screening for risk factors associated with eating disorders and T1D.[2] Health care teams working with adolescent

Table 8.III.1 Warning Signs for Eating Disorders in T1D

Unexplained elevations in A1C values

Repeated problems with DKA

Extreme concerns about weight and body shape

Excessive exercise (sometimes accompanied or followed by frequent hypoglycemia)

Unusually low-calorie meal plans

Amenorrhea

and adult women with diabetes should be alert to patterns that could indicate the presence of disturbed eating behaviors (see Table 8.III.1). However, these problems cannot be used as a sole diagnostic indicator. Further screening and evaluation by a mental health professional with experience in eating disorders is required.

Women with eating disorders can be quite ashamed about their struggle, resulting in well-hidden eating disorder behaviors. It is important to use sensitive, open-ended questions constructed to increase the clinician's understanding of the patient's situation without the risk of unintentionally educating the patient about these dangerous behaviors. For example, such questions may include:

■ How do you feel about your body size?
■ What do you think of your recommended meal plan?
■ Do you ever take more or less insulin than recommended in order to have an impact on your weight?[23]

Early detection and intervention for disturbed eating behavior in the context of T1D is important and requires an effective and efficient screening tool. The Diabetes Eating Problem Survey (DEPS-R) is a validated 16-item questionnaire designed to detect disordered eating in T1D. It was validated in a cohort of 13- to 19-year-olds with T1D, and takes approximately 10 minutes to administer. The validation of the DEPS-R is an important contribution to the field, however, it has not yet been validated in adult populations.[24] Until that time, clinicians should note that a positive response to a single, straightforward question: "Do you take less insulin than you should?" was shown to be associated with increased eating disorder symptoms and mortality risk in women with T1D.[21]

Alternatively, those interested in screening adults may also consider using the DEPS-R despite the fact that it has not yet been validated in this age group or may wish to consider other, validated eating disorder screening tools used in populations without diabetes. In those cases where a non-diabetes–specific screening tool raises concern about a possible eating disorder, Young-Hyman and Davis recommend that someone who understands T1D treatment evaluate the patient.[25] In this way, questionnaire items that may overlap between eating disorders and diabetes treatment recommendations may be teased apart and potentially better understood.

MANAGEMENT

Insulin restriction becomes a more significant problem in older adolescents, perhaps as parental supervision of insulin administration decreases. It becomes more common and potentially worse in severity and frequency throughout early adulthood.[15] Once the pattern of frequent and habitual insulin restriction becomes entrenched, the cycle of negative feelings about body image, shape, and weight; chronically elevated blood sugars; depression, anxiety, and shame; and poor diabetes self-care can be complex and difficult to treat.

A multidisciplinary team approach to treatment is considered the standard of care for both eating disorders and diabetes treatment.[26,27] Treating a patient with these two comorbidities requires a team that includes an endocrinologist, a nurse educator, a nutritionist with eating disorder or diabetes training, and a psychologist or social worker to provide weekly individual therapy. Depending on the severity of related psychiatric conditions like depression and anxiety, a psychiatrist for psychopharmacologic evaluation and treatment should also be consulted. Team members should communicate frequently to maintain congruent treatment goals. When such a comprehensive team cannot be constructed, as many team members as possible should be included. Often, the most difficult member to find is a mental health specialist with both eating disorders and diabetes treatment experience. It is important for diabetes clinicians to have a referral network of mental health providers they respect. One of these should be an eating disorder specialist who is willing to collaborate with the diabetes team in order to learn the unique ways that diabetes contributes to the patient's struggle.[28]

Patients may require a medical or psychiatric inpatient hospitalization until they are medically stable and appropriate for outpatient treatment. Early in the treatment, monthly appointments with a team endocrinologist or nurse educator may be necessary to maintain medical stability; monthly appointments with the nutritionist are also recommended. Laboratory tests (especially A1C and electrolytes) and weight checks should occur routinely at medical appointments. It is unlikely that intensive glycemic management of diabetes is an appropriate *early* treatment goal for a person with T1D and an eating disorder. The treatment team must be willing to collaboratively establish small goals that the patient feels are realistic. An essential first goal is the patient's agreement to maintain medical safety. For example, this goal may be as small (but clinically meaningful) as agreeing to routinely take basal insulin doses or checking for ketones for DKA prevention.

Helping patients to identify and anticipate possible treatment challenges can help to solidify the treatment relationship and possibly decrease the risk of treatment drop out. The first challenge most patients face is weight gain associated with improved blood glucose. If they have been routinely restricting insulin and are dehydrated at the start of treatment, patients need to be reassured that this weight gain is related to fluid retention, sometimes referred to as *insulin edema*. Because these patients are exquisitely sensitive to body shape and weight changes, edema just as they are starting to see blood glucose improvements can be frightening. They may reveal that this fluid retention was a precursor to relapse in the past. Once fluid levels have stabilized, the treatment team must seriously address the patients' ongoing concerns about weight gain. When patients attempt to lower their blood glucose ranges and experience unwanted weight gain, their frustrated attempts to lose the weight may again raise their risk of relapse.

Some patients report that recurrent hypoglycemia is another potential risk factor for relapse. They may fear that treating hypoglycemic reactions can trigger them into episodes of binge eating. Other patients worry about taking in the extra calories associated with treating hypoglycemia. It may be helpful to anticipate with patients that treating hypoglycemia can trigger a feeling of overeating and concerns about weight gain. To reduce this risk, it can be useful to educate patients about fast portion-controlled treatments for hypoglycemia like glucose gels or tablets, which may be less tempting to overeat.

The risks above underscore the importance of ongoing and frequent communication between the patient and the diabetes team to promote gradual blood glucose progress and try to prevent relapse into insulin restriction.

FUTURE CLINICAL RESEARCH/FILLING THE GAPS

Recent research shows that patients who endorse insulin restriction may and do get better over time.[14] The key factors that helped them achieve success have yet to be identified. To date, no treatment outcome studies have examined treatment efficacy for eating disorders in T1D. However, there are several empirically supported treatments for eating disorders without diabetes. Perhaps these treatments can be adapted to incorporate the unique aspects presented by T1D and then examined for efficacy. In a similar vein, treatments aimed at promoting family comanagement of diabetes treatment tasks and decreasing diabetes-related family conflict have already been shown to promote improved diabetes outcomes in children and teens with T1D.[29] Perhaps related approaches could be evaluated as they may be used to diminish the risk of developing eating disturbances. Finally, diabetes-specific screening tools may need to be used more routinely in practice in order to then be able to evaluate potential eating disorder prevention programs for this vulnerable population.

CONCLUSION

Eating disorders in T1D represent a women's health issue that conveys risk of severe diabetes complications—both acute and long-term. The gold standard for both eating disorders treatment and diabetes treatment involves a multidisciplinary team working in collaboration with each other and with the patient to insure that mutually agreed upon treatment goals are pursued. The risk of edema, weight gain, and hypoglycemia early in treatment may be decreased by frequently reviewing blood glucose patterns and making insulin adjustments as needed. Over the course of time and with greater medical stability, treatment goals can build toward increasing doses of insulin, more frequent blood glucose monitoring, achieving lower blood glucose ranges, and greater flexibility in meal planning. Frequent communication and support can also help to establish and reinforce realistic expectations for blood glucose improvements. Such messages may help patients to maintain motivation and decrease the risk of treatment drop out.[30] As mentioned above, treatment outcome studies as well as investigations of potential programs aimed at prevention are seriously needed. These are the future research areas one needs to target, in order to best meet the needs of patients with disordered eating and T1D.

REFERENCES

1. Colton P, Olmsted M, Daneman D, Rydall A, Rodin G: Disturbed eating behavior and eating disorders in preteen and early teenage girls with type 1 diabetes: a case-controlled study. *Diabetes Care* 27:1654–1659, 2004
2. Olmsted MP, Colton PA, Daneman D, Rydall AC, Rodin GM: Prediction of the onset of disturbed eating behavior in adolescent girls with type 1 diabetes. *Diabetes Care* 31:1978–1982, 2008
3. Polonsky WH, Anderson BJ, Lohrer PA, Aponte JE, Jacobson AM, Cole CF: Insulin omission in women with IDDM. *Diabetes Care* 17:1178–1185, 1994
4. Jones JM, Lawson ML, Daneman D, Olmsted MP, Rodin G: Eating disorders in adolescent females with and without type 1 diabetes: cross sectional study. *BMJ* 320:1563–1566, 2000
5. Peveler RC, Bryden KS, Neil HA, Fairburn CG, Mayou RA, Dunger DB, Turner HM: The relationship of disordered eating habits and attitudes to clinical outcomes in young adult females with type 1 diabetes. *Diabetes Care* 28:84–88, 2005
6. de Groot M, Anderson R, Freedland KE, Clouse RE, Lustman PJ: Association of depression and diabetes complications: a meta-analysis. *Psychosom Med* 63:619–630, 2001
7. Domargard A, Sarnblad S, Kroon M, Karlsson I, Skeppner G, Aman J: Increased prevalence of overweight in adolescent girls with type 1 diabetes mellitus. *Acta Paediatr* 88:1223–1228, 1999
8. Diabetes Control and Complications Trial Research Group: The effect of intensive treatment of diabetes on the development and progression of long-term complications in insulin-dependent diabetes mellitus. *N Engl J Med* 329:977–986, 1993
9. DCCT Research Group: Weight gain associated with intensive therapy in the diabetes control and complications trial. *Diabetes Care* 11:567–573, 1988
10. Influence of intensive diabetes treatment on body weight and composition of adults with type 1 diabetes in the Diabetes Control and Complications Trial. *Diabetes Care* 24:1711–1721, 2001
11. Thompson CJ, Cummings JF, Chalmers J, Gould C, Newton RW: How have patients reacted to the implications of the DCCT? *Diabetes Care* 19:876–879, 1996
12. Daneman D, Olmsted M, Rydall A, Maharaj S, Rodin G: Eating disorders in young women with type 1 diabetes: prevalence, problems and prevention. *Horm Res* 50:79–86, 1998
13. Markowitz JT, Lowe MR, Volkening LK, Laffel LMB: Self-reported history of overweight and its relationship to disordered eating in adolescent girls with type 1 diabetes. *Diabet Med* 26:1165–1171, 2009
14. Goebel-Fabbri AE, Anderson B, Fikkan J, Franko DL, Pearson K, Weinger K: Improvement and emergence of insulin restriction in women with type 1 diabetes. *Diabetes Care* 34:545–550, 2011
15. Colton PA, Olmsted MP, Daneman D, Rydall AC, Rodin GM: Natural history and predictors of disturbed eating behaviour in girls with type 1 diabetes. *Diabet Med* 24:424–429, 2007

16. Goebel-Fabbri AE, Fikkan J, Connell A, Vangsness L, Anderson BJ: Identification and treatment of eating disorders in women with type 1 diabetes mellitus. *Treat Endocrinol* 1:155–162, 2002
17. Young-Hyman D, Laffel L, Markowitz J, Norman J, Muir A, Lindsley K: Eating disorder risk (EDR) at time of youth T1D diagnosis (Abstract). *Diabetes* 60 (Suppl. 1):A226, 2011
18. Rydall AC, Rodin GM, Olmsted MP, Devenyi RG, Daneman D: Disordered eating behavior and microvascular complications in young women with insulin-dependent diabetes mellitus. *N Engl J Med* 336:1849–1854, 1997
19. Bryden KS, Neil A, Mayou RA, Peveler RC, Fairburn CG, Dunger DB: Eating habits, body weight, and insulin misuse: a longitudinal study of teenagers and young adults with type 1 diabetes. *Diabetes Care* 22:1956–1960, 1999
20. Verrotti A, Catino M, De Luca FA, Morgese G, Chiarelli F: Eating disorders in adolescents with type 1 diabetes mellitus. *Acta Diabetol* 36:21–25, 1999
21. Goebel-Fabbri AE, Franko DL, Pearson K, Anderson BJ, Weinger K: Insulin restriction and associated morbidity and mortality in women with type 1 diabetes. *Diabetes Care* 31:415–419, 2008
22. Svensson M, Engstrom I, Aman J: Higher drive for thinness in adolescent males with insulin-dependent diabetes mellitus compared with healthy controls. *Acta Pediatr* 92:114-117, 2003
23. Criego A, Crow S, Goebel-Fabbri AE, Kendall D, Parkin C: Eating disorders and diabetes: screening and detection. *Diabetes Spectrum* 22:143–146, 2009
24. Markowitz JT, Butler DA, Volkening LK, Antisdel JE, Anderson B, Laffel LM: Brief screening tool for disordered eating in Diabetes. *Diabetes Care* 33:495–500, 2010
25. Young-Hyman, DL, Davis, CL: Disordered eating behavior in individuals with diabetes: Importance of context, evaluation, and classification. *Diabetes Care* 33:683–689, 2010
26. Mitchell J, Pomeroy, C, Adson, DE: Managing medical complications. In *Handbook for Treatment of Eating Disorders.* Garner D, Garfinkel, PE, Eds. New York, Guilford Press, 1997, p. 383–393
27. *Diagnostic and Statistical Manual of Mental Disorders.* Washington, DC, American Psychiatric Association, 1994
28. Goebel-Fabbri AE, Polonsky W, Uplinger N, Gerkin S, Mangham D, Moxness, R, Taylor D, Parkin C: Outpatient management of eating disorders in type 1 diabetes. *Diabetes Spectrum.* 22:147–152, 2009
29. Nansel TR, Anderson BJ, Laffel LM, Simons-Morton BG, Weissberg-Benchell J, Wysocki T, Iannotti RJ, Holmbeck GN, Hood KK, Lochrie AS: A multisite trial of a clinic-integrated intervention for promoting family management of pediatric type 1 diabetes: feasibility and design. *Pediatr Diabetes* 2008 [published online before print 20 August]
30. Wolpert HA, Anderson BJ: Metabolic control matters: why is the message lost in the translation? The need for realistic goal-setting in diabetes care. *Diabetes Care* 24:1301–1303, 2001

9

Monitoring for Diabetes
I. Monitoring

David C. Klonoff, MD, FACP

INTRODUCTION

The introduction of self-monitoring of blood glucose (SMBG) methods in the early 1980s was one of the breakthroughs in monitoring diabetes control that made intensive treatment aimed at normalizing blood glucose (BG) and hemoglobin A1C (A1C) levels possible. Over the past 30 years, improvements in the accuracy, speed, and ease of use of BG meters have helped to maintain SMBG as a cornerstone of management.

The current recommendation of the ADA in their 2012 Standards of Care for SMBG is that SMBG should be carried out three or more times daily for patients using multiple insulin injections or insulin pump therapy.[1] This statement, as well as others in the current ADA standards, applies to both type 1 and type 2 diabetes (T1D and T2D). It is well known that T1D and T2D differ in certain fundamental ways, and different clinical recommendations for SMBG in individuals with T1D and T2D are indicated in many cases. Data suggest that A1C is lower in patients with T1D as BG monitoring frequency increases although there is individual variation in response.[2,3] Moreover, people with T1D have higher rates of severe hypoglycemia compared to those with T2D and may require additional continuous monitoring of glucose levels. Measures in addition to glucose, such as A1C, are usually performed every 3 months in people with T1D, to help assess adequacy of therapy. Additional tests exist, such as fructosamine, glycated albumin, 1, 5-anhydroglucitol, or advanced glycated end products, but the routine monitoring of these parameters has not been established.

SELF-MONITORING OF BG

Introduction

SMBG is an important part of the self-management of T1D. It is not an intervention but is a tool for data accumulation. SMBG has four purposes:

1. Protect a patient by allowing immediate confirmation of low or high BG levels;
2. Self-treat high or low glucose levels by adjusting therapy to reach target A1C levels;

DOI: 10.2337/9781580404785ch09s1

3. Educate about the effects of diet, exercise, and other factors on BG levels;
4. Motivate healthy behavior.

SMBG allows a patient to identify fasting, preprandial, and postprandial hyperglycemia; identify hypoglycemia; detect glycemic excursions; and get immediate feedback about the effect of food choices, activity, stress, and insulin dosing on glycemic control.[4] There are four essential principles that health care professionals need to apply when prescribing self-monitoring of BG to patients with diabetes, listed in Table 9.I.1.

SMBG is a tool for patients that empowers improved day-to-day self-care.[5] This tool provides the greatest benefits when patients and health care professionals collaborate and use the information to make treatment decisions. Patients require education on when to test and how to respond to the information. Health care professionals require education, in some cases, so they can provide their patients with useful algorithms to improve glycemic control. If a patient brings a log to a physician's office and the physician neglects to explain how this information pertains to care decisions or if the physician does not study the results, then the patient will often feel discouraged and curtail the testing frequency.[6]

SAFETY

Avoiding Transmission of Blood-Borne Viral Pathogens

Safe BG monitoring requires attention to three factors, including: *1*) avoiding transmission of blood-borne viral pathogens from patient to patient, *2*) avoiding community exposure to sharps and other medical waste, and *3*) minimizing finger trauma due to lancing. These issues affect the safety of the self-testing patients, other diabetes patients, and the entire community including individuals without diabetes.

The Centers for Disease Control (CDC) has reported 20 outbreaks of hepatitis B (HBV) due to unsafe BG monitoring practices since 1990.[7,8] These incidents involved hospitalized inpatients, long-term care patients, or assisted living facility patients. Based on these known episodes of blood-borne viruses being inadvertently transferred in settings where two or more patients are being tested by

Table 9.I.1 The Four Essential Principles when Prescribing SMBG

1. Monitoring can only improve outcomes if patients actually use the monitors as prescribed.

2. The purpose of real-time monitoring is to adjust treatment in real time—not just to enter data into a log.

3. Health care professionals must educate their patients about what to do with the monitored data.

4. To maximize benefits from SMBG, smart monitors with telemedicine capabilities can be used to store, transmit, and analyze data, recommend therapy, or send alerts.

Table 9.I.2 Settings Where Patients Receive Assisted Monitoring of Blood Glucose[9]

1.	Hospitals
2.	Nursing homes
3.	Assisted living facilities
4.	Prisons
5.	Home health care
6.	Medical practitioners' offices or clinics
7.	Diabetes research laboratories
8.	Health fairs
9.	Schools
10.	Children's camps
11.	Shelters

others, a new term was coined in 2010 to describe the practice of assisting others with BG monitoring. The new term for this practice is *assisted monitoring of blood glucose*, or AMBG.[9] Settings where patients receive AMBG and where shared paraphernalia might be used are listed in Table 9.I.2.

Subsequently, the Food and Drug Administration (FDA), CDC, and Centers for Medicare & Medicaid Services (CMS) each published guidelines recommending avoiding the use of reusable blood-lancing devices and point-of-care blood-testing devices on more than one person, as well as changing gloves between patients.[10–13] These practices are summarized in Table 9.I.3.[11]

In late 2010, the FDA specified that BG monitors must be labeled as intended for either single-patient use, multiple-patient use, or both. If a system is intended

Table 9.I.3 Recommendations by FDA and CDC for Safe Performance of AMBG[9]

1. Lancing devices should never be used for more than one person. Only auto-disabling, single-use lancing devices should be used for assisted BG monitoring in multiple patients.

2. Point-of-care blood testing devices such as BG meters should be used only on one patient and not shared. If dedicating BG meters to a single patient is not possible, the meters must be properly cleaned and disinfected after every use following the guidelines provided in device labeling.

3. Health care personnel should change gloves between patients, even if patient-dedicated testing devices and single-use self-disabling lancing devices are used.

for multiple users, then the labeling should clearly state that only auto-disabling, single-use lancing devices should be used with this system and that the monitor should be disinfected between patients.[11] In 2012, the CDC reported an increased risk for acute HBV among adults with diagnosed diabetes. This association might be due to the frequent practice of AMBG in diabetes patients. AMBG can be a risk factor for transmission of HBV if proper precautions are not taken.[14]

The Advisory Committee on Immunization Practices (ACIP) is a group of experts in fields associated with immunization who have been selected by the secretary of the U.S. Department of Health and Human Services to provide advice and guidance to the secretary, the assistant secretary for health, and the CDC on the control of vaccine-preventable diseases.[15] The outbreaks of HBV prompted the Hepatitis Vaccines Work Group of ACIP to evaluate the risk for HBV infection among all adults with diagnosed diabetes. Based on the group's findings, in 2011 ACIP recommended that all previously unvaccinated adults aged 19 through 59 years with diabetes (both T1D and T2D) be vaccinated against HBV immediately after a diagnosis of diabetes is made. ACIP also recommended that unvaccinated adults aged ≥60 years with diabetes be vaccinated at the discretion of the treating clinician after assessing their risk and the likelihood of an adequate immune response to vaccination.[16]

Avoiding Community Exposure to Sharps and Other Medical Waste

Needles, syringes, and lancets, following use, are usually incinerated or treated and disposed of in landfills.[17,18] CDC has estimated that 25.8 million people in the U.S. have diabetes (although 25% are unaware that they have it) and that 63.4% of adults with diabetes in the U.S. test at least once daily.[19,20] Assuming that children with diabetes perform SMBG at least as frequently as adults, then this means that over 12 million BG strips and lancets are used daily. CDC has also estimated that in the U.S. at least 26% of patients with diabetes use insulin.[19] Assuming two injections per patient per day, then approximately 10 million injections are administered daily to insulin users, which is an additional daily environmental burden of approximately 10 million needles and syringes.[21]

Two sharps recycling programs are the Coalition for Safe Community Needle Disposal and BD ecoFinity Life Cycle Solution (BD).[22,23] The former is a collaboration of businesses, community groups, nonprofit organizations, and government that promotes public awareness and solutions for safe disposal of needles, syringes, and other sharps in the community. The latter is a joint private program between BD and Waste Management, which recycles medical waste and uses the material to manufacture new sharps containers. In 2011, the FDA launched a new website for patients and caregivers on the safe disposal of needles and other sharps (http://www.fda.gov/MedicalDevices/ProductsandMedicalProcedures/HomeHealthandConsumer/ConsumerProducts/Sharps/ucm20025647.htm).[24] The website is intended to help people understand the public health risks created by improperly disposing of used sharps and learn how users should safely dispose of them.

Minimizing Finger Trauma Due to Lancing

Alternate site testing to obtain blood from the forearms, thighs, and palms has been proposed because these methods cause less pain.[25] Sampling from alternate sites, compared to finger-stick testing, tends to produce less blood volume, but many modern monitors can provide readings from small volumes. This procedure should not be performed on the forearms or thighs if a self-monitored BG test is needed immediately after a meal or after exercise, if hypoglycemia is suspected, or if rapid fluctuations in glycemia are suspected because rapidly changing BG levels might lag at an alternate site.[26–28]

A study of lancing device features reported six factors that may mitigate pain, which are listed in Table 9.I.4.[29] In addition to pain, poor wound healing will decrease motivation for self-testing of BG. Both pain and poor wound healing can be decreased if patients can receive instruction about proper lancing from a diabetes educator.[30] Patients might choose not to switch to a dedicated stand-alone, so-called pain-free lancing system because of the added cost of switching to a new product instead of reusing lancets and the inconvenience of carrying a separate device.[31]

Analytical Accuracy

BG monitors can be classified based upon their analytical accuracy or their clinical accuracy. Two analytical performance standards for BG monitors are expected to be revised and released shortly: *1*) International Organization for Standardization (ISO) 15197 for in vitro diagnostic systems specifies requirements for BG monitoring systems, and *2*) Clinical Laboratory Standards Institute (CLSI) POCT 12-A3: Point of Care Blood Glucose Testing in Acute and Chronic Care Facilities; Approved Guideline–Third Edition (formerly C30-A2). The FDA currently approves BG monitors if they meet the analytical accuracy criteria as defined by ISO 15197. ISO specifies that for approval of a point-of-care BG monitor, 95% of glucose results must be for glucose <75 mg/dl to within 15 mg/dl of reference and for glucose >75 mg/dl to within 20% of reference.[32] The FDA has also announced plans to revise its own guidelines soon for analytical accuracy of BG monitors, and these may or may not be the same as the upcoming ISO standards.

Table 9.I.4 Six Factors That Mitigate Lancing Pain[27]

1. Shallow lancet penetration
2. Fast lancing speed
3. Sharp tip and cutting edges
4. Smooth lancet surface
5. Steady motion (no vibrations/jolts)
6. Skin fixation at lancet interface

Clinical Accuracy

Another metric for assessing accuracy of a BG monitor defines clinical accuracy. Each data point (representing both the BG monitor value and the reference value) can be classified into a performance zone, which permits data sets to be defined on the basis of the percentage of data points which fall into each category. Clinical accuracy metrics are intended to describe outlier data points in terms of whether their degree of inaccuracy will lead to untoward clinical consequences and if so, the severity of the consequences.[33,34] These error grids assign a performance zone for each data point based on the effect on the clinical action and if so then how the clinical outcome will be affected.[35] Error grids are intended to allow interpretation of the seriousness of outlier data points, which result in altered clinical action, and for regulatory classification of the performance of specific BG monitors as clinically acceptable or unacceptable.

At this time, regulatory agencies have not formally proposed clinical scenarios for applying error grids or standards for defining what percentage of data points must fall into the highest performance zone or zones to be defined as providing adequate clinical accuracy.[36] This type of tool could potentially be used in the future by regulatory agencies to identify highly performing monitors with respect to clinical accuracy or determine whether a specific BG monitor should be allowed to enter or remain on the market.

Effectiveness of SMBG in T1D

SMBG is a basic part of the treatment of T1D. This tool for monitoring patients was part of the intensive intervention arm of the DCCT and since then it has been accepted as a basic management component of T1D. Only a single randomized controlled trial has assessed the effect on A1C of a structured intervention focused on SMBG in T1D patients. In that Norwegian study, A1C levels in the intervention and control groups were similar: 8.65 ± 0.10 in the intervention group and 8.61 ± 0.09 in the control group. The control group was stable, with comparable A1C values at study start and study end, 8.61 vs. 8.84% ($P = 0.12$). In the intervention group, the A1C fell from 8.65 to 8.2%. At study end at 9 months the significant decrease in A1C in the intervention group ($P <0.05$) was net 0.6% lower compared with the change in the control group ($P <0.05$)[37]. Several observational studies have linked SMBG testing with lower A1C levels, but there is a possibility in these types of studies the subjects who were adherent to follow SMBG recommendations were also the same types of subjects who were engaged with many other healthy lifestyle recommendations.[38-41] Only a randomized controlled trial can separate the effects of SMBG being an epiphenomenon of widely increased adherence. The practice is so well accepted that it will be difficult to design any ethical future trials of SMBG in T1D to include non-SMBG.

Assessing Glycemic Control with SMBG and A1C Measurements

A1C is an important measure of mean glycemic exposure over the previous 2–3 months, but this analyte does not provide information about glucose levels at specific times of day. SMBG adds valuable information to A1C levels because it indicates trends in BG levels before meals, after meals, at bedtime, and in the middle of the night, postmeal BG levels, and day-to-day changes in glucose levels. Even with acceptable mean glycemic levels as assessed by A1C, recurrent episodes of hypoglycemia or hyperglycemia can only be elucidated by glucose monitoring.[42] SMBG, unlike A1C levels, provides information that allows patients to immediately adjust their food intake, exercise pattern, or insulin dosage. To maximize the benefit of SMBG as an adjunct to A1C testing, the health care professional should provide patients with a structured format containing the appropriate times to test and algorithmic responses to various BG levels.[6] It is also valuable to review patients' techniques for testing because analytical errors in testing can lead to inaccurate readings.

Emerging Technologies for SMBG

Electrochemistry. BG monitors that are currently used break down glucose molecules and then measure the current that is generated from electrons that are liberated in the reaction using electrochemistry or colorimetry. First-generation monitors use oxygen as a catalytic mediator. This type of monitor can have accuracy problems if the patient is hypoxemic. Second-generation monitors use synthetic mediators to mediate electron transfer. With this type of monitor, the mediator can diffuse away from the electrode, leaving oxygen to be the reactive species, as with a first-generation monitor. Third-generation monitors permit direct electron transfer between the enzyme and the electrode monitors. With this type of monitor there can be excessively slow diffusion from glucose across the enzyme molecule to the electrode.[43] Nonenzymatic methods for measuring glucose are under development. These are potential fourth-generation monitors that promote direct conversion of glucose by glucose adsorbing to a metal[44] or carbon (such as diamond or nanotubule material) electrode in the absence of an enzyme.[45] Nanoporous materials with high surface-to-volume ratios are facilitating advances in glucose sensor technology.

Fluorescence glucose sensing. Implanted fluorescing nano-optodes are being developed for subcutaneous injection, like tattoos, to fluoresce in proportion to the ambient interstitial fluid glucose concentration following interrogation with an ultraviolet light source. The fluorescence glucose-sensing sensors can be tuned to show the greatest changes in signal at any chosen level, including in the hypoglycemic range, which would make this technology potentially very sensitive for measuring glucose levels very accurately in the presence of high or low glucose concentrations. It is not known how long a batch of fluorescing molecules will maintain their fluorescent response proportionate to the glucose concentration.[46]

Noninvasive monitoring. Noninvasive optical methods are being developed to measure glucose using either optical spectroscopic measurement of skin,[47,48] rotation of polarized light in the anterior chamber,[49] measurement of exhaled volatile organic compounds in breath,[50] or glucose measurement in tears.[51] A novel approach to measuring glucose qualitatively could involve measuring the physiological response to hypoglycemia irrespective of the absolute quantitative glucose concentration. Hypoglycemia-associated EEG changes could be detected by an automated mathematical algorithm, which is being developed for subjects exposed to insulin-induced hypoglycemia; the EEG changes usually occurred before cognitive testing could detect the hypoglycemia.[52] A recognition algorithm for an EKG-enabled detection system is being developed to serve as an adjunct method for noninvasive overnight monitoring for hypoglycemia events in young people with T1D.[53] These EEG and EKG methods measure the brain's and heart's response to hypoglycemia and can allow correction of hypoglycemia at an early stage, before a BG measurement would be clearly diagnostic of end-organ hypoglycemia.

All of the proposed noninvasive methods will need to be subjected to intensive testing during periods of both stable and dynamically changing glucose levels. Studies will be needed of their performance ranges, lag times during periods of rapid fluctuations, and accuracy in the presence of high concentrations of analytes known to produce interference with electrochemical methods.

A1C

Introduction

A1C is a stable hemoglobin variant formed by a nonenzymatic attachment of glucose to the N-terminal valine of the β chain of hemoglobin.[54] A1C is the best measure of mean glycemia over the previous 3 months and is the best predictive marker for the risk of microvascular complications of diabetes. Many quality assurance programs use A1C to assess the quality of diabetes care. In 2009 an international expert committee appointed by the ADA, the EASD (European Association for the Study of Diabetes), and the IDF (International Diabetes Federation) concluded that the A1C test can be used to diagnose diabetes with a cut point of ≥6.5% for the diagnosis.[55]

Although the average lifespan of an erythrocyte is approximately 120 days, a large change in mean BG is accompanied by a change in A1C within a matter of 1–2 weeks, not 3–4 months. Recent glycemic levels contribute relatively more to the A1C level than earlier glycemic levels. The mean BG level in the 30 days immediately preceding the blood sampling (days 0–30) contributes approximately 50% to the final A1C level; however, the mean BG level of days 90–120 contributes only ~10%.[56]

Racial and Ethnic Differences

A1C levels may be impacted by factors other than mean glycemia. Increasing age and smoking are associated with higher A1C levels.[57] Racial or ethnic differences in A1C levels have been observed in three populations of subjects of multiple racial and ethnic backgrounds both before and after adjusting for factors that can affect glycemia. These three populations were: *1)* participants in the Third National Health and Nutrition Examination Survey (NHANES) who had not been treated for diabetes, *2)* subjects with impaired glucose tolerance in the Diabetes Prevention Program, and *3)* and subjects with relatively poorly controlled T2D whose baseline A1C exceeded 7.0% in the DURABLE study of Basal vs. Lispro Mix 75/25 Insulin Efficacy Trial.[58–60] The mean A1C level that was measured for each racial or ethnic group in these three studies is presented in Table 9.I.5. In all three studies, both before and after adjusting for variables that might be related to the differences in A1C, the mean A1C remained higher in non-Caucasian groups than in Caucasians.[58–60]

Another analysis of NHANES data showed that prevalence of retinopathy (the complication on which A1C and glucose cut points for diabetes were based) begins to increase at lower A1C levels in blacks than in whites.[61] An analysis of the Atherosclerosis Risk in Communities Study suggested that African Americans did indeed have higher levels of A1C when controlled for fasting plasma glucose; however, they also had higher levels of fructosamine and glycated albumin, and lower levels of 1,5-dihydroglucitol (which is inversely related to postprandial hyperglycemia). These authors suggested that African Americans (who are at higher risk of diabetes complications) truly have higher glycemia than whites.[62]

Any condition that shortens erythrocyte survival or decreases mean erythrocyte age may falsely lower A1C test results. Acute blood loss and hemolytic anemia are associated with this phenomenon. Vitamins C and E therapy can also falsely lower test results, possibly by inhibiting hemoglobin glycation; iron deficiency anemia falsely increases test results.[63]

Glycation Gap

A *glycation gap* is the difference between the mean glycemia described by A1C and that predicted from fructosamine levels. This measure has been described and attributed to fast glycation by some individuals or members of some groups

Table 9.I.5 Racial and Ethnic Differences in A1C Levels

Racial/Ethnic Group	No Diabetes (n = 7,974)[53]	Impaired Glucose Tolerance (n = 3,819)[54]	Moderately Poorly Controlled T2D (n = 2,094)[55]
Caucasian	4.93	5.80	8.9
Hispanic	5.05	5.89	9.4
Asian	—	5.96	9.2
Native American	—	5.96	9.4*
African-American	5.16	6.19	9.0

In all three populations after adjusting for variables that might be related to the differences in A1C, the mean A1C was higher in the non-Caucasian groups than in Caucasians. (No diabetes: *P* <0.01; impaired glucose tolerance: *P* <0.001; moderately poorly controlled diabetes: *P* <0.002.)

* = Other races including Native American, Inuit, and mixed racial

such that these people will have higher A1C levels and more complications than those who glycate at slower rates. The concept of a glycation gap supports the idea that another factor, besides the nonenzymatic attachment of glucose to hemoglobin, reflects the mean glucose concentration over the preceding 8–12 weeks and correlates with the risk for developing vascular complications in diabetes.[64] The best method to measure glycemia can only be determined when an in vitro test of glycation will be developed. In addition, a similar concept to the glycation gap is the *hemoglobin glycation index*, which is the difference between the observed A1C and the A1C level that is predicted from mean BG levels. Whether these two alternate (to A1C) measures of glycation are independent predictors of the risks of microvascular and cardiovascular complications is unclear, and these tests are not widely accepted currently.[65] Development of a new reference test of tissue glycation will help document differences in A1C levels between individuals with similar mean glycemic levels that are not accounted for by corresponding differences in glycemia but instead might be due to different glycabilities of hemoglobin between individuals. Proof of variable glycability as a risk factor might then lead to new therapies for susceptible individuals to prevent vascular complications of diabetes.

Hemoglobinopathies

All known human genetic variation data for hemoglobin has been collected and documented in the HbVar database of hemoglobin variants and thalassemia mutations.[66] Over 1,100 hemoglobin variants have been identified to date.[67] Many of these hemoglobinopathies can cause false results in A1C determinations depending on the type of assay that is used, including those that are the most frequently encountered: HbC, HbS, HbE or HbD trait, and elevated levels of HbF.[68,69] Hemoglobinopathies can cause false elevations or false depressions of A1C levels. However, manufacturers of A1C assays have responded by developing assays that are not significantly affected by the most common hemoglobin variants; 95% of assays in the U.S. now fall into this category (www.ngsp.org/interf.asp). For individuals with hemoglobinopathies and altered red cell survival time, one can measure fructosamine or glycated albumin (see below).

Correlation of A1C with Mean Glycemia

The A1c-Derived Average Glucose Study Group (ADAG) suggested that A1C can be translated into an estimated average glucose value for most adult patients. ADAG developed a linear regression analysis equation linking A1C and AG values AG (mg/dl) = 28.7 × A1C – 46.7, R(2) = 0.84, (*P* < 0.0001) to calculation of an estimated average glucose (eAG) for A1C values. The relationship between the A1C and estimated average glucose levels can be found in Table 9.I.6.

The equation was robust across subgroups stratified by age, gender, diabetes type, race or ethnicity, and smoking status. The regression equation for A1C and average glucose (AG) using only the CGM results to calculate AG was AG by

Table 9.I.6 Relationship between Measured A1C Level and Estimated Average Glucose (eAG) Level[65]

A1C (%)	eAG (mg/dl)	eAG (mmol/l)
5	97	5.4
6	126	7.0
7	154	8.6
8	183	10.2
9	212	11.8
10	240	13.4
11	269	14.9
12	298	16.5

CGM = 28.0 × A1C − 36.9 (R^2 = 0.82, $P < 0.0001$); the regression equation for A1C and AG using only the seven-point finger-stick results to calculate AG was AG by 7-POINT = 29.1 × A1C − 50.7 (R^2 = 0.82, $P < 0.0001$). The difference between these two formulae for the two slopes and the two intercepts combined was not statistically significant (P = 0.11).[70] Other studies using CGM data as the basis of calculating average glucose have not found such a robust relationship and have concluded that this equation introduces unwanted error. The ADAG study group went on to demonstrate that A1C and mean BG show stronger associations with cardiovascular disease risk factors than do postprandial glycemia or glucose variability in persons with diabetes, which is a blow to the concept that variability is a key independent risk factor for adverse outcomes, although this study did not account for cardiovascular outcomes, but rather risk factors.[71] A study of the relationship between AG and A1C using CGM in children showed much more variability than was seen in the ADAG study.[72]

Reporting Methods of A1C

There are currently three choices for reporting A1C. First is the traditional method that expresses A1C as a percentage to one decimal point of total hemoglobin, based on linear regression calculations. This method is popular in the U.S. and uses the same numbers that were used in the Diabetes Complications and Control Study. Second is the Standard International (SI) Unit method that expresses A1C as a ratio of millimoles of hemoglobin A1C to moles of hemoglobin A. This method is popular in Europe. Third is a compromise method that uses neither the U.S. units nor the European units and expresses A1C as an estimated average glucose level. This method is not popular anywhere but is accepted for use as a patient education tool. Many countries are currently reporting A1C in both percent and millimole per mole units, and at this time it is not clear whether an international consensus will be reached on a reporting standard.[73] The master equations that link the U.S. (National Glycohemoglobin Standardization Program [NGSP]) and international (International Federation of Clinical Chemistry [IFCC]) methods are: NGSP (in percent) = (0.09148 × IFCC) + 2.152 and IFCC (in mmol A1C/mol Hb) = (10.93 × NGSP) – 23.50.[74]

NATIONAL GLYCOHEMOGLOBIN STANDARDIZATION PROGRAM

The NGSP began in 1996. At that time, right after the DCCT study was completed, there was a lack of comparability of A1C test results among methods and laboratories and that represented an obstacle to implementing guidelines for diabetes care. The NGSP was formed to enable laboratories to report DCCT/UKPDS-traceable GHb/A1C results. NGSP also works with the College of American Pathologists to develop proficiency-testing requirements for A1C testing. Finally, because the IFCC has developed a reference system for A1C that facilitates traceability, the NGSP works with IFCC to maintain traceability to the IFCC network via ongoing sample comparisons.[75]

FRUCTOSAMINE, GLYCATED ALBUMIN, AND 1,5-ANHYDROGLUCITOL

Three additional analytes besides A1C (fructosamine, glycated albumin, and 1,5-anhydroglucitol) have been touted as useful for reflecting shorter term changes in glycemia than A1C can detect. These tests have not been validated for long-term outcomes as has A1C, and there is little information in the literature about how to titrate patients on the basis of changes in these three analytes. Evidence suggesting the usefulness of all three in specific situations, including a small amount of evidence of a correlation with long-term complications, can nevertheless be found in the literature.[76]

The protein that circulates in the highest concentration in blood is hemoglobin. A1C represents glycated hemoglobin molecules. Other circulating plasma proteins, such as fructosamine, can also be glycated. The largest component of plasma proteins is albumin. An assay for glycated albumin measures the principal component of fructosamine. Serum fructosamine has been advocated as an alternate test to A1C when hemoglobinopathies or disorders of red blood survival are present, to obtain a look at mean glycemia free from interferences present in the A1C method. Because the lifespan of albumin and other molecules is much shorter than that of a red blood cell, a RBC, fructosamine can reflect changes in glycemia over a period of 2–3 weeks. Nevertheless, fructosamine has been disappointing to date in its reproducibility and its correlation to mean glycemia. Other than occasionally in gestational diabetes, this test is seldom ordered.[77]

Serum glycated albumin is the main constituent of fructosamine and in theory this assay would be more specific and useful than fructosamine, especially in states where glycemia is fluctuating rapidly and where A1C readings are not expected to be reliable. At this time there is no standardized reference method for this analyte. In states of rapid albumin turnover or decreased albumin levels, there is no generally agreed upon method for correcting the level of this analyte. This test might prove useful for following mean glycemia in patients with chronic renal failure.[78]

1,5-anhydroglucitol (1,5-AG) is a marker of very short-term glycemic control. This monosaccharide molecule competes with glucose for reabsorption in the kidneys. 1,5-AG is rapidly depleted when BG levels exceed the renal threshold for glucosuria. 1,5-AG detects rapid changes in frequency and severity of elevated glucose levels (but not hypoglycemic episodes) over a period of about one week, which is too short a time span for A1C, fructosamine, or glycated albumin to change by much. Postprandial BG has been claimed to be an independent risk factor for macrovascular complications, even in the presence of normal A1C levels. 1,5-AG has been proposed as an appropriate indicator to detect and screen for postprandial hyperglycemia. There is a concern that changes in the dietary intake of this molecule could affect its circulating levels.[79] Recently, a comparison of A1C, fructosamine, glycated albumin, and 1,5-AG demonstrated that all four measures of mean glycemia had a similar degree of correlation with CGM-measured mean glucose (absolute r value = 0.50 – 0.56) and with hyperglycemic area under the curve below 180 mg/dl, which bodes well for these three new analytes to possibly become well-accepted.[80]

OTHER MARKERS

Advanced glycation end products (AGEs) have been associated with the development of diabetic complications. Dermal AGEs might be sensitive biomarkers for the risk of developing diabetes and related complications. AGEs can fluoresce when they are exposed to infrared light and can be measured noninvasively by optical spectroscopy. A device to measure dermal fluorescence might be useful to identify people who are at increased risk of developing diabetes or its complications and such technology is being developed.[81] Skin fluorescence in women with gestational diabetes does not differ from that of normal pregnancy probably because there is insufficient time to accumulate AGEs in gestational diabetes.[82]

Many have hypothesized that glycemic variability is linked to the development of vascular complications in diabetes. There is no generally agreed upon metric for glycemic variability. The greater the mean level of glycemia, the greater the amount of glycemic variability that is present. Distinguishing the effect of mean glycemia from the isolated effect of variability has not been possible to date, but the correlation of large numbers of BG levels along with a yet-to-be-developed formula will potentially lead to a measurement that can become a target for treatment to decrease the incidence of complications in diabetes. For glycemic variability to become an independent treatment target two gaps must be filled. First, there must be a demonstration that glycemic variability is mechanistically linked to a measurable physiologic change, which is in turn linked to either a complication, a surrogate endpoint for a complication, or even a risk factor for a complication. Second, an intervention will need to be developed and experimentally proven to reduce or eliminate the physiological abnormality which is linked to glycemic variability.

TELEMEDICINE

Data management systems are now being increasingly used to manage and preserve SMBG and other types of physiological data as well as to provide and analyze this data for health care professionals. Four trends in automatic data management from BG monitors are presented in Table 9.I.7.

It is expected that in the future data from a BG monitor will be sent automatically, directly, and wirelessly to a server and then back to the smart phone. Software applications for smart phones are becoming increasingly ubiquitous.[83] Hardware extensions to smart phones will extend the monitoring capabilities of these devices to a point at which they might become an essential part of diabetes treatment. Remote monitoring will also be applicable to other types of remote sensors of physiological monitors, and the measurements will be combined into a multimeasure report or even a single blended metric for viewing and taking action. Future monitoring devices will need to be compatible with each other to avoid electromagnetic interference and data dropout.[84] As more and more devices become connected with the web, medical monitors will be part of this technological revolution.

FUTURE CLINICAL RESEARCH/FILLING THE GAPS

The gaps in clinical research for monitoring exist in the understanding of:

1. How can we best define glycemic variability (GV)?
2. What is the clinical significance of developing high GV?

Table 9.I.7 Trends in Automatic Telemetric Management of Glucose Data

1. All medical devices are synchronized with an atomic clock.
2. Data is automatically time stamped.
3. Data is automatically stored.
4. Glucose data is assimilated into a profile containing other real-time physiological data.
5. Data is analyzed and displayed containing tables, graphics.
6. Data is automatically transmitted to the health care provider, the patient, and/or caregivers.
7. Data is accompanied by specific management recommendations delivered through decision support software.

3. How can GV be decreased using SMBG as a tool without causing hypoglycemia?
4. Does lowering the GV levels improve clinical outcomes?

There are also knowledge gaps regarding other analytes for monitoring diabetes, in that we need additional information about:

Hemoglobin A1C

1. Which factors, other than mean glycemia, lead to glycation?
2. How can hemoglobin variants, which may interfere with hemoglobin A1C assays and lead to falsely elevated or depressed A1C levels, be identified in the routine assessment of mean glycemia?
3. Some people may have higher A1Cs than others for the same level of mean glycemia. Should there be different A1C standards for various ages, racial, and ethnic populations? Or should there be a one-size-fits-all treatment target?

Other Analytes

1. What is the role of fructosamine and glycated albumin, and how do we test for these analytes? The role of these analytes in diabetes management is currently not defined except in the presence of hemoglobinopathies or red blood cell disorders.
2. The role of the shorter duration (vs. A1C) measures of mean glycemia has not been determined for clinical situations. For example, these tests provide unique information, but the utility of prognostic test results that change every few weeks is questionable since the typical follow-up visit for diabetes patients is every few months. Health care professionals would have to review the test results more often with their patients. Otherwise, they would need a structured response to out-of-target mean glycemic values. More frequent mean glycemia results may be too much information for health care providers to assimilate. In addition, the increased frequency of patient contact might be too time consuming or costly for the health care professional and for the patient.

How to Fill the Gaps?

The knowledge gaps for the role or benefits of any glycemic tests that provide real-time results and enable real-time responses by a patient (such as SMBG, real-time CGM, or home testing of A1C) will require clinical trials with clearly defined clinical endpoints. Self-tested analytes, which by definition is a test of a behavioral intervention, will require randomized controlled trials using cluster randomization of sites rather than the more commonly used individual randomization of subjects.[4] For example, if an intervention subject is directly exposed to a control subject in the same waiting room or indirectly exposed by sharing the same treating professional staff, then the benefits of a robust intervention may inadvertently bias the control subject. The control subject might then increase testing frequency so that the difference between treatment and control groups will be washed out by this contamination of controls. In cluster randomization trials, controls and intervention subjects do not meet. Their caregivers cannot be biased by positive results in intervention subjects (e.g., occasionally encourage controls to partake in the study intervention with a greater frequency). If the investigator knows the intervention that the subject is receiving (e.g., active intervention, base treatment, or dummy treatment or placebo), then there is a possibility that the investigator will treat intervention subjects differently from control subjects. The inadvertent treatment biases may cause outcome differences between the two groups, separate from the actual intervention.

CONCLUSION

Monitoring A1C and other analytes provides vital information to patients and health care professionals on short-term and long-term physiologic perturbations that require treatment adjustments. These tests provide the most benefit in guiding management if the information is collected and used in a structured format. The advantages of glycemic control are now well established. Monitoring glucose and other analytes permits patients to stay on track and achieve target levels of glycemia. Even as standards of care for monitoring are constantly evolving, the capabilities of current monitors are also constantly increasing. This cycle of new technology followed by outcomes research to fill the knowledge gaps, again followed by newer technology, promises to usher in a new era of diabetes technology to benefit those living with diabetes.

REFERENCES

1. American Diabetes Association: Standards of medical care in diabetes: 2012. *Diabetes Care* 35 (Suppl. 1):S11–S63, 2012
2. Ziegler R, Heidtmann B, Hilgard D, Hofer S, Rosenbauer J, Holl R; for the DPV-Wiss-Initiative: Frequency of SMBG correlates with HbA1c and acute complications in children and adolescents with type 1 diabetes. *Pediatr Diabetes* 12:11–17, 2011
3. Karter AJ, Parker MM, Moffet HH, Spence MM, Chan J, Ettner SL, Selby JV: Longitudinal study of new and prevalent use of self-monitoring of blood glucose. *Diabetes Care* 29:1757–1763, 2006
4. Klonoff DC, Bergenstal R, Blonde L, Boren SA, Church TS, Gaffaney J, Jovanovic L, Kendall DM, Kollman C, Kovatchev BP, Leippert C, Owens DR, Polonsky WH, Reach G, Renard E, Riddell MC, Rubin RR, Schnell O, Siminiero LM, Vigersky RA, Wilson DM, Wollitzer AO: Consensus report of the coalition for clinical research–self-monitoring of blood glucose. *J Diabetes Sci Technol* 2:1030–1053, 2008
5. Chatzimarkakis J: Why patients should be more empowered: a European perspective on lessons learned in the management of diabetes. *J Diabetes Sci Technol* 4:1570–1573, 2010
6. Klonoff DC, Blonde L, Cembrowski G, Chacra AR, Charpentier G, Colagiuri S, Dailey G, Gabbay RA, Heinemann L, Kerr D, Nicolucci A, Polonsky

W, Schnell O, Vigersky R, Yale JF: Consensus report: the current role of self-monitoring of blood glucose in non-insulin-treated type 2 diabetes. *J Diabetes Sci Technol* 5:1529–1548, 2011

7. Thompson ND, Perz JF: Eliminating the blood: ongoing outbreaks of hepatitis B virus infection and the need for innovative glucose monitoring technologies. *J Diabetes Sci Technol* 3:283–288, 2009

8. Counard CA, Perz JF, Linchangco PC, Christiansen D, Ganova-Raeva L, Xia G, Jones S, Vernon MO: Acute hepatitis B outbreaks related to fingerstick blood glucose monitoring in two assisted living facilities. *J Am Geriatr Soc* 58:306–311, 2010

9. Klonoff DC, Perz JF: Assisted monitoring of blood glucose: special safety needs for a new paradigm in testing glucose. *J Diabetes Sci Technol* 4:1027–1031, 2010

10. Food and Drug Administration: Fingerstick devices to obtain blood specimens: initial communication: risk of transmitting bloodborne pathogens. Reusable fingerstick (blood lancing) devices and point of care (POC) blood testing devices (e.g., blood glucose meters, PT/INR anticoagulation meters, cholesterol testing devices). Available at http://www.fda.gov/Safety/MedWatch/SafetyInformation/SafetyAlertsforHumanMedicalProducts/ucm224135.htm. Accessed 11 October 2012

11. Letter to manufacturers of blood glucose monitoring systems listed with the FDA. Available at http://www.fda.gov/MedicalDevices/Productsand MedicalProcedures/InVitroDiagnostics/ucm227935.htm. Accessed 11 October 2012

12. Infection prevention during blood glucose monitoring and insulin administration. Available at http://www.cdc.gov/injectionsafety/blood-glucose-monitoring.html. Accessed 16 June 2012

13. Point of care devices and infection control in nursing homes. Available at http://www.cms.gov/Medicare/Provider-Enrollment-and-Certification/SurveyCertificationGenInfo/downloads/SCLetter10_28.pdf. Accessed 11 October 2012

14. Reilly ML, Schillie SF, Smith E, Poissant T, Vonderwahl CW, Gerard K, Baumgartner J, Mercedes L, Sweet K, Muleta D, Zaccaro DJ, Klevens RM, Murphy TV: Increased risk of acute hepatitis B among adults with diagnosed diabetes mellitus. *J Diabetes Sci Technol* 2012. In press

15. Advisory Committee on Immunization Practices (ACIP). Available at http://www.cdc.gov/vaccines/acip/about.html. Accessed 11 October 2012

16. Centers for Disease Control and Prevention (CDC): Use of hepatitis B vaccination for adults with diabetes mellitus: recommendations of the Advisory Committee on Immunization Practices (ACIP). *MMWR Morb Mortal Wkly Rep* 60:1709–1711, 2011

17. Pfützner A, Musholt PB, Malmgren-Hansen B, Nilsson NH, Forst T: Analysis of the environmental impact of insulin infusion sets based on loss of resources with waste. *J Diabetes Sci Technol* 5:843–847, 2011

18. Krisiunas E: Waste disposal in the 21st century and diabetes technology: a little coffee (cup) or beer (can) with that insulin infusion (set). *J Diabetes Sci Technol* 5:851–852, 2011

19. National diabetes fact sheet, 2011. Available at http://www.cdc.gov/diabetes/pubs/pdf/ndfs_2011.pdf. Accessed 11 October 2012

20. Self-monitoring of blood glucose among adults with diabetes—United States, 1997–2006. *MMWR* Morb Mortal Wkly Rep 56:1133–1137, 2007. Available at http://www.cdc.gov/mmwr/preview/mmwrhtml/mm5643a3.htm#tab1. Accessed 11 October 2012

21. Klonoff DC: Improving the safety of blood glucose monitoring. *J Diabetes Sci Technol* 5:1307–1311, 2011

22. Available at http://www.safeneedledisposal.org. Accessed 28 October 2012

23. Available at http://www.bd.com/ecofinity. Accessed 28 October 2012

24. Available at http://www.fda.gov/MedicalDevices/ProductsandMedical Procedures/HomeHealthandConsumer/ConsumerProducts/Sharps/ucm20025647.htm. Accessed 11 October 2012

25. Jacoby JM: An analysis of alternate site tests to improve patient compliance with self-monitoring of blood glucose. *J Diabetes Sci Technol* 4:911–912, 2010

26. Ellison JM, Stegmann JM, Colner SL, Michael RH, Sharma MK, Ervin KR, Horwitz DL: Rapid changes in postprandial blood glucose produce concentration differences at finger, forearm, and thigh sampling sites. *Diabetes Care* 25:961–964, 2002

27. Kempe KC, Budd D, Stern M, Ellison JM, Saari LA, Adiletto CA, Olin B, Price DA, Horwitz DL: Palm glucose readings compared with fingertip readings under steady and dynamic glycemic conditions, using the OneTouch Ultra Blood Glucose Monitoring System. *Diabetes Technol Ther* 7:916–926, 2005

28. Rosenthal M: Alternate-site testing. Haven't got time for the pain. *Diabetes Self Manag* 28:26–27, 2011

29. Kocher S, Tshiananga JK, Koubek R: Comparison of lancing devices for self-monitoring of blood glucose regarding lancing pain. *J Diabetes Sci Technol* 3:1136–1143, 2009

30. Heinemann L, Boecker D: Lancing: quo vadis? *J Diabetes Sci Technol* 5:966–981, 2011

31. Lekarcyk J, Ghiloni S: Analysis of the comparison of lancing devices for self-monitoring of blood glucose regarding lancing pain. *J Diabetes Sci Technol* 3:1144–1145, 2009

32. 24 ISO 15197. Available at http://www.iso.org/iso/iso_catalogue/catalogue_tc/catalogue_detail.htm?csnumber=54976. Accessed 11 October 2012

33. Clarke WL, Cox D, Gonder-Frederick LA, Carter W, Pohl SL: Evaluating clinical accuracy of systems for self-monitoring of blood glucose. *Diabetes Care* 10:622–628, 1987

34. Parkes JL, Slatin SL, Pardo S, Ginsberg BH: A new consensus error grid to evaluate the clinical significance of inaccuracies in the measurement of blood glucose. *Diabetes Care* 23:1143–1148, 2000

35. Klonoff DC: The need for clinical accuracy guidelines for blood glucose monitors. *J Diabetes Sci Technol* 6:1–4, 2012

36. Krouwer JS, Cembrowski GS: Towards more complete specifications for acceptable analytical performance: a plea for error grid analysis. *Clin Chem Lab Med* 49:1127–1130, 2011

37. Skeie S, Kristensen GBB, Carlsen S, Sandberg S: Self-monitoring of blood glucose in type 1 diabetes patients with insufficient metabolic control: focused self-monitoring of blood glucose intervention can lower glycated hemoglobin A1C. *J Diabetes Sci Technol* 3:83–88, 2009
38. Strowig SM, Raskin P: Improved glycemic control in intensively treated type 1 diabetic patients using blood glucose meters with storage capability and computer-assisted analyses. *Diabetes Care* 21:1694–1698, 1998
39. Levine BS, Anderson BJ, Butler DA, Antisdel JE, Brackett J, Laffel LM: Predictors of glycemic control and short-term adverse outcomes in youth with type 1 diabetes. *J Pediatr* 139:197–203, 2001
40. Haller MI, Stalvey MS, Silverstein JH: Predictors of control of diabetes: monitoring may be the key. *J Pediatr* 144: 660–661, 2004
41. Karter AJ, Ackerson LM, Darbinian JA, D'Agostino RB Jr, Ferrara A, Liu J, Selby JV: Self-monitoring of blood glucose levels and glycemic control: the Northern California Kaiser Permanente Diabetes registry. *Am J Med* 111:1–9, 2001
42. Dailey G: Assessing glycemic control with self-monitoring of blood glucose and hemoglobin A(1c) measurements. *Mayo Clin Proc* 82:229–235; quiz 236, 2007
43. Toghill KE, Compton RG: Electrochemical non-enzymatic glucose sensors: a perspective and an evaluation. *Int J Electrochem Sci* 5:1246–1301, 2010
44. Zhang Y, Su L, Manuzzi D, de los Monteros HV, Jia W, Huo D, Hou C, Lei Y: Ultrasensitive and selective non-enzymatic glucose detection using copper nanowires. *Biosens Bioelectron* 31:426–432, 2012
45. Bo X, Ndamanisha JC, Bai J, Guo L: Nonenzymatic amperometric sensor of hydrogen peroxide and glucose based on Pt nanoparticles/ordered mesoporous carbon nanocomposite. *Talanta* 82:85–91, 2010
46. Balaconis MK, Billingsley K, Dubach MJ, Cash KJ, Clark HA: The design and development of fluorescent nano-optodes for in vivo glucose monitoring. *J Diabetes Sci Technol* 5:68–75, 2011
47. Alexeeva NV, Arnold MA: Impact of tissue heterogeneity on noninvasive near-infrared glucose measurements in interstitial fluid of rat skin. *J Diabetes Sci Technol* 4:1041–1054, 2010
48. Dingari NC, Barman I, Kang JW, Kong CR, Dasari RR, Feld MS: Wavelength selection-based nonlinear calibration for transcutaneous blood glucose sensing using Raman spectroscopy. *J Biomed Opt* 16:087009, 2011
49. Purvinis G, Cameron BD, Altrogge DM: Noninvasive polarimetric-based glucose monitoring: an in vivo study. *J Diabetes Sci Technol* 5:380–387, 2011
50. Minh TD, Blake DR, Galassetti PR: The clinical potential of exhaled breath analysis for diabetes mellitus. *Diabetes Res Clin Pract* 97:195–205, 2010. Epub 10 Mar 2012
51. Baca JT, Finegold DN, Asher SA: Tear glucose analysis for the noninvasive detection and monitoring of diabetes mellitus. *Ocul Surf* 5:280–293, 2007
52. Juhl CB, Højlund K, Elsborg R, Poulsen MK, Selmar PE, Holst JJ, Christiansen C, Beck-Nielsen H: Automated detection of hypoglycemia-induced EEG changes recorded by subcutaneous electrodes in subjects with type 1 diabetes–the brain as a biosensor. *Diabetes Res Clin Pract* 88:22–28, 2010

53. Skladnev VN, Ghevondian N, Tarnavskii S, Paramalingam N, Jones TW: Clinical evaluation of a noninvasive alarm system for nocturnal hypoglycemia. *J Diabetes Sci Technol* 4:67–74, 2010

54. Liu G, Khor SM, Iyengar SG, Gooding JJ. Development of an electrochemical immunosensor for the detection of HbA1c in serum. *Analyst* 137:829–832, 2012

55. The International Expert Committee. Report on the role of the A1C assay in the diagnosis of diabetes. *Diabetes Care* 32:1327–1334, 2009

56. Goldstein DE, Little RR, Lorenz RA, Malone JI, Nathan D, Peterson CM, Sacks DB: Tests of glycemia in diabetes. *Diabetes Care* 27:1761–1773, 2004

57. Higgins T, Cembrowski G, Tran D, Lim E, Chan J: Influence of variables on hemoglobin A1C values and nonheterogeneity of hemoglobin A1C reference ranges. *J Diabetes Sci Technol* 3:644–648, 2009

58. Saaddine JB, Fagot-Campagna A, Rolka D, Narayan KM, Geiss L, Eberhardt M, Flegal KM: Distribution of HbA(1c) levels for children and young adults in the U.S. Third National Health and Nutrition Examination Survey. *Diabetes Care* 25:1326–1330, 2002

59. Herman WH, Ma Y, Uwaifo G, Haffner S, Kahn SE, Horton ES, Lachin JM, Montez MG, Brenneman T, Barrett-Connor E: Diabetes Prevention Program Research Group: Differences in A1C by race and ethnicity among patients with impaired glucose tolerance in the Diabetes Prevention Program. *Diabetes Care* 30:2453–2457, 2007

60. Herman WH, Dungan KM, Wolffenbuttel BH, Buse JB, Fahrbach JL, Jiang H, Martin S. Racial and ethnic differences in mean plasma glucose, hemoglobin A1C, and 1,5-anhydroglucitol in over 2000 patients with type 2 diabetes. *J Clin Endocrinol Metab* 94:1689–1694, 2009

61. Tsugawa Y, Mukamal KJ, Davis RB, Taylor WC, Wee CC: Should the hemoglobin A1C diagnostic cutoff differ between blacks and whites? A cross-sectional study. *Ann Intern Med* 157:153–159, 2012.

62. Selvin E, Steffes MW, Ballantyne CM, Hoogeveen RC, Coresh J, Brancati FL: Racial differences in glycemic markers: a cross-sectional analysis of community-based data. *Ann Intern Med* 154:303–309, 2011.

63. Sacks DB, Arnold M, Bakris GL, Bruns DE, Horvath AR, Kirkman MS, Lernmark A, Metzger BE, Nathan DM: Guidelines and recommendations for laboratory analysis in the diagnosis and management of diabetes mellitus. *Clin Chem* 57:e1–e47, 2011

64. Rodriguez-Segade S, Rodriguez J, García Lopez JM, Casanueva FF, Camiña F: Estimation of the glycation gap in diabetic patients with stable glycemic control. *Diabetes Care* 2012. Epub ahead of print

65. Lachin JM, Genuth S, Nathan DM, Rutledge BN: The hemoglobin glycation index is not an independent predictor of the risk of microvascular complications in the Diabetes Control and Complications Trial. *Diabetes* 56:1913–1921, 2007

66. Giardine B, Borg J, Higgs DR, Peterson KR, Philipsen S, Maglott D, Singleton BK, Anstee DJ, Basak AN, Clark B, Costa FC, Faustino P, Fedosyuk H, Felice AE, Francina A, Galanello R, Gallivan MV, Georgitsi M, Gibbons RJ, Giordano PC, Harteveld CL, Hoyer JD, Jarvis M, Joly P, Kanavakis E, Kollia P, Menzel S, Miller W, Moradkhani K, Old J, Papachatzopoulou

A, Papadakis MN, Papadopoulos P, Pavlovic S, Perseu L, Radmilovic M, Riemer C, Satta S, Schrijver I, Stojiljkovic M, Thein SL, Traeger-Synodinos J, Tully R, Wada T, Waye JS, Wiemann C, Zukic B, Chui DH, Wajcman H, Hardison RC, Patrinos GP: Systematic documentation and analysis of human genetic variation in hemoglobinopathies using the microattribution approach. *Nat Genet* 43:295–301, 2011
67. Available at http://globin.bx.psu.edu/hbvar/menu.html. Accessed 16 June 2012
68. Jain N, Kesimer M, Hoyer JD, Calikoglu AS: Hemoglobin Raleigh results in factitiously low hemoglobin A1C when evaluated via immunoassay analyzer. *J Diabetes Complicat* 25:14–18, 2011
69. Available at http://www.ngsp.org/interf.asp. Accessed 11 October 2012
70. Nathan DM, Kuenen J, Borg R, Zheng H, Schoenfeld D, Heine RJ: Translating the A1C assay into estimated average glucose values. *Diabetes Care* 31:1473–1478, 2008
71. Borg R, Kuenen JC, Carstensen B, Zheng H, Nathan DM, Heine RJ, Nerup J, Borch-Johnsen K, Witte DR: ADAG Study Group: HbA$_1$(c) and mean blood glucose show stronger associations with cardiovascular disease risk factors than do postprandial glycaemia or glucose variability in persons with diabetes: the A1C-Derived Average Glucose (ADAG) study. *Diabetologia* 54:69–72, 2011
72. Diabetes Research in Children Network (DirecNet) Study Group, Wilson DM, Kollman: Relationship of A1C to glucose concentrations in children with type 1 diabetes: assessments by high-frequency glucose determinations by sensors. *Diabetes Care* 31:381–385, 2008
73. Hare MJ, Shaw JE, Zimmet PZ: Current controversies in the use of haemoglobin A1C. *J Intern Med* 271: 227–236, 2012; doi: 10.1111/j.1365-2796.2012.02513.x
74. Weykamp C, John WG, Mosca A: A review of the challenge in measuring hemoglobin A1C. *J Diabetes Sci Technol* 3:439–445, 2009
75. Little RR, Rohlfing CL, Sacks DB: National Glycohemoglobin Standardization Program (NGSP) Steering Committee: Status of hemoglobin A1C measurement and goals for improvement: from chaos to order for improving diabetcs care. *Clin Chem* 57:205–214, 2011
76. Selvin E, Francis LM, Ballantyne CM, Hoogeveen RC, Coresh J, Brancati FL, Steffes MW: Nontraditional markers of glycemia: associations with microvascular conditions. *Diabetes Care* 34:960–967, 2011
77. Foo JP, Mantzoros CS: The quest for the perfect biomarker of long-term glycemia: new studies, new trials and tribulations. *Metabolism* 60:1651–1654, 2011
78. Kim JK, Park JT, Oh HJ, Yoo DE, Kim SJ, Han SH, Kang SW, Choi KH, Yoo TH: Estimating average glucose levels from glycated albumin in patients with end-stage renal disease. *Yonsei Med J* 53:578–586, 2012
79. Dungan KM, Buse JB, Largay J, Kelly MM, Button EA, Kato S, Wittlin S: 1,5-anhydroglucitol and postprandial hyperglycemia as measured by continuous glucose monitoring system in moderately controlled patients with diabetes. *Diabetes Care* 29:1214–1219, 2006
80. Beck R, Steffes M, Xing D, Ruedy K, Mauras N, Wilson DM, Kollman C: Diabetes Research in Children Network (DirecNet) Study Group:

The interrelationships of glycemic control measures: HbA1c, glycated albumin, fructosamine, 1,5-anhydroglucitrol, and continuous glucose monitoring. *Pediatr Diabetes* 12:690–695, 2011

81. Ediger MN, Olson BP, Maynard JD: Noninvasive optical screening for diabetes. *J Diabetes Sci Technol* 3:776–780, 2009

82. de Ranitz-Greven WL, Bos DC, Poucki WK, Visser GH, Beulens JW, Biesma DH, de Valk HW: Advanced glycation end products, measured as skin autofluorescence, at diagnosis in gestational diabetes mellitus compared with normal pregnancy. *Diabetes Technol Ther* 14:43–49, 2012

83. Rao A, Hou P, Golnik T, Flaherty J, Vu S: Evolution of data management tools for managing self-monitoring of blood glucose results: a survey of iPhone applications. *J Diabetes Sci Technol* 4:949–957, 2010

84. Paul N, Kohno T, Klonoff DC: A review of the security of insulin pump infusion systems. *J Diabetes Sci Technol* 5:1557–1562, 2011

II. Continuous Glucose Monitoring

William V. Tamborlane, MD

While SMBG remains a mainstay of diabetes management, this method of glucose monitoring only provides patients with intermittent, single point-in-time snapshots of glucose levels. In patients with T1D, the readings often miss marked and sustained hyperglycemic excursions immediately after meals during the day and the frequent occurrence of asymptomatic hypoglycemia while patients are asleep at night. Due in part to the limitations of SMBG, too many patients with diabetes who are treated with insulin fail to achieve treatment goals, and the frequency of hypoglycemia remains unacceptably high. Consequently, the introduction of the first devices for the continuous measurement of interstitial glucose levels more than 10 years ago was hailed as the most important breakthrough in diabetes technology in the new millennium.

Real-time continuous glucose monitoring (RT-CGM) provides patients and clinicians with glucose measurements at 1–5 min intervals. These data can be used for immediate and retrospective adjustments of treatment regimens. Retrospective analysis of nocturnal glucose profiles on glucose sensor data provides an opportunity to optimize basal insulin replacement. Daytime profiles can assist in determining and adjusting carbohydrate-to-insulin ratios and correction doses of insulin. Real-time sensor data and hyperglycemia alarms allow patients to make immediate corrections rather than to wait for the next regularly scheduled BG meter test. Hypoglycemia alarms can help prevent catastrophic nighttime events.

It seemed intuitive that a perfect, nonintrusive, accurate, and easy-to-use CGM device would be of great benefit to patients. However, the first generation of FDA-approved devices was relatively inaccurate, difficult to use, and either provided data only for short-term retrospective analysis or was too difficult and uncomfortable to use. While still a challenge to use, the newer generation of RT-CGM systems provided better accuracy, functionality, and patient tolerance. These improvements paved the way for a series of randomized clinical trials aimed at gathering level A evidence regarding the actual benefits of CGM. Table 9.II.1 summarizes key features of the two current CGM devices marketed in the U.S.

ADA 2012 CLINICAL PRACTICE RECOMMENDATIONS FOR CGM

The current ADA recommendations regarding CGM reflect the limitations in the published evidence regarding the efficacy of CGM. They indicate that CGM:

Table 9.II.1 Features of the RT-CGM Systems

	DexCom Seven® Plus	Medtronic MiniMed Paradigm® Real-time Revel System or Guardian® Real Time
Range of glucose values	40 to 400 mg/dl	40 to 400 mg/dl
Update of glucose values	Every 5 min	Every 5 min
Sensor duration	Up to 168 h (7 days)⁺	Up to 72 h (3 days)⁺
Sensor length, angle, and gauge	13mm, 45 degrees, 26 gauge	12mm, 45–60 degrees, 23 gauge
Transmitter size	1.5" × 0.9" × 0.4"	1.4" × 1.1" × 0.3"
Number of components to wear or carry	Receiver, transmitter, and home glucose meter	Receiver, transmitter, and home glucose meter
Warm-up period before glucose readings displayed	2 h	2 h
Required frequency of calibration	2 times a day (every 12 h)	2 times a day (every 12 h)
Available alarms	High and low glucose alarms	High and low glucose alarms; predicted high and low glucose alarms; rate of change alarms
Glucose display graphs	1-, 3-, 6-, 12-, and 24-h	3-, 6-, 12-, and 24-h
Trending arrows	Yes	Yes
Capacity to enter events	Insulin, meals, exercise, and health	Insulin, meals, exercise
FDA approval status	Age 18 years and older with blood sugar testing using a home glucose meter	Age 7 years and older with blood sugar testing using a home glucose meter

- In conjunction with intensive insulin regimens may be a useful tool to lower A1C levels in selected adults (age ≥25 years) with T1D;
- May be helpful in lowering A1C levels in younger adults, adolescents, and children ≥8 years of age, but the evidence is less strong;
- May be a supplemental tool to SMBG in patients with hypoglycemia unawareness or frequent hypoglycemic episodes.

In the sections below, the results of studies that led to these recommendations will be reviewed in greater detail. More recent data that have been published in this rapidly evolving area of clinical and translational research will also be presented.

JDRF CGM STUDY GROUP RANDOMIZED CLINICAL TRIALS

Study Design

In 2006, JDRF formed the JDRF CGM Study Group, a consortium of 10 leading adult and pediatric endocrinology centers in the United States. As summarized in Table 9.II.2, the group designed two concurrent, nearly identical randomized trials to evaluate the CGM devices in two cohorts of patients: the primary cohort with A1C levels $\geq$7.0% and the secondary cohort with A1C <7.0%.[1,2]

Major Findings

- A1C levels in the primary cohort: there was a significant improvement in A1C levels with CGM in subjects $\geq$25 years of age (mean between group difference in change 0.53%; P <0.001) but not in the younger (8 to <15 or 15 to <25 years old) age-groups.
- In the primary cohort, the improvements in A1C levels that were achieved in the CGM group during the first 6 months were maintained during the 6-month extension study and A1C levels remained at 6.4% in the CGM group in the secondary cohort.
- In the secondary cohort exposure to biochemical hypoglycemia (i.e., average minutes per day with sensor values $\leq$70 and $\leq$60 mg/dl) was reduced by 33 and 50%, respectively, in the sensor group but was unchanged in the control group.
- In the secondary cohort, CGM use also helped patients maintain target A1C levels; A1C levels remained <7.0% in 88% of CGM subjects vs. 63% of control subjects.
- As suggested in earlier CGM trials, the success of CGM was closely related to the frequency of device use. Across all age groups in the primary cohort, CGM use for 6–7 days/week was associated with a $\geq$0.5% reduction in A1C values.
- Increased number of BG meter tests per day was a predictor of frequent CGM use during the study, as was the frequency of CGM use during the first month of the study.[3]
- In both cohorts, lower A1C levels during the 6 months of the study did not result in an increase in severe hypoglycemic rates compared to controls.
- CGM outcomes were similar in patients receiving CSII and multiple daily injection (MDI) therapy.

Table 9.II.2 JDRF CGM Trial

Cohort	n	A1C	Primary Outcome	CGM
Primary	322	Baseline 7–10%	A1C change at 6 months	Stratified in age-groups (years): 8 to ≤15 15 to ≤25 >25
Secondary	129	Baseline <7%	Exposure to biochemical hypoglycemia, assessed by CGM profiles	No age stratification

Other Findings

- The greatest discrepancy in scores on the CGM satisfaction scale between frequent and infrequent users pertained to items in the hassles subscale; namely, the infrequent users perceived the CGM devices much more difficult to use than the frequent users; whereas the perceived benefits of CGM were similar.[4]
- Scores on other questionnaires showed no adverse effects of CGM on quality of life and a slight lessening of hypoglycemia fear.[5]
- Subjects who experienced a severe hypoglycemic event in the 6 months prior to the study and females were more likely to experience a severe hypoglycemic event during the study.[6]
- In a post-hoc analysis of children and adolescents (8–17 years of age), patients using the CGM device ≥6 days/week lowered A1C levels by 0.9% from baseline to 6 months and this improvement was sustained for the full 12 months if 6–7 day/week use was sustained. Unfortunately, only 21% of the subjects were able to maintain ≥6 days/week CGM use for the entire 12-month study period Those who stopped using CGM frequently during the second 6 months lost the A1C benefit.[7]
- Long-term projections on the benefits of lowering A1C levels in adults in the primary cohort and of maintaining target A1C levels in the secondary cohort indicate that CGM is cost effective and could be cost saving if the requirement to confirm sensor reading by additional meter tests were eliminated.[8]

STAR 3 STUDY

A number of previous studies have compared the efficacy of CSII versus MDI and CGM versus SMBG. Star 3 was the first study that examined whether and to what extent switching from SMBG and multiple daily injections directly to CGM and insulin pump therapy (also called sensor-augmented pump [SAP] therapy) might improve metabolic control in patients who had elevated A1C levels during treatment with MDI and SMBG.[9] Star 3 is also notable because it remains the largest (485 subjects, age ≥8 years) and longest (12 months) randomized clinical trial involving CGM that has been completed thus far. The most important findings were:

1. Reduction in A1C levels was clinically and statistically significantly greater in the SAP versus the MDI/SMBG treatment group (between group difference –0.6%, *P* <0.0001).
2. Differences in A1C between SAP and the MDI/SMBG group were similar in adult and pediatric patients and in preadolescents and adolescents.[10]
3. Greater proportion of adult and pediatric patients in the SAP group achieved target A1C levels recommended by the ADA.
4. Rates of severe hypoglycemia and DKA were low and did not differ between treatment groups.
5. This was one of the few randomized clinical trials where the pediatric subset of patients in the treatment arm using CGM achieved lower A1C values than the treatment arm that employed SMBG.

OTHER STUDY IN WELL-CONTROLLED T1D PATIENTS

A multicenter European/Israeli study of well-controlled children (ages 10–17 years) and adults with T1D whose A1C levels were <7.5% showed that 6 months of CGM use markedly reduced the time spent in hypoglycemia <63 mg/dl and lowered A1C by 0.3%.[11]

NEGATIVE PEDIATRIC STUDIES

■ The ONSET study was a pediatric trial that compared the use of SAP in newly diagnosed patients with use of insulin pump without CGM in 160 patients No significant difference was observed between the two groups in A1C levels (SAP 7.4% and pump/SMBG 7.6%) after 12 months.[12]

■ The Diabetes Research in Children Network (DirecNet) carried out a randomized clinical trial of CGM versus SMBG monitoring in 146 children with T1D aged 4–9 years. No improvement in metabolic control was achieved and only 41% of these young children were using CGM on 6–7 days/week at the end of the study (6 months).[13]

■ DirecNet also carried out a CGM pilot study in 23 young children with T1D who were <4 years of age. A1C values were unchanged after 6 months and only ~50% of families used CGM 6–7 days/week. Nevertheless, parental satisfaction with CGM was high in the group as a whole, suggesting that parents were primarily using CGM in this age group to prevent hypoglycemia.[14]

ENDOCRINE SOCIETY CGM PRACTICE GUIDELINES FOR ADULTS WITH T1D

In October 2011 the Endocrine Society published updated CGM practice guidelines for adults with T1D.[15] The major recommendations are listed below:

■ Use of RT-CGM devices is recommended for adult patients with T1D who have A1C levels ≥7.0%, and who have demonstrated they can use these devices on a nearly daily basis in order to lower A1C levels.

■ Use of RT-CGM devices is recommended for adult patients with T1D who have A1C levels <7.0%, and who have demonstrated they can use these devices on a nearly daily basis in order to maintain target A1C levels and reduce exposure to biochemical hypoglycemia.

■ It is suggested that intermittent use of CGM systems designed for short-term retrospective analysis may be of benefit in adult patients with diabetes whose clinicians:
1. Worry about dawn phenomenon, and postprandial hyperglycemia or
2. Experiment with important changes in their diabetes regimen (such as instituting new insulin or switching from MDI to pump therapy). These devices represent an alternative for patients who cannot safely and effectively take advantage of the information provided to them by RT-CGM.

INTERNATIONAL CONSENSUS PANEL GUIDELINES FOR CGM IN PEDIATRIC PATIENTS WITH T1D

In 2012, an international panel of pediatric diabetologists published guidelines for use of CGM in children and adolescents with T1D.[16]
Indications for CGM use in pediatrics:

■ RT-CGM can be used effectively for lowering A1C and reducing glucose variability in the pediatric population with T1D without increasing the frequency of severe hypoglycemia.

■ RT-CGM can be used effectively for shortening the time spent in hypoglycemia in the pediatric population with T1D.

■ The effectiveness of RT-CGM in the pediatric population with T1D is significantly related to the amount of sensor use. Therefore, efforts for increased adherence with sensor use are paramount in this age group.

■ SAP treatment is effective in lowering A1C levels in children and adolescents with T1D who have elevated A1C values on MDI therapy using standard BG monitoring.

■ Intermittent, retrospective, or real-time CGM may be useful in children and adolescents with T1D to detect the dawn phenomenon, postprandial hyperglycemia, asymptomatic and nocturnal hypoglycemia, and in evaluating the effects of major changes in treatment regimens.

This panel also made a number of recommendations regarding practical aspects of using CGM in children and adolescents.

Patient Education:

- Initial and ongoing education is needed regarding the lag time and need to confirm CGM glucose results with standard SMBG prior to insulin administration, and when it is possible and clinically safe, prior to treatment of hypoglycemia.
- Initial and ongoing education is needed regarding the optimal approach. The timing of sensor calibration should help ensure optimal sensor performance.
- Initial and ongoing education is needed regarding sensor site care with attention to using sensors according to manufacturers' recommendations, including the need for finger-stick blood sugars for all treatment decisions.

Utility of intermittent use of CGM in pediatric patients:

- Detection of nocturnal hypoglycemia or hyperglycemia (e.g., dawn phenomenon)
- Individuals in whom the causes of persistently high A1C levels are unclear for detection of hyperglycemic peaks not identified by SMBG.
- Making changes to patients' diabetes treatment regimen (e.g., changing of insulin type or switching from MDI to CSII or vice versa).
- Special situations, such as: sport, eating outside the home, trying new foods; traveling or driving; or patients with severe fear of hypoglycemia.
- Cystic fibrosis–related diabetes
- Monitoring glycemia in research settings

PRACTICAL REALITIES

At the 2012 Advanced Technologies and Treatments for Diabetes (ATTD) meeting in Barcelona, Spain, the T1D Exchange Clinical Registry group presented their data on CGM use in patients with T1D who were receiving their care at one of the 67 adult and pediatric diabetes treatment centers enrolled in the registry. As shown in Table 9.II.3, a small minority of patients was currently using CGM. Many of those patients were not using CGM frequently enough to be of clinical benefit and few patients were downloading data for retrospective

Table 9.II.3 Use of CGM by Patients Enrolled in the T1D Exchange Clinic Registry

Patient age	1–25 Years	>25 Years
% currently using CGM	2–3%	14%
% using CGM 6–7 days/week	<40%	~60%
% downloading data	~20%	~40%

analysis. It is also discouraging to know that the number of patients who had tried and then abandoned CGM use outnumbered current users by two to one.

HOPE FOR THE FUTURE: CLOSED-LOOP INSULIN DELIVERY

Despite advances in diabetes therapeutics, including the introduction of insulin analogs and the development of smart insulin pumps, too many patients fail to achieve target A1C levels. Moreover, in those patients who are able to achieve very strict control of their diabetes, results of CGM studies confirm the belief that no treatment of T1D will ever eliminate the risk of severe hypoglycemia until there are closed-loop systems that automatically control insulin delivery rates based on RT-CGM. All three elements of an artificial pancreas system (insulin pumps, RT-CGM, and controller algorithms to regulate insulin delivery) are already available. The drive to develop such systems has helped to forge partnerships between academic clinical investigators in Australia, Europe, and North America, agencies and organizations such as NIH and the JDRF, and industry.

The main obstacle that must be overcome before closed-loop systems become a practical reality for the treatment of T1D at home is to have redundant safeguards in place that will prevent the overdelivery of insulin due to a system malfunction. While automatically turning up insulin delivery to prevent hyperglycemia presents a potentially devastating safety risk, turning off a pump for a relatively short period of time to limit the extent and duration of hypoglycemia presents an attractive first step on the path to an artificial pancreas. Medtronic has taken that step with the Veo, an integrated sensor-augmented pump (iSAP) which automatically suspends the basal infusion of insulin for 2 h when the patient's glucose sensor values cross a low glucose threshold and the patient does not respond to the system alarm. Other iSAP systems with low glucose suspend (LGS) features are currently in the pipeline.

Several lines of evidence indicate that incorporation of LGS capability into an iSAP system would be particularly useful in lowering the risk of seizures and other severe hypoglycemia events, especially while the patient is asleep during the night, when severe hypoglycemia risk is highest. Nighttime poses a triple threat of hypoglycemia for T1D patients due to the loss of plasma epinephrine responses to hypoglycemia during deep sleep, delayed glucose lowering effects of exercise on the prior afternoon, and fixed doses of insulin delivery at night.[17] It is especially noteworthy that a recent case series described four T1D patients who were wearing a CGM on a night in which they had a hypoglycemic seizure.[18] In each case, low sensor glucose levels preceded the seizure for several hours before the actual event, providing a window for prevention[18] by an LGS-equipped device by automatically suspending the basal insulin infusion. Years ago, our group at Yale demonstrated that interrupting an insulin pump's basal infusion for 2 h in the middle of the night was associated with a modest rise in BG without any meaningful increase in serum β-hydroxybutyrate levels.[19] Moreover, our patients regularly disconnect their pumps for up to 2 h for sport, swimming, and other activities without any adverse consequences.

The Veo pump is approved for use in Australia, Canada, and Europe, but the Food and Drug Administration has not yet approved the sale of LGS-equipped pumps in the U.S. The results of recent clinical use studies of this system have shown that LGS is well accepted by patients It is safe and effective at reducing duration of hypoglycemia. The next step is to utilize the LGS function to prevent hypoglycemic events by suspending the basal insulin infusion based on a projected low due to a rapid rate of fall of sensor glucose levels. Ultimately, closed-loop systems for home use will need to be easily managed by patients, adaptable to the challenges of human physiology during normal daily activities and due to changes in insulin sensitivity, and protective against errors that lead to insulin overinfusion. It now seems likely that such a mechanical solution to the problems of managing T1D will be achieved before a cell-based biological solution.

GAPS ACCORDING TO THE EDITORS

1. There is a need for improved continuous glucose monitoring systems that have greater accuracy and can serve as replacement for traditional BG monitoring systems.
2. There is a need to design, implement, and evaluate approaches to integrate CGM into routine diabetes management, particularly for young patients with T1D who are likely to discontinue CGM use.
3. There is a need to provide better training and reimbursement for health care professionals to work with patients and families for CGM implementation and sustained use.
4. There is substantial need for ongoing investigations to create a closed-loop artificial pancreas system to reduce glycemic excursions while minimizing patient input.

REFERENCES

1. Juvenile Diabetes Research Foundation Continuous Glucose Monitoring Study Group: Continuous glucose monitoring and intensive treatment of type 1 diabetes. *N Engl J Med* 359:1464–1476, 2008
2. Juvenile Diabetes Research Foundation Continuous Glucose Monitoring Study Group: The effect of continuous glucose monitoring in well-controlled type 1 diabetes. *Diabetes Care* 32:1378–1383, 2009
3. Juvenile Diabetes Research Foundation Continuous Glucose Monitoring Study Group: Factors predictive of use and of benefit from continuous glucose monitoring in type 1 diabetes. *Diabetes Care* 32:1947–1953, 2009
4. Juvenile Diabetes Research Foundation Continuous Glucose Monitoring Study Group; Tansey M, Laffel L, Cheng J, Beck R, Coffey J, Huang E, Kollman C, Lawrence J, Lee J, Ruedy K, Tamborlane W, Wysocki T, Xing D on behalf of Juvenile Diabetes Research Foundation Continuous Glucose Monitoring Study Group: Satisfaction with continuous glucose monitoring in adults and youth with type 1 diabetes. *Diabetic Med* 28:1118–1122, 2011
5. Juvenile Diabetes Research Foundation Continuous Glucose Monitoring Study Group: Quality of life measures in children and adults with type 1 diabetes: the Juvenile Diabetes Research Foundation Continuous Glucose Monitoring Randomized Trial. *Diabetes Care* 33:2175–2177, 2010

6. Juvenile Diabetes Research Foundation Continuous Glucose Monitoring Study Group: Factors predictive of severe hypoglycemia in type 1 diabetes: analysis from the JDRF Continuous Glucose Monitoring Randomized Control Trial dataset. *Diabetes Care* 34:586–590, 2011

7. Juvenile Diabetes Research Foundation Continuous Glucose Monitoring Study Group: Continuous glucose monitoring in youth with type 1 diabetes: 12-month follow up of the JDRF Continuous Glucose Monitoring Randomized Trial. *Diabetes Technol Ther* 12:507–515, 2010

8. Juvenile Diabetes Research Foundation Continuous Glucose Monitoring Study Group: The cost-effectiveness of continuous glucose monitoring in type 1 diabetes. *Diabetes Care* 33:1269–1274, 2010

9. Bergenstal RM, Tamborlane WV, Ahmann A, Buse J, Dailey G, Davis SN, Joyce C, Perkins BA, Willi SM, Wood M, for the STAR 3 Study Group: Effectiveness of sensor-augmented insulin pump therapy in type 1 diabetes. *N Engl J Med* 363:311–320, 2010

10. Slover RH, Welsh JB, Criego A, Weinzimer SA, Willi SM, Wood MA, Tamborlane WV: Effectiveness of sensor-augmented pump therapy in children and adolescents with type 1 diabetes in the STAR 3 Study. *Pediatr Diabetes* 13:6–11, 2012

11. Battelino T, Phillip M, Bratina N, Nimri R, Oskarsson P, Bolinder J: Effect of continuous glucose monitoring on hypoglycemia in type 1 diabetes. *Diabetes Care* 34:1–6, 2011

12. Kordonouri O, Pankowska E, Rami B, Kapellen T, Coutant R, Hartmann R, Lange K, Knip M, Danne T: Sensor-augmented pump therapy from diagnosis of childhood type 1 diabetes: results of the Paediatric Onset Study (ONSET) after 12 months of treatment. *Diabetologia* 53:2487–2495, 2010

13. Diabetes Research in Children Network (DirecNet) Study Group: A randomized clinical trial to assess the efficacy and safety of real-time continuous glucose monitoring in the management of type 1 diabetes in young children (4 to <10 year olds). *Diabetes Care* 35:204–210, 2012

14. Diabetes Research in Children Network (DirecNet) Study Group: Feasibility of prolonged continuous glucose monitoring in toddlers with type 1 diabetes. *Pediatr Diabetes* 13:294–300, 2012

15. Klonoff DC (Chair), Buckingham B, Christiansen JS, Montori VM, Tamborlane WV, Vigersky RA, Wolpert H: Continuous glucose monitoring: an Endocrine Society clinical practice guideline. *J Clin Endocrinol Metab* 96:2968–2979, 2011

16. Phillip M, Danne T, Shalitin S, Buckingham B, Laffel, Tamborlane W, Battelino T, for the Consensus Forum Participants: Use of continuous glucose monitoring in the pediatric age group. *Pediatr Diabetes* 13:215–228, 2012

17. Tamborlane WV: Triple jeopardy for hypoglycemia on nights following exercise in youth with type 1 diabetes. *J Clin Endocrinol Metab* 92:815–816, 2007

18. Buckingham B, Wilson DM, Lecher T, Hanas R, Kaiserman K, Cameron F: Duration of nocturnal hypoglycemia before seizures. *Diabetes Care* 31:2110–2112, 2008

19. Attia N, Jones TW, Holcombe J, Tamborlane WV: Comparison of human regular insulin and lispro insulin after interruption of CSII and in the treatment of acutely decompensated IDDM. *Diabetes Care* 21:817–821, 1998

10

Nutrition

Laurie A. Higgins, MS, RD, LDN, CDE, and Mary Ziotas Zacharatos, RD, CDE, CDN, LD

INTRODUCTION

Healthy nutrition is critically important in the management of individuals with type 1 diabetes (T1D). Historically, the diet for T1D patients restricted higher carbohydrate meals and discouraged snacks and desserts. In recent decades, greater understanding of physiology has enabled liberalization of the diet. The advent of multiple daily insulin injections and insulin pump therapy has allowed greater freedom in food choices and timing. However, this has required that T1D individuals become ever more sophisticated about carbohydrate counting and dosing insulin for anticipated food consumption as well as dosing if additional carbohydrates are consumed.

This chapter is not meant to discuss general nutrition principles or weight-loss approaches. Rather, it is meant to review very specific issues related to nutrition and T1D management. General nutrition principles apply, but the goal is to address specific T1D concerns. Since nutrition issues are similar between the pediatric and adult populations, all points will apply to both groups. Specific differences will be noted.

STANDARDS OF CARE

The goals of Medical Nutrition Therapy (MNT) established by the American Diabetes Association (ADA) are:[1,2]

1. Attain and maintain
   - Optimal blood glucose levels,
   - A lipid profile that reduces macrovascular disease risk,
   - Blood pressure levels that reduce the risk of vascular disease.
2. Prevent and treat chronic diabetes complications by modifying nutrient intake and lifestyle.
3. Address individual nutritional needs taking into account personal and cultural preference and willingness to change.
4. Maintain the pleasure of eating by only limiting the foods when indicated by scientific evidence.

Attaining these goals necessitates continual evaluation to ensure they address age-specific and developmental requirements. Providers need to create a unique nutrition therapy plan for each patient that takes the patient's eating preferences, behavior, and life stage into account as well as each patient's ability to implement and follow the nutrition therapy.

Achieving these goals requires synchronizing food, insulin dosage, and activity. For example, it is difficult to improve the effectiveness of an insulin-to-carbohydrate ratio (I:C) if patients with T1D do not accurately count carbohydrates or follow an outdated food plan. T1D patients benefit from regular nutritional assessment and education. Patients reap significant benefits in overall health when nutrition is incorporated in their annual diabetes goals. Very young children, who have frequently changing caloric requirements, and the elderly, who may have changing medical needs, often benefit from more frequent, quarterly nutrition assessments and follow-up. T1D patients with concurrent medical issues (e.g., celiac disease) may require frequent and ongoing nutrition support.

EVIDENCE TO SUPPORT BENEFITS OF MEDICAL NUTRITION THERAPY

MNT studies in T1D patients are difficult to perform. Shorter studies, in controlled settings, provide a limited understanding of the true impact of nutritional interventions. Longer-term, outpatient studies give insight into dietary practices in the real world, but much of the control over the content of the diet and insulin administration is lost. Still, a number of clinical trials have been performed in people with T1D. A summary of the results is presented in Table 10.1

Specific Studies

The Dose Adjusted for Normal Eating (DAFNE) trial, conducted in the United Kingdom, evaluated whether a 5-day course teaching adjustments of mealtime insulin based on planned carbohydrate intake could improve both glycemia and quality of life in T1D individuals.[3] The insulin regimen was determined first, followed by a consistent meal matched to the timing of insulin action. Individuals were either taught how to determine mealtime bolus insulin doses based on desired carbohydrate intake on a meal-to-meal basis or attended the training 6 months later. In the group receiving the DAFNE training, their A1C levels were improved by 1% (with no significant increase in severe hypoglycemia), they noted positive effects on quality of life and were satisfied with treatment, and they had improved psychological well-being. The results in the treatment group occurred despite an increase in insulin injections (but not in total insulin amount) and an increase in blood glucose monitoring compared with the control subjects.

A follow-up (mean ~4 years) of the original subjects showed a mean A1C improvement of 0.4% from baseline, remaining significant but less than the 12-month levels. Quality of life improvements were well maintained over ~4 years.[4] Another follow-up report examined changes in food and eating practices in the DAFNE trial participants after changing to flexible, intensive insulin therapy. Investigators were concerned that T1D individuals, if given the option to adjust insulin doses based on carbohydrate intake, would overeat or select unhealthy food choices. These concerns were unfounded, as individuals using flexible, intensive insulin therapy did not overeat or choose unhealthy options. Instead, many of the subjects reported making few dietary changes and, in some cases, reported being more rigid in their dietary habits.[5]

Table 10.1 Clinical Trials in T1D Patients

	Population/Type of Study	Study Length	Nutrition Therapy Intervention	A1C and Other Outcomes
Delahanty 1993	n = 623/ observational	Quarterly visits during DCCT (average 4.1 years)	Intensive MNT; exchange lists; CHO counting	A1C reduction 0.9% (P < 0.001)
DAFNE Study Group 2002	n = 169/RCT	5-day course (follow-up at 6 months)	Advanced CHO counting; I:C ratios	A1C ↓ 1.0% (P < 0.0001), ↑ dietary freedom (P < 0.0001) and overall quality of life (P < 0.01)
Sämann 2005	n = 1,592/time series	5-day classes (follow-up at 3 years)	CHO counting; I:C ratios	A1C: ↓ 0.7% (P < 0.001), severe hypoglycemia: ↓0.2 events/ patient-year (P < 0.001)
Lowe 2008	n = 82 individuals with T1D and 55 with T2D	Intensive self-management course (follow-up at 12 months)	Carb counting: I:C ratios	A1C: ↓ 0.6% and ↑ empowerment and quality of life
Scavone 2010	n = 256 adults	4-week nutritional education program vs. not (followed for 9 months)	Carb counting; I:C ratios	A1C reduction of 0.4% compared to control, less hypoglycemia, less insulin
Laurenzi 2011	n = 61 adults	Carb counting education vs. control (followed for 24 weeks)	Carb counting	If used carb counting consistently A1C reduction of − 0.35%, overall no change. Improved diabetes-related quality of life

CHO, carbohydrate. Adapted from American Diabetes Association,[10] Academy of Nutrition and Dietetics,[13] Scavone et al.,[98] and Laurenzi et al.[99]

A German group reported a lower A1C level (1.5%) 1 year after a 5-day intensive training course. Trained dietitians and nurse educators taught matching insulin doses to dietary choices while maintaining blood glucose levels near normal.[6] Improvements lasted 3 years without increasing the risk of hypoglycemia.[7] In Australia, dietitians and doctors teaching carbohydrate counting and insulin dose adjustment to T1D or type 2 diabetes (T2D) patients also revealed good results. Participants reported an A1C drop from 8.7% to 8.1% at 12 months.[8]

The Diabetes Control and Complications Trial (DCCT) examined the role of nutrition in achieving glycemic control and found four behaviors associated with a clinically significant reduction in A1C (0.9%): adherence to the prescribed meal and snack plan, adjusting insulin dose in response to meal size, prompt treatment of hyperglycemia, and avoiding overtreatment of hypoglycemia.[9]

MNT AND INSULIN MANAGEMENT

Food plans must be individualized to meet food preferences, eating schedules, physical activity patterns, and cultural influences. Education on the basic diabetes nutrition concepts should begin promptly after diagnosis and be reviewed regularly to encourage adherence. Basic concepts of a food plan should be taught to young children in a developmentally appropriate manner, with specific details given to parents, other family members, and caretakers. Older children and adolescents are often capable of understanding the basics of a meal plan but require parental support and guidance for adherence.

Based on DCCT results, ADA recommends intensive insulin therapy for all T1D patients, using basal and bolus insulin to reproduce or mimic normal physiological insulin secretion: 1) using multiple-dose insulin injections or insulin pump therapy; 2) matching prandial I:C intake, premeal blood glucose, and anticipated activity; and 3) using insulin analogs, especially if hypoglycemia is a concern.[10] The basal and prandial insulin should closely approximate physiologic insulin patterns.

Insulin therapy should be tailored to the individual's usual eating and physical activity pattern, with insulin doses adjusted according to the carbohydrate content of meals and snacks. For planned exercise, insulin doses can be adjusted; for unplanned exercise, extra carbohydrates may be needed.[11] (See chapter 12, Insulin, and chapter 11, Physical Activity.)

Achieving nutrition-related goals requires a well-coordinated team effort that involves the patient in the decision-making process. The complex nutrition issues require a registered dietitian (RD) knowledgeable in T1D and skilled in implementing nutrition therapy to lead nutrition management.[10] However, all team members, including physicians and nurses, should be knowledgeable about nutrition therapy and support its implementation.[11]

The Academy of Nutrition and Dietetics (Acad Nutr Diet) Evidence-based Nutrition Practice Guidelines (EBNPG) state: "MNT plays a crucial role in managing diabetes and reducing the potential complications related to poor glycemic, lipid, and blood pressure control."[12,13] Carbohydrate intake and available insulin primarily determine postprandial glucose levels. Therefore, insulin doses must be adjusted to match carbohydrate intake for those who take mealtime (prandial) insulin or are on CSII. Comprehensive nutrition education and counseling should teach how to interpret blood glucose monitoring patterns and nutrition-related medication management. People using flexible insulin dosing should understand the relationship and coordination of their basal-bolus insulin plan (insulin action) with the blood glucose–raising effect of carbohydrate intake. T1D patients on fixed insulin doses should eat consistent meals and snacks at similar times each day that contain the same amount of carbohydrates, since carbohydrate consistency has shown improved glycemic control.[11,13]

Frequency of MNT

It is recommended that an initial series of three to four encounters with an RD lasting from 45 to 90 min begin at the diagnosis for diabetes or at first referral to an RD for MNT and should be completed within 3 to 6 months.[12,13] The RD should determine whether additional MNT encounters are needed and, if so, provide for continued care.[12,13] At least one follow-up encounter is recommended annually to reinforce lifestyle changes and to evaluate and monitor outcomes that indicate the need for changes in MNT or medication(s).[12,13] Researchers found in the DAFNE program that nutrition support at 6 months was crucial for continued motivation in following an I:C plan.[14] Chapter 7 (Diabetes Self-Management Education) further discusses the need for continued intervention and support to promote the sustainability of changes in health-related behaviors.

PEDIATRICS

Normal Growth and Development

Children and adolescents require adequate calories for normal growth and development. Thus, growth must be monitored and recorded every 3 months (http://www.cdc.gov/growthcharts).[15,16] Table 10.2 lists approximate caloric requirements for children and adolescents based on sex, age, and activity level.[17] Children need guidance to select appropriate amounts and types of food to sustain normal growth. Nutrition assessment tools such as 24-h recall, 3-day food records, and food frequency questionnaires can be used in conjunction with a computer nutrient analysis program to determine usual nutrient intake. Once calorie and nutrient needs are established, they can be adjusted to accommodate growth or prevent accelerated weight gain.

At diagnosis, many children and adolescents have T1D-associated weight loss, which must be restored with insulin, hydration, and adequate caloric intake. In youth, weight loss or insufficient weight gain at diagnosis usually requires additional calories to promote catch-up growth. Because energy requirements change with age, physical activity, and growth rate, an evaluation of height, weight, BMI, and nutrition plan should be constantly monitored.

Chronic undertreatment with insulin and long-standing poor diabetes control often leads to poor growth and weight loss. Overtreatment with insulin can lead to excessive weight gain. Impaired linear growth or poor weight gain should raise suspicion for other related autoimmune diseases such as hypothyroidism and celiac disease, and behaviors such as disordered eating behaviors or insulin omission.

Height and weight evaluations at each clinic visit will allow for early recognition of any deviations from the norm, which then can be promptly evaluated and treated.[16]

Medical Nutrition Therapy

When young children and adolescents are diagnosed with T1D, their lives are profoundly impacted by diabetes and require consideration when devising a diabetes medical management plan and providing nutrition recommendations. The following checklist (Table 10.2) can help when designing an appropriate nutrition plan. Nutrition guidance should be individualized for the patient and family's needs and taught in such a way that considers learning theory, behavior change, patient engagement, and other factors that impact understanding and implementing the recommendations. (See chapters 7, Diabetes Self-Management Education, and 8, Psychosocial Issues in Type 1 Diabetes, for further discussion on these important considerations.)

Table 10.2 Nutrition Recommendations Redistributed: Calories from Macronutrients

Calorie Sources	Requirements for Growth, Based on Nutrition Assessment		
Acceptable Macronutrient Distribution Range (AMDR) % of energy			
	Children 1–3 Years of Age	Children 4–18 Years of Age	Adults
Carbohydrate	45–65%	45–65%	45–65%
Protein	5–20%	10–30%	10–35%
Fat	30–40%	25–35%	20–35%
Fiber			
1–3 years of age	19 g/day		
4–8 years of age		25 g/day	
9–13 years of age			
Males		31 g/day	
Females		26 g/day	
14–50 years of age			
Males			38 g/day
Females			26 g/day
Fiber Daily Reference Intake = 14g fiber/1,000 kcals after 12 months of age			

Adapted from Institute of Medicine[24,100] and Slavin[101]

Nutrition education and counseling. Nutrition therapy for children and adolescents should be initiated at diagnosis and continued regularly. One model for educating families at diagnosis is to begin with survival skills. An RD with expertise in both pediatric nutrition and T1D should educate the family. Nutrition therapy should be part of the team's initial education, with close and frequent follow-up after diagnosis. The child or adolescent should be seen by an RD at least annually to evaluate height, weight, BMI, and the food plan. Young children require more frequent evaluations.[16]

Age components of nutrition education and counseling. The challenges of nutrition education for children and adolescents are often age related and require consideration of the child's specific nutrition and developmental needs. Below is a summary of the specific characteristics to consider when working with different age groups:

Toddlers

- Variable appetites
- Eat small, frequent meals
- Prone to food jags/selective eating, resulting in food battles with parents
- Daycare providers need instruction on diabetes management

Preschool/school age

- More consistent growth and nutrition intake
- Usually eat three meals and snacks between meals
- Begin to be involved in organized sports and physical education class
- School personnel need understanding and training in diabetes management

Adolescents

- Variable schedules/more inconsistency/sleeping in on weekends
- Often working and going to school
- Peer influence on food choices
- More responsible for food choices and diabetes self-care
- More likely to miss shots or boluses
- Alcohol use needs to be discussed
- School personnel need understanding and training in diabetes management
- Skipping meals
- Potential eating disorders

Nutrition therapy goals and recommendations for youth. Nutrition therapy goals for children and adolescents with T1D include achievement and maintenance of glucose, lipid, and blood pressure goals to prevent or slow chronic complications from arising and to prevent and treat acute complications.[11,16] These goals and recommendations apply specifically to youth and their unique needs. Nutrient recommendations are based on requirements for all healthy children and adolescents because there is no research on the nutrient requirements for children and adolescents with diabetes.[16] Therefore, youth and their families should be encouraged to follow the Dietary Guidelines for Americans, 2010, which out-line general nutrition recommendations for all youth ≥2 years of age.[17] Depending on age, sex, and activity level, those recommendations include a daily intake of:

- 3–10 oz of grains
- 1–2.5 cups of fruit
- 1.5–4 cups of vegetables
- 3–7 oz protein foods
- 2–3 cups of dairy

Youth with diabetes fail to meet their nutrition goals (see Table 10.1).[18–21] They consume more total and saturated fat than recommended and inadequate amounts of fruits, vegetables, and grains.[18,19,22] The SEARCH for Diabetes in Youth study, the largest study conducted on youth, found that only 6.5% of the cohort (1,697 youth) met ADA recommendations of <10% of energy for satu-rated fat, and <50% met recommendations for total fat, vitamin E, fiber, fruits, vegetables, and grains.[19]

YOUNG ADULTS AND OLDER

A similar approach to MNT is used with those older than the pediatric patient: individualized food plans based on nutritional, physical and medical needs, food preferences, schedule, access to food, and ability to learn and follow a food plan as well as ability to adjust insulin based on food intake. People who are now living alone, either as a young adult or older individual, may be unfamiliar with pur-chasing and preparing food and may require some of these basic skills in order to appropriately follow a food plan.

For older individuals with T1D, there are unique nutritional considerations yet there are few studies specifically addressing this age group. Those with long-standing disease may have gastrointestinal complications and alterations in taste that create nutritional challenges. Additionally, dental issues can make it difficult to eat normally, and thus alterations in food choices may be required. Medications that cause gastrointestinal side effects in a patient should be reduced or avoided. Other comorbid conditions such as hypertension, dyslipidemia, and renal insuf-ficiency may require dietary modifications such as low sodium, lower cholesterol, and lower potassium diets, respectively.

It is remarkable how changes due to aging may affect one's ability to eat nutri-tiously and enjoy food. For example, it is estimated that at age 70 years people have 70% fewer taste buds than at age 30 years and this may lead older individuals to increase their use of salt and sugar to improve taste satisfaction.[23] Loss of smell, vision, hearing, and touch additionally affect food choices.[23] When gastrointes-tinal function is compromised, a review of medications and food intake should be taken. Constipation can be alleviated, in some, with a liberal fluid intake and adequate dietary fiber.[23] Consuming foods labeled sugar free yet containing sugar alcohols may cause gastrointestinal distress. These should be decreased or elimi-nated, yet replacement foods should be discussed so appropriate substitutions are recommended.

Hospitalization rates increase in older individuals and weight loss can occur from both acute and chronic illness. Thus, it is important to help older patients achieve an appropriate balance: a healthy and nutritious diet designed to maintain a healthy weight with their food preferences and habits formed over a lifetime. Periodic nutritional reassessment of weight and burden of illness as well as changing functional status and ability to obtain healthy food should be undertaken.

Physical activity is strongly encouraged for the elderly population; however, providers must take the patient's overall health into consideration. (See chapters 11 and 18.)

MACRONUTRIENT CONSIDERATIONS

Rigid approaches to T1D food planning are no longer used. Most RDs aim to normalize the food plan to increase the overall acceptance of healthy food choices. This allows individuals to monitor carbohydrate intake using carbohydrate counting. Blood glucose monitoring helps assess the I:C ratio. According to the ADA 2008 nutrition position statement, it is unlikely that an optimal mix of macronutrients for the diabetic diet exists.[11] The dietary reference intakes (DRIs) of the Institute of Medicine (IOM) for an adult healthy eating pattern may be helpful.[24] The DRI acceptable macronutrient distribution ranges are 45–65% (carbohydrate), 10–35% (protein), 20–35% (fat), and of total energy (see Table 10.2). The IOM also states that regardless of the macronutrient distribution, total energy intake must be appropriate for weight management. The macronutrient mix should be adjusted to meet the metabolic goals and individual preferences of the patient with diabetes.[10]

A 2012 ADA systematic review of the literature on macronutrients, food groups, and eating patterns in diabetes management concluded that different macronutrient distributions may lead to improvement in glycemic or cardiovascular disease (CVD) risk factors, but different approaches to medical nutrition therapy and eating patterns may equally be as effective.[25] RDs should encourage T1D patients to consume macronutrients based on DRIs, since there is insufficient evidence supporting ideal percentages of dietary macronutrients.[12,13]

The *Dietary Guidelines for Americans, 2010*, includes healthy food options that accommodate cultural, ethnic, traditional, and personal preferences and consider food costs and availability. Although healthy eating patterns widely vary, key elements exist: generous vegetables and fruits, focusing on whole grains, various protein foods in moderation, limited amounts of foods high in added sugars, and more oils than solid fats. The benefits of healthy eating patterns are seen in the Dietary Approaches to Stop Hypertension (DASH), a Mediterranean-style eating pattern, and vegetarianism.[26]

Carbohydrates

Sugars, starches, and fibers, rather than simple or complex carbohydrates, are the preferred names for carbohydrate categories, since these terms reflect the chemical composition of the carbohydrates.[17] The DRIs set a recommended dietary allowance (RDA) of at least 130 g of carbohydrates/day for adults and children.[24] This is based on the estimated average requirement for carbohydrate ingestion that will provide the brain with adequate glucose without drawing additional glucose from protein or triglycerides stored in the fat cells (100 g/day), and allows a 15% coefficient of variation for variable brain glucose utilization. The RDA is equal to the estimated average requirement plus twice the coefficient of variation to cover the needs of 97–98% of individuals. Thus, the RDA is at least 130% of the estimated average requirement, or at least 130 g/day of carbohydrate. The ADA notes: "Although brain fuel needs can be met on lower-carbohydrate diets, long-term metabolic effects of very-low-carbohydrate diets are unclear, and such diets eliminate many foods that are important sources of energy, fiber, vitamins, and minerals and that are important in dietary palatability."[10]

Carbohydrate intake. Many have thought that individuals with T1D should avoid sugars (especially sucrose and even naturally occurring sugars), assuming that sugars were rapidly absorbed and therefore aggravated hyperglycemia, and suggested replacement with starch. Starches or complex carbohydrates were thought to break down more slowly, thus producing a slower, steadier rise in blood glucose levels. This thinking began to change with research in 1977 that showed the glycemic response to potatoes was a little higher than that of dextrose.[27]

Recent research has consistently shown that sucrose and other sugars, when consumed separately or as a part of a meal or snack, do not have a greater impact on blood glucose levels as compared to other carbohydrates.[28] Investigators replaced 45 g (~20% of calories) of starch with 45 g of sucrose for 6 weeks, with no significant differences in glycemic or lipid responses in T1D and T2D subjects.[29] Fructose has a lower glycemic response than glucose if an individual is not insulin deficient.[30] The lower response may be caused by its slow rate of absorption and its rapid removal by the liver and storage as glycogen rather than conversion to glucose.[31] Sucrose-containing foods can be substituted for other carbohydrates in the meal plan or, if added to the meal plan, covered with insulin.[11,28]

In DCCT subjects receiving intensive treatment, a lower carbohydrate (37%) intake and higher total (45%) and saturated (17%) fat intakes were associated with worse glycemic control at year 5 compared to a higher carbohydrate (56%) intake (A1C values of 7.5 versus 7.0%, respectively). This finding was independent of exercise and BMI.[32] The authors surmise that carbohydrate content is less critical than the total and saturated fat content, to which it is usually inversely related. It is suggested that high-fat meals may interfere with insulin signaling, resulting in a transient increase in insulin resistance,[33] and that lower-fat diets reduce basal free-fatty acid concentrations and improve peripheral insulin sensitivity in T1D.[34]

A eucaloric diet higher in carbohydrate and lower in fat was compared to one lower in carbohydrate and higher in monounsaturated fatty acids (MUFAs) to determine dietary effects on CVD risk factors. After 6 months, other than decreased plasminogen activator inhibitor 1 and weight gain in the lower-carbohydrate/MUFA group, there was no significant difference between the groups. This suggests that if individuals choose to lower carbohydrate intake, the calories should be replaced with unsaturated fats (vs. saturated fats), with special attention to total energy intake.[35]

Carbohydrate types (recommendations for those with all types of diabetes). In studies where sucrose was substituted for isocaloric amounts of starch, the Acad Nutr Diet EBNPG concluded: "If persons with diabetes choose to eat foods containing sucrose, the sucrose-containing foods can be substituted for other carbohydrate foods. Sucrose intakes of 10–35% of total energy do not have a negative effect on glycemic or lipid level responses when substituted for isocaloric amounts of starch."[12,13] The ADA also concluded that: "Sucrose-containing foods can be substituted for other carbohydrates in the meal plan, or, if added to the food/meal plan, covered with insulin or other glucose-lowering medications."[11] However, in general, it is recommended that avoiding excess energy and sugar intake promotes a healthier eating pattern. The DGAC suggests limited adding sugar intake to ≤25% of total calories because consuming added sugars at or above this level is more likely to result in poor intakes of essential nutrients.[17] For many, consuming this maximum limit can be a very high intake of sugar. For example, for a daily energy intake of ~2,000 kcal, this would be equal to ~31 tsp of added sugars (500 calories or 125 g of carbohydrate). The average daily intake in the U.S. is ~22 tsp sugar (~350 calories, 88 g of carbohydrate). (For comparison: one 12-oz can of cola contains ~9 tsp [~140–150 calories, 35–40 g of carbohydrate]). People with T1D are often made to feel guilt if they choose foods with added sugars. Knowing the total carbohydrate content, including sugars, can assist T1D individuals to make appropriate, enjoyable food choices while maintaining glycemic control. Some recommend that women eat or drink no more than 100 kcal/day from added sugars and men no more than 150 kcal/day.[36]

High fructose corn syrup. High fructose corn syrup is composed of either 42% or 55% fructose and has a similar composition to table sugar (sucrose). The above sucrose recommendations also apply to high fructose corn syrup and would be included in the overall sugar intake. High fructose corn syrup does not differ uniquely from sucrose and other nutritive sweeteners in metabolic effects (glucose, insulin, and triglycerides), subjective effects (hunger, satiety, and energy intake at subsequent meals), and adverse effects such as weight gain.[37]

Fiber and whole grains. The Acad Nutr Diet EBNPG evaluated the effect of fiber intake on glycemic and lipid outcomes in those with diabetes and concluded: "While diets containing 44 to 50 g fiber daily are reported to improve glycemia in persons with diabetes, more usual intakes (up to 24 g/day) have not shown beneficial effects on glycemia. Fiber intake recommendations are similar for patients with diabetes and for the general public (DRI: 14 g/1,000 kcal)."[12,13,38] Guidelines recommend including foods containing 25–30 g fiber/day, emphasizing soluble fiber sources (7–13 g) due to fiber's beneficial effect on lipids.

The ADA also recommends that those with diabetes choose various soluble and insoluble fiber-containing foods such as legumes, fiber-rich cereals (≥5 g fiber/serving), fruits, vegetables, and whole-grain products due to the vitamins, minerals, and other substances important for good health. Of note, it is difficult to meet dietary fiber recommendations with a low-carbohydrate intake.[17]

Whole-grain foods are equally as important as fiber in reducing CVD risk. Whole-grain foods contain fiber, minerals, vitamins, phenolic compounds, phytoestrogens, and other unmeasured constituents, which have shown to lower blood pressure and serum lipids, improve glucose and insulin metabolism and endothelial function, and alleviate oxidative stress and inflammation in the general population.[39] In a prospective study of 7,822 women with T2D, intake of cereal fiber, whole grain, and bran were inversely associated with all-cause and CVD mortality during a 26-year follow-up.[39] Bran intake had the strongest association, but germ intake was not associated with all-cause or CVD mortality.

Glycemic index or glycemic load. Glycemic index (GI) measures the relative area under the glucose curve after consuming 50 g digestible carbohydrate compared with 50 g of a standard food, either glucose or white bread. The GI index does not measure how rapidly blood glucose levels increase after eating different types of carbohydrate-containing foods, thus high-GI foods do not necessarily peak quicker compared to low-GI food. Studies comparing different types of low- and high-GI foods and glucose in people without diabetes showed that glucose peaks occurred consistently at ~30 min, regardless of whether the food had a low-, medium-, or high-GI, with a modest difference in glucose peak values between high- and low-GI foods.[40] Contrary to popular belief, low-GI foods did not cause a slower rise in blood glucose, nor did they produce an extended, sustained glucose response. It is recommended that if individuals want to use the GI as a method of meal planning, they should be advised on the conflicting evidence of effectiveness and that research studies used various definitions of GI and different food components.[12,13]

The estimated glycemic load of foods, meals, and eating patterns is calculated by multiplying the GI by the carbohydrate amount in each food, and then adding all the individual food values in the meal. The glycemic load index is primarily used in epidemiological research since the extensive calculations make it impractical for meal-planning purposes or prandial insulin dosing.

Nonnutritive sweeteners and sugar alcohols. Five nonnutritive sweeteners have been approved by the Food and Drug Administration (FDA): aspartame, saccharine, acesulfame K, neotame, and sucralose. Stevia is approved as Generally Recognized As Safe (GRAS). The FDA also sets a sweetener Acceptable Daily Intake (ADI), namely the level one may safely consume daily over a lifetime without incurring risk. The ADI is usually 1/100th of the amount shown to be safe in animal toxicology studies. All nonnutritive sweeteners undergo rigorous scrutiny in preliminary human studies (including people with diabetes and pregnant women), prior to wider public consumption.[11] The Acad Nutr Diet EBNPG state that nonnutritive sweeteners alone do not affect glycemic responses, but some products contain energy and carbohydrate from other foods, which need to be accounted for.[12,13]

FDA-approved reduced-calorie sweeteners include sugar alcohols (polyols) such as erythritol, isomalt, lactitol, maltitol, mannitol, sorbitol, xylitol, tagatose, and hydrogenated starch hydrolysates. They have lower postprandial glucose responses than sucrose or glucose, and, on average, contain about 2 cal/g. There is no evidence that the sugar alcohol will reduce energy intake, glycemia, or weight. While safe, they may cause diarrhea, especially in children.[11]

Protein

The Acad Nutr Diet EBNPG and the ADA have insufficient evidence to recommend changing the usual protein intake of 15–20% of total daily energy intake for T1D or T2D individuals with normal renal function.[11,13] Individuals who consume excessive amounts of protein-rich foods high in saturated fatty acids, those who have insufficient protein intake (less than the RDA of 0.8 g good-quality protein/kg body weight/day or on average ~10% of energy intake), or those with diabetic nephropathy need to consult with their health care provider and dietitian, as the recommendations may differ.

Studies on protein intake in T1D individuals are limited. A standard lunch (450 kcal) was compared with a protein-added lunch (an additional 200 kcal). The early glucose response was similar, but the late glucose response (2–5 h) was slightly increased and required 3–4 units of additional insulin for those with higher protein intake. However, the total insulin requirement over the 5 h was not increased.[41] Larger than usual amounts of protein may modestly increase postprandial glucose levels and may require slightly higher prandial insulin. If less protein than usual is consumed, insulin doses may also need to be decreased. Perhaps the best assumption is that prandial bolus insulin doses cover the carbohydrates and the basal insulin doses cover the protein consumed. Generally, an individual's protein intake is fairly consistent, and extra insulin is only required when excessive protein is consumed. If lean proteins without fat (e.g., egg whites, skinless chicken) are consumed, additional insulin may not be needed, as protein alone does not necessarily delay glucose release into the blood stream. There is no evidence that suggests protein slows carbohydrate absorption, contributes to sustained glucose elevations, or aids in hypoglycemia treatment.[42]

Dietary Fat

There is no evidence that dietary fats slow glucose absorption and delay peak glycemic response after carbohydrate consumption. A study of T2D subjects showed that adding varying amounts of fat (5, 15, 30, or 50 g butter) to a 50 g carbohydrate meal (potato) resulted in similar postprandial mean glucose area response.[43] In another study, 50 g potato alone or with 100 g butter or 80 g olive oil was compared (discrepancy in amounts of fats was due to the 20% water content of the butter), and the addition of both fats had no effect on glucose or insulin postprandial responses.[44] In T1D subjects, adding 200 kcal (22 g fat) to a standard meal did not affect glucose response or insulin requirements.[41] Therefore, these limited studies show that the addition of fat appears to have minimal effect on postprandial glucose.

The effects of trans fatty acids on CVD risk are due to their positive association with LDL cholesterol, the effect on inflammatory processes, and their interference with fat metabolism. The reverse association is seen with HDL cholesterol. The majority of trans fatty acids come from commercial hydrogenation of unsaturated fats, but ~1–2% (<2% of total energy intake) is found naturally in the gastrointestinal tracts of ruminant animals, ending up in meats and dairy products. The DGAC concluded that avoiding industrial trans fats is important, while leaving small amounts of ruminant trans fats in the diet.[17]

The DGAC studied the effects of dietary cholesterol. From a review of 16 studies published since 1991, the committee concluded that consumption of one egg/day is not associated with CVD risk or stroke in healthy adults, but eating seven or more eggs/week was associated with increased risk. Omega-3 fatty acids (Ω-3) from fish or from supplements have been shown to reduce adverse CVD outcomes in people with and without diabetes. A Cochrane Systematic Review and a second systematic review and meta-analysis concluded that Ω-3 supplementation in T2D subjects lowers triglyceride levels but may raise LDL cholesterol and have no effect on glycemic control or fasting insulin.[45,46] In the ORIGIN Trial, an RCT performed in over 12,000 T2D individuals, supplementation with 1 g of Ω-3 fatty acids daily did not reduce CVD events compared to placebo.[47]

The Acad Nutr Diet EBNPG reviews research on CVD prevention and treatment in people with diabetes. Its guidelines recommend that cardioprotective nutrition interventions start in the initial nutrition therapy encounters, since both glycemic control and cardioprotective nutrition interventions improve the lipid profile, reduce CVD risk, and improve CVD outcomes.[12,13] Nutrition interventions include reducing saturated and trans fatty acids and dietary cholesterol and improving blood pressure. (See chapter 16.II, Microvascular Complications.)

Micronutrients

There are no adequately controlled studies that link pathogenesis of carbohydrate intolerance to trace elements.[48,49] Although animal studies have suggested that deficiencies in many of the trace elements—including zinc, chromium, magnesium, copper, manganese, and vitamin B6—may lead to glucose intolerance, the evidence is not definitive. Animal laboratory diets, in comparison to human diets, can be easily manipulated. Thus, animal study results should not be extrapolated to humans without validating the findings in human pilot studies.

In studies with individuals with T1D, trace-metal and water-soluble vitamin urinary losses are increased during uncontrolled hyperglycemia and glycosuria. Therefore, the micronutrient effect may depend on the degree of glucose tolerance. Also, the micronutrient effect on insulin secretion is biphasic. Low vitamin concentrations may stimulate insulin secretion, and high concentrations may have an inhibitory effect.

In human studies, dietary micronutrient amounts are often unknown. To further confuse the micronutrient role and diabetes, serum or tissue content of certain elements—copper, manganese, iron, and selenium—can be higher in people with diabetes than in control subjects without diabetes. On the other hand, serum ascorbic acid (vitamin C), B vitamins, and vitamin D may be lower in individuals with diabetes, whereas vitamins A and E have been reported to be normal or increased.

Regardless, micronutrients are intimately involved in carbohydrate or glucose metabolism, insulin release, and insulin sensitivity. Unfortunately, this information is frequently extrapolated beyond what the research supports. The ADA recommends that individuals optimize food choices in meal plans to meet RDA and DRI intakes for all micronutrients.[10]

ALCOHOL

Earlier studies in T1D subjects showed no acute effect on blood glucose levels with moderate alcohol intake with meals. Further studies reported associations with late-onset hypoglycemia.[50] Possible causes include inhibition of gluconeogenesis, reduced hypoglycemia awareness due to cerebral effects of alcohol, or impaired counterregulatory responses to hypoglycemia. A study with men with T1D who consumed wine in the evening (0.75 g alcohol/kg body weight; ~20 oz for a 70-kg individual) resulted in hypoglycemia treatment being required after breakfast.[51] Growth hormone levels were significantly reduced, but no other differences in insulin or other hormone levels were reported.[51] Similarly, in T1D adults, hypoglycemia (blood glucose 50 mg/dl) resulted in lower peak growth hormone levels compared to placebo; however, this study was also associated with a decrease in insulin sensitivity.[52] In a study similar to the men's wine study, T1D individuals drank either orange juice or vodka with their evening meal. Continuous glucose monitoring data showed that individuals who drank alcohol (0.85 g alcohol/kg body weight) had more than twice as many hypoglycemic episodes throughout the next 24 h than those who drank orange juice.[53]

In T1D subjects, both mild alcohol intoxication and hypoglycemia (blood glucose ~43 mg/dl) were associated with deteriorating reaction time and other cognitive function tests, and total impairment was greater when both were experienced together.[54] The authors emphasized that individuals must test blood glucose levels before driving. They should not drive when mildly hypoglycemic, even if asymptomatic.

Elevated total ketone body concentrations are characteristic of both diabetic ketoacidosis (DKA) and alcoholic ketoacidosis (AKA). However, compared to AKA, DKA is characterized by a higher glucose concentration and lower β-hydroxybutyrate:acetoacetate and lactate:pyruvate ratios. Hormonal profiles are similar with decreased insulin levels and elevated levels of counterregulatory hormones.[55] T1D subjects who liberally consumed alcohol at lunchtime had elevated postprandial β-hydroxybutrate levels vs. suppressed levels with placebo.[56] The authors propose that binge drinking may increase the risk of significant ketosis, especially with erratic insulin administration, and recommend that patient education materials highlight these potential problems.

Adolescents, in particular, must be instructed on alcohol and its potential hypoglycemic effects, and on responsible drinking. Adolescents who drive should be instructed on blood glucose monitoring before driving and on carrying a carbohydrate source with them at all times in case hypoglycemia should occur.

In summary, moderate alcohol (one drink/day or less for women and two drinks/day or less for men) consumption appears to have minimal, if any, acute effects on glucose levels and insulin need, but patients must be aware of the occurrence of late-onset hypoglycemia, likely due to alcohol-related growth hormone reduction. Thus, alcohol should be consumed with food.[11] Also, patients should repeatedly self-monitor blood glucose levels after drinking alcohol to assess if hypoglycemia treatment is needed. The additive effect of alcohol and hypoglycemia on cognitive function highlights the urgency of avoiding alcohol when planning to drive.

CARBOHYDRATE COUNTING

Carbohydrate counting is a meal-planning method based on the principle that all types of carbohydrate (except fiber) are digested, with the majority being absorbed into the bloodstream as glucose molecules. The total carbohydrate consumed has a greater effect on blood glucose elevations than the specific type consumed. There are two main methods of meal planning: an I:C ratio to adjust prandial insulin for variable carbohydrate intake (physiological insulin regimen) or a consistent carbohydrate meal plan when using a fixed insulin regimen.

The most widely used method of meal planning for youth with T1D is carbohydrate counting. Rigid meal plans have been replaced with more flexible ones, matching insulin to the child's nutrition (carbohydrate) intake. For people who have difficulty with carbohydrate counting, simplified, healthy eating meal-planning guidelines are recommended. Which method a child uses will depend on the insulin regimen and the family's skill level. Often, the youth will start a basal-bolus insulin regimen (multiple daily injections [MDIs]) and then transition to an insulin pump, if desired. Nutritional recommendations will be made based on a child's age and eating patterns.

To accurately count carbohydrate amounts, children and their families are taught how to read the nutrition facts on food labels for total carbohydrate grams. Families should measure or weigh foods periodically to reinforce accurate portion sizes, and thus accurate carbohydrate content, so the correct insulin dose can be taken. There are books, websites, and smartphone applications that provide carbohydrate content for unlabeled foods. Families should have easy access to one of these resources to accurately estimate carbohydrates. Some school districts are displaying carbohydrate information for school breakfasts and lunches, facilitating carbohydrate counting; if not displayed, the information is available from the school lunch program.

Because accurate carbohydrate counting is essential for accurate insulin dosing, researchers have evaluated carbohydrate-counting accuracy in the pediatric population. Research in children, adolescents, and their parents indicates that individuals may not be accurately estimating the carbohydrates. In one study, parents of 4- to 12-year-old children overestimated carbohydrate intake of their children by an average of 120% of the nutrition database calculated intake.[57] Another study found that adolescents either significantly over- or underestimated carbohydrate content of 23 of 32 individual foods presented as real foods or food models.[58] Lastly, a study conducted in the United Kingdom and Australia found that adolescents estimated carbohydrates within 10–15 g of the actual amount for 73% of meals presented.[59] These authors concluded that adolescents carbohydrate count reasonably well, but if accuracy was defined more stringently (within 10 g of the actual amount), then many estimates would have been inaccurate. Additional research is needed to help determine the best strategies for helping children, adolescents, and their families enhance their carbohydrate-counting skills and potentially improve glycemic control.

Fixed Carbohydrate Meal Plan

Both children and adults using fixed daily insulin doses must use a carbohydrate-counting meal-planning approach or some other method of quantifying carbohydrate intake to maintain day-to-day consistency, both in the timing and quantity of food intake. Alternatives to carbohydrate counting include *1)* the plate method, and *2)* preplanned menus. Accuracy in portion sizes remains important, and creative education is encouraged to promote accuracy, such as using beverage glasses, plates, and bowls that have lines or patterns that guide serving (portion) sizes.

Food Factors Affecting Glycemic Control

Postprandial hyperglycemia involves more than knowing how to count carbohydrates. Many T1D patients struggle to understand why their blood glucose levels dramatically fluctuate on a daily basis despite eating consistent carbohydrate grams. One explanation may be due to inadequate education on how to accurately dose prandial insulin and quantify carbohydrate intake.[60] The CDC reports that only 55.7% of people with diabetes participate in a diabetes self-management education (DSME) class, suggesting that many patients never receive formal instructions on meal planning, such as carbohydrate counting, to enable accurate quantification of carbohydrate intake.[61] Consequently, they may either under- or overdose prandial insulin requirements. An accurate prandial insulin dose to actual food (carbohydrate grams) intake is a critical component of basal-bolus insulin therapy.

Aside from correct carbohydrate counting, several extrinsic and intrinsic variables affect glycemic control. Extrinsic factors, such as macronutrient distribution of the meal, fasting or preprandial blood glucose level, available insulin, antecedent exercise, and degree of insulin resistance may influence the impact of carbohydrates on the postprandial response.[11] Additionally, intrinsic variables include type and source of carbohydrate, the physical form of the food (e.g., whole food vs. juice), starch type (e.g., amylopectin vs. amylose), method of food preparation (e.g., baking vs. frying), cooking time and amount of heat and moisture used, degree of processing, and ripeness of food.[11] Individuals can use information from self-monitoring of blood glucose (SMBG) and continuous glucose sensors to better learn how both the extrinsic and intrinsic variables affect their glycemic control.

Meal-Planning Approaches and Tools

Other than carbohydrate counting, meal-planning approaches such as the glycemic index also have been studied. Australian researchers developed a food insulin index, a physiological basis for ranking foods according to insulin demand for 120 single foods.[62] They concluded that the relative insulin demand evoked by mixed meals consumed by lean healthy subjects is best predicted by a physiological index (food insulin index) based on integrating insulin responses to isoenergetic portions of single foods. Eating patterns that provoke less insulin secretion may be helpful in managing diabetes. In 2011, another Australian study compared a novel algorithm based on the food insulin index for estimating mealtime insulin dose to carbohydrate counting in T1D adults using CSII.[63] The study concluded that, when compared with carbohydrate counting, the food insulin index algorithm improved acute postprandial glycemia in well-controlled T1D subjects. The authors acknowledge that clinical application of these findings is not currently feasible, since the food insulin index does not presently appear on food labels and the food insulin index database includes only ~120 foods.

Another group collected data on food intake, physical activity, insulin administration, and blood glucose test results in T1D patients using self-administered questionnaires.[64] Sixty-four percent of the participants incorrectly estimated their prandial insulin, revealing that optimal prandial insulin dosing is not easy and requires continuous assessment and related education and support, even after a long duration of diabetes.

Insulin dosing aids such as bolus insulin calculation cards and dosing guides have been developed to reduce potential calculation errors.[65-67] Bolus calculators with personalized insulin-dosing algorithms can be programmed in a wide range of devices, such as personal digital assistants (PDAs), smartphone applications, or insulin pumps.[68,69]

The Diabetes Interactive Diary is an automatic carbohydrate and insulin bolus calculator installed on a mobile phone, using patient-physician communication via text messages. When compared with a standard carbohydrate-counting education program, the Diabetes Interactive Diary was as effective as a traditional carbohydrate-counting education program, without an increased hypoglycemia risk.[70] Technology has reduced education time while significantly improving treatment satisfaction and several quality-of-life dimensions. Adaptive aids are popular with the tech-savvy but may be useful for those with health literacy and numeracy concerns, such as young children or adults who cannot perform complex mathematical equations required for intensive insulin therapy.[71] Technology may allow more people with insulin-requiring diabetes to have access to diabetes self-management tools, education, and support.

Factors That may Affect Long-Term Adherence to Carbohydrate Counting

Three studies have explored the food and eating practices of T1D subjects who converted to flexible intensive insulin therapy (FIIT) as part of the DAFNE course.[5,14,72] Ironically, in efforts to simplify food choices for easier carbohydrate estimation, patients may rely on prepackaged foods, with higher saturated fats and salt, but with nutrition labels, rather than calculate the carbohydrate content for fresh fruits, vegetables, and other unprocessed items that do not have food labels. FIIT participants also expressed anxieties about miscalculating carbohydrate amounts and injecting the wrong dose. This caused participants to eat the same foods repeatedly, limiting intake of new foods or foods with difficult-to-determine carbohydrate content. Some participants intentionally choose low- or no-carbohydrate foods to simplify prandial dose calculations. Despite formal intensive insulin therapy classes, many subjects feared hypoglycemia when matching mealtime insulin to desired food (carbohydrate) intake.[5] These data raise factors that need to be addressed during initial and ongoing nutrition therapy. Strategies are needed to successfully sustain this therapy on a daily basis.[72]

One study interviewed DAFNE program participants at 6 weeks and 6 and 12 months on assimilating course principles.[14] Subjects initially (6 weeks) felt support from other participants, for example, by sharing experiences. However, after 6 months, subjects valued support from responsive health care professionals that focused on collaborative decision making. The investigators concluded that diabetes educators must clearly communicate to participants that FIIT principles take time (perhaps over 12 months). Support at 6 months appeared to be an important timeframe for subjects, since motivation at this point was lowest for many.

People with insulin-requiring diabetes may also diligently perform dose calculations using their individualized algorithms when beginning intensive insulin therapy.[68] However, adherence to the ongoing determination of the prandial insulin dose may become relaxed as the individual with diabetes gains familiarity with the self-adjustment of the insulin. As time passes, there may be the tendency to begin to approximate premeal doses by titrating insulin based on the standard or usual carbohydrate content of the meal. In addition, many people with insulin-requiring diabetes may actually be hesitant to take on the responsibility of increasing or decreasing their insulin doses on the basis of their carbohydrate intake and premeal blood glucose level.[68]

ADDITIONAL CONSIDERATIONS

Disordered Eating Behaviors, Eating Disorders, and Other Age-Related Concerns

Body image and weight-management issues in T1D adolescents and young adults with T1D may lead to eating disorders and disordered eating behaviors (see chapter 8, Psychosocial Issues in Type 1 Diabetes). It is unclear if there is an increased prevalence of diagnosable eating disorders and disordered eating behaviors in T1D patients compared with the general population. Some studies show a higher rate in T1D patients, while others have found the same or lower rates.[73] Estimates in T1D adolescent and young adult females range from 3.8 to 27.5% for patients classified as bulimic or having binge eating disorder. When insulin omission is considered purging, the estimate is as high as 38–40%. The presence of eating disorders has been associated with increases in retinopathy, neuropathy, transient lipid abnormalities, hospitalizations for diabetic ketoacidosis, and poor short-term metabolic control. Adolescents with diabetes should be screened regularly for signs of potential eating issues and concerns with weight and body image as well as insulin omission. After screening, issues can be addressed and action can be taken to prevent the development of an eating disorder, which is very complicated to treat especially when it coexists with T1D. Warning signs that suggest an eating disorder in adolescents include inadequate weight gain or growth, significant weight loss without illness, suboptimal overall glycemic control, and recurrent diabetic ketoacidosis. If signs of disordered eating and weight or body image concerns are present, they need to be addressed; referral to a dietitian and psychotherapist or psychologist is recommended. If a patient is at high risk of an eating disorder, the patient should be referred to an eating disorder program for an assessment and treatment, if necessary.

Finally, adolescents with diabetes may experiment with alternative eating patterns, such as vegetarianism or nutritional supplement use. Practical information on these topics will enable adolescents to make wise choices for their health.

NUTRITION THERAPY FOR CELIAC DISEASE AND T1D

Celiac disease (CD) is an important entity to consider since those with T1D are also at increased risk for developing CD. Individuals diagnosed with both CD and T1D should seek the care of an RD familiar with the nutritional management of both entities. The RD should also provide comprehensive support and education about gluten-free diets (GFD).

The Gluten-Free Diet

Since nutritional deficiencies have been reported with long-term GFD, comprehensive nutrition assessments must be done to ensure adequate nutrient intake.[74,75] A GFD can be extremely challenging, since ongoing monitoring of ingredients in foods and food processing are intricate parts of nutrition interventions.

For newly diagnosed children and adults with CD, studies report that adherence to a gluten-free eating pattern results in significant improvements in serum Hb, iron, zinc, and calcium, as a result of intestinal healing and improved absorption. However, adherence to the gluten-free eating pattern may result in a diet that is high in fat and low in carbohydrates, fiber, iron, folate, niacin, vitamin B_{12}, calcium, phosphorus, and zinc. A small number of adult studies show a trend toward weight gain after diagnosis.[76]

Several studies report that patients with CD (treated and untreated) are more likely to experience gastrointestinal symptoms such as diarrhea, constipation, abdominal pain and bloating, nausea or vomiting, reduced gut motility, and delayed gastric emptying than healthy control subjects. However, long-term adherence to a GFD has been shown to reduce the prevalence of these symptoms.[76]

Implementing the Gluten-Free Diet

A GFD can be more expensive than a normal diet and requires extensive, repeated counseling and RD instruction. Patients with CD must be meticulous label readers and knowledgeable about food processing, preparation, and handling practices to avoid cross-contamination with gluten-containing grains. As little as 10 mg gluten (1/50th a slice of bread) can cause significant mucosal inflammation in some individuals. Therefore, it is recommended that contaminating gluten should be kept to <50 mg/day in the treatment of CD.[77] Gluten-free grains, seeds, and flours may inadvertently become contaminated; therefore, food manufacturers are urged to test gluten-free products for contamination using validated testing methods.[78] The FDA has proposed that gluten-free products contain <20 parts/million gluten using validated testing methods. Unfortunately, this testing would be voluntary. Prescription and over-the-counter medications, vitamins, minerals and supplements, and nonfood items such as play dough may also contain gluten.

Studies evaluating the impact of gluten-free diets on T1D have shown conflicting results, with some showing no change in A1C levels in either children or adults,[79-86] while others have shown improvements in A1C.[87-91] One study noted a worse A1C in children.[92] This indicates that with education and support, patients can successfully implement the CD and T1D food plans to maintain or improve A1C levels.

Bone Health

Osteoporosis and osteopenia are the most common complications of undiagnosed or untreated CD. Studies examining bone mineral density (BMD) levels in adolescents and children with CD and T1D have shown conflicting results, with some reporting lower BMD in patients with CD and T1D[93,94] and another finding no difference.[95] One pediatric study stratified BMD results according to GFD adherence, showing individuals who adhere strictly have the same BMD as T1D control subjects, but those with poor compliance to the GFD resulted in lower BMD.[96] Pediatric patients who followed a GFD had improvement in BMD and bone mineral apparent density Z scores.[94] An adult study identified lower BMD in T1D and undiagnosed CD.[97]

CONCLUSION

Medical nutrition therapy and insulin dosing is the crux of T1D management. There are limited randomized, well-controlled clinical trials evaluating nutrition and T1D; however, many general principles apply and have been presented. Whether an individual meticulously counts carbohydrates and adjusts each mealtime insulin dose, or "guesstimates" portions, T1D management always involves extensive nutrition knowledge. Critical to any success is the involvement of an RD well versed in T1D management. This is true whether treating a child or an adult. Clearly a team approach is needed and other health care providers should be familiar with medical nutrition therapy, but the RD is the key resource. With appropriate guidance, ongoing support and encouragement, individuals with T1D and their families can succeed at learning and applying medical nutrition therapy, improve diabetes control, minimize long-term complications, and enjoy a higher quality of life.

Gaps in Nutritional Education and Support for People with T1D

1. Include documentation of food intake and fixed meals in drug and device studies to better understand impact of food, combinations of food, and timing of meals.
2. Undertake more research on best method for teaching carbohydrate counting that creates sustainable impact on diabetes management.
3. Initiate research on eating patterns to identify those that optimize glucose management; include evaluation of random eating patterns vs. consistent eating patterns.
4. Develop real-time tools for assisting patients in estimating carbohydrate count of a meal or snack.
5. Continue to work on ways to better identify and treat nutritional issues in those with T1D and eating disorders, CD, and various subgroups such as the elderly and the obese.

REFERENCES

1. Pastors JG, Franz MJ: Effectiveness of medical nutrition therapy in diabetes. In *American Diabetes Association Guide to Nutrition Therapy for Diabetes*. 2nd ed. Franz MJ, Evert AB, Eds. Alexandria, VA, American Diabetes Association, 2012, p. 1–18
2. American Diabetes Association. Clinical Practice Recommendations 2012. *Diabetes Care* 35 (Suppl. 1):S1–S110, 2012
3. DAFNE Study Group: Training in flexible, intensive insulin management to enable dietary freedom in people with type 1 diabetes: Dose Adjustment for Normal Eating (DAFNE) randomised controlled trial. *BMJ* 325:746, 2002
4. Speight J, Amiel SA, Bradley C, Heller S, Oliver L, Roberts S, Rogers H, Taylor C, Thompson G: Long-term biomedical and psychosocial outcomes following DAFNE (Dose Adjustment For Normal Eating) structured education to promote intensive insulin therapy in adults with sub-optimally controlled type 1 diabetes. *Diabetes Res Clin Pract* 89:22–29, 2010. Epub 18 April 2010
5. Lawton J, Rankin D, Cooke DD, Clark M, Elliot J, Heller S: UK NIHR DAFNE Study Group: Dose Adjustment for Normal Eating: a qualitative longitudinal exploration of the food and eating practices of type 1 diabetes patients converted to flexible intensive insulin therapy in the UK. *Diabetes Res Clin Pract* 91:87–93, 2011. Epub 3 December 2010
6. Pieber TR, Brunner GA, Schnedl WJ, Schattenberg S, Kaufmann P, Krejs GJ: Evaluation of a structured outpatient group education program for intensive insulin therapy. *Diabetes Care* 18:625–630, 1995
7. Sämann A, Mühlhauser I, Bender R, Kloos Ch, Müller UA: Glycaemic control and severe hypoglycaemia following training in flexible, intensive insulin therapy to enable dietary freedom in people with type 1 diabetes: a prospective implementation study. *Diabetologia* 48:1965–1970, 2005. Epub 18 August 2005
8. Lowe J, Linjawi S, Mensch M, James K, Attia J: Flexible eating and flexible insulin dosing in patients with diabetes: results of an intensive self-management course. *Diabetes Res Clin Pract* 80:439–443, 2008. Epub 18 March 2008
9. Delahanty LM, Halford BN: The role of diet behaviors in achieving improved glycemic control in intensively treated patients in the Diabetes Control and Complications Trial. *Diabetes Care* 16:1453–1458, 1993
10. American Diabetes Association: Standards of medical care in diabetes—2012. *Diabetes Care* 35 (Suppl. 1):S11–S63, 2012; doi:10.2337/dc12-s011
11. American Diabetes Association: Nutrition recommendations and interventions for diabetes. *Diabetes Care* 31 (Suppl. 1):S61–S78, 2008; doi: 10.2337/dc08-S061
12. Franz MJ, Powers MA, Leontos C, Holzmeister LA, Kulkarni K, Monk A, Wedel N, Gradwell E: The evidence for medical nutrition therapy for type 1 and type 2 diabetes in adults. *J Am Diet Assoc* 110:1852–1889, 2010
13. Academy of Nutrition and Dietetics: Diabetes Mellitus Type 1 & 2 Evidence-Based Nutrition Practice Guideline, 2008. Available at http://andevidencelibrary.com/topic.cfm?cat=3252. Accessed 30 October 2012

14. Casey D, Murphy K, Lawton J, White FF, Dineen S: A longitudinal qualitative study examining the factors impacting on the ability of persons with T1DM to assimilate the Dose Adjustment for Normal Eating (DAFNE) principles into daily living and how these factors change over time. *BMC Public Health* 11:672, 2011
15. Centers for Disease Control and Prevention: Growth Charts, 2010. Available at http://www.cdc.gov/growthcharts. Accessed 30 October 2012
16. Silverstein J, Klingensmith G, Copeland K, Plotnick L, Kaufman F, Laffel L, Deeb L, Grey M, Anderson B, Holzmeister LA, Clark N: American Diabetes Association: Care of children and adolescents with type 1 diabetes: a statement of the American Diabetes Association. *Diabetes Care* 28:186–212, 2005
17. Dietary Guidelines Advisory Committee: Report of the Dietary Guidelines Advisory Committee on the Dietary Guidelines for Americans, 2010, to the Secretary of Agriculture and the Secretary of Health and Human Services. Washington, DC, U.S. Department of Agriculture, Agricultural Research Service, 2010
18. Helgeson VS, Viccaro L, Becker D, Escobar O, Siminerio L: Diet of adolescents with and without diabetes: trading candy for potato chips? *Diabetes Care* 29:982–987, 2006
19. Mayer-Davis EJ, Nichols M, Liese AD, Bell RA, Dabelea DM, Johansen JM, Pihoker C, Rodriguez BL, Thomas J, Williams D: SEARCH for Diabetes in Youth Study Group: Dietary intake among youth with diabetes: the SEARCH for Diabetes in Youth Study. *J Am Diet Assoc* 106:689–697, 2006
20. Patton SR, Dolan LM, Powers SW: Dietary adherence and associated glycemic control in families of young children with type 1 diabetes. *J Am Diet Assoc* 107:46–52, 2007
21. Overby NC, Flaaten V, Veierød MB, Bergstad I, Margeirsdottir HD, Dahl-Jørgensen K, Andersen LF: Children and adolescents with type 1 diabetes eat a more atherosclerosis-prone diet than healthy control subjects. *Diabetologia* 50:307–316, 2007. Epub 29 November 2006
22. Overby NC, Margeirsdottir HD, Brunborg C, Andersen LF, Dahl-Jørgensen K: The influence of dietary intake and meal pattern on blood glucose control in children and adolescents using intensive insulin treatment. *Diabetologia* 50:2044–2051, 2007. Epub 9 August 2007
23. McLaughlin S: Considerations in caring for older persons with diabetes. In *Handbook of Diabetes Medical Nutrition Therapy*. Powers MA, Ed. Gaithersburg, MD, Aspen Publishers, Inc., 1996, p. 527–546
24. Institute of Medicine: *Dietary Reference Intakes for Energy, Carbohydrate, Fiber, Fat, Fatty Acids, Cholesterol, Protein, and Amino Acids*. Washington, DC, National Academies Press, 2002
25. Wheeler ML, Dunbar SA, Jaacks LM, Karmally W, Mayer-Davis EJ, Wylie-Rosett J, Yancy WS Jr: Macronutrients, food groups, and eating patterns in the management of diabetes: a systematic review of the literature, 2010. *Diabetes Care* 35:434–445, 2012
26. U.S. Department of Agriculture, U.S. Department of Health and Human Services: *Dietary Guidelines for Americans, 2010*. 7th ed. Washington, DC, U.S. Government Printing Office, 2010

27. Crapo PA, Reaven G, Olefsky J: Postprandial plasma-glucose and insulin responses to different complex carbohydrates. *Diabetes* 26:1178, 1977

28. Academy of Nutrition and Dietetics: Diabetes mellitus type 1 & 2 evidence-based nutrition practice guideline, 2008. Available at http://andevidenceli-brary.com/topic.cfm?cat=3252. Accessed 30 October 2012

29. Peterson DB, Lambert J, Gerring S, Darling P, Carter RD, Jelfs R, Mann JL: Sucrose in the diet of diabetic patients–just another carbohydrate? *Diabetologia* 29:216–220, 1986

30. Uusitupa MI: Fructose in the diabetic diet. *Am J Clin Nutr* 59 (Suppl.):753S–757S, 1994

31. Rumessen JJ, Gudmand-Høyer E: Absorption capacity of fructose in healthy adults. Comparison with sucrose and its constituent monosaccharides. *Gut* 27:1161–1168, 1986

32. Delahanty LM, Nathan DM, Lachin JM, Hu FB, Cleary PA, Ziegler GK, Wylie-Rosett J, Wexler DJ: Diabetes Control and Complications Trial/Epidemiology of Diabetes: Association of diet with glycated hemoglobin during intensive treatment of type 1 diabetes in the Diabetes Control and Complications Trial. *Am J Clin Nutr* 89:518–524, 2009. Epub 23 December 2008

33. Savage DB, Petersen KF, Shulman GI: Disordered lipid metabolism and the pathogenesis of insulin resistance. *Physiol Rev* 87:507–520, 2007

34. Rosenfalck AM, Almdal T, Viggers L, Madsbad S, Hilsted J: A low-fat diet improves peripheral insulin sensitivity in patients with type 1 diabetes. *Diabet Med* 23:384–392, 2006

35. Strychar I, Cohn JS, Renier G, Rivard M, Aris-Jilwan N, Beauregard H, Meltzer S, Bélanger A, Dumas R, Ishac A, Radwan F, Yale JF: Effects of a diet higher in carbohydrate/lower in fat versus lower in carbohydrate/higher in monounsaturated fat on postmeal triglyceride concentrations and other cardiovascular risk factors in type 1 diabetes. *Diabetes Care* 32:1597–1599, 2009. Epub 18 June 2009

36. Johnson RK, Appel LJ, Brands M, Howard BV, Lefevre M, Lustig RH, Sacks F, Steffen LM, Wylie-Rosett J: on behalf of the American Heart Association Nutrition Committee of the Council on Nutrition, Physical Activity, and Metabolism and the Council on Epidemiology and Prevention: AHA Scientific Statement: Dietary sugars intake and cardiovascular health: a scientific statement from the American Heart Association. *Circulation* 120:1011–1020, 2009

37. Fitch C, Keim KS; Academy of Nutrition and Dietetics: Position of the Academy of Nutrition and Dietetics: use of nutritive and nonnutritive sweeteners. *J Acad Nutr Diet* 112:739–758, 2012. Epub 25 April 2012

38. Franz MJ, Powers MA, Leontos C, Holzmeister LA, Kulkarni K, Monk A, Wedel N, Gradwell E: The evidence for medical nutrition therapy for type 1 and type 2 diabetes in adults. *J Am Diet Assoc* 110:1852–1889, 2010

39. He M, van Dam RM, Rimm E, Hu FB, Qi L: Whole-grain, cereal fiber, bran, and germ intake and the risks of all-cause and cardiovascular disease-specific mortality among women with type 2 diabetes mellitus. *Circulation* 121:2162–2168, 2010. Epub 10 May 2010

40. Brand-Miller JC, Stockmann K, Atkinson F, Petocz P, Denyer G: Glycemic index, postprandial glycemia, and the shape of the curve in healthy subjects:

analysis of a database of more than 1,000 foods. *Am J Clin Nutr* 89:97–105, 2009. Epub 3 December 2008

41. Peters AL, Davidson MB: Protein and fat effects on glucose responses and insulin requirements in subjects with insulin-dependent diabetes mellitus. *Am J Clin Nutr* 58:555–560, 1993

42. Franz MJ: Protein and diabetes: much advice, little research. *Curr Diab Rep* 2:457–464, 2002

43. Gannon MC, Ercan N, Westphal SA, Nuttall FQ: Effect of added fat on plasma glucose and insulin response to ingested potato in individuals with NIDDM. *Diabetes Care* 16:874–880, 1993

44. Thomsen C, Storm H, Holst JJ, Hermansen K: Differential effects of saturated and monounsaturated fats on postprandial lipemia and glucagon-like peptide 1 responses in patients with type 2 diabetes. *Am J Clin Nutr* 77:605–611, 2003

45. Hartweg J, Perera R, Montori V, Dinneen S, Neil HA, Farmer A: Omega-3 polyunsaturated fatty acids (PUFA) for type 2 diabetes mellitus. *Cochrane Database Syst Rev* CD003205, 2008

46. Hartweg J, Farmer AJ, Holman RR, Neil A: Potential impact of omega-3 treatment on cardiovascular disease in type 2 diabetes. *Curr Opin Lipidol* 20:30–38, 2009

47. Bosch J, Gerstein HC, Dagenais GR, Díaz R, Dyal L, Jung H, Maggiono AP, Probstfield J, Ramachandran A, Riddle MC, Rydén LE, Yusuf S: ORIGIN Trial Investigators: n-3 fatty acids and cardiovascular outcomes in patients with dysglycemia. *N Engl J Med* 367:309–318, 2012. Epub 11 June 2012

48. Mooradian AD, Failla M, Hoogwerf B, Maryniuk M, Wylie-Rosett J: Selected vitamins and minerals in diabetes. *Diabetes Care* 17:464–479, 1994

49. Mooradian AD, Morley JE: Micronutrient status in diabetes mellitus. *Am J Clin Nutr* 45:877–895, 1987

50. Franz MJ: Diabetes mellitus: considerations in the development of guidelines for the occasional use of alcohol. *J Am Diet Assoc* 83:147–152, 1983

51. Turner BC, Jenkins E, Kerr D, Sherwin RS, Cavan DA: The effect of evening alcohol consumption on next-morning glucose control in type 1 diabetes. *Diabetes Care* 24:1888–1893, 2001

52. Kerr D, Cheyne E, Thomas P, Sherwin R: Influence of acute alcohol ingestion on the hormonal responses to modest hypoglycaemia in patients with type 1 diabetes. *Diabet Med* 24:312–316, 2007

53. Richardson T, Weiss M, Thomas P, Kerr D: Day after the night before: influence of evening alcohol on risk of hypoglycemia in patients with type 1 diabetes. *Diabetes Care* 28:1801–1802, 2005

54. Cheyne EH, Sherwin RS, Lunt MJ, Cavan DA, Thomas PW, Kerr D: Influence of alcohol on cognitive performance during mild hypoglycaemia; implications for type 1 diabetes. *Diabet Med* 21:230–237, 2004

55. Umpierrez GE, DiGirolamo M, Tuvlin JA, Isaacs SD, Bhoola SM, Kokko JP: Differences in metabolic and hormonal milieu in diabetic- and alcohol-induced ketoacidosis. *J Crit Care* 15:52–59, 2000

56. Kerr D, Penfold S, Zouwail S, Thomas P, Begley J: The influence of liberal alcohol consumption on glucose metabolism in patients with type 1 diabetes: a pilot study. *QJM* 102:169–174, 2009. Epub 19 December 2008

57. Mehta SN, Quinn N, Volkening LK, Laffel LM: Impact of carbohydrate counting on glycemic control in children with type 1 diabetes. *Diabetes Care* 32:1014–1016, 2009. Epub 24 February 2009

58. Bishop FK, Maahs DM, Speigel G, Owen D, Klingensmith GJ, Bortsov A, Thomas J, Mayer-Davis EJ: The Carbohydrate Counting in Adolescents With Type 1 Diabetes (CCAT) Study. *Diabetes Spectrum* 22:56–62, 2009; doi: 10.2337/diaspect.22.1.56

59. Smart CE, Ross K, Edge JA, King BR, McElduff P, Collins CE: Can children with type 1 diabetes and their caregivers estimate the carbohydrate content of meals and snacks? *Diabet Med* 27:348–353, 2010

60. Boukhors Y, Rabasa-Lhoret R, Langelier H, Soultan M, Lacroix A, Chiasson JL: The use of information technology for the management of intensive insulin therapy in type 1 diabetes mellitus. *Diabetes Metab* 29:619–627, 2003

61. Centers for Disease Control and Prevention: National Diabetes Fact Sheet, 2011. Atlanta, GA, Centers for Disease Control and Prevention, 2011

62. Bao J, de Jong V, Atkinson F, Petocz P, Brand-Miller JC: Food insulin index: physiologic basis for predicting insulin demand evoked by composite meals. *Am J Clin Nutr* 90:986–992, 2009. Epub 26 August 2009

63. Bao J, Gilbertson HR, Gray R, Munns D, Howard G, Petocz P, Colagiuri S, Brand-Miller JC: Improving the estimation of mealtime insulin dose in adults with type 1 diabetes: the Normal Insulin Demand for Dose Adjustment (NIDDA) study. *Diabetes Care* 34:2146–2151, 2011

64. Ahola AJ, Mäkimattila S, Saraheimo M, Mikkilä V, Forsblom C, Freese R, Groop PH: FinnDIANE Study Group: Many patients with type 1 diabetes estimate their prandial insulin need inappropriately. *J Diabetes* 2:194–202, 2010. doi: 10.1111/j.1753-0407.2010.00086.x

65. Anderson DG: Multiple daily injections in young patients using the ezy-BICC bolus insulin calculation card, compared to mixed insulin and CSII. *Pediatr Diabetes* 10:304–309, 2009. Epub 5 December 2008

66. Chiarelli F, Tumini S, Morgese G, Albisser AM: Controlled study in diabetic children comparing insulin-dosage adjustment by manual and computer algorithms. *Diabetes Care* 13:1080–1084, 1990

67. Kaufman FR, Halvorson M, Carpenter S: Use of a plastic insulin dosage guide to correct blood glucose levels out of the target range and for carbohydrate counting in subjects with type 1 diabetes. *Diabetes Care* 22:1252–1257, 1999

68. Gross TM, Kayne D, King A, Rother C, Juth S: A bolus calculator is an effective means of controlling postprandial glycemia in patients on insulin pump therapy. *Diabetes Technol Ther* 5:365–369, 2003

69. Pańkowska E, Błazik M: Bolus calculator with nutrition database software, a new concept of prandial insulin programming for pump users. *J Diabetes Sci Technol* 4:571–576, 2010

70. Rossi MC, Nicolucci A, Di Bartolo P, Bruttomesso D, Girelli A, Ampudia FJ, Kerr D, Ceriello A, Mayor Cde L, Pellegrini F, Horwitz D, Vespasiani G: Diabetes Interactive Diary: a new telemedicine system enabling flexible diet and insulin therapy while improving quality of life: an open-label, international, multicenter, randomized study. *Diabetes Care* 33:109–115, 2010. Epub 6 October 2009

71. Wolff K, Cavanaugh K, Malone R, Hawk V, Gregory BP, Davis D, Wallston K, Rothman RL: The Diabetes Literacy and Numeracy Education Toolkit (DLNET): materials to facilitate diabetes education and management in patients with low literacy and numeracy skills. *Diabetes Educ* 35:233–236, 238–241, 244–245, 2009. Epub 24 February 2009

72. Rankin D, Cooke DD, Clark M, Heller S, Elliott J, Lawton J: UK NIHR DAFNE Study Group: How and why do patients with type 1 diabetes sustain their use of flexible intensive insulin therapy? A qualitative longitudinal investigation of patients' self-management practices following attendance at a Dose Adjustment for Normal Eating (DAFNE) course. *Diabet Med* 28:532–538, 2011. doi: 10.1111/j.1464-5491.2011.03243.x

73. Young-Hyman DL, Davis CL: Disordered eating behavior in individuals with diabetes: importance of context, evaluation, and classification. *Diabetes Care* 33:683–689, 2010

74. Thompson T, Dennis M, Higgins LA, Lee AR, Sharrett MK: Gluten-free diet survey: are Americans with coeliac disease consuming recommended amounts of fibre, iron, calcium and grain foods? *J Hum Nutr Diet* 18:163–169, 2005

75. Hallert C, Grant C, Grehn S, Grännö C, Hultén S, Midhagen G, Ström M, Svensson H, Valdimarsson T: Evidence of poor vitamin status in coeliac patients on a gluten-free diet for 10 years. *Aliment Pharmacol Ther* 16:1333–1339, 2002

76. Academy of Nutrition and Dietetics: Celiac disease evidence analysis project, 2009. Available at http://www.adaevidencelibrary.com/topic.cfm?cat=3055. Accessed 30 October 2012

77. Catassi C, Fabiani E, Iacono G, D'Agate C, Francavilla R, Biagi F, Volta U, Accomando S, Picarelli A, De Vitis I, Pianelli G, Gesuita R, Carle F, Mandolesi A, Bearzi I, Fasano A: A prospective, double-blind, placebo-controlled trial to establish a safe gluten threshold for patients with celiac disease. *Am J Clin Nutr* 85:160–166, 2007

78. Thompson T, Lee AR, Grace T: Gluten contamination of grains, seeds, and flours in the United States: a pilot study. *J Am Diet Assoc* 110:937–940, 2010

79. Saukkonen T, Väisänen S, Akerblom HK, Savilahti E: Childhood Diabetes in Finland Study Group: Coeliac disease in children and adolescents with type 1 diabetes: a study of growth, glycaemic control, and experiences of families. *Acta Paediatr* 91:297–302, 2002

80. Saadah OI, Zacharin M, O'Callaghan A, Oliver MR, Catto-Smith AG: Effect of gluten-free diet and adherence on growth and diabetic control in diabetics with coeliac disease. *Arch Dis Child* 89:871–876, 2004

81. Rami B, Sumnik Z, Schober E, Waldhör T, Battelino T, Bratanic N, Kürti K, Lebl J, Limbert C, Madacsy L, Odink RJ, Paskova M, Soltesz G: Screening detected celiac disease in children with type 1 diabetes mellitus: effect on the clinical course (a case control study). *J Pediatr Gastroenterol Nutr* 41:317–321, 2005

82. Hansen D, Brock-Jacobsen B, Lund E, Bjørn C, Hansen LP, Nielsen C, Fenger C, Lillevang ST, Husby S: Clinical benefit of a gluten-free diet in type 1 diabetic children with screening-detected celiac disease: a

population-based screening study with 2 years' follow-up. *Diabetes Care* 29:2452–2456, 2006

83. Valletta E, Ulmi D, Mabboni I, Tomasselli F, Pinelli L: Early diagnosis and treatment of celiac disease in type 1 diabetes. A longitudinal, case-control study. *Pediatr Med Chir* 29:99–104, 2007

84. Goh VL, Estrada DE, Lerer T, Balarezo F, Sylvester FA: Effect of gluten-free diet on growth and glycemic control in children with type 1 diabetes and asymptomatic celiac disease. *J Pediatr Endocrinol Metab* 23:1169–1173, 2010

85. Abid N, McGlone O, Cardwell C, McCallion W, Carson D: Clinical and metabolic effects of gluten free diet in children with type 1 diabetes and coeliac disease. *Pediatr Diabetes* 12:322–325, 2011. doi: 10.1111/j.1399-5448.2010.00700.x. Epub 29 March 2011

86. Fröhlich-Reiterer EE, Kaspers S, Hofer S, Schober E, Kordonouri O, Pozza SB, Holl RW: Diabetes Patienten Verlaufsdokumentationssystem-Wiss Study Group: Anthropometry, metabolic control, and follow-up in children and adolescents with type 1 diabetes mellitus and biopsy-proven celiac disease. *J Pediatr* 158:589–593, e2, 2011. Epub 4 November 2010

87. Amin R, Murphy N, Edge J, Ahmed ML, Acerini CL, Dunger DB: A longitudinal study of the effects of a gluten-free diet on glycemic control and weight gain in subjects with type 1 diabetes and celiac disease. *Diabetes Care* 25:1117–1122, 2002

88. Sanchez-Albisua I, Wolf J, Neu A, Geiger H, Wäscher I, Stern M: Coeliac disease in children with type 1 diabetes mellitus: the effect of the gluten-free diet. *Diabet Med* 22:1079–1082, 2005

89. Depczynski B: Coeliac disease and its relation to glycaemic control in adults with type 1 diabetes mellitus. *Diabetes Res Clin Pract* 79:e10, 2008. Epub 6 August 2007

90. Leeds JS, Hopper AD, Hadjivassiliou M, Tesfaye S, Sanders DS: High prevalence of microvascular complications in adults with type 1 diabetes and newly diagnosed celiac disease. *Diabetes Care* 34:2158–2163, 2011. Epub 12 September 2011

91. Kaspers S, Kordonouri O, Schober E, Grabert M, Hauffa BP, Holl RW: German Working Group for Pediatric Diabetology: Anthropometry, metabolic control, and thyroid autoimmunity in type 1 diabetes with celiac disease: a multicenter survey. *J Pediatr* 145:790–795, 2004

92. Sun S, Puttha R, Ghezaiel S, Skae M, Cooper C, Amin R: North West England Paediatric Diabetes Network: The effect of biopsy-positive silent coeliac disease and treatment with a gluten-free diet on growth and glycaemic control in children with type 1 diabetes. *Diabet Med* 26:1250–1254, 2009

93. Diniz-Santos DR, Brandão F, Adan L, Moreira A, Vicente EJ, Silva LR: Bone mineralization in young patients with type 1 diabetes mellitus and screening-identified evidence of celiac disease. *Dig Dis Sci* 53:1240–1245, 2008. Epub 16 October 2007

94. Artz E, Warren-Ulanch J, Becker D, Greenspan S, Freemark M: Seropositivity to celiac antigens in asymptomatic children with type 1 diabetes mellitus: association with weight, height, and bone mineralization. *Pediatr Diabetes* 9:277–284, 2008. Epub 7 May 2008

95. Simmons JH, Klingensmith GJ, McFann K, Rewers M, Taylor J, Emery LM, Taki I, Vanyi S, Liu E, Hoffenberg EJ: Impact of celiac autoimmunity on children with type 1 diabetes. *J Pediatr* 150:461–466, 2007

96. Valerio G, Spadaro R, Iafusco D, Lombardi F, Del Puente A, Esposito A, De Terlizzi F, Prisco F, Troncone R, Franzese A: The influence of gluten free diet on quantitative ultrasound of proximal phalanxes in children and adolescents with type 1 diabetes mellitus and celiac disease. *Bone* 43:322–326, 2008. Epub 18 April 2008

97. Lunt H, Florkowski CM, Cook HB, Whitehead MR: Bone mineral density, type 1 diabetes, and celiac disease. *Diabetes Care* 24:791–792, 2001

98. Scavone G, Manto A, Pitocco D, Gagliardi L, Caputo S, Mancini L, Zaccardi F, Ghirlanda G: Effect of carboydrate counting and medical nutritional therapy on glycaemic control in type 1 diabetic subjects: a pilot study. *Diabet Med* 27:477–479, 2010

99. Laurenzi A, Bolla AM, Panigoni G, Doria V, Uccellatore A, Peretti E, Saibene A, Galimberti G, Bosi E, Scavini M: Effects of carbohydrate counting on glucose control and quality of life over 24 weeks in adult patients with type 1 diabetes on continuous subcutaneous insulin infusion. *Diabetes Care* 34:823–827, 2011

100. Institute of Medicine: *Dietary Reference Intakes: The Essential Guide to Nutrient Requirements*. Washington, D.C., National Academies Press, 2006

101. Slavin JL: Position of the American Dietetic Association: health implications of dietary fiber. *J Am Diet Assoc* 108:1716–1731, 2008

11

Physical Activity: Regulation of Glucose Metabolism, Clinical Management Strategies, and Weight Control

Sheri R. Colberg, PhD, and Michael C. Riddell, PhD

OVERVIEW OF THE BENEFITS OF EXERCISE AND TYPES OF EXERCISE

INTRODUCTION

Engaging in regular physical activity is an effective measure to protect against a number of health risks across all ages. Physical activity is known to reduce the risk of coronary heart disease, stroke, osteoporosis, and some cancers in the general population.[1] Moreover, increased physical activity reduces the likelihood of developing obesity, osteoarthritis, and low back pain, while improving mental health.[1] Considerable evidence exists for the health benefits of regular physical activity for people with type 1 diabetes (T1D).[2] These health benefits include:

- Increased cardiovascular and cardiorespiratory fitness
- Muscle strength
- Maintenance of insulin sensitivity
- Weight control
- Reduced cardiovascular risk profile
- Improved sense of well-being
- Reduced morbidity and mortality

It is also critical to note that increased physical activity is strongly associated with psychological and social well-being in adolescents with T1D.[3] Unfortunately, older patients and females with diabetes tend to be less physically active, spending only ~3.5 days/week doing 60 min of physical activity.[3]

Impact of Exercise on Future Complications and Mortality

Although regular aerobic activity or resistance training may not necessarily improve overall glycemic management, as measured by glycated hemoglobin (A1C) or fasting glycemia, it appears to reduce all-cause mortality in those with T1D.[2,4] One seminal cohort study of people with T1D found that 7-year mortality was 50% lower in those reporting ~2,000 kilocalories (kcal) of weekly physical activity (equivalent to 7 h/week of brisk walking) compared to those

DOI: 10.2337/9781580404785ch11

reporting <1,000 kcal of activity.[4] The estimated increase in longevity with regular exercise is estimated to be ~10 years, the same value by which diabetes is estimated to lower life expectancy.[5] The reason why glycemic control is not always improved, in spite of the fact that glycemia acutely decreases with most types of exercise, may be related to rebound hyperglycemia or inappropriate modifications to diet and insulin regimens in anticipation of exercise and in recovery, or both. The reduction in insulin requirements resulting from regular exercise appears to range between 6% to over 15%.[6,7] In theory, regular physical activity should help prevent diabetes-related complications through beneficial effects on insulin sensitivity, blood pressure, lipid levels, endothelial function, and possibly glycemic control. In one large epidemiological study of 628 individuals with T1D, males (but not females) who reported higher levels of historical physical activity had a significantly lower prevalence of nephropathy and neuropathy, but not retinopathy.[8] Regular aerobic exercise increases cardiorespiratory fitness in both T1D and type 2 diabetes (T2D) and may limit the development of diabetic peripheral neuropathy and perhaps microvascular and macrovascular disease, although definitive evidence is lacking in this regard.[9–11]

THE MAJOR CLASSIFICATIONS OF ACTIVITY AND TYPES OF FITNESS

Physical activity is a broad term that encompasses all forms of body movement that substantially increase energy expenditure.[12] Exercise may be considered one form of physical activity that is often structured and performed for improved physical fitness or pleasure. *Sedentarism* is a term used to characterize the behavior of people accumulating less than 30 min of activity daily (or <1.5 Metabolic Equivalents of Tasks [METs]-h/day).[13] Sedentary behavior has been associated with poor glycemic management in both adult and pediatric populations of T1D.[3,14,15] As mentioned, however, regular exercise training has not been shown to universally improve glycemic control in the vast majority of studies in patients with T1D, perhaps because of the difficulties in making appropriate insulin or carbohydrate adjustments for exercise.

The terms *aerobic* and *anaerobic* are commonly used to define the two major forms of physical activity that can be performed. These two types of activity can have very divergent effects on glycemia in patients with T1D.[16] In brief, aerobic activities may be defined as ones that produce rhythmic, repeated, and continuous movements of the same large muscle groups for at least 5–10 min at a time. *Aerobic fitness* refers to the body's ability to transport and use oxygen during prolonged strenuous exercise or work.[12] In contrast, anaerobic or resistance activities use muscular strength to move a weight or work against a resistant load; a sprinting activity may be primarily fueled through anaerobic metabolic pathways as well. *Anaerobic fitness* refers to the body's ability to produce energy without the use of oxygen.[12]

Physical fitness refers to a physiologic state of well-being that allows one to meet the demands of daily living (health-related physical fitness) or that provides the basis for sports performance (performance-related physical fitness) or both.[12] Health-related physical fitness involves the components of physical fitness related to health status, including cardiovascular fitness, musculoskeletal fitness, body composition, and metabolism.[12] All these components of fitness are important for patients with T1D for optimal health and performance.[17]

Physical fitness can be assessed through well-established appraisal protocols, used by qualified exercise professionals, from organizations like the American College of Sports Medicine (http://www.acsm.org/). These assessments are designed to evaluate the individual components of health-related physical fitness, including body composition, aerobic fitness, and musculoskeletal fitness (muscular strength, muscular endurance, power, and flexibility). Exercise and fitness assessment is beyond the scope of this review, but interested readers may refer to a recent text that includes sections on exercise stress testing in patients with diabetes.[18] Table 11.1 lists general terms and definitions of fitness activities, while Table 11.2 gives some metabolic equivalents of a variety of common physical activities.

In general, the overall fitness of an individual with T1D may be somewhat impaired compared to age-matched controls, but patients have achieved all levels of competitive stature including national, professional, and Olympic status.[19-21] Poor glycemic control in T1D is associated with reduced fitness.[21,22] Highly trained individuals with T1D who are in good control can achieve the same cardiopulmonary exercise responses as trained subjects without diabetes, but these responses are clearly reduced by poor glucose control.[23,24] Importantly, all forms of exercise are deemed reasonably safe for anyone with T1D, particularly if there is no evidence of underlying micro- and macrovascular disease. However,

Table 11.1 General Terms and Definitions

Term	Definition
Metabolic Equivalent of Tasks (METs)	Ratio of the metabolic rate of an activity relative to the resting metabolic rate; 1 MET is defined as 1 kcal/kg/h and is comparable to the energy cost of sitting quietly.
	1 MET is approximately 3.5 ml/kg/min.
Sedentarism	Term used to characterize the behavior of persons accumulating less than 30 min of activity daily (or <1.5 MET-h/day).[13]
Aerobic exercise	Body's ability to transport and use oxygen during prolonged strenuous exercise or work (e.g., running or bicycling).[12]
Anaerobic exercise	Body's ability to produce energy without the use of oxygen (e.g., resistance training, such as weight lifting).[12]
Physical fitness	Physiologic state of well-being that allows one to meet the demands of daily living (health-related physical fitness) or that provides the basis for sport performance (performance-related physical fitness), or both.[12]
Health-related physical fitness	Components of physical fitness related to health status, including cardiovascular fitness, musculoskeletal fitness, body composition and metabolism.[12]

Table 11.2 METs of Some Physical Activities

Physical Activity	METs
Light-Intensity Activities	**< 3**
Sleeping	0.9
Watching television	1.0
Walking 2.5 mph (4 km/h)	2.9
Moderate-Intensity Activities	**3–6**
Walking 3.4 mph (5.5 km/h)	3.6
Bicycling <10 mph (16 km/h), leisure, to work or for pleasure	4.0
Vigorous-Intensity Activities	**> 6**
Jogging, general	7.0
Calisthenics (e.g., pushups, situps, pullups, jumping jacks), heavy, vigorous effort	8.0
Jumping rope	10.0

appropriate pre-exercise screening is warranted using available physical activity clearance algorithms.[25]

RECOMMENDED PHYSICAL ACTIVITY LEVELS FOR INDIVIDUALS WITH T1D

Children and Adolescents

Infants, toddlers, and preschoolers (0–4 years). Common sense more than empiric research supports the recommendations for physical activity for children from birth to age 5 years with T1D. In general, infants' activity is based upon their interactions with caregivers who provide the infants with opportunities to explore movement and their surroundings. The physical activity of infants supports their development; active play, along with interactions with adults, enhances the infants' well-being and physical and emotional development. Toddlers should participate in at least 30 min of physical activity daily, often with unstructured play lasting more than 30 min at a time. In fact, toddlers should not be sedentary for more than 60 min at one time (except during sleep) in order to encourage their motor skill development. Toddlers will likely engage in indoor and outdoor activities that promote development of their large muscles and gross motor skills, utilizing either structured or unstructured physical activities. Preschoolers should have at least 60 min of structured physical activity daily, along with several hours of unstructured play each day. As with toddlers, preschoolers should generally not be sedentary for more than 60 min at a time (except for sleep). The physical activity of preschoolers continues to help them develop motor skills and enhances their socialization.

The caregivers and parents of infants, toddlers, and preschoolers contribute to the overall health and well-being of these young children by promoting physical activity with both structured and unstructured play. Just like older children, for every 30 min of physical activity, the young child with T1D will require additional carbohydrate intake in order to prevent severe hypoglycemia. It is difficult to adjust insulin in advance of activity in young children due to the unpredictable nature of the exercise. In general, 5–10 g/30–60 min of physical activity will be needed for young children, depending upon the child's initial blood sugar and intensity of the exercise. It is important for the supervising adults to check the young child's blood glucose levels frequently as these young children are unable to convey symptoms of hypoglycemia. Thus, it is recommended to check blood glucose levels both before and after physical activity and to generally begin periods of exercise with glucose levels of 150–200 mg/dl in toddlers and preschoolers.

Young children (5–11 years) and adolescents (12–17 years). For health benefits, it is generally recommended that all children (aged 5–11 years) and youth (aged 12–17 years) accumulate at least 60 min of moderate- to vigorous-intensity mixed aerobic and anaerobic physical activity daily (420 min/week).[1,26,27] This recommendation appears appropriate for youth with T1D, although it can clearly increase the risk for hypoglycemia.[28] More physical activity likely provides greater health benefits, helping to limit high blood cholesterol, high blood pressure, metabolic syndrome, obesity, low bone density, and depression, although the risk for injury does increase.[27] Being physically active with T1D, compared with being sedentary with the disease, is expected to improve cholesterol levels, blood pressure, body composition, bone density, cardiorespiratory and musculoskeletal fitness, and various aspects of mental health and well-being.[2] These recommendations appear particularly suitable for children and adolescents with T1D since physical activity patterns in youth track into adulthood. As cardiovascular disease (CVD) is the major cause of early mortality and morbidity in diabetes it is important to begin these activity patterns in childhood and adolescence.[29,30]

To summarize, the recommendations for daily exercise in all children and adolescents with T1D are expected to include:

■ At least 60 min of accumulated physical activity every day
■ Vigorous-intensity aerobic activities at least 3 days/week
■ Activities that strengthen muscle and bone at least 3 days/week each

Children and youth should be physically active daily as part of play, games, sports, transportation, recreation, physical education, or planned exercise in the context of family, school, and community activities (e.g., volunteer, employment). This should be achieved above and beyond the incidental physical activities accumulated in the course of daily living. Reducing sedentary time is convincingly associated with a favorable cardiovascular profile, and several expert panels recommend limiting leisure screen time to <2 h/day.[26]

For school-aged children and youth who are physically inactive, doing amounts below the recommended levels (such as 30 min/day instead of 60 min/day) likely provides some health benefits, compared with being completely sedentary. The benefits of exercise are highlighted by the finding that sedentary youth with T1D have higher A1C levels compared with active youth.[3,15,27] Interestingly, extensive media consumption is a significant risk factor for poor metabolic control in youth with diabetes, irrespective of socioeconomic status and physical activity.[31] For sedentary youth, it may be appropriate to start with smaller amounts of physical activity and gradually increase duration, frequency, and intensity as a stepping stone to meeting the guidelines.

These guidelines for daily physical activity, which should include vigorous aerobic and muscle-strengthening activities, may be considered ambitious for young persons with T1D, given their potential fear of hypoglycemia and sometimes sedentary nature.[3,32] A large sample of children and adolescents with T1D (23,251 youth ages 3–18 years) found that ~45% of this cohort was generally sedentary (i.e., <30 min of continuous physical activity per week, excluding school sports), with only 37% of the cohort having regular physical activity for 30 min 1–2 times/week.[33] However, this study also found that A1C levels were lower in patients with higher frequencies of physical activity and that blood lipid profiles were more favorable compared to those who were sedentary. Interestingly, multiple regression analysis revealed that regular physical activity was one of the most important factors influencing A1C levels.[33] Other studies[34-36] have found that more frequent exercise is associated with lower A1C levels, although a number of exercise training studies have found no relationship,[7,37-40] perhaps because appropriate insulin and carbohydrate adjustments for exercise were not in place.

Adults (18–64 Years)

To achieve health benefits, adults ages 18–64 years should accumulate at least 150 min of moderate- to vigorous-intensity aerobic physical activity per week, in bouts of 10 min or more.[26,41] It is also beneficial to add muscle- and bone-strengthening activities that use major muscle groups, at least 2 days/week. Although the total energy expenditure should be ~1,000 kcal/week of physical activity, the American College of Sports Medicine has stated that health benefits occur with energy expenditures as low as 500 kcal/week, with additional benefits occurring at higher levels.[41] In other words, according to the ACSM guidelines, some is good and more is better in most cases.[41]

Adults with T1D can meet recommended guidelines through planned exercise sessions, transportation, recreation, sports, or occupational demands, in the context of family, work, volunteer, and community activities. This should be achieved above and beyond the incidental physical activities accumulated in the course of daily living.[42] Following these guidelines can reduce the risk of premature death, coronary heart disease, stroke, hypertension, colon cancer, breast cancer, and osteoporosis, and improve fitness, body composition, and indicators of mental health.[26] The potential benefits far exceed the potential risks associated with physical activity, even in people with T1D.[25] Physical activity appears to lower cardiovascular mortality risk at all levels of glycemic control.[43] For those who are initially physically inactive, doing amounts below the recommended levels can provide some health benefits. For these adults, it is appropriate to start with smaller amounts of physical activity and then gradually increase the duration, frequency, and intensity as a stepping stone to meeting these guidelines.[1,44]

Older Adults (≥65 Years)

To achieve health benefits and improve functional abilities, adults ages 65 years and older should accumulate at least 150 min of moderate- to vigorous-intensity aerobic physical activity per week, in bouts of 10 min or more.[1,45] It is also beneficial to add muscle- and bone-strengthening activities that use major muscle groups, at least 2 days/week. [1,45]

While the exercise guidelines for adults also apply to older adults, there are some additional ones that apply only to older adults (with or without T1D): [1,45]

- When older adults cannot do 150 min of moderate-intensity aerobic activity a week because of chronic conditions, they should be as physically active as their abilities and conditions allow.
- Recommend exercises that maintain or improve balance, particularly if they are at risk of falling.
- Determine their level of effort for physical activity relative to their level of fitness.
- Those with chronic conditions should understand whether and how their conditions affect their ability to do regular physical activity safely.

Older adults can meet these guidelines through the same means as younger adults (i.e., increased activities of daily living) to reduce the risk of comorbid disease and premature death, maintain functional independence and mobility, as well as improve fitness, body composition, bone health, cognitive function, and indicators of mental health.[1,45] The potential benefits exceed the potential risks associated with physical activity, even for older adults with diabetes.[25] These guidelines may be appropriate for older adults with frailty or other comorbid conditions; however, individuals with health issues should consult a health professional to understand the types and amounts of physical activity appropriate for them based on their exercise capacity and specific health risks or limitations.[25]

REGULATION OF GLUCOSE METABOLISM

Effect of Physical Activity on Metabolic Control

Acute impact. Acutely, exercise can have wide-ranging effects on glycemia, likely because several variables influence glucose homeostasis during the activity. The intensity, duration, and timing of the activity as well as the familiarity of the exercise performed and the associated stress hormones of exercise and/or competition all impact glucose homeostasis.[46] In general, low- to moderate-intensity aerobic activities (walking, jogging, racquet sports) promote a decrease in glycemia during the activity, while high-intensity aerobic or anaerobic activities (such as sprint running, sprint cycling, etc.) can cause an increase in glycemia. Activities that combine some anaerobic and aerobic activities tend to have a moderating effect on glycemia.[47] Resistance exercise (i.e., weight lifting) is associated with less decline in glycemia compared to aerobic exercise; if resistance exercise is performed before aerobic exercise, then the drop in blood glucose may be attenuated somewhat compared to doing them in reverse order.[48]

Importantly, the glycemic response to aerobic exercise has some degree of reproducibility within an individual with T1D, as long as many of the variables known to impact glucose homeostasis are held constant (such as pre-exercise meal, insulin dose, and the exercise task itself).[49] Unfortunately, the glycemic response differs markedly from patient to patient even if the relative exercise intensity and timing are identical, thereby making universal guidelines for the prevention of exercise-associated dysglycemia difficult.[49–52]

Lipid levels and blood pressure. Regular physical activity may be considered the best nonpharmacological and most cost-effective approach for maintaining optimal lipid and blood pressure levels. Reductions in lipid levels, increased C-reactive protein (CRP) level, and increased plasminogen activator inhibitor-1 (PAI-1) levels are thought to play a role in the maintenance of an inflammatory state and in the development of cardiovascular disease. Elevations in PAI-1 are also linked with muscle dysfunction in rodent models of T1D.[53] Importantly, individuals who are physically trained have improvements in lipid profile and lower PAI-1 levels compared to sedentary individuals.[54] Lifestyle intervention improves lipid profiles and lowers PAI-1 levels in patients with T2D, according to the Look AHEAD study.[55] A majority of other studies of physical activity and T1D show a beneficial effect on lipid levels.[33,35,56–63] Studies lasting up to 4 months demonstrate increases in HDL-cholesterol by 8–14%, reductions in LDL-cholesterol by 8–14% and triacylglycerols by 13–15%.[2] In general, the improvements in lipid profile appear independent of changes in glycemic control and weight and are more evident in those with a poor initial lipid profile.[2]

Evidence that regular exercise improves blood pressure levels in T1D is equivocal, with some studies showing a small improvement (2–3% reduction)[35,58] and others no effect.[56,60] However, these studies typically had small numbers of young subjects who did not have elevated blood pressure levels. A large cross-sectional study found a small effect of physical activity levels on the risk of having elevated diastolic blood pressure.[33]

Exercise Intensity or Type and Hormonal Responses to Physical Activity

The metabolic regulation of glucose homeostasis during exercise is complex and regulated by several hormonal and nonhormonal factors (e.g., contraction-mediated changes in insulin sensitivity). In general, more strenuous aerobic activities utilize more blood glucose as fuel.[64] In the postabsorptive state, the liver is the key organ responsible for glucose production during exercise to help maintain glucose supply to the working muscles and the central nervous system. Glucose production by the liver in individuals without diabetes increases ~2–3-fold during low- to moderate-intensity exercise.[65,66] At higher exercise intensities, glucose production via the liver exceeds its uptake into the periphery because of elevations in catecholamines, and hyperglycemia ensues.[67] Blood glucose utilization also increases with the duration of exercise as muscle glycogen levels decline.[66] When liver glycogen levels become depleted, or if glucose production is impaired because of elevations in circulating insulin levels, then hypoglycemia and fatigue develops, even in people without diabetes.[68,69] In general, the glucose disappearance from the circulation is similar in individuals with T1D and those without diabetes, as long as the T1D patients are well-insulinized.[70] However, it may be that T1D patients rely more heavily on muscle glycogen as a fuel during exercise and have a somewhat limited capacity to oxidize orally ingested glucose as an energy source, particularly if they are underinsulinized.[71–73] As described below, despite near normal substrate utilization during exercise, the maintenance of euglycemia is challenging for the patient with T1D.

Figure 11.1 illustrates a simplified schematic of the regulation of glucose homeostasis during exercise in healthy people or in people with diabetes who have taken the correct amount of insulin for exercise and who have normal glucose counterregulatory responses to exercise. Figure 11.1 also illustrates the mechanisms for exercise-associated hypoglycemia or hyperglycemia. A number of neuroendocrine mechanisms normally exist to defend against hypoglycemia, both at rest and during exercise. Interestingly, the hormonal responses to hypoglycemia and prolonged exercise are nearly identical. During exercise or hypoglycemia, insulin secretion diminishes while increases in glucagon, catecholamines, growth hormone, and cortisol occur.[74] However, the normal counterregulatory hormone response to exercise is amplified by simultaneous hypoglycemia in individuals without diabetes, thereby helping to augment glucose production by the liver and limit glucose uptake into working muscle. These hormonal changes during exercise help to maintain fuel supply to the central nervous system and protect against hypoglycemia.[75,76] Unfortunately, the counterregulatory response to hypoglycemia (both at rest and during exercise) and to exercise performed after a bout of hypoglycemia is impaired in patients with T1D.[77] The reciprocal effects of antecedent hypoglycemia and antecedent exercise on glucose counterregulation are described in the following sections.

Metabolic Dysregulation During Physical Activity

Hypoglycemia. Hypoglycemia during physical activity occurs typically when circulating insulin levels are too high during the activity (i.e., too much insulin on board), although the exact mechanisms for the high risk for hypoglycemia during exercise in T1D are likely complex and multifactorial. In rare circumstances, hypoglycemia can also occur when hepatic glycogen stores are exhausted because of prolonged fasting or exercise, even in those who do not have diabetes and with low circulating insulin levels.[78] Even if it does not suppress hepatic glycogen mobilization, relative hyperinsulinemia during exercise may also increase peripheral glucose uptake (into exercising muscle and other tissues) and may reduce hepatic gluconeogenesis, thereby contributing to hypoglycemia risk.[79] An additional factor that contributes to increased risk for exercise-associated hypoglycemia is the deficiency in glucose counterregulation to exercise or to hypoglycemia, which can occur during the activity.[80] Thus, for individuals with T1D, the inability to reduce circulating insulin concentrations at the onset of exercise because the insulin has already been injected or infused prior to the activity, as well as other factors, contributes to the high risk for exercise-associated hypoglycemia.

Due to increased blood flow and circulatory responses, exercise itself may increase insulin absorption kinetics.[81] Even if mealtime bolus insulin has not been injected or infused in the hours prior to exercise, it is still possible to have exercise-associated hypoglycemia, likely because basal insulin levels tend to be higher than what would normally occur during physical activity in people without diabetes.[82] Indeed, one of the challenges clinically is that basal–bolus therapy is

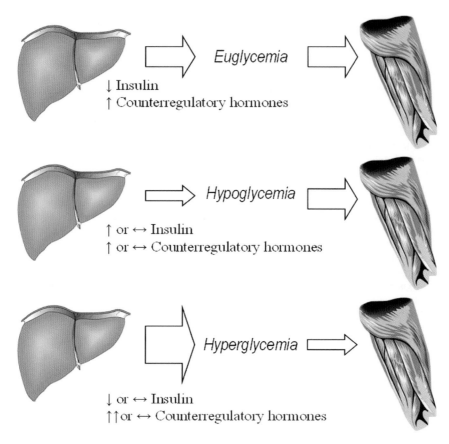

Euglycemia

↓ Insulin
↑ Counterregulatory hormones

Hypoglycemia

↑ or ↔ Insulin
↑ or ↔ Counterregulatory hormones

Hyperglycemia

↓ or ↔ Insulin
↑↑ or ↔ Counterregulatory hormones

Figure 11.1 Glucose homeostasis during exercise in nondiabetes and T1D. Upper panel: In nondiabetic individuals and in individuals with T1D who have reduced their insulin levels in anticipation of exercise and who have normal glucose counterregulatory responses to exercise, glucose production by the liver matches glucose uptake into working muscle and euglycemia is maintained. Middle panel: In people with T1D who have relatively high insulin levels because of the timing of exercise (and because insulin dose reductions in anticipation of exercise have not occurred) or who have defective glucose counterregulatory responses, hypoglycemia results from insufficient glucose production relative to glucose disposal. Bottom panel: In people with T1D who have not taken enough insulin or who are experiencing elevations in catecholamine or cortisol levels because of competition stress or because of very high-intensity exercise (>75% Vo_{2max}), glucose production exceeds peripheral glucose disposal and hyperglycemia ensues. Reprinted with permission from the publisher.[16]

normally titrated initially to sedentary days, rather than to days in which habitual activity occurs. This may be problematic for patients who are routinely active, as they will inevitably require either additional energy in the form of carbohydrates or reductions in basal–bolus insulin, or both, on days in which increased physical activity occurs.

During exercise, relative hyperinsulinemia may limit the effect of glucagon on hepatic glucose production and promote increases in peripheral glucose disposal, thereby reducing circulating levels rapidly.[83] Since the total amount of glucose in the circulation is only ~4 g and because exercise increases glucose utilization rates five- to sixfold above rest, hypoglycemia can ensue within minutes if circulating insulin levels are not adjusted for the activity or if exogenous carbohydrates are not consumed.[84,85] In addition to relative hyperinsulinemia, a failure in glucagon response during exercise or during hypoglycemia may also exist if a recent episode of exercise or hypoglycemia occurred.[80] Finally, other factors such as an impaired adrenergic response to hypoglycemia during exercise or a reduced level of liver glycogen because of recent hypoinsulinemia may contribute to exercise-associated hypoglycemia.[86,87] Based on euglycemic clamp studies of adolescents with T1D, it would appear that insulin sensitivity is elevated during exercise and immediately in recovery and again hours later.[88] This biphasic increase in the glucose requirements to maintain euglycemia may predict the risk for postexercise hypoglycemia. Indeed, the glycemic nadir after exercise appears to be about 7–11 h after the end of exercise.[89–94]

Hyperglycemia. The development of hyperglycemia during and after exercise may occur for a number of reasons. First, the high likelihood of hypoglycemia caused by exercise may force individuals to consume excessive carbohydrates before and following exercise. Second, the fear of hypoglycemia may promote an overly aggressive reduction in insulin dose before the activity, with some individuals omitting insulin administration altogether. Third, the stress of competition may increase catecholamine and cortisol levels, which leads to greater glucose production by the liver and limited peripheral glucose disposal. Finally, brief periods of intense aerobic or anaerobic activities promote dramatic increases in catecholamine release, which would normally be compensated for by increased insulin secretion in the individual without diabetes.[95] This latter phenomenon caused by intense exercise has been shown to particularly aggravate postexercise hyperglycemia in people with T1D, even if insulin is administered during recovery.[96]

With respect to the second reason given, individuals using pump therapy may find that discontinuing insulin infusion (i.e., pump disconnect) during exercise may cause hyperglycemia, particularly if the activity is prolonged.[97] Strategies to limit exercise-associated hyperglycemia, based on limited experimental data, are described in the following section.

Effects of glycemia on maximal oxidative capacity and performance. Maintenance of normal glucose homeostasis during exercise in people with T1D is challenging for a number of physiological and psychosocial or behavioral reasons. Behaviorally, a fear of hypoglycemia caused by exercise may promote hyperglycemia, while at the same time, the sophisticated hormonal regulatory system that maintains euglycemia during the activity is often defective when disease is long-standing.[32,83] Thus, many patients are exercising when blood glucose levels are suboptimal; this may affect exercise and sports performance. Moreover, a number of physiological processes may be compromised by prolonged suboptimal glycemic control.

If impairment in physical work capacity exists in patients with T1D, it would appear to be related to the level of glycemic control. For example, two studies report that physical capacities are inversely related to the level of metabolic control, as measured by A1C.[22,98] It is unclear, however, if a reduced work capacity in youth with T1D is a result of poorer oxygenation of muscle or a lower amount of muscle capillarization, or if poorer metabolic control is a function of lower amounts of habitual physical activity.[99–101]

Studies investigating muscular strength and endurance capacity in individuals with T1D have shown mixed results, although a generalized myopathy does exist if glycemic control is poor.[102] Fatigue is a common complaint in diabetes, particularly at the time of diagnosis or with elevated glycemia.[103,104] Surprisingly, the effect of T1D on exercise endurance capacity is not clear. Compared to controls, patients with T1D have been reported to have both impaired[105] and enhanced[106] endurance capacity during relatively brief bouts of intense exercise. Ratings of perceived exertion during prolonged aerobic exercise have been reported to be higher in boys with T1D compared to controls without diabetes.[107] During prolonged aerobic exercise, those with T1D who are under reasonable glycemic control have a higher glycolytic flux and rely more on muscle glycogen utilization, thereby resulting in premature fatigue.[71,108] Exercising while hyperglycemic has been shown to increase reliance on muscle glycogen compared to exercising while euglycemic, and the individual who is exercising while hypoinsulinemic and hyperglycemic would be prone to early dehydration and acidosis, all factors that might promote early fatigue.[109,110] A diet rich in carbohydrate (~60% of total energy) for 3 weeks has been shown to increase glycemia and insulin requirements, reduce muscle glycogen levels, and lower exercise capacity compared to a lower carbohydrate diet (50% of total energy) in athletes with diabetes.[111] Moreover, increasing blood glucose levels to 288 mg/dl (16 mmol/l) has been shown to reduce isometric muscle strength, but not maximal isokinetic muscle strength, compared with strength measured at normal glycemia.[112] This reduction in isometric strength might play a role in the development of early fatigue during certain types of resistance and anaerobic activities.

If individuals with T1D are actively engaged in regular exercise and are under reasonable glycemic control, then they can achieve elite level performance. One German study of 10 middle-aged long-distance triathletes with T1D followed over 3 years showed that overall endurance performance was normal, despite documented hyperglycemia during the early part of a race, then hypoglycemia during the marathon leg.[113] Another study found that good glycemic control, as measured by A1C, was associated with a normal peak cardiopulmonary exercise response and performance, while suboptimal control was associated with deterioration in athletic performance.[23]

The degree to which acute blood glucose levels influence sports skill performance or exercise performance has also been examined.[107,114–116] In one study of prepubertal boys with T1D ($n = 16$), lowering the insulin dose prior to exercise to reduce the likelihood of hypoglycemia did not influence aerobic capacity during cycling compared to the usual insulin dose.[114] In eight endurance-trained adults with T1D, elevating blood glucose levels from 95 to 225 mg/dl (5.3 mmol/l to 12.4 mmol/l) failed to change peak power output or other physiological end points, such as lactate, heart rate, or respiratory exchange ratio.[116] In another study, compared with hyperglycemia or euglycemia, exercise capacity was reduced and ratings of perceived exertion increased with hypoglycemia in a group of youth with T1D, although the research investigators (not the subjects) always stopped the exercise for possible safety reasons.[52] Another study demonstrated that the oral administration of dextrose at 1g/kg body mass 30 min before cycling exercise (55–60% Vo_{2max}) results in a 12% improvement in cycling performance time compared with placebo, perhaps as euglycemia is facilitated and because working muscles are provided more fuel for oxidation.[117,118] A sports camp field study of 28 youth with T1D found that the ability to carry out fundamental sports skills was shown to be markedly reduced by mild hypoglycemia of 55 mg/dl (3 mmol/l) compared with either euglycemia or hyperglycemia of 300 mg/dl (~17 mmol/l).[115] Importantly, this finding of significantly impaired sports performance with hypoglycemia appeared universally across nearly all subjects and is similar to the well-documented detrimental effects of hypoglycemia on cognitive processing.[119]

Profound or sustained hyperglycemia also likely impairs endurance performance in those with T1D, although the evidence for this statement is somewhat limited. Prolonged hyperglycemia with low insulin levels would be expected to lower muscle glycogen levels, reduce muscle strength, and predispose the individual to dehydration and electrolyte imbalance.[120] Exercising while hyperglycemic has been shown to increase the reliance on muscle glycogen as a fuel source and limit the capacity to switch from carbohydrate to lipid as an energy source.[109] Thus, overall, evidence suggests that optimal glycemic control and regular exercise may be needed to maximize muscle strength and endurance performance.

Hypoglycemia Associated with Physical Activity

Hypoglycemia risk. Hypoglycemia is the most common negative side effect of exercise, ranging from mild to life threatening in severity. The incidence of hypoglycemia during or after a single bout of moderate-intensity exercise in children and adolescents with T1D is reported to be as high as 30%.[121] Based on a small sample of athletes with T1D attending a vigorous sports camp, ~7% of an individual's time will be spent in a hypoglycemia and about 11% in hyperglycemia.[92] In extreme cases, hypoglycemia during exercise or sports can be detrimental to performance, cause premature fatigue, and result in loss of consciousness during the activity and permanent organ damage.[115,122,123]

A number of factors appear to increase the risk for exercise-associated hypoglycemia, including the timing of the exercise, the duration and intensity of the activity, and having experienced an episode of hypoglycemia in the previous 24–48 h. Limited evidence also suggests that unfamiliarity with the activity may also increase the risk, while endurance training may lower risk.[124] As mentioned, normally, at the onset of exercise, insulin secretion is lowered and levels drop in the portal circulation rapidly.[77] This drop in portal insulin sensitizes the liver to glucagon, thereby increasing glucose production via glycogen breakdown. Since exercise often occurs in a time frame of 0–4 h after insulin administration, patients taking regular or rapid-acting insulin analogs are typically exercising when circulating insulin levels are simply too high, relatively speaking, for aerobic exercise.[125] In these situations, corrections in insulin dosage and/or additional carbohydrates are typically needed.

People with T1D have multiple impairments in the counterregulatory response to hypoglycemia and exercise, placing then at high risk for severe hypoglycemia (i.e., hypoglycemia requiring assistance from another). After the first few years of onset of diabetes, the glucagon response to hypoglycemia is typically diminished or lost, although its response to exercise may still be intact.[86,126,127] Increases in epinephrine are also blunted in people with T1D both during exercise and hypoglycemia.[86] Even if counterregulatory responses to hypoglycemia (and to exercise) occur, excessive exogenous insulin administration by the patient can blunt hepatic glucose production and increase peripheral glucose disposal, thereby resulting in rapid hypoglycemia.[77,86] Other factors such as inadequate carbohydrate intake, failure to monitor blood glucose levels, exercise in warm environments, prolonged exercise activities, and unfamiliarity with the exercise activity may also increase risk. Finally, a vicious cycle appears to exist between exercise and hypoglycemia in which antecedent hypoglycemia or exercise cause reduced neuroendocrine, metabolic, and symptom responses to subsequent hypoglycemia or exercise.[80] For more details on the proposed mechanisms of this vicious cycle, the interested reader may refer to an excellent review article.[74]

Hypoglycemia treatment. Hypoglycemia treatment during exercise depends on its severity and whether the individual plans to continue exercising. Mild to moderate hypoglycemia can generally be treated with 15–20 g of simple carbohydrate (or ~0.3 g carbohydrate/kg body mass) using glucose tablets, soft drinks, dextrose gels, or juice.[128] It is recommended that the carbohydrate source be low in fat to increase the rate of absorption. Individuals should check glucose levels again after 15 min and retreat if glucose levels have not elevated to a normal range. In situations in which exercise is to be continued, higher amounts of fast-acting carbohydrate should be consumed, along with a lower glycemic index snack once euglycemia is attained. In the postexercise period, a meal containing complex carbohydrate should be consumed, with an appropriate (albeit likely reduced) amount of bolus insulin so that muscle and liver glycogen stores may be repleted.

Hypoglycemia prevention. The risk for exercise-associated hypoglycemia is greatest during prolonged moderate- to high-intensity aerobic exercise, particularly if circulating insulin levels are elevated during the activity. Intermittent high-intensity exercise may pose less risk for hypoglycemia because of the associated increases in catecholamine levels.[129] Performing resistance exercise before aerobic exercise helps limit the risk of hypoglycemia compared with performing aerobic before resistance exercise.[48] The carbohydrates eaten to enhance glycogen storage and replacement before and after physical activity are frequently different from the ones used to rapidly treat a hypoglycemic event, since hyperglycemia prevention is also a concern.

The ADA guidelines on exercise and T1D published in 1994 recommended consuming 10–15 g of carbohydrate to prevent exercise-induced hypoglycemia.[130] However, findings of recent research estimate that 40 g of a liquid glucose supplement may be necessary to prevent hypoglycemia during and after 1 h of late postprandial exercise in people using rapid-acting analog (lispro) in basal–bolus therapy.[131] Even higher amounts of glucose may be needed if peak insulin levels are in circulation and hepatic glucose production is at a minimum. For example, one study in youth with diabetes showed that matching glucose intake with endogenous carbohydrate utilization (~1 g carbohydrate/kg body mass/h) prevented blood glucose levels from dropping during 60 min of exercise.[52] To estimate carbohydrate utilization in youth who differ in size and energy expenditure based on the activity, a table of exercise exchanges (ExCarbs) may be a useful starting point (see Table 11.3).[46,132] It is important to note that the carbohydrate requirements progressively decreased when 1 h of exercise was performed 1, 2.5, 4, and 5.5 h after a meal preceded by an injection of a standard dose (1 U/kg) of regular insulin.[133]

Table 11.3 Total Amount of Carbohydrates Utilized during 30 Min of Various Sporting Activities of Children Weighing Differing Amounts. These values can be used to estimate the amount of additional carbohydrate that could be consumed for 30 min of a given sport when peak insulin levels are high and if no reductions in insulin were made in anticipation of the activity.

	Body Mass, lb (kg)		
	44 (20)	88 (40)	132 (60)
Basketball	23	45	68
Cycling			
moderate	7	11	18
heavy	10	18	27
Skating	18	36	54
Running			
moderate	17	30	41
heavy	30	41	55
Soccer	17	32	48
Swimming			
breaststroke	14	27	52
Tennis	11	19	28

Even if insulin adjustments are not made in anticipation of the activity, patients will be able to exercise if they consume extra carbohydrates to compensate. For example, consuming a carbohydrate beverage (6% carbohydrate solution) before the start of exercise (~1.0 g carbohydrate/kg body mass/h of exercise), without taking any additional insulin, is effective in limiting the drop in glycemia during prolonged exercise in youth with T1D.[52] Based on one study, consuming fast-acting carbohydrate (dextrose) is preferable to those with a lower glycemic index (i.e., isomaltulose) for the prevention of hypoglycemia.[134]

However, there is no clear consensus on the amount of additional carbohydrate required to limit exercise-associated hypoglycemia. Recommendations for carbohydrate consumption before or during exercise in T1D individuals range from amounts based on pre-exercise blood glucose concentration to amounts based on exercise duration (e.g., 20–60 g every 30 min) or body mass (1–2 g/kg body mass).[117,132,135–138] Based on these and other studies, it is clear that the carbohydrate requirements to prevent hypoglycemia need to be individualized based on the size of the individual, the energy expenditure of the activity, and the type of insulin regimen that the patient is on.

Insulin Adjustments

Reductions in insulin administration are effective in preventing hypoglycemia during exercise in individuals with T1D, although the reductions in insulin levels range between 10 and 90%, based on several factors including the type of insulin used and the type and timing of the exercise performed.[139–142] Although it is generally recommended that exercise be avoided in the 2-h window after rapid-acting insulin is injected because of an increased risk for hypoglycemia, the administration of a reduced dose of rapid-acting insulin by 25–75% along with the ingestion of carbohydrates within this window of elevated risk is effective in limiting dysglycemia.[46,134,140,142] A useful starting point, Table 11.4 is based on a study that describes bolus reductions in insulin dose, taking into consideration the duration and intensity of the activity.

Hyperglycemia Associated with Physical Activity

Hyperglycemia risk. Although exercise is typically associated with hypoglycemia, it can also induce hyperglycemia because of increases in stress hormones

Table 11.4 Guidelines for the Reduction of the Premeal Insulin Dose in Relation to the Intensity and Duration of Exercise (for Activities Performed within 90 Min of a Meal)[140]

Intensity of aerobic exercise	30 min of exercise	60 min of exercise
Mild (~25% of maximal aerobic capacity)	25%	50%
Moderate (~50% of maximal aerobic capacity)	50%	75%
Heavy (~75% of maximal aerobic capacity)	75%	—

caused either by vigorous exercise or by the stress of competition.[16] In some cases, hyperglycemia may result from excessive carbohydrate intake or because insulin was withheld in an attempt to prevent hypoglycemia. On occasion, illness or a block in an insulin pump infusion set can also promote hyperglycemia. Excessive pre-exercise carbohydrate consumption provokes mild to moderate hyperglycemia pre-exercise, but this usually resolves once the exercise begins.[143] Moreover, if a high-glycemic carbohydrate (i.e., dextrose) is ingested just prior to vigorous exercise, it can increase the risk for postexercise hyperglycemia.[134] In any case, if hyperglycemia occurs in association with elevations in ketone levels, the exercise should be postponed until these are resolved, as exercise may exacerbate the condition.[130,144]

Hyperglycemia Treatment

Treatment of hyperglycemia at the time of exercise is challenging since insulin sensitivity may be elevated because of exercise-mediated increases in GLUT-4 translocation in skeletal muscle.[145] Although no studies have been conducted to date, correction of hyperglycemia with small amounts of rapid-acting insulin analogs via injection or infusion may be desirable to help prevent dehydration and impaired sports performance. In these situations, about half the normal insulin correction factor should be used and frequent glucose monitoring should be encouraged. Hydration is also an important consideration as individuals may be prone to rapid dehydration because of the combined effects of exercise and polyuria.

Hyperglycemia Prevention

No current guidelines exist for the prevention of exercise-associated hyperglycemia caused by vigorous exercise and the associated increases in catecholamine levels. If the exercise duration is short (i.e., <30 min), it may be safer to attempt to correct any hyperglycemia following exercise rather than to try to prevent it by taking more insulin before the activity. Some limited laboratory data suggest that a doubling in circulating insulin levels immediately postexercise, relative to the pre-exercise state, may be needed.[95] The occurrence of postexercise hyperglycemia is less dramatic following prolonged aerobic exercise if a low-glycemic–index carbohydrate is consumed prior to exercise, rather than dextrose; however, the risk for hypoglycemia during the exercise may be marginally increased.[134]

Use of Technology

Blood glucose monitors. Frequent self-monitoring of blood glucose (SMBG) is critical to better understand the glycemic responses to exercise and to try to limit the amount of dysglycemia. Prior to exercise, it is recommended to take at least two glucose measurements, spaced 15–30 min apart, so that directional changes in glucose can be determined.[130] Knowing that glucose is stable at 110 mg/dl before exercise likely requires a different strategy than seeing that it has dropped from 215 mg/dl to 100 mg/dl in the last 30 min. It is also recommended to test blood glucose levels every 30 min during the activity so that carbohydrate and insulin intake strategies can be modified if needed. Blood glucose monitoring in late recovery is also recommended as increased insulin sensitivity typically occurs 7–11 h later in recovery (often during sleep).[88]

Insulin pumps. Insulin pump devices (see chapter 12) offer a number of advantages and disadvantages for the active individual with T1D.[46,146,147] In general, pump users can adjust both the bolus insulin and the basal rate infusion before, during, and after exercise, thereby offering more flexibility in insulin dosing compared to fixed insulin injections. The insulin pump can be suspended or disconnected during exercise, if required. One major advantage is that basal insulin reductions following exercise can occur automatically during discrete hours during sleep (i.e., bedtime to 3 a.m.) to help prevent nocturnal hypoglycemia.[94] Internal calculators can be used to estimate the amount of on board insulin during the activity and can help prevent excessive insulin dosing at meal times.[148] In contrast, however, insulin pumps may interfere or be damaged during contact sports and there may be an increased risk for rapid development of hyperglycemia and ketosis if the pump is disconnected or if the infusion set is blocked. Indeed, postexercise hyperglycemia often occurs if the pump is removed (or if the infusion is reduced to zero) for exercise.[97] Insulin infusion sets may become displaced in conditions of heavy perspiration or water exposure (e.g., swimming) and skin irritation may result at the site of infusion, although strategies exist to help ameliorate these issues.

Continuous glucose monitoring (CGM). A number of relatively small studies have examined the utility of using CGM (see chapter 12) with exercise. In most studies, CGM has been demonstrated to accurately track the change in glycemia during exercise in patients with T1D.[91,149,150] However, real-time CGM tends to overestimate blood glucose levels if hypoglycemia is developing, likely because of the 10–20 min time delay in equilibrium between interstitial fluid and capillary glucose.[147] In one study, CGM was shown to be effective in detecting between ~65–70% of exercise-induced hypoglycemia, depending on the number of calibrations that were used (3 vs. 4/day).[151] Similarly, during vigorous exercise, CGM may fail to capture hyperglycemia if the changes are rapid.[152]

Real-time CGM use may help reduce the fear of exercise-associated hypoglycemia if directional arrows and alerts are used.[153] CGM may be very useful in situations in which SMBG is impractical (e.g., cycling road racing) or impossible, such as with scuba diving and when subjects are sleeping, to help reveal nocturnal hypoglycemia.[93,154] CGM may hold the promise of preventing hyperglycemia altogether during sports by keeping users more aware of their glucose concentrations and thus better prepared to take preventative actions. Indeed, a new carbohydrate intake algorithm designed to be used with glucose directional alters has been shown effective in preventing hypoglycemia altogether in a T1D youth sports camp setting.[155] Since glucose changes during exercise can be rapid, increasing the low-glucose-alert alarms from ~3.5 to 5.5 confers additional protection against exercise-induced hypoglycemia, without promoting false alarms.[156]

EXERCISE WITH COMPLICATIONS OR OTHER HEALTH CONDITIONS

Relative and Absolute Contraindications

The ADA and others have stressed the importance of appropriate screening procedures to clear patients for participation in exercise.[157–164] For patients with T1D, all of the diabetes-associated complications (microvascular and macrovascular disease) place the individual at a theoretically elevated risk for an adverse event caused by exercise, although actually documenting adverse events as a result of exercise in this population has been challenging.[25] Nonetheless, a number of precautions are warranted.

Coronary artery disease or stroke. Due to their elevated risk for macrovascular and microvascular disease (see chapter 16), patients with T1D who have had diabetes >10–15 years should undergo screening before starting a new program of unaccustomed vigorous activity (>6 METs).[25,165] However, no exercise restrictions should be placed on already active patients or on patients previously sedentary who are age <30 years or on patients age >30 years with no apparent complications. Pre-exercise screening is recommended for those who have been living with the disease for >10–15 years and who are age >30 years and should be conducted by a physician and or a qualified exercise professional (i.e., ACSM Certified Exercise Physiologist). Any symptoms of exercise intolerance (exhaustion, symptoms of poor perfusion, etc.) should be followed up, possibly with an exercise stress test or cardiac imaging or both. Traditional and nontraditional symptoms of cardiovascular disease requiring diagnostic follow-up are:

- Difficulty completing usual tasks
- Dyspnea with minimal exertion
- Unusual lack of energy
- Shoulder pain with a history similar to bursitis and related to activity
- Dizziness with activity
- Easy fatigability
- Neck or jaw discomfort
- Upper back pain

For previously sedentary persons with T1D age >30 years (and with diabetes duration ≥10 years) or with any diabetes-related complications (micro- or macrovascular) exercise programming of activities more vigorous than brisk walking should be suspended pending medical follow-up that may include exercise stress testing for the evaluation of CVD.[166] If CVD is stable, then mild- to moderate-intensity exercise may be considered safe and effective in limiting disease morbidity.

Since those with diabetes who are more physically active have much less risk for a cardiovascular event than those with disease who are sedentary, the consensus is that the risks of exercise are outweighed by the numerous benefits, as long as certain precautions are taken.[25,167] It is important to note that not all persons with T1D should be considered at high risk for CVD, particularly if they are in good glycemic control.[168]

Retinopathy. The effect of exercise on retinal damage (see chapter 16) in those with either background or proliferative retinopathy is unclear, but there is concern that increases in blood pressure or jarring movements, or both, at the latter stages of disease progression may facilitate retinal hemorrhage.[169] During a 10-year, exercise-based outpatient program for individuals with diabetes (both T1D and T2D) who had multiple complications at baseline, there was a 10% occurrence of retinal hemorrhage temporally related to exercise (3 of 30 patients who had baseline retinopathy).[170] It is important to note that events occurred only when the exercise was more vigorous than what had been prescribed by their exercise professional and the occurrences of retinal hemorrhage in nonactive patients with retinopathy was not provided for comparison.[170]

Other prospective cohort studies in humans with existing retinopathy have not shown an increased risk of retinopathy progression or of vitreous hemorrhage as a result of increased participation in team sports and exercise in patients with background retinopathy.[159,171,172] Moreover, several cross-sectional[8,173] and two retrospective observational studies[174,175] show no association between exercise participation and the risk of worsening retinopathy in people with T1D. Some evidence from one of these cross-sectional studies even supports the notion that increased physical activity participation might delay the development of retinopathy, at least in females.[172] These limited data suggest that exercise participation does not influence the risk of developing diabetic retinopathy if exercise is performed appropriately (i.e., not causing an excessive hypertensive response). Nonetheless, because of the fear that an increase in blood pressure associated with heavy exercise might cause retinal hemorrhaging and since prolonged exercise might increase growth hormone levels, both of which are associated with the development of retinopathy, persons with advanced retinopathy are frequently advised to avoid strenuous activities that increase blood pressure above 170 mm Hg systolic.[176,177]

In a National Institutes of Health consensus panel report, it was stated that "activities that require straining and breath holding" increase ocular risk of retinal detachment and vitreous hemorrhage as a result of elevations in blood pressure.[178] Accordingly, the panel does not endorse certain activities, such as weight lifting, for persons with diabetes with evidence of retinopathy. This expert opinion–based recommendation is controversial, however, since resistance exercise using moderate weight training (e.g., three sets at a moderate level using the major muscle groups) appears to be associated with lower blood pressure response compared to typical aerobic activities like stair climbing.[96] Given the preceding evidence, authors of various organizations have generally recommended moderate-intensity exercise (aerobic and resistance) but advised against vigorous exercise for those with severe nonproliferative or proliferative retinopathy.[158,163,177,179]

Neuropathy (peripheral and autonomic) or amputation. Distal sensory polyneuropathy (see chapter 16) occurs in several motor and sensory nerves in patients with long-standing disease and may be associated with movement difficulties, weakness, pain, and the loss of peripheral sensation. Peripheral neuropathy is linked to increased risk of foot ulceration and poor wound healing, causing amputation. Several aspects of exercise safety are of consideration for people with neuropathy, including their cardiovascular impairment, their risk of foot ulcerations, and their risk of falls. Unfortunately, clinical trials measuring the beneficial effects and adverse events associated with exercise in patients with neuropathy are limited.

Increased physical activity participation appears to dramatically lower the risk of developing peripheral neuropathy.[8,10] Little evidence proves that exercise worsens diabetic neuropathy. In fact, two studies observed that increased exercise participation actually decreased foot-ulceration risk in persons with diabetes who were also diagnosed with neuropathy.[180,181] However, some laboratory-based evidence suggests that abrupt increases in activity may increase the short-term risk of ulceration because of increased plantar pressures.[164,181] Moreover, with increased physical activity, there is likely an increased risk for falls and injury and, thus, supervised exercise may be advisable in higher risk individuals.

Nephropathy. Existing evidence does not support the avoidance of physical activity for patients with diabetic kidney disease (see chapter 16), although some precautions may be warranted.[182,183] Those with early nephropathy, who typically have low exercise tolerance, should probably avoid vigorous exercise, although mild- to moderate-intensity exercise is thought to be beneficial.[183] Individuals with end-stage renal disease have very low exercise tolerance, low aerobic capacity (Vo_{2max} <20 ml × kg^{-1} × min^{-1}), decreased cardiac output, blunted heart rate response to exercise, anemia, and decreased oxygen extraction.[184] These individuals need special care when being prescribed exercise and should be under close supervision, although mild and moderate aerobic exercise done during dialysis treatments has shown to increase fitness levels and exercise compliance.[185] Cardiovascular complications are also common in individuals with nephropathy, although little evidence exists that exercise triggers any adverse events.[186–189] As special care may be needed in these individuals with advanced disease, including erythropoietin administration, supervised exercise programs are recommended for those with advanced kidney disease.[25,186,188]

A summary of the recommended pre-exercise assessment strategies for patients with T1D at different ages is found in Table 11.5.

SPECIAL CONSIDERATIONS

Hydration

Due to potentially greater water losses with hyperglycemia, exercisers with T1D must focus on staying adequately hydrated before, during, and after any physical activity.[190] Starting several hours before exercise, individuals should take in normal amounts of fluids and meals to attain a state of euhydration prior to exercising, particularly if they have recently experienced hyperglycemia, either acutely or chronically.[190] According to the American College of Sports Medicine, the goal of fluid intake during exercise is to prevent excessive dehydration (>2% body weight loss from water deficit) and electrolyte imbalances.[191] Hydration state at the start of exercise, sweating rates, and environmental conditions all affect fluid requirements during physical activity.[191] Individual sweat rates can be estimated by measuring body weight before and after exercise. Excessive weight loss indicates a dehydrated state and should be prevented, whereas weight gain

Table 11.5 Pre-Exercise Assessment and Strategies for Adults with T1D*

	Age <30 Years	Age >30 Years and No Other Risk Factors	Age >30 Years and Duration of Diabetes >10 Years and/or Risk Factors
Cardiac evaluation	Not needed	Evaluate on a case-by-case basis, particularly in those who are sedentary prior to starting exercise.	Physician assessment for exercise greater than brisk walking in those who are unaccustomed to vigorous physical activity
Retinopathy (routine screening)	Moderate-intensity exercise (aerobic and resistance) is acceptable, but vigorous exercise should not be undertaken without clearance by an eye care specialist for those with severe nonproliferative or proliferative retinopathy. This is particularly true for exercises that raise systolic BP above 170 mmHg or activities that require straining and breath holding.		
Nephropathy (CKD stage 4 or 5)	Generally not an issue	Rarely an issue but if present send for evaluation by a nephrologist. May need to avoid strenuous exercise	If present, nephrologist should evaluate. Individuals often on multiple medications, which can limit exercise tolerance
Neuropathy—loss of protective sensation and/or high-risk foot	Usually not an issue, if present, podiatrist should evaluate and fit with special shoes as needed.		If present, podiatrist should evaluate and fit with special shoes as indicated. Evaluate for risk of falls and fractures and structure exercise accordingly.
Osteoporosis	Rarely a problem	If present, weight-bearing exercise is helpful. Exercise should be tailored to avoid falls and fractures.	

* As expected in the management of diabetes, individualize the need to assess exercise tolerance for adults with T1D.

from excess fluid intake during activities may lead to hyponatremia and should also be avoided.[192] During exercise, consuming beverages containing electrolytes and carbohydrates can provide benefits over water alone under certain circumstances, such as when carbohydrate is needed to prevent hypoglycemia and during more prolonged activities.[192–194] After exercise, the goal is simply to replace any fluid or electrolyte deficit, which can usually be accomplished with water intake and a healthy diet. Whole milk and sports drinks that are designed for both quick and long-lasting nutrient replenishment (including carbohydrates) can also be used by anyone with T1D to lower the risk of late-onset hypoglycemia associated with prior exercise.[195,196]

Extreme Athletic Events

Despite the challenges presented by participation in long-duration athletic events, many individuals with T1D are currently training for and participating in such events. Research in this area is lacking, but a handful of studies have attempted to investigate the metabolic and hormonal effects of more extreme athletic participation in such individuals.

In an early study on T1D and distance running, researchers examined the metabolic and hormonal effects of a 3-h marathon training run.[197] In that study, insulin was withheld for 16–26 h before the start of the run, although participants ate a normal breakfast 2.5 h before. Blood glucose levels decreased during the 3-h run, and postexercise ketosis was elevated compared to controls without diabetes. Counterregulatory hormone secretion was found to be normal (or even elevated) in response to hypoglycemia during a long-distance run in these reasonably well-controlled, well-trained subjects with T1D but without long-term complications. Similarly, a study of nine males with T1D during a 75-km cross-country skiing race reported that insulin dose reductions of 30–40% before the event resulted in hyperglycemia during the early part of the race, but near normoglycemia during the remainder, likely attributable to several-fold increases in counterregulatory hormone levels.[198] In another study, on the day of a marathon, runners with T1D reduced prerace insulin doses by an average of 26% and ingested 130 g of carbohydrate before, 91 g during, and 115 g after the race.[199]

More recently, a study involving 14 male amateur athletes with T1D treated with insulin analogs examined responses to participation in two consecutive editions of the same half-marathon.[124] For the half-marathon day, athletes reduced total insulin doses by 18.3% the first year, but only by 14.2% the second; basal insulin was reduced by 23.3% and 20.4% and short-acting insulin at breakfast prior to the competition by 31.7% and 15.3% in years 1 and 2, respectively. Athletes also consumed more carbohydrates during the event the second year (49.0 g vs. 59.1 g), with fewer glycemic excursions. Thus, athletes with T1D who are treated using insulin analogs alone may choose to make a lesser insulin reduction compared to traditional guidelines and slightly increase carbohydrate supplementation (amount and timing) to effectively balance blood glucose levels during long-distance competitions.

Others have shown reduced postmarathon insulin needs and increased insulin clearance, resulting in a decreased insulin availability that may allow enhanced muscle lipid utilization and spare glucose after long-duration exercise.[200] However, in another study, after successfully managed marathon running, insulin sensitivity was not increased despite low glycogen content and enhanced glycogen synthase activity after marathon, likely due to increased lipid oxidation.[199] Also examined were pre-exercise insulin reductions on consequent metabolic and dietary patterns for 24 h after a bout of running in individuals with T1D.[141] Participants self-administered 100%, 75%, 50%, or 25% of their full, rapid-acting insulin dose immediately before consuming a meal and 2 h before completing 45 min of moderate running. Initially blood glucose levels were little affected; levels were highest 3 h postexercise with the lowest dose (25%) of rapid-acting insulin, which was maintained over the rest of the 24-h period despite less energy and carbohydrate intake. Based on this study, one can conclude that greater reductions in mealtime insulin may result in greater protection during the activity but may also result in a greater likelihood for postexercise hyperglycemia.

Researchers have also studied use of continuous glucose monitoring systems (CGMS) during and after marathon participation to determine whether asymptomatic episodes of hypo- and hyperglycemia can be more effectively identified.[201] Although such systems are limited in their ability to detect rapid changes in blood glucose levels (see above section on CGM), use of CGMS may help to identify asymptomatic hypoglycemia or hyperglycemia during and after a long distance run. The system may also be helpful in improving understanding about the individual changes of glucose during and after a marathon and may protect against hypoglycemic or hyperglycemic periods in future races. Of note, individuals with insulin-treated diabetes are advised not to undertake prolonged intensive exercise after severe hypoglycemia due to increased risk of acute damage to skeletal muscle and to organs such as the liver, risk of severe neuroglycopenia, and the induction of seizures.[123]

Physical Education Classes and After-School and Team Sports

The goals for most physical education classes are to engage children and adolescents in healthy activities so that students can learn about and achieve the health and fitness benefits of exercise and to help develop some basic motor skills (throwing, catching, running, jumping, etc.) (see chapter 18, Schools). Participating in a 30–45 min physical education class also helps achieve at least a portion of their recommended daily physical activities and helps them learn the importance of communication and teamwork with their friends, peers, and teachers. It is also important for young people to be engaged in such activities early in life so that their participation as adults can be fostered. However, for the child or adolescent with T1D and the caregiver participation in physical activity can be challenging because of the possibility for glucose instability (hypoglycemia or hyperglycemia). The International Society for Pediatric and Adolescent Diabetes encourages participation in physical activity classes for students with diabetes and the American Diabetes Association publishes guidelines on diabetes care in school and day care settings.[202]

Obviously, participation in vigorous exercise during physical education classes can precipitate hypoglycemia, even if the activity is for just 30 min. For students with diabetes, participation in physical education classes and team sports requires communication and collaboration between the student, his or her health care provider, parents, the school nurse, the physical education instructor, and the team coach. A diabetes care plan should be in place for the child or teen and should include specific instructions for physical activity. The Juvenile Diabetes Foundation (http://www.jdrf.org/) has a useful checklist of actions for the physical education instructor or coach:

- Encourage exercise and participation in physical activities and sports for students with diabetes as you would for other students.
- Treat the student with diabetes the same as other students, except in meeting his or her medical needs (remember to respect the student's right to privacy and confidentiality).

- Make sure blood glucose monitoring equipment is available at all activity sites, and encourage the student to keep personal supplies readily accessible.
- Always allow the student to check blood glucose levels.
- Understand and be aware that hypoglycemia can occur during and after physical activity and that a change in the student's behavior could be a symptom of blood glucose changes.
- Be prepared to recognize and respond to the signs and symptoms of hypoglycemia and hyperglycemia, and when a blood sugar event occurs, take initial actions in accordance with the student's school plan.
- To treat hypoglycemia, provide the student with immediate access to a fast-acting form of glucose. Consider taping three or four glucose tablets or hard candies to a clipboard or include them in the first aid pack at physical activities, practices, and games.
- Communicate with the school nurse or trained diabetes personnel or both regarding any observations or concerns about the student.

Students with diabetes should be responsible for wearing a medic alert ID tag at all times. Students and their teachers should be equipped with fast-acting carbohydrate snacks at all times and instructed on the appropriate treatment of hypoglycemia (15 g of carbohydrate; wait 15 min and retest and retreat if necessary). If reductions in pre-exercise insulin are not performed in anticipation of physical education, then carbohydrate intake at a rate of 1 g carbohydrate/kg body mass/h can be implemented. If blood glucose is already elevated prior to the class (>8–11 mmol/l) then additional carbohydrate may not be required. As with other types of activity, vigorous activity during school should be avoided if glucose is markedly elevated (>14 mmol/l) in the presence of moderate or higher levels of ketones.

Parents, teachers, and the patient with T1D should be educated as to the symptoms of hypoglycemia, the individualized action plan for prevention and treatment of hypoglycemia, and for potential emergencies (loss of consciousness).

Camps for Kids

Camping provides young people with diabetes and their families with a unique opportunity to share with and learn from others with diabetes, often in a physically demanding setting (see chapter 18, Camps). Some studies suggest that a camp experience may improve a child's psychosocial status and levels of glycemic control, although it should be expected that the experience may increase day-to-day glycemic variability.[203–206] Based on retrospective analysis of camp medical records, it is estimated that an empiric 10% reduction in basal insulin appears reasonable upon arrival to camp, as nearly equal numbers of children required dose increases as dose decreases as camp progressed.[207] In one study of campers, treatment in a camp setting with 0.3 g of fast-acting carbohydrate (glucose tablets, hard candy, or orange juice) was shown to be effective in resolving hypoglycemia within 15 min in most children.[208] Guidelines for the staffing and management of diabetes camps can be found through numerous sources including the ADA.[209,210]

Scuba Diving

Individuals with T1D were once dissuaded from participating in scuba diving, primarily due to concern that hypoglycemia during immersion would be
likely to occur and difficult to treat. The National Association of Underwater
Instructors (www.naui.org) still prevents individuals with T1D from obtaining
certification to dive through their organization, whereas the Professional Association of Diving Instructors (www.padi.com) allows individuals with T1D to
be certified. The Divers Alert Network (www.diversalertnetwork.org) reports
that many active divers have T1D and that the majority of such divers do not
experience dive-related hypoglycemia.[211] The United Kingdom is supportive of
allowing persons with T1D to scuba dive, as long as certain precautions are taken
(http://www.ukdiving.co.uk/information/medicine/diabetes.htm). Indeed, recent
evidence suggests that scuba diving can be undertaken safely by well-controlled,
experienced, and complication-free individuals with T1D, assuming that appropriate precautionary measures are taken. Important precautions to help prevent
hypoglycemia include the use of a rigorous protocol of serial predive blood glucose measurements to determine glucose levels and rates of change before entering the water.[212] Some authors recommend a glycemic goal of 200–250 mg/dl
(11–13.75 mmol/l) before immersion with a significant reduction of insulin doses
(by 30%) and the availability of rapid-acting carbohydrates either on hand or
on board.[213] These affirmative results resulted in the French diving federation
(FESSM) now allowing individuals with T1D to dive with some restrictive quali-
fication requirements: dives must be within the safety curve (no decompression
curve), in >14°C water, within depths limited to 6–20 meters, and with mandatory
guidance by a diving instructor.

During a simulated dive to 27 meters in a hyperbaric chamber, well-controlled
adults with T1D who were free of long-term complications were able to effectively
self-regulate blood glucose levels to avoid hypoglycemia.[214] However, long-term
complications of diabetes (such as diabetic proliferative retinopathy) may need to
be excluded before a diver with diabetes may be permitted to dive.[215] In addition,
it may be advantageous for divers to use CGM to help limit hypoglycemia.[154] In
a CGM-related study, 117 dives were undertaken by 24 adults, half with T1D;
hypoglycemia (<70 mg/dl) was detected using CGM in six individuals and on
nine occasions, but in none of these cases were hypoglycemic symptoms present
during or immediately after diving.[154] The number of hypoglycemic episodes, 10
min prediving or immediately postdiving, were related to the duration of diabetes,
percentage of SMBG values below target (<72 mg/dl), and total duration below
low limit (<70 mg/dl). These results led to the conclusion that well-informed,
well-controlled individuals with T1D can dive safely and that the use of CGM and
repetitive self-monitoring of blood glucose on a schedule allows identification of
individuals who are suitable for diving. Use of CGM under diving conditions has
also been reported to be reliable and reasonably accurate.[216]

Practical diving guidelines include:

- Blood glucose levels should be >150 mg/dl before the dive, and the dive
  should occur following a meal.
- If the blood glucose is <150 mg/dl, 5 g of glucose should be consumed
  for every 25 mg <150 mg/dl. Carbohydrates in the form of simple

sugars, such as fruit juice, milk, or glucose tablets or liquid, should be ingested.
- The diver should carry liquid sugar in the wet suit during the dive and use as needed.
- The diver should measure blood glucose after the dive and ingest glucose as needed.
- The diver should always dive with a companion who understands how to recognize and treat a hypoglycemic reaction. When under water, divers should have a prearranged means to communicate the likely incidence of hypoglycemia.
- Glycemic control should be stable during the days of planned diving.
- Alcohol should not be consumed 24 h before or during the diving activities.[217]

Treatment of Overweight and Obesity with Physical Activity

Engaging in regular physical activity generally lowers overall insulin requirements and reduces the risk of weight gain associated with excess insulin use.[218–222] In rats with alloxan-induced T1D, intensive insulin treatment induces insulin resistance by impairing glucose metabolism–related mechanisms in muscle and liver (i.e., by increasing insulin resistance).[223] With the expectation that insulin resistance develops in hyperinsulinized diabetic patients as well, the authors of that study suggested using insulin-sensitizer approaches (like increased physical activity) to effectively treat T1D.

In adults without diabetes, exercise has been shown to have beneficial effects on body fatness in the absence of prescribed dietary change, with a progressive loss of body fat associated with higher exercise energy expenditures in both men and women.[224] Even greater free-living activity energy expenditure (such as walking, household chores, and work-related physical activity) can aid in weight loss and weight maintenance.[225] Similarly, in individuals with T1D, physical activity can improve insulin action, albeit acutely, and potentially lower insulin requirements and body weight. For example, in one study involving 13 previously sedentary individuals with T1D (ages 13–30 years), engaging in either 12 weeks of aerobic or resistance exercise training lowered their insulin needs, waist circumference, and post-training blood glucose levels, although their A1C levels were not significantly improved.[7] Moreover, all adolescents with T1D can benefit from combined aerobic and strength training undertaken twice weekly for 20 weeks, which results in lower daily insulin requirements, improved physical fitness, and an enhanced sense of well-being.[226] Similar training has also been shown to reduce cardiovascular risk and insulin resistance risk factors in diabetic adolescent girls.[227] Exercise truly is a powerful medicine for anyone with T1D, especially if overweight or obese from insulin use.

AREAS FOR FUTURE RESEARCH

A number of key research areas still need development in the area of exercise and T1D. These include:

- What are the health benefits of resistance training for patients with T1D?
- What is the impact of exercise in various environments on the pharmacokinetics and pharmacodynamics of rapid-acting and long-acting insulin analogs?
- What are the appropriate insulin adjustments for resistance and anaerobic type exercise that results in hyperglycemia?
- What are the appropriate postexercise basal rate adjustments to limit postexercise hyperglycemia in the pump-treated patient?
- What should be the low-glucose suspend level for sensor-augmented, pump-treated patients engaged in physical activity?
- What is the appropriate insulin dose adjustment (correction) for postexercise hyperglycemia in the patient on a multiple daily injection regimen?
- What is the optimal feeding strategy to prevent exercise-associated hypoglycemia (type of carbohydrate, timing of ingestion, and dosage)?
- What other noninsulin adjustment strategies help to prevent exercise-associated hypoglycemia (e.g., caffeine, protein supplementation, glucagon stimulants or agonists, adrenergic agonists, etc.)?
- What are the optimal approaches to prevent severe nocturnal hypoglycemia?
- What limitations, if any, should be placed on individuals wishing to perform extreme or higher risk activities (scuba, skydiving, Ironman, etc.)?
- What are the optimal insulin-adjustment and nutritional strategies to help facilitate weight (fat) loss via increased physical activity in T1D?

REFERENCES

1. Physical Activity Guidelines Advisory Committee: *Physical Activity Guidelines Advisory Committee Report*. U.S. Department of Health and Human Services, 2008
2. Chimen M, Kennedy A, Nirantharakumar K, Pang TT, Andrews R, Narendran P: What are the health benefits of physical activity in type 1 diabetes mellitus? A literature review. *Diabetologia* 55:542–551, 2012
3. Aman J, Skinner TC, de Beaufort CE, Swift PG, Aanstoot HJ, Cameron F; Hvidoere Study Group on Childhood Diabetes: Associations between physical activity, sedentary behavior, and glycemic control in a large cohort of adolescents with type 1 diabetes: the Hvidoere Study Group on Childhood Diabetes. *Pediatr Diabetes* 10:234–239, 2009
4. Moy CS, Songer TJ, LaPorte RE, Dorman JS, Kriska AM, Orchard TJ, Becker DJ, Drash AL: Insulin-dependent diabetes mellitus, physical activity, and death. *Am J Epidemiol* 137:74–81, 1993
5. Soedamah-Muthu SS, Fuller JH, Mulnier HE, Raleigh VS, Lawrenson RA, Colhoun HM: All-cause mortality rates in patients with type 1 diabetes mellitus compared with a non-diabetic population from the UK general practice research database, 1992-1999. *Diabetologia* 49:660–666, 2006
6. Koivisto VA, Yki-Jarvinen H, DeFronzo RA: Physical training and insulin sensitivity. *Diabetes Metab Rev* 1:445–481, 1986
7. Ramalho AC, de Lourdes Lima M, Nunes F, Cambui Z, Barbosa C, Andrade A, Viana A, Martins M, Abrantes V, Aragao C, Temistocles M: The effect

of resistance versus aerobic training on metabolic control in patients with type-1 diabetes mellitus. *Diabetes Res Clin Pract* 72:271–276, 2006

8. Kriska AM, LaPorte RE, Patrick SL, Kuller LH, Orchard TJ: The association of physical activity and diabetic complications in individuals with insulin-dependent diabetes mellitus: the Epidemiology of Diabetes Complications Study—VII. *J Clin Epidemiol* 44:1207–1214, 1991

9. Balducci S, Iacobellis G, Parisi L, Di Biase N, Calandriello E, Leonetti F, Fallucca F: Exercise training can modify the natural history of diabetic peripheral neuropathy. *J Diabetes Complicat* 20:216–223, 2006

10. Nielsen PJ, Hafdahl AR, Conn VS, Lemaster JW, Brown SA: Meta-analysis of the effect of exercise interventions on fitness outcomes among adults with type 1 and type 2 diabetes. *Diabetes Res Clin Pract* 74:111–120, 2006

11. Waden J, Forsblom C, Thorn LM, Saraheimo M, Rosengard-Barlund M, Heikkila O, Lakka TA, Tikkanen H, Groop PH; FinnDiane Study Group: Physical activity and diabetes complications in patients with type 1 diabetes: the Finnish Diabetic Nephropathy (FinnDiane) Study. *Diabetes Care* 31:230–232, 2008

12. Bouchard C, Shephard RJ: Physical activity, fitness, and health: the model and key concepts. In *Physical Activity, Fitness and Health:International Proceedings and Consensus Statement.* Bouchard C, Shephard RJ, Stephens T, Eds. Champaign, IL, Human Kinetics, 1994, p. 77–88

13. Hart TL, Craig CL, Griffiths JM, Cameron C, Andersen RE, Bauman A, Tudor-Locke C: Markers of sedentarism: the joint Canada/U.S. Survey of health. *J Phys Act Health* 8:361–371, 2011

14. Bernardini AL, Vanelli M, Chiari G, Iovane B, Gelmetti C, Vitale R, Errico MK: Adherence to physical activity in young people with type 1 diabetes. *Acta Biomed* 75:153–157, 2004

15. Waden J, Tikkanen H, Forsblom C, Fagerudd J, Pettersson-Fernholm K, Lakka T, Riska M, Groop PH; FinnDiane Study Group: Leisure time physical activity is associated with poor glycemic control in type 1 diabetic women: the FinnDiane study. *Diabetes Care* 28:777–782, 2005

16. Riddell MC, Perkins BA: Type 1 diabetes and exercise: part I: applications of exercise physiology to patient management during vigorous activity. *Can J Diab* 30:63–71, 2006

17. Sigal R, Kenny G, Oh P, Perkins BA, Plotnikoff RC, Prud'homme D, Riddell MC: Physical activity and diabetes. Canadian Diabetes Association Clinical Practice Guidelines Expert Committee. Canadian Diabetes Association 2008 clinical practice guidelines for the prevention and management of diabetes in Canada. *Can J Diab* 32:S37–S39, 2008

18. Evans CH, White RD: *Exercise Testing for Primary Care and Sports Medicine Physicians.* New York, Springer, 2009

19. Niranjan V, McBrayer DG, Ramirez LC, Raskin P, and Hsia CC: Glycemic control and cardiopulmonary function in patients with insulin-dependent diabetes mellitus. *Am J Med* 103:504–513, 1997

20. Komatsu WR, Gabbay MA, Castro ML, Saraiva GL, Chacra AR, de Barros Neto TL, Dib SA: Aerobic exercise capacity in normal adolescents and those with type 1 diabetes mellitus. *Pediatr Diabetes* 6:145–149, 2005

21. Williams BK, Guelfi KJ, Jones TW, Davis EA: Lower cardiorespiratory fitness in children with type 1 diabetes. *Diabet Med* 28:1005–1007, 2011
22. Poortmans JR, Saerens P, Edelman R, Vertongen F, Dorchy H: Influence of the degree of metabolic control on physical fitness in type I diabetic adolescents. *Int J Sports Med* 7:232–235, 1986
23. Baldi JC, Cassuto NA, Foxx-Lupo WT, Wheatley CM, Snyder EM: Glycemic status affects cardiopulmonary exercise response in athletes with type I diabetes. *Med Sci Sports Exerc* 42:1454–1459, 2010
24. Baldi JC, Hofman PL: Does careful glycemic control improve aerobic capacity in subjects with type 1 diabetes? *Exerc Sport Sci Rev* 38:161–167, 2010
25. Riddell MC, Burr J: Evidence-based risk assessment and recommendations for physical activity clearance: diabetes mellitus and related comorbidities. *Appl Physiol Nutr Metab* 36 (Suppl. 1):S154–S189, 2011
26. Janssen I, Leblanc AG: Systematic review of the health benefits of physical activity and fitness in school-aged children and youth. *Int J Behav Nutr Phys Act* 7:40, 2010
27. Expert Panel on Integrated Guidelines for Cardiovascular Health and Risk Reduction in Children and Adolescents and National Heart, Lung, and Blood Institute: Expert panel on integrated guidelines for cardiovascular health and risk reduction in children and adolescents: summary report. *Pediatrics* 128 (Suppl. 5):S213–S256, 2011
28. Rachmiel M, Buccino J, Daneman D: Exercise and type 1 diabetes mellitus in youth; review and recommendations. *Pediatr Endocrinol Rev* 5:656–665, 2007
29. Kelder SH, Perry CL, Klepp KI, Lytle LL: Longitudinal tracking of adolescent smoking, physical activity, and food choice behaviors. *Am J Public Health* 84:1121–1126, 1994
30. Astrup AS: Cardiovascular morbidity and mortality in diabetes mellitus: prediction and prognosis. *Dan Med Bull* 58:B4152, 2011
31. Galler A, Lindau M, Ernert A, Thalemann R, Raile K: Associations between media consumption habits, physical activity, socioeconomic status, and glycemic control in children, adolescents, and young adults with type 1 diabetes. *Diabetes Care* 34:2356–2359, 2011
32. Brazeau AS, Rabasa-Lhoret R, Strychar I, Mircescu H: Barriers to physical activity among patients with type 1 diabetes. *Diabetes Care* 31:2108–2109, 2008
33. Herbst A, Kordonouri O, Schwab KO, Schmidt F, Holl RW; DPV Initiative of the German Working Group for Pediatric Diabetology Germany: Impact of physical activity on cardiovascular risk factors in children with type 1 diabetes: a multicenter study of 23,251 patients. *Diabetes Care* 30:2098–2100, 2007
34. Durak EP, Jovanovic-Peterson L, Peterson CM: Randomized crossover study of effect of resistance training on glycemic control, muscular strength, and cholesterol in type I diabetic men. *Diabetes Care* 13:1039–1043, 1990
35. Zoppini G, Carlini M, Muggeo M: Self-reported exercise and quality of life in young type 1 diabetic subjects. *Diabetes Nutr Metab* 16:77–80, 2003
36. Salem MA, Aboelasrar MA, Elbarbary NS, Elhilaly RA, Refaat YM: Is exercise a therapeutic tool for improvement of cardiovascular risk factors in adolescents with type 1 diabetes mellitus? A randomised controlled trial. *Diabetol Metab Syndr* 2:47, 2010

37. Zinman B, Zuniga-Guajardo S, Kelly D: Comparison of the acute and long-term effects of exercise on glucose control in type I diabetes. *Diabetes Care* 7:515–519, 1984
38. Raile K, Kapellen T, Schweiger A, Hunkert F, Nietzschmann U, Dost A, Kiess W: Physical activity and competitive sports in children and adolescents with type 1 diabetes. *Diabetes Care* 22:1904–1905, 1999
39. Roberts L, Jones TW, Fournier PA: Exercise training and glycemic control in adolescents with poorly controlled type 1 diabetes mellitus. *J Pediatr Endocrinol Metab* 15:621–627, 2002
40. Harmer AR, Chisholm DJ, McKenna MJ, Morris NR, Thom JM, Bennett G, Flack JR: High-intensity training improves plasma glucose and acid-base regulation during intermittent maximal exercise in type 1 diabetes. *Diabetes Care* 30:1269–1271, 2007
41. Garber CE, Blissmer B, Deschenes MR, Franklin BA, Lamonte MJ, Lee IM, Nieman DC, Swain DP; American College of Sports Medicine: American College of Sports Medicine position stand. Quantity and quality of exercise for developing and maintaining cardiorespiratory, musculoskeletal, and neuromotor fitness in apparently healthy adults: guidance for prescribing exercise. *Med Sci Sports Exerc* 43:1334–1359, 2011
42. Warburton DE, Nicol CW, Bredin SS: Prescribing exercise as preventive therapy. *CMAJ* 174:961–974, 2006
43. Reddigan JI, Riddell MC, Kuk JL: The joint association of physical activity and glycaemic control in predicting cardiovascular death and all-cause mortality in the US population. *Diabetologia* 55:632–635, 2012
44. Physical Activity Guidelines Advisory Committee: Report, 2008. To the secretary of health and human services. Part A: executive summary. *Nutr Rev* 67:114–120, 2009
45. Tremblay MS, Warburton DE, Janssen I, Paterson DH, Latimer AE, Rhodes RE, Kho ME, Hicks A, Leblanc AG, Zehr L, Murumets K, Duggan M: New Canadian physical activity guidelines. *Appl Physiol Nutr Metab* 36:36–46, 47–58, 2011
46. Chu L, Hamilton J, Riddell MC: Clinical management of the physically active patient with type 1 diabetes. *Phys Sportsmed* 39:64–77, 2011
47. Guelfi KJ, Ratnam N, Smythe GA, Jones TW, Fournier PA: Effect of intermittent high-intensity compared with continuous moderate exercise on glucose production and utilization in individuals with type 1 diabetes. *Am J Physiol Endocrinol Metab* 292:E865–E870, 2007
48. Yardley JE, Kenny GP, Perkins BA, Riddell MC, Malcolm J, Boulay P, Khandwala F, Sigal RJ: Effects of performing resistance exercise before versus after aerobic exercise on glycemia in type 1 diabetes. *Diabetes Care* 35:669–675, 2012
49. Caron D, Poussier P, Marliss EB, Zinman B: The effect of postprandial exercise on meal-related glucose intolerance in insulin-dependent diabetic individuals. *Diabetes Care* 5:364–369, 1982
50. Temple MY, Bar-Or O, Riddell MC: The reliability and repeatability of the blood glucose response to prolonged exercise in adolescent boys with IDDM. *Diabetes Care* 18:326–332, 1995
51. Riddell MC, Bar-Or O, Ayub BV, Calvert RE, Heigenhauser GJ: Glucose ingestion matched with total carbohydrate utilization attenuates

hypoglycemia during exercise in adolescents with IDDM. *Int J Sport Nutr* 9:24–34, 1999
52. Kilbride L, Charlton J, Aitken G, Hill GW, Davison RC, McKnight JA: Managing blood glucose during and after exercise in type 1 diabetes: reproducibility of glucose response and a trial of a structured algorithm adjusting insulin and carbohydrate intake. *J Clin Nurs* 20:3423–3429, 2011
53. Krause MP, Moradi J, Nissar AA, Riddell MC, Hawke TJ: Inhibition of plasminogen activator inhibitor-1 restores skeletal muscle regeneration in untreated type 1 diabetic mice. *Diabetes* 60:1964–1972, 2011
54. Lira FS, Rosa JC, Lima-Silva AE, Souza HA, Caperuto EC, Seelaender MC, Damaso AR, Oyama LM, Santos RV: Sedentary subjects have higher PAI-1 and lipoproteins levels than highly trained athletes. *Diabetol Metab Syndr* 2:7, 2010
55. Belalcazar LM, Ballantyne CM, Lang W, Haffner SM, Rushing J, Schwenke DC, Pi-Sunyer FX, Tracy RP; Look Action for Health in Diabetes Research Group: Metabolic factors, adipose tissue, and plasminogen activator inhibitor-1 levels in type 2 diabetes: findings from the look AHEAD study. *Arterioscler Thromb Vasc Biol* 31:1689–1695, 2011
56. Wallberg-Henriksson H, Gunnarsson R, Henriksson J, DeFronzo R, Felig P, Ostman J, Wahren J: Increased peripheral insulin sensitivity and muscle mitochondrial enzymes but unchanged blood glucose control in type I diabetics after physical training. *Diabetes* 31:1044–1050, 1982
57. Yki-Jarvinen H, DeFronzo RA, Koivisto VA: Normalization of insulin sensitivity in type I diabetic subjects by physical training during insulin pump therapy. *Diabetes Care* 7:520–527, 1984
58. Lehmann R, Kaplan V, Bingisser R, Bloch KE, Spinas GA: Impact of physical activity on cardiovascular risk factors in IDDM. *Diabetes Care* 20:1603–1611, 1997
59. Mosher PE, Nash MS, Perry AC, LaPerriere AR, Goldberg RB: Aerobic circuit exercise training: effect on adolescents with well-controlled insulin-dependent diabetes mellitus. *Arch Phys Med Rehabil* 79:652–657, 1998
60. Laaksonen DE, Atalay M, Niskanen LK, Mustonen J, Sen CK, Lakka TA, Uusitupa MI: Aerobic exercise and the lipid profile in type 1 diabetic men: a randomized controlled trial. *Med Sci Sports Exerc* 32:1541–1548, 2000
61. Rigla M, Sanchez-Quesada JL, Ordonez-Llanos J, Prat T, Caixas A, Jorba O, Serra JR, de Leiva A, Perez A: Effect of physical exercise on lipoprotein(a) and low-density lipoprotein modifications in type 1 and type 2 diabetic patients. *Metabolism* 49:640–647, 2000
62. Fuchsjager-Mayrl G, Pleiner J, Wiesinger GF, Sieder AE, Quittan M, Nuhr MJ, Francesconi C, Seit HP, Francesconi M, Schmetterer L, Wolzt M: Exercise training improves vascular endothelial function in patients with type 1 diabetes. *Diabetes Care* 25:1795–1801, 2002
63. Valerio G, Spagnuolo MI, Lombardi F, Spadaro R, Siano M, Franzese A: Physical activity and sports participation in children and adolescents with type 1 diabetes mellitus. *Nutr Metab Cardiovasc Dis* 17:376–382, 2007
64. Coggan AR: Plasma glucose metabolism during exercise in humans. *Sports Med* 11:102–124, 1991
65. Wahren J, Felig P, Ahlborg G, Jorfeldt L: Glucose metabolism during leg exercise in man. *J Clin Invest* 50:2715–2725, 1971

66. Bergeron R, Kjaer M, Simonsen L, Bulow J, Galbo H: Glucose production during exercise in humans: a-hv balance and isotopic-tracer measurements compared. *J Appl Physiol* 87:111–115, 1999

67. Purdon C, Brousson M, Nyveen SL, Miles PD, Halter JB, Vranic M, Marliss EB: The roles of insulin and catecholamines in the glucoregulatory response during intense exercise and early recovery in insulin-dependent diabetic and control subjects. *J Clin Endocrinol Metab* 76:566–573, 1993

68. Coggan AR, Coyle EF: Reversal of fatigue during prolonged exercise by carbohydrate infusion or ingestion. *J Appl Physiol* 63:2388–2395, 1987

69. Coggan AR, Coyle EF: Effect of carbohydrate feedings during high-intensity exercise. *J Appl Physiol* 65:1703–1709, 1988

70. Raguso CA, Coggan AR, Gastaldelli A, Sidossis LS, Bastyr EJ 3rd, Wolfe RR: Lipid and carbohydrate metabolism in IDDM during moderate and intense exercise. *Diabetes* 44:1066–1074, 1995

71. Krzentowski G, Pirnay F, Pallikarakis N, Luyckx AS, Lacroix M, Mosora F, Lefebvre PJ: Glucose utilization during exercise in normal and diabetic subjects: the role of insulin. *Diabetes* 30:983–989, 1981

72. Riddell MC, Bar-Or O, Schwarcz HP, Heigenhauser GJ: Substrate utilization in boys during exercise with [13C]-glucose ingestion. *Eur J Appl Physiol* 83:441–448, 2000

73. Robitaille M, Dube MC, Weisnagel SJ, Prud'homme D, Massicotte D, Peronnet F, Lavoie C: Substrate source utilization during moderate intensity exercise with glucose ingestion in Type 1 diabetic patients. *J Appl Physiol* 103:119–124, 2007

74. Younk LM, Mikeladze M, Tate D, Davis SN: Exercise-related hypoglycemia in diabetes mellitus. *Expert Rev Endocrinol Metab* 6:93–108, 2011

75. Sotsky MJ, Shilo S, Shamoon H: Regulation of counterregulatory hormone secretion in man during exercise and hypoglycemia. *J Clin Endocrinol Metab* 68:9–16, 1989

76. Zinker BA, Allison RG, Lacy DB, Wasserman DH: Interaction of exercise, insulin, and hypoglycemia studied using euglycemic and hypoglycemic insulin clamps. *Am J Physiol* 272: E530–E542, 1997

77. Camacho RC, Galassetti P, Davis SN, Wasserman DH: Glucoregulation during and after exercise in health and insulin-dependent diabetes. *Exerc Sport Sci Rev* 33:17–23, 2005

78. Karelis AD, Smith JW, Passe DH, Peronnet F: Carbohydrate administration and exercise performance: what are the potential mechanisms involved? *Sports Med* 40:747–763, 2010

79. Chokkalingam K, Tsintzas K, Snaar JE, Norton L, Solanky B, Leverton E, Morris P, Mansell P, Macdonald IA: Hyperinsulinaemia during exercise does not suppress hepatic glycogen concentrations in patients with type 1 diabetes: a magnetic resonance spectroscopy study. *Diabetologia* 50:1921–1929, 2007

80. Briscoe VJ, Tate DB, Davis SN: Type 1 diabetes: exercise and hypoglycemia. *Appl Physiol Nutr Metab* 32:576–582, 2007

81. Berger M, Halban PA, Assal JP, Offord RE, Vranic M, Renold AE: Pharmacokinetics of subcutaneously injected tritiated insulin: effects of exercise. *Diabetes* 28 (Suppl. 1):53–57, 1979

82. Edelmann E, Staudner V, Bachmann W, Walter H, Haas W, Mehnert H: Exercise-induced hypoglycaemia and subcutaneous insulin infusion. *Diabet Med* 3:526–531, 1986

83. Wasserman DH: Berson award lecture 2008 four grams of glucose. *Am J Physiol Endocrinol Metab* 296:E11–E21, 2009

84. Wasserman DH: Regulation of glucose fluxes during exercise in the postabsorptive state. *Annu Rev Physiol* 57:191–218, 1995

85. Francescato MP, Carrato S: Management of exercise-induced glycemic imbalances in type 1 diabetes. *Curr Diabetes Rev* 7:253–263, 2011

86. Schneider SH, Vitug A, Ananthakrishnan R, Khachadurian AK: Impaired adrenergic response to prolonged exercise in type I diabetes. *Metabolism* 40:1219–1225, 1991

87. Cline GW, Rothman DL, Magnusson I, Katz LD, Shulman GI: 13C-nuclear magnetic resonance spectroscopy studies of hepatic glucose metabolism in normal subjects and subjects with insulin-dependent diabetes mellitus. *J Clin Invest* 94:2369–2376, 1994

88. McMahon SK, Ferreira LD, Ratnam N, Davey RJ, Youngs LM, Davis EA, Fournier PA, Jones TW: Glucose requirements to maintain euglycemia after moderate-intensity afternoon exercise in adolescents with type 1 diabetes are increased in a biphasic manner. *J Clin Endocrinol Metab* 92:963–968, 2007

89. Diabetes Research in Children Network (DirecNet) Study Group; Tsalikian E, Kollman C, Tamborlane WB, Beck RW, Fiallo-Scharer R, Fox L, Janz KF, Ruedy KJ, Wilson D, Xing D, Weinzimer SA: Prevention of hypoglycemia during exercise in children with type 1 diabetes by suspending basal insulin. *Diabetes Care* 29:2200–2204, 2006

90. Iscoe KE, Campbell JE, Jamnik V, Perkins BA, Riddell MC: Efficacy of continuous real-time blood glucose monitoring during and after prolonged high-intensity cycling exercise: spinning with a continuous glucose monitoring system. *Diabetes Technol Ther* 8:627–635, 2006

91. Diabetes Research in Children Network (DirecNet) Study Group: Impaired overnight counterregulatory hormone responses to spontaneous hypoglycemia in children with type 1 diabetes. *Pediatr Diabetes* 8:199–205, 2007

92. Iscoe KE, Corcoran M, Riddell MC: High rates of nocturnal hypoglycemia in a unique sports camp for athletes with type 1 diabetes: lessons learned from continuous glucose monitoring. *Can J Diab* 32:182–189, 2008

93. Maran A, Pavan P, Bonsembiante B, Brugin E, Ermolao A, Avogaro A, Zaccaria M: Continuous glucose monitoring reveals delayed nocturnal hypoglycemia after intermittent high-intensity exercise in nontrained patients with type 1 diabetes. *Diabetes Technol Ther* 12:763–768, 2010

94. Taplin CE, Cobry E, Messer L, McFann K, Chase HP, Fiallo-Scharer R: Preventing post-exercise nocturnal hypoglycemia in children with type 1 diabetes. *J Pediatr* 157:784–8.e1, 2010

95. Marliss EB, Vranic M: Intense exercise has unique effects on both insulin release and its roles in glucoregulation: implications for diabetes. *Diabetes* 51 (Suppl. 1):S271–S283, 2002

96. Sigal RJ, Purdon C, Fisher SJ, Halter JB, Vranic M, Marliss EB: Hyperinsulinemia prevents prolonged hyperglycemia after intense exercise in insulin-dependent diabetic subjects. *J Clin Endocrinol Metab* 79:1049–1057, 1994

97. Delvecchio M, Zecchino C, Salzano G, Faienza MF, Cavallo L, De Luca F, Lombardo F: Effects of moderate-severe exercise on blood glucose in type 1 diabetic adolescents treated with insulin pump or glargine insulin. *J Endocrinol Invest* 32:519–524, 2009
98. Huttunen NP, Kaar ML, Knip M, Mustonen A, Puukka R, Akerblom HK: Physical fitness of children and adolescents with insulin-dependent diabetes mellitus. *Ann Clin Res* 16:1–5, 1984
99. Ditzel J, Standl E: The problem of tissue oxygenation in diabetes mellitus. *Acta Med Scand Suppl* 578:59–68, 1975
100. Kivela R, Silvennoinen M, Touvra AM, Lehti TM, Kainulainen H, Vihko V: Effects of experimental type 1 diabetes and exercise training on angiogenic gene expression and capillarization in skeletal muscle. *FASEB J* 20:1570–1572, 2006
101. Robertson K, Adolfsson P, Scheiner G, Hanas R, Riddell MC: Exercise in children and adolescents with diabetes. *Pediatr Diabetes* 10 (Suppl. 12):154–168, 2009
102. Krause MP, Riddell MC, Hawke TJ: Effects of type 1 diabetes mellitus on skeletal muscle: clinical observations and physiological mechanisms. *Pediatr Diabetes* 12:345–364, 2011
103. Surridge DH, Erdahl DL, Lawson JS, Donald MW, Monga TN, Bird CE, Letemendia FJ: Psychiatric aspects of diabetes mellitus. *Brit J Psychiat* 145:269–276, 1984
104. Van der Does FE, De Neeling JN, Snoek FJ, Kostense PJ, Grootenhuis PA, Bouter LM, Heine RJ: Symptoms and well-being in relation to glycemic control in type II diabetes. *Diabetes Care* 19:204–210, 1996
105. Almeida S, Riddell MC, Cafarelli E: Slower conduction velocity and motor unit discharge frequency are associated with muscle fatigue during isometric exercise in type 1 diabetes mellitus. *Muscle Nerve* 37:231–240, 2008
106. Andersen H: Muscular endurance in long-term IDDM patients. *Diabetes Care* 21:604–609, 1998
107. Riddell MC, Bar-Or O, Gerstein HC, Heigenhauser GJ: Perceived exertion with glucose ingestion in adolescent males with IDDM. *Med Sci Sports Exerc* 32:167–173, 2000
108. Crowther GJ, Milstein JM, Jubrias SA, Kushmerick MJ, Gronka RK, Conley KE: Altered energetic properties in skeletal muscle of men with well-controlled insulin-dependent (type 1) diabetes. *Am J Physiol Endocrinol Metab* 284:E655–E62, 2003
109. Magee MF, Bhatt BA: Management of decompensated diabetes: diabetic ketoacidosis and hyperglycemic hyperosmolar syndrome. *Crit Care Clin* 17:75–106, 2001
110. Jenni S, Oetliker C, Allemann S, Ith M, Tappy L, Wuerth S, Egger A, Boesch C, Schneiter P, Diem P, Christ E, Stettler C: Fuel metabolism during exercise in euglycaemia and hyperglycaemia in patients with type 1 diabetes mellitus—a prospective single-blinded randomised crossover trial. *Diabetologia* 51:1457–1465, 2008
111. McKewen MW, Rehrer NJ, Cox C, Mann J: Glycaemic control, muscle glycogen and exercise performance in IDDM athletes on diets of varying carbohydrate content. *Int J Sports Med* 20:349–353, 1999

112. Andersen H, Schmitz O, Nielsen S: Decreased isometric muscle strength after acute hyperglycaemia in type 1 diabetic patients. *Diabet Med* 22:1401–1407, 2005
113. Boehncke S, Poettgen K, Maser-Gluth C, Reusch J, Boehncke WH, Badenhoop K: Endurance capabilities of triathlon competitors with type 1 diabetes mellitus. *Dtsch Med Wochenschr* 134:677–682, 2009
114. Heyman E, Briard D, Dekerdanet M, Gratas-Delamarche A, Delamarche P: Accuracy of physical working capacity 170 to estimate aerobic fitness in prepubertal diabetic boys and in 2 insulin dose conditions. *J Sports Med Phys Fitness* 46:315–321, 2006
115. Stettler C, Jenni S, Allemann S, Steiner R, Hoppeler H, Trepp R, Christ ER, Zwahlen M, Diem P: Exercise capacity in subjects with type 1 diabetes mellitus in eu- and hyperglycaemia. *Diabetes Metab Res Rev* 22:300–306, 2006
116. Kelly D, Hamilton JK, Riddell MC: Blood glucose levels and performance in a sports camp for adolescents with type 1 diabetes mellitus: a field study. *Int J Pediatr* 2010: 216167. E-pub Aug 2, 2010
117. Ramires PR, Forjaz CL, Strunz CM, Silva ME, Diament J, Nicolau W, Liberman B, Negrao CE: Oral glucose ingestion increases endurance capacity in normal and diabetic (type I) humans. *J Appl Physiol* 83:608–614, 1997
118. Riddell MC, Bar-Or O, Hollidge-Horvat M, Schwarcz HP, Heigenhauser GJ: Glucose ingestion and substrate utilization during exercise in boys with IDDM. *J Appl Physiol* 88:1239–1246, 2000
119. Gonder-Frederick LA, Zrebiec JF, Bauchowitz AU, Ritterband LM, Magee JC, Cox DJ, Clarke WL: Cognitive function is disrupted by both hypo- and hyperglycemia in school-aged children with type 1 diabetes: a field study. *Diabetes Care* 32:1001–1006, 2009
120. Jimenez CC, Corcoran MH, Crawley JT, Guyton Hornsby W, Peer KS, Philbin RD, Riddell MC: National athletic trainers' association position statement: management of the athlete with type 1 diabetes mellitus. *J Athl Train* 42:536–545, 2007
121. Tansey MJ, Tsalikian E, Beck RW, Mauras N, Buckingham BA, Weinzimer SA, Janz KF, Kollman C, Xing D, Ruedy KJ, Steffes MW, Borland TM, Singh RJ, Tamborlane WV; Diabetes Research in Children Network (DirecNet) Study Group: The effects of aerobic exercise on glucose and counterregulatory hormone concentrations in children with type 1 diabetes. *Diabetes Care* 29:20–25, 2006
122. Mendez-Villanueva A, Fernandez-Fernandez J, Bishop D: Exercise-induced homeostatic perturbations provoked by singles tennis match play with reference to development of fatigue. *Br J Sports Med* 41:717–722, discussion 722, 2007
123. Graveling AJ, Frier BM: Risks of marathon running and hypoglycaemia in type 1 diabetes. *Diabet Med* 27:585–588, 2010
124. Murillo S, Brugnara L, Novials A: One year follow-up in a group of half-marathon runners with type-1 diabetes treated with insulin analogues. *J Sports Med Phys Fitness* 50:506–510, 2010
125. Tuominen JA, Karonen SL, Melamies L, Bolli G, Koivisto VA: Exercise-induced hypoglycaemia in IDDM patients treated with a short-acting insulin analogue. *Diabetologia* 38:106–111, 1995

126. Gerich JE, Langlois M, Noacco C, Karam JH, Forsham PH: Lack of glucagon response to hypoglycemia in diabetes: evidence for an intrinsic pancreatic alpha cell defect. *Science* 182:171–173, 1973
127. Zander E, Schulz B, Chlup R, Woltansky P, Lubs D: Muscular exercise in type I-diabetics. II. Hormonal and metabolic responses to moderate exercise. *Exp Clin Endocrinol* 85:95–104, 1985
128. American Diabetes Association: Standards of medical care in diabetes: 2012. *Diabetes Care* 35 (Suppl. 1):S11–S63, 2012
129. Guelfi KJ, Jones TW, Fournier PA: New insights into managing the risk of hypoglycaemia associated with intermittent high-intensity exercise in individuals with type 1 diabetes mellitus: implications for existing guidelines. *Sports Med* 37:937–946, 2007
130. Wasserman DH, Zinman B: Exercise in individuals with IDDM. *Diabetes Care* 17:924–937, 1994
131. Dube MC, Weisnagel SJ, Prud'homme D, Lavoie C: Exercise and newer insulins: how much glucose supplement to avoid hypoglycemia? *Med Sci Sports Exerc* 37:1276–1282, 2005
132. Riddell MC, Iscoe KE: Physical activity, sport, and pediatric diabetes. *Pediatr Diabetes* 7:60–70, 2006
133. Francescato MP, Geat M, Fusi S, Stupar G, Noacco C, Cattin L: Carbohydrate requirement and insulin concentration during moderate exercise in type 1 diabetic patients. *Metabolism* 53:1126–1130, 2004
134. Bracken RM, Page R, Gray B, Kilduff LP, West DJ, Stephens JW, Bain SC: Isomaltulose improves glycaemia and maintains run performance in type 1 diabetes. *Med Sci Sports Exerc* 2011
135. American College of Sports Medicine and American Diabetes Association joint position statement: Diabetes mellitus and exercise. *Med Sci Sports Exerc* 29:i–vi, 1997
136. Gallen I: Exercise in type 1 diabetes. *Diabet Med* 20 (Suppl. 1):2–5, 2003
137. Steppel JH, Horton ES: Exercise in the management of type 1 diabetes mellitus. *Rev Endocr Metab Disord* 4:355–360, 2003
138. De Feo P, Di Loreto C, Ranchelli A, Fatone C, Gambelunghe G, Lucidi P, Santeusanio F: Exercise and diabetes. *Acta Biomed* 77 (Suppl. 1):14–17, 2006
139. Rabasa-Lhoret R, Bourque J, Ducros F, Chiasson JL: Guidelines for premeal insulin dose reduction for postprandial exercise of different intensities and durations in type 1 diabetic subjects treated intensively with a basal-bolus insulin regimen (ultralente-lispro). *Diabetes Care* 24:625–630, 2001
140. Mauvais-Jarvis F, Sobngwi E, Porcher R, Garnier JP, Vexiau P, Duvallet A, Gautier JF: Glucose response to intense aerobic exercise in type 1 diabetes: maintenance of near euglycemia despite a drastic decrease in insulin dose. *Diabetes Care* 26:1316–1317, 2003
141. West DJ, Morton RD, Bain SC, Stephens JW, Bracken RM: Blood glucose responses to reductions in pre-exercise rapid-acting insulin for 24 h after running in individuals with type 1 diabetes. *J Sports Sci* 28:781–788, 2010
142. West DJ, Stephens JW, Bain SC, Kilduff LP, Luzio S, Still R, Bracken RM: A combined insulin reduction and carbohydrate feeding strategy 30 min before running best preserves blood glucose concentration after exercise

through improved fuel oxidation in type 1 diabetes mellitus. *J Sports Sci* 29:279–289, 2011

143. Sane T, Helve E, Pelkonen R, Koivisto VA: The adjustment of diet and insulin dose during long-term endurance exercise in type 1 (insulin-dependent) diabetic men. *Diabetologia* 31:35–40, 1988

144. Berger M, Berchtold P, Cuppers HJ, Drost H, Kley HK, Muller WA, Wiegelmann W, Zimmerman-Telschow H, Gries FA, Kruskemper HL, Zimmermann H: Metabolic and hormonal effects of muscular exercise in juvenile type diabetics. *Diabetologia* 13:355–365, 1977

145. Klip A, Marette A, Dimitrakoudis D, Ramlal T, Giacca A, Shi ZQ, Vranic M: Effect of diabetes on glucoregulation. From glucose transporters to glucose metabolism in vivo. *Diabetes Care* 15:1747–1766, 1992

146. Perkins BA, Riddell MC: Type 1 diabetes and exercise: part II: using the insulin pump to maximum advantage. *Can J Diab* 30:72–80, 2006

147. Riddell MC, Perkins BA: Exercise and glucose metabolism in persons with diabetes mellitus: perspectives on the role for continuous glucose monitoring. *J Diabetes Sci Technol* 3:914–923, 2009

148. Zisser H, Robinson L, Bevier W, Dassau E, Ellingsen C, Doyle FJ, Jovanovic L: Bolus calculator: a review of four "smart" insulin pumps. *Diabetes Technol Ther* 10:441–444, 2008

149. Wilson DM, Beck RW, Tamborlane WV, Dontchev MJ, Kollman C, Chase P, Fox LA, Ruedy KJ, Tsalikian E, Weinzimer SA; DirecNet Study Group: The accuracy of the FreeStyle Navigator continuous glucose monitoring system in children with type 1 diabetes. *Diabetes Care* 30:59–64, 2007

150. Iscoe KE, Riddell MC: Continuous moderate-intensity exercise with or without intermittent high-intensity work: effects on acute and late glycaemia in athletes with type 1 diabetes mellitus. *Diabet Med* 2011

151. Diabetes Research In Children Network (Direcnet) Study Group; Buckingham BA, Kollman C, Beck R, Kalajian A, Fiallo-Scharer R, Tansey MJ, Fox LA, Wilson DM, Weinzimer SA, Ruedy KJ, Tamborlane WV: Evaluation of factors affecting CGMS calibration. *Diabetes Technol Ther* 8:318–325, 2006

152. Davey RJ, Ferreira LD, Jones TW, Fournier PA: Effect of exercise-mediated acidosis on determination of glycemia using CGMS. *Diabetes Technol Ther* 8:516–518, 2006

153. Davey RJ, Stevens K, Jones TW, Fournier PA: The effect of short-term use of the Guardian RT continuous glucose monitoring system on fear of hypoglycaemia in patients with type 1 diabetes mellitus. *Prim Care Diabetes* 6:35–39, 2012

154. Adolfsson P, Ornhagen H and Jendle J: The benefits of continuous glucose monitoring and a glucose monitoring schedule in individuals with type 1 diabetes during recreational diving. *J Diabetes Sci Technol* 2:778–784, 2008

155. Riddell MC, Milliken J: Preventing exercise-induced hypoglycemia in type 1 diabetes using real-time continuous glucose monitoring and a new carbohydrate intake algorithm: an observational field study. *Diabetes Technol Ther* 13:819–825, 2011

156. Iscoe KE, Davey RJ, Fournier PA: Increasing the low-glucose alarm of a continuous glucose monitoring system prevents exercise-induced hypoglycemia without triggering any false alarms. *Diabetes Care* 34:e109, 2011

157. Bernbaum M, Albert SG, Cohen JD: Exercise training in individuals with diabetic retinopathy and blindness. *Arch Phys Med Rehabil* 70:605–611, 1989
158. Graham C, Lasko-McCarthey P: Exercise options for persons with diabetic complications. *Diabetes Educ* 16:212–220, 1990
159. Albert SG, Bernbaum M: Exercise for patients with diabetic retinopathy. *Diabetes Care* 18:130–132, 1995
160. Draznin MB: Type 1 diabetes and sports participation: strategies for training and competing safely. *Phys Sportsmed* 28:49–56, 2000
161. Chipkin SR, Klugh SA, Chasan-Taber L: Exercise and diabetes. *Cardiol Clin* 19:489–505, 2001
162. Flood L, Constance A: Diabetes and exercise safety. *Am J Nurs* 102:47–55, quiz 56, 2002
163. Kanade RV, van Deursen RW, Harding K, Price P: Walking performance in people with diabetic neuropathy: benefits and threats. *Diabetologia* 49:1747–1754, 2006
164. Colberg SR, Sigal RJ, Fernhall B, Regensteiner JG, Blissmer BJ, Rubin RR, Chasan-Taber L, Albright AL, Braun B; American College of Sports Medicine; American Diabetes Association: Exercise and type 2 diabetes: the American College of Sports Medicine and the American Diabetes Association: joint position statement executive summary. *Diabetes Care* 33:2692–2696, 2010
165. Nathan DM, Cleary PA, Backlund JY, Genuth SM, Lachin JM, Orchard TJ, Raskin P, Zinman B; Diabetes Control and Complications Trial/Epidemiology of Diabetes Interventions and Complications (DCCT/EDIC) Study Research Group: Intensive diabetes treatment and cardiovascular disease in patients with type 1 diabetes. *N Engl J Med* 353:2643–2653, 2005
166. Hughes BC, White RD: Testing in special populations. In *Exercise Testing for Primary Care and Sports Medicine*. New York, Springer-Verlag, 2005, p. 55–77
167. Gill JM, Malkova D: Physical activity, fitness and cardiovascular disease risk in adults: interactions with insulin resistance and obesity. *Clin Sci* (Lond) 110:409–425, 2006
168. Konduracka E, Gackowski A, Rostoff P, Galicka-Latala D, Frasik W, Piwowarska W: Diabetes-specific cardiomyopathy in type 1 diabetes mellitus: no evidence for its occurrence in the era of intensive insulin therapy. *Eur Heart J* 28:2465–2471, 2007
169. Aiello LP, Cahill MT and Wong JS: Systemic considerations in the management of diabetic retinopathy. *Am J Ophthalmol* 132:760–776, 2001
170. Schneider SH, Khachadurian AK, Amorosa LF, Clemow L, Ruderman NB: Ten-year experience with an exercise-based outpatient life-style modification program in the treatment of diabetes mellitus. *Diabetes Care* 15:1800–1810, 1992
171. Cruickshanks KJ, Moss SE, Klein R, Klein BE: Physical activity and proliferative retinopathy in people diagnosed with diabetes before age 30 yr. *Diabetes Care* 15:1267–1272, 1992
172. Cruickshanks KJ, Moss SE, Klein R, Klein BE: Physical activity and the risk of progression of retinopathy or the development of proliferative retinopathy. *Ophthalmology* 102:1177–1182, 1995

173. Samanta A, Burden AC, Jagger C: A comparison of the clinical features and vascular complications of diabetes between migrant Asians and Caucasians in Leicester, U.K. *Diabetes Res Clin Pract* 14:205–213, 1991
174. LaPorte RE, Dorman JS, Tajima N, Cruickshanks KJ, Orchard TJ, Cavender DE, Becker DJ, Drash AL: Pittsburgh Insulin-Dependent Diabetes Mellitus Morbidity and Mortality Study: physical activity and diabetic complications. *Pediatrics* 78:1027–1033, 1986
175. Orchard TJ, Dorman JS, Maser RE, Becker DJ, Ellis D, LaPorte RE, Kuller LH, Wolfson SK Jr, Drash AL: Factors associated with avoidance of severe complications after 25 yr of IDDM. Pittsburgh Epidemiology of Diabetes Complications Study I. *Diabetes Care* 13:741–747, 1990
176. Aiello LP, Wong J, Cavallerano JD, Bursel SE, Aiken LM: Retinopathy. In *Handbook of Exercise in Diabetes.* Ruderman NB, Devlin JT, Schneider SH, Kriska AM, Eds. Alexandria, VA, American Diabetes Association, 2002, p. 401–413
177. Jawa A, Kcomt J, Fonseca VA: Diabetic nephropathy and retinopathy. *Med Clin North Am* 88:1001–1036, xi, 2004
178. National Institutes of Health: Consensus Development Conference on Diet and Exercise in Non-Insulin-Dependent Diabetes Mellitus. National Institutes of Health. *Diabetes Care* 10:639–644, 1987
179. Sigal RJ, Kenny GP, Wasserman DH, Castaneda-Sceppa C: Physical activity/exercise and type 2 diabetes. *Diabetes Care* 27:2518–2539, 2004
180. Lemaster JW, Reiber GE, Smith DG, Heagerty PJ, Wallace C: Daily weight-bearing activity does not increase the risk of diabetic foot ulcers. *Med Sci Sports Exerc* 35:1093–1099, 2003
181. Armstrong DG, Lavery LA, Holtz-Neiderer K, Mohler MJ, Wendel CS, Nixon BP, Boulton AJ. Variability in activity may precede diabetic foot ulceration. *Diabetes Care* 27:1980–1984, 2004
182. Headley SA, Germain MJ, Braden GL: Nephropathy: advanced. In *Handbook of Exercise in Diabetes.* Ruderman NB, Devlin JT, Schneider SH, Kriska AM, Eds. Alexandria, VA, American Diabetes Association, 2002, p. 451–462
183. Mogensen CE: Nephropathy: early. In *Handbook of Exercise in Diabetes.* Ruderman NB, Devlin JT, Schneider SH, Kriska AM, Eds. Alexandria, VA, American Diabetes Association, 2002, p. 433–449
184. Evans N, Forsyth E: End-stage renal disease in people with type 2 diabetes: systemic manifestations and exercise implications. *Phys Ther* 84:454–463, 2004
185. Oh-Park M, Fast A, Gopal S, Lynn R, Frei G, Drenth R, Zohman L: Exercise for the dialyzed: aerobic and strength training during hemodialysis. *Am J Phys Med Rehabil* 81:814–821, 2002
186 Painter PL: Exercise in end-stage renal disease. *Exerc Sport Sci Rev* 16:305–339, 1988
187. Moore GE, Painter PL, Brinker KR, Stray-Gundersen J, Mitchell JH: Cardiovascular response to submaximal stationary cycling during hemodialysis. *Am J Kidney Dis* 31:631–637, 1998
188. Painter PL, Hector L, Ray K, Lynes L, Dibble S, Paul SM, Tomlanovich SL, Ascher NL: A randomized trial of exercise training after renal transplantation. *Transplantation* 74:42–48, 2002

189. Painter PL, Hector L, Ray K, Lynes L, Paul SM, Dodd M, Tomlanovich SL, Ascher NL: Effects of exercise training on coronary heart disease risk factors in renal transplant recipients. *Am J Kidney Dis* 42:362–369, 2003

190. Burge MR, Garcia N, Qualls CR, Schade DS: Differential effects of fasting and dehydration in the pathogenesis of diabetic ketoacidosis. *Metabolism* 50:171–177, 2001

191. American College of Sports Medicine; Sawka MN, Burke LM, Eichner ER, Maughan RJ, Montain SJ, Stachenfeld NS: American College of Sports Medicine position stand: exercise and fluid replacement. *Med Sci Sports Exerc* 39:377–390, 2007

192. Tamis-Jortberg B, Downs DA Jr, Colten ME: Effects of a glucose polymer sports drink on blood glucose, insulin, and performance in subjects with diabetes. *Diabetes Educ* 22:471–487, 1996

193. Hubing KA, Bassett JT, Quigg LR, Phillips MD, Barbee JJ, Mitchell JB: Exercise-associated hyponatremia: the influence of pre-exercise carbohydrate status combined with high volume fluid intake on sodium concentrations and fluid balance. *Eur J Appl Physiol* 111:797–807, 2011

194. Peacock OJ, Thompson D, Stokes KA: Voluntary drinking behaviour, fluid balance and psychological affect when ingesting water or a carbohydrate-electrolyte solution during exercise. *Appetite* 58:56–63, 2012

195. Hernandez JM, Moccia T, Fluckey JD, Ulbrecht JS, Farrell PA: Fluid snacks to help persons with type 1 diabetes avoid late onset postexercise hypoglycemia. *Med Sci Sports Exerc* 32:904–910, 2000

196. Perrone C, Laitano O, Meyer F: Effect of carbohydrate ingestion on the glycemic response of type 1 diabetic adolescents during exercise. *Diabetes Care* 28:2537–2538, 2005

197. Meinders AE, Willekens FL, Heere LP: Metabolic and hormonal changes in IDDM during long-distance run. *Diabetes Care* 11:1–7, 1988

198. Koivisto VA, Sane T, Fyhrquist F, Pelkonen R: Fuel and fluid homeostasis during long-term exercise in healthy subjects and type I diabetic patients. *Diabetes Care* 15:1736–1741, 1992

199. Tuominen JA, Ebeling P, Vuorinen-Markkola H, Koivisto VA: Post-marathon paradox in IDDM: unchanged insulin sensitivity in spite of glycogen depletion. *Diabet Med* 14:301–308, 1997

200. Tuominen JA, Ebeling P, Koivisto VA: Exercise increases insulin clearance in healthy man and insulin-dependent diabetes mellitus patients. *Clin Physiol* 17:19–30, 1997

201. Cauza E, Hanusch-Enserer U, Strasser B, Ludvik B, Kostner K, Dunky A, Haber P: Continuous glucose monitoring in diabetic long distance runners. *Int J Sports Med* 26:774–780, 2005

202. American Diabetes Association; Clarke W, Deeb LC, Jameson P, Kaufman F, Klingensmith G, Schatz D, Silverstein JH, Siminerio LM: Diabetes care in the school and day care setting. *Diabetes Care* 35 (Suppl. 1):S76–S80, 2012

203. Choleau C, Aubert C, Cahane M, Reach G: High day-to-day glucose variability: a frequent phenomenon in children and adolescents with type 1 diabetes attending summer camp. *Diabetes Metab* 34:46–51, 2008

204. Ruzic L, Sporis G, Matkovic BR: High volume-low intensity exercise camp and glycemic control in diabetic children. *J Paediatr Child Health* 44:122–128, 2008

205. Santiprabhob J, Likitmaskul S, Kiattisakthavee P, Weerakulwattana P, Chaichanwattanakul K, Nakavachara P, Peerapatdit T, Nitiyanant W: Glycemic control and the psychosocial benefits gained by patients with type 1 diabetes mellitus attending the diabetes camp. *Patient Educ Couns* 73:60–66, 2008

206. Wang YC, Stewart S, Tuli E, White P: Improved glycemic control in adolescents with type 1 diabetes mellitus who attend diabetes camp. *Pediatr Diabetes* 9:29–34, 2008

207. Miller AR, Nebesio TD and Dimeglio LA: Insulin dose changes in children attending a residential diabetes camp. *Diabet Med* 28:480–486, 2011

208. McTavish L, Wiltshire E: Effective treatment of hypoglycemia in children with type 1 diabetes: a randomized controlled clinical trial. *Pediatr Diabetes* 12:381–387, 2011

209. American Diabetes Association: Management of diabetes at diabetes camps. *Diabetes Care* 22:167–169, 1999

210. Ciambra R, Locatelli C, Suprani T, Pocecco M: Management of diabetes at summer camps. *Acta Biomed* 76 (Suppl. 3):81–84, 2005

211. Dear Gde L, Pollock NW, Uguccioni DM, Dovenbarger J, Feinglos MN, Moon RE: Plasma glucose responses in recreational divers with insulin-requiring diabetes. *Undersea Hyperb Med* 31:291–301, 2004

212. Bonomo M, Cairoli R, Verde G, Morelli L, Moreo A, Grottaglie MD, Brambilla MC, Meneghini E, Aghemo P, Corigliano G, Marroni A: Safety of recreational scuba diving in type 1 diabetic patients: the Deep Monitoring programme. *Diabetes Metab* 35:101–107, 2009

213. Lormeau B, Sola A, Tabah A, Chiheb S, Dufaitre L, Thurninger O, Bresson R, Lormeau C, Attali JR, Valensi P: Blood glucose changes and adjustments of diet and insulin doses in type 1 diabetic patients during scuba diving (for a change in French regulations). *Diabetes Metab* 31:144–151, 2005

214. Edge CJ, Grieve AP, Gibbons N, O'Sullivan F, Bryson P: Control of blood glucose in a group of diabetic scuba divers. *Undersea Hyperb Med* 24:201–207, 1997

215. Edge CJ, St Leger Dowse M, Bryson P: Scuba diving with diabetes mellitus: the UK experience 1991-2001. *Undersea Hyperb Med* 32:27–37, 2005

216. Adolfsson P, Ornhagen H and Jendle J: Accuracy and reliability of continuous glucose monitoring in individuals with type 1 diabetes during recreational diving. *Diabetes Technol Ther* 11:493–497, 2009

217. Kruger DF, Owen SK, Whitehouse FW: Scuba diving and diabetes. Practical guidelines. *Diabetes Care* 18:1074, 1995

218. Influence of intensive diabetes treatment on body weight and composition of adults with type 1 diabetes in the Diabetes Control and Complications Trial. *Diabetes Care* 24:1711–1721, 2001

219. Ferriss JB, Webb D, Chaturvedi N, Fuller JH, Idzior-Walus B; EURODIAB Prospective Complications Group: Weight gain is associated with improved glycaemic control but with adverse changes in plasma lipids and blood pressure in type 1 diabetes. *Diabet Med* 23:557–564, 2006

220. Jacob AN, Salinas K, Adams-Huet B, Raskin P: Potential causes of weight gain in type 1 diabetes mellitus. *Diabetes Obes Metab* 8:404–411, 2006
221. Conway B, Miller RG, Costacou T, Fried L, Kelsey S, Evans RW, Orchard TJ: Temporal patterns in overweight and obesity in Type 1 diabetes. *Diabet Med* 27:398–404, 2010
222. Brown RJ, Wijewickrama RC, Harlan DM, Rother KI: Uncoupling intensive insulin therapy from weight gain and hypoglycemia in type 1 diabetes. *Diabetes Technol Ther* 13:457–460, 2011
223. Okamoto MM, Anhe GF, Sabino-Silva R, Marques MF, Freitas HS, Mori RC, Melo KF, Machado UF: Intensive insulin treatment induces insulin resistance in diabetic rats by impairing glucose metabolism-related mechanisms in muscle and liver. *J Endocrinol* 211:55–64, 2011
224. Elder SJ, Roberts SB: The effects of exercise on food intake and body fatness: a summary of published studies. *Nutr Rev* 65:1–19, 2007
225. Weinsier RL, Hunter GR, Desmond RA, Byrne NM, Zuckerman PA, Darnell BE: Free-living activity energy expenditure in women successful and unsuccessful at maintaining a normal body weight. *Am J Clin Nutr* 75:499–504, 2002
226. D'hooge R, Hellinckx T, Van Laethem C, Stegen S, De Schepper J, Van Aken S, Dewolf D, Calders P: Influence of combined aerobic and resistance training on metabolic control, cardiovascular fitness and quality of life in adolescents with type 1 diabetes: a randomized controlled trial. *Clin Rehabil* 25:349–359, 2011
227. Heyman E, Toutain C, Delamarche P, Berthon P, Briard D, Youssef H, Dekerdanet M, Gratas-Delamarche A: Exercise training and cardiovascular risk factors in type 1 diabetic adolescent girls. *Pediatr Exerc Sci* 19:408–419, 2007

12

Insulin

I. Insulin

PEDIATRICS

Jane Lee Chiang, MD, and Georgeanna J. Klingensmith, MD

ADULTS

Irl B. Hirsch, MD

INTRODUCTION

Normal Physiology

The normal pancreas deftly releases basal insulin, superimposed with bursts of insulin for rising glucose levels associated with food intake, life stressors, and medications. Insulin is secreted into the portal system, which clears half of the insulin. Those afflicted with type 1 diabetes (T1D) have near-absolute deficiency of endogenous insulin secretion due to β-cell destruction. Therefore, exogenously administered insulin must attempt to mimic the critical role played by the normal pancreas.

Historical Perspective

Banting and Best's discovery of insulin in 1921 enabled the use of animal-based soluble (regular) insulin to treat individuals with T1D. Six decades later, human insulin, made by recombinant DNA technology, replaced animal-based insulin. This dramatic technology breakthrough enabled purification of insulin (less than one part per million of impurities), resulting in reduced insulin antibodies, fewer insulin allergies, and near elimination of injection site lipoatrophy.

In characterizing insulin, we need to review its actions. *Pharmacokinetics* is the profile of insulin measured in blood after subcutaneous injection. *Pharmacodynamics* is the time required for insulin to move glucose into cells. Pharmacodynamics is a longer time interval than pharmacokinetics and is measured by performing euglycemic insulin clamps. Both terms are measured as time to onset, peak, and duration of action and are influenced by the injected insulin dose.

Insulin Terminology

Below are commonly used terms for insulin management

- *Analog insulins (rapid-acting analog [RAA] and long-acting analog [LAA])* are altered forms of insulin (i.e., not human or animal) made by recombinant

DNA techniques. The Food and Drug Administration (FDA) refers to them as *insulin receptor ligands*, but they are commonly referred to as insulin analogs.

■ Non-*analog insulins* (e.g., *regular and NPH*). Regular insulin (U-100 standard) is recombinant human insulin, stabilized, and is considered a short-acting insulin. NPH insulin is regular insulin complexed with protamine to form hexamers, which does not bind to insulin receptors, and therefore must slowly dissociate back into its monomeric form to be effective. Thus, its action is prolonged, and it is considered an intermediate-acting insulin. It may be used as a sort of basal insulin.

■ *Basal insulin* provides the maintenance level required to maintain glucose in a target range when food is not consumed and prevents unrestrained hepatic gluconeogenesis, hyperglycemia, and subsequent ketosis.

■ *Prandial insulin* is given at (or preferably before) mealtime to prevent the postmeal rise in blood glucose by allowing peripheral glucose disposal by the muscles.

■ *Nutritional (vs. prandial) insulin* is used when calories are provided continuously via tube feeds, parenterally (TPN).

■ *Correction* (or *supplemental*) *insulin* refers to additional insulin needed to correct pre- or postmeal hyperglycemia to target levels. Correction is usually RAA and rarely regular insulin.

■ *Insulin sensitivity factor* (*ISF*, or *correction factor*) refers to how much one unit of insulin will lower plasma glucose.

■ *Insulin-to-carbohydrate (I:C) ratio* refers to the carbohydrate grams covered by one unit of prandial insulin to maintain plasma glucose.

■ *Lag time* refers to the time between prandial insulin dose and the meal start.

■ *Active insulin (insulin on board [IOB])* refers to the remaining insulin activity (see pharmacodynamic) when considering a correction dose.

FUNDAMENTALS OF INSULIN MANAGEMENT

In healthy individuals with normal insulin sensitivity and oral intake, basal and prandial insulin each account for about 50% of the total daily dose. Basal insulin provides constant background coverage, and the bolus component covers food consumption and corrects high blood glucoses. Previously, insulin was dosed twice daily (usually before breakfast and before dinner), and was known as *conventional insulin therapy* (CIT). Although this method was simple and required limited injections, nocturnal hypoglycemia (midnight to 4 a.m.) and early morning (4–8 a.m.) and later afternoon (3–6 p.m.) hyperglycemia were not infrequent. In addition, the Diabetes Control and Complications Trial Research Group (DCCT) proved that twice-daily insulin (CIT) targeted to higher glycemic targets was not as effective as *multiple daily injections* (MDI) or *continuous subcutaneous insulin infusion* (CSII) therapy (i.e., insulin pumps) targeted to normal blood glucose levels.[1] The introductions of both widespread home blood glucose monitoring and MDI with 4–6 daily insulin injections (or with insulin pump therapy) have enabled a more physiologic method of insulin delivery.

This *basal-bolus* therapy is now considered standard therapy and, when combined with frequent blood glucose monitoring (and with increasing frequency, continuous glucose monitoring [CGM]), is considered *intensified diabetes management*. Importantly, a target A1C will not be specified with intensified diabetes management, since that needs to be individualized based on age, duration of diabetes, hypoglycemia unawareness history, and other factors.

INSULIN TYPES

Regular human insulin and neutral protamine Hagedorn (NPH, combined with protamine to delay absorption and duration) were long the mainstays of T1D management. However, insulin development has evolved to include a vast array of choices, including three LAAs or basal analogs (insulin glargine, detemir, and degludec [under development]) and RAAs (insulin lispro, insulin aspart, and insulin glulisine) (see Figures 12.I.1 and 12.I.2, and Table 12.I.1). We will not address U-500 regular insulin, since it is rarely used in T1D.[2]

Basal Insulin

Insulin *glargine* and *detemir* are the currently available LAAs. They are engineered to gradually dissociate to delay insulin absorption into the blood stream. *Degludec* insulin is an ultralong-acting basal insulin analog currently under development.[3,4] Detemir and degludec are bound to albumin, prolonging their activity in the circulation. Detemir lasts 14–20 hours. Glargine is effective 20–24 hours. Degludec lasts over 24 hours, with longer durations seen with larger doses. The long effective activity and limited peak in these insulins make them especially effective as basal insulins since the risk of hypoglycemia, especially nocturnal hypoglycemia, is decreased compared to NPH. Basal insulin dosing is titrated to achieve a target fasting blood glucose value while avoiding premeal or nocturnal hypoglycemia.

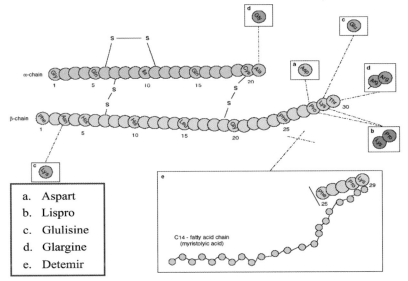

Figure 12.I.1 Adaptations of native human insulin. Reprinted from Miles and Acerini[13], with permission from the publisher.

Glargine is often given once a day (starting dose 0.2–0.4 units/kg of body weight). In older children and adults, it is usually most effective if given 2–4 h after dinner with the dose titrated upwards until a target fasting blood glucose (BG) is obtained. In children (<10 years of age) and some geriatric (≥65 years old) patients, a morning dose of glargine may prevent early morning hypoglycemia since young children are insulin sensitive and may require little exogenous insulin in the early morning hours.

Detemir may be initiated as daily insulin. If there is evidence of waning insulin action (i.e., hyperglycemia hours prior to the scheduled detemir dose), adding a second dose is usually effective in establishing stable basal glycemia. We recommend dividing it into 12 equal hourly doses. This waning insulin effect makes detemir an attractive option for morning administration in children (<8–10 years old).

Degludec has been shown to provide an action of beyond 24 h allowing the development of a steady state insulin action when given daily at a consistent time. Of note, as of the time this book went to press, degludec is not available for commercial use.

As a precaution with all LAAs, it is difficult to adjust the insulin dose for occasional and intermittent changes in daily activities. If using LAAs, it is important to develop strategies to adjust carbohydrate intake and alter prandial insulin doses to prevent hypoglycemia during and after additional physical exercise.

A steady state assessment of basal insulin can be helpful. With LAA therapy, the morning fasting glucose should be in range and ideally an individual should be able to skip a meal without significant hypoglycemia. Individuals should perform a basal rate check by missing the breakfast meal on a morning after the bedtime glucose was in range and no bedtime snack was eaten. The basal rate check should include a glucose value at the usual breakfast time and at a later awakening time (if schedules are erratic). This is particularly important in individuals with variable weekly schedules, especially teens and young adults who tend to sleep in on weekends or nonworkdays.

It is important to emphasize that the bedtime blood glucose levels should be within target range. Occasionally, high bedtime blood glucose levels may not come down overnight and may remain elevated in the morning. If the blood glucose remains elevated, a small correction dose needs to be given, even when skipping breakfast. Teenagers often sleep through breakfast, so a blood glucose check followed by a small correction dose is recommended for fasting hyperglycemia. We do not recommend increasing the basal dose, as this will bring the fasting glucose level too low. Often, patients receive too much basal insulin when they do not understand that the primary issue is starting too high at bedtime. Therefore, ensuring that nighttime glucose levels are within target is critical. Patients who consistently miss meals and have erratic glucose levels despite aggressive MDI should consider CSII. Furthermore, due to changes in basal insulin requirements overnight (e.g., midnight to 4 a.m.) compared to early morning (4–8 a.m.), it may not be possible to replace basal insulin well without CSII. This can be easily seen with frequent glucose monitoring overnight and early morning, especially when skipping breakfast. The use of a diagnostic CGM may be helpful to determine if basal insulin changes are needed to better control overnight glycemia or if CSII would be a better option.

Intermediate-Acting Insulin

For nonanalog insulins (NPH and regular), the injection site is a major contributor to pharmacokinetics and pharmacodynamics. NPH is an intermediate-acting insulin, but may also be used as a basal insulin. Its onset of action, peak time, and duration of action is less predictable than with the LAAs, so the risk for unexpected hypoglycemia is greater with NPH vs. LAA insulin. NPH is often recommended for twice-daily dosing: prebreakfast and predinner or prebedtime. NPH peaks between 4–10 hours, so giving NPH in the evening increases the risk of nocturnal hypoglycemia compared to a LAA. Likewise the variable timing of the peak may cause unexpected hypoglycemia during the day. NPH increases hypoglycemic risk, so a lower percent of the total daily dose (TDD) is given as the basal dose when using NPH.

Since NPH peaks, a steady state assessment (basal check) is more difficult and a meal or snack may be required at the expected peak time of NPH action. Intermittent determination of blood glucose profiles prior to and 2–3 hours after meals throughout the day and night or a diagnostic 3–6 day CGM assessment may help in assessing the appropriate NPH dose.

We strongly discourage the use of NPH for individuals requiring more intensive diabetes management or for those at greater risk of hypoglycemia (e.g., young children and older adults). In general, we do not recommend NPH for T1D. We would reserve it for certain circumstances (i.e., those with or without insurance >18 years of age who cannot afford analog insulin and cannot get it provided by insulin companies).

Prandial Insulin

Short-acting insulin. Zinc atoms added to regular insulin causes insulin dimers to form hexamers and delay absorption until the hexamers disassociate. Regular insulin is less expensive, but the delayed action leads to greater postprandial glucose excursions unless the dose is given 20–40 min prior to the meal. For example, if insulin absorption is unusually rapid, then hypoglycemia may occur prior to food absorption, or if it unusually delayed, then it may occur 3–4 h postmeal. Regular insulin is preferred to RAA in patients with delayed gastric absorption, such as those with gastroparesis or those taking pramlintide. It is also used for IV insulin infusions. Like NPH, regular insulin is not preferable and is recommended for certain circumstances (e.g., those with or without insurance >18 years of age who cannot afford analog insulin and cannot get it provided by insulin companies).

RAAs. Insulin lispro, aspart, and glulisine are RAAs that are structurally engineered to dissociate and be absorbed more rapidly. The advantages of the RAAs (vs. regular insulin) include quicker onset of action and less postprandial glycemic peak. The shorter duration of RAA often results in less postabsorptive hypoglycemia. This is true particularly at night when the risk of hypoglycemia is greatest.

Mixed Insulins

We do not recommend the use of mixed insulins unless the individual or family is unable to mix insulins. In addition, the individual must always eat consistent

Table 12.I.1 Insulins[2,5]

Insulin preparations available in the U.S.	Trade Names	Onset of Action	Peak Action	Duration
Rapid-acting	Insulin lispro (Humalog)			
	Insulin aspart (Novolog)	5–15 min	30–90 min	4–6 h
	Insulin glulisine (Apidra)			
Short-acting	Regular (Humulin R)	30–60 min	2–3 h	8–10 h
	Regular (Novolin R)			
Intermediate-acting	NPH (Humulin)	2–4 h	4–10 h	12–18 h
	NPH (Novolin)			
Long-acting	Glargine (Lantus)	2–4 h	None	20–24 h
	Detemir (Levemir)			14–24 h
Combinations	Humalog 75/25 (75 NPH/25 lispro)			
	Humalog 50/50 (50 NPH/50 lispro)	5–15 min	Dual	12–20 h
	Novolog 70/30 (70 NPH/30 aspart)			

carbohydrates for each meal. In children, fixed mixed insulins are used only in adolescents who refuse to take more than two daily doses of insulin and will not mix insulins. Another option is to free mix analog RAA and NPH in the morning and RAA and LAA in the evening.

PRINCIPLES OF INSULIN MANAGEMENT

1. Basal insulin accounts for ~50% of total daily dose:
   i. LAA (insulin glargine, detemir, degludec) or NPH if LAA is not an option
2. Prandial insulin accounts for remaining ~50%:
   i. RAA or short-acting regular insulin (if RAA is not an option, or high-fat foods are frequently consumed) before meals and snacks (when required)
   ii. Calculated by I:C ratio or short-acting insulin (~20% prebreakfast, ~10% prelunch, or ~20% predinner)

It was hoped that RAAs would enable simultaneous food consumption with dosing; unfortunately, depending on the carbohydrates consumed, a large post-prandial glucose peak may still occur. Several studies have shown the lag time should be at least 10–20 min depending on the premeal blood glucose.

INSULIN DOSING PRINCIPLES

Starting Dose

The starting insulin dose is usually based on weight, with doses ranging from 0.4 to 1.0 units/kg/day of total insulin with higher amounts during puberty. Most clinicians start at 0.5 units/kg/day when the patient is metabolically stable, higher if immediately after presentation in ketoacidosis.

I:C Ratios

The insulin amount for a given amount of carbohydrates varies, but most adult patients require an I:C ratio of 1 unit/8 g (1:8) to 1:20. In adolescents, it is not uncommon for the I:C ratio to be 1:5, while in very young children (aged <6 years) the I:C may be as low as 1:50. A food diary over several days providing the insulin doses given, the food and grams of carbohydrate eaten, with glucose levels before and 2–3 h after meals will assist in determining the I:C ratio.

Various formulas have been developed as a starting place (e.g., 1,700 or 1,800/ TDD = how many mg/dl 1 unit of insulin will drop the blood glucose when the glucose control is excellent on this daily dose). When considering the insulin dose, one must know the glucose target. For example:

Target blood glucose = 120 mg/dl before meals
Target blood glucose = 150 mg/dl at bedtime

- If prebreakfast glucose = 220 mg/dl and an ISF of 50
  Then 220 (current) – 120 (target) = 100/50 = 2 units of RAA at breakfast
- If prebedtime glucose = 220 mg/dl and an ISF of 50
  Then 220 (current) – 150 (target) = 70/50 = 1.4 units of RAA at nighttime
  However, at bedtime, it would be 1.4 units (most insulin pens could only give 1.0) due to the higher target.

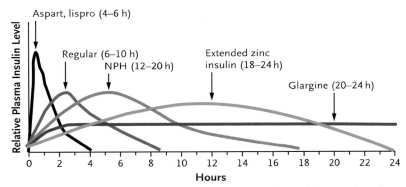

Figure 12.I.2 Approximate pharmacokinetic profiles of human insulin and insulin analogs.[6] Reprinted with permission from the publisher.

Insulin Stacking

Insulin stacking must be factored when considering prandial insulin dosing. From the pharmacodynamic times above, the RAAs last 4–6 h, meaning if a full correction dose is provided within this time frame, insulin stacking may lead to hypoglycemia. We minimize this problem by having patients subtract the amount of estimated IOB from their correction dose. Patients using MDI can see IOB from a graph provided to them.[6]

INSULIN REGIMENS

A typical MDI regimen provides the basal insulin component as LAA insulin either once or twice daily. The usual treatment plan begins with a once daily basal insulin and progresses to a BID regimen if adequate basal therapy is not achieved with daily LAA. The prandial component is usually RAA. The dose is determined by the amount needed to correct the high blood glucose plus the dose required for meals, which is determined by the I:C ratio. The doses may be individually calculated, or with a bolus dose calculator. Sometimes, a constant carbohydrate diet is recommended (i.e., fixed insulin dose and fixed amount of carbohydrate for each meal).

If using NPH, it is recommended for twice daily dosing, prebreakfast and predinner or bedtime. Since NPH peaks at 4–10 h, giving NPH in the evening increases nocturnal hypoglycemic risk compared to using LAA. Likewise the variable peak timing may cause unexpected hypoglycemia during the day. Because of the increased hypoglycemic risks with NPH, a lower percent of the total daily dose (TDD) is given as the basal portion when NPH (vs. LAA) is used. (See NPH description above.)

NPH given in 3–4 lower doses daily may decrease the unpredictable hypoglycemic risk and establishe a more consistent basal profile. If NPH is used as basal insulin, modern dosing recommends the following:

- Morning: NPH (20–30% of TDD) and prandial regular or RAA insulin
- Lunch: RAA. This is based on the morning NPH dose, peak NPH time, and frequent BG monitoring.
- Evening: NPH (15–20% of TDD) predinner or prebedtime (more common) and bolus regular or RAA insulin
- If an afternoon snack is taken, a prandial dose is usually required for optimal glycemic control.

Some NPH insulin regimens recommend prandial dosing with regular insulin and NPH as a single dose in the evening before bed. This plan is more effective if regular insulin is used for the prandial insulin because of its longer duration versus RAA. While more economical, this regimen is less reliable due to the unpredictable actions of both regular and NPH insulin. It is not recommended for individuals requiring more intensive diabetes management or for those at greater risk from hypoglycemia including children and older adults.

METHODS OF INSULIN ADMINISTRATION

Disposable pens and cartridges currently aid patients in measuring and administering insulin and facilitate compliance. There are many options with pens and pen needles (partial listing: disposable or durable, half or whole units, and with or without memory). Mixing insulins is currently rarely done since the basal-bolus regimens offer more flexibility and allow tailoring the dosing to the current glucose value. LAA insulins should not be mixed with other insulins, although there are reports in the literature indicating this is safe and does not alter glucose values compared to injecting separately. NPH may be mixed with rapid- or short-acting insulins. Fixed mixtures are also available commercially; however, none allow daily variation in dosing for variable glucose levels.

In considering needles, there are two factors to consider. The first factor is the thickness or gauge (higher gauge = thinner needle). The thickest gauge is 28 and 32 is the thinnest. Most people prefer thinner gauges, which do not clinically alter glucose control. For large doses a thicker gauge is preferable due to the ease in administering the insulin (pen or syringe).

The second consideration is the needle length. We initially thought that obese patients require longer needles, but that has not been shown to be true, at least to a BMI of 40 kg/m.[2,7] Needle lengths can vary from 4 mm to 12.7 mm, with most patients preferring shorter needles.[8,9] Syringe and pen needle manufacturers suggest needles be used only once, since sterility cannot be guaranteed with multiple usage, which also risks needle bending. There are data that suggest dosage may be affected if the pen needle is left in place. The needle also needs to be recapped after each use.

Pens offer an advantage over syringes with *1)* more consistent dosing when multiple caregivers provide insulin dosing, *2)* larger numbers than on syringes and an audible click as the dose is dialed in for visually impaired individuals, and *3)* frequently greater comfort since the pen needle does not go through the stopper on the insulin vial, making the needle sharper for injection. In children, school personnel may require insulin administration with a pen to minimize dosing errors. Parents also prefer the consistency of the pen if the child is away from both home and parental supervision.

There are pens that deliver 0.5-unit doses, one beginning with 0.5 unit and another beginning with 1.5 units. Both of these options use insulin cartridges and a nondisposable pen unit. Otherwise, individuals requiring 0.5-unit dosing will need to use syringes, which have 0.5-unit markings that allow administration of whole or 0.5-unit doses. Basal insulin is available in vials for use with syringes, or in disposable pens that administer insulin in 1-unit increments.

An insulin pump or CSII is an effective way to deliver insulin. It is discussed in detail in the next section of this chapter.

SPECIAL CIRCUMSTANCES FOR INSULIN DOSING

Remission or Honeymoon

Within 3 days to 3 weeks after diagnosis and initiation of insulin therapy, the patient generally enters a remission phase. This is thought to be due to β-cell recovery from glucotoxicity. During this phase, stable glucose levels allow low insulin requirements. Insulin doses for meals may decrease to very low levels. Active individuals may require very little to no insulin. But it is unclear if a small amount of basal insulin during this time is important for maintaining β-cell function and for reinforcing the need for continued glucose surveillance. The predominant opinion is that maintenance of some insulin therapy is important.

Newborns and Infants

If feasible, children aged <1 year to 18 months of age should begin CSII therapy as soon as possible after diagnosis. Infants <6–9 months of age will benefit from CSII initiation while hospitalized for the initial diagnosis. There is little data comparing trials of injection therapy vs. pump therapy in these very young children. However, if anecdotal reports in infants and data supporting CSII in young children (aged <6 years) apply, then one could extrapolate that CSII use should be supported in very young children (<18 months of age). Children diagnosed with T1D prior to 6 months of age (neonatal diabetes) should be evaluated for monogenic causes of diabetes, which may be more effectively and safely treated with sulfonylurea drugs.

School-Age Children

Please refer to chapters 5 and 18 for comprehensive information about school-age children.

Geriatrics

There is extreme heterogeneity within the older adult population: ranging from highly functional and independent to requiring significant assistance in managing their diabetes (see chapter 18). Hypoglycemia is a significant concern, particularly if there is concomitant cerebrovascular disease or coronary artery disease. Dosing may be more complex when comorbidities become more common and physical activity often becomes more sporadic. An important concern is related to mental status declines, often making many diabetes self-management decisions impractical. This is particularly relevant for patients using CSII. Basic diabetes management mistakes, including forgetting to test blood glucose or bolus insulin dosing, become more common. Worse is the forgetful patient who neglects to check if a bolus was given and inadvertently administers a second bolus. Like other aspects of aging, diabetes self-management may become more difficult without assistance from a care provider. Losing independence, after decades of self-care, is a difficult situation. This has to be first addressed by removing the CSII, particularly for those patients requiring frequent hospitalizations or a skilled nursing facility.

Sick Days or Illness

Please refer to chapter 5 for sick days or illness.

Insulin Resistance

While T1D is due to insulin deficiency secondary to β-cell destruction, the so-called global obesity epidemic has impacted those with T1D. If an individual has T1D, plus obesity, and a strong family history of type 2 diabetes, then insulin resistance may occur. Additional treatment with insulin sensitizers such as metformin may be useful. There is also increasing evidence that insulin resistance commonly occurs in T1D even in the absence of overweight or obesity.

Insulin Allergies

Allergic reactions to insulin are rare, with reactions being transient or due to artifacts. Patients, especially those with atopy, may have a local or systemic allergy to insulin, protamine, or the low pH of glargine insulin. Inadvertent intradermal injections or localized allergic reactions may cause burning, erythema, and urticaria at the injection site. If the symptoms persist despite proper injection techniques, then patients should switch brands or use antihistamines, or both. Patients should be treating accordingly, if true anaphylaxis or severe asthma occurs, and be considered for insulin desensitization.[5]

ALTERNATIVE INSULIN DELIVERY SYSTEMS

Pulmonary insulin delivery was first reported in 1925. Approximately 10–30% of inhaled insulin is absorbed into the circulation and appeared to be well tolerated. Studies have demonstrated that inhaled insulin is more rapidly absorbed than subcutaneous regular insulin and as quickly as rapid-acting insulin (lispro or aspart). Its duration is longer than rapid-acting insulin and similar to regular insulin. The bioavailability of inhaled insulin relative to subcutaneous regular insulin is ~10%. The first pulmonary insulin (Exubera®) was available from 2006–2007 but was withdrawn by the manufacturer in late 2007 for non-medical reasons. Technosphere (Afrezza®) is a monomeric, dry powder insulin with an onset of action of 10–15 min and a duration of 3–4 h.[10,11] It is currently undergoing phase III studies in both T1D (NCT01445951) and type 2 diabetes (NCT01451398) patients to demonstrate efficacy and safety of inhaled insulin, with results expected in the next 1–2 years.[12]

Peritoneal insulin, with an implantable insulin pump, has been used for the last 20 years in research settings. Intraperitoneal insulin is rapidly and predictably absorbed into the portal circulation, simulating physiologic insulin delivery and absorption. Clinical studies have demonstrated that implantable pumps are safe and effective for attaining glycemic control and reducing severe hypoglycemia. This route also avoids peripheral hyperinsulinemia and the theoretical risk of atherosclerosis.[5]

FILLING THE GAPS/CONCLUSION

On January 11, 1922, Leonard Thompson received an injection of "thick brown muck," also known as insulin. Since then, extraordinary progress in insulin development and delivery has enabled T1D patients to have healthy, productive lives. Despite the advancements in the insulin field, T1D remains a burden to many, and gaps in our insulin formulations and understanding of insulin therapy remain. The following are areas where more clinical research is needed:

1. Better, flatter, more predictable basal insulins
2. Faster prandial insulins (both faster in and faster out), which will also work with CSII
3. Better, more comfortable insulin needles and CSII infusion devices
4. Insulin pens that electronically communicate with another device such as a meter or smartphone with easy downloading

5. A glucose responsive insulin, i.e., an insulin injected infrequently (e.g., once daily) that is attached to a protein and is released when glucose levels rise
6. Insulin coformulations, with the most obvious candidates: pramlintide (known to be effective in T1D) and GLP-1 analogues (definitive T1D data still pending)

While some of these ideas for insulin therapy may seem far off in the future, it must be remembered how quickly we have seen vast improvements in our current insulin formulations and treatment strategies. While the ultimate goal is to eliminate insulin therapy for all patients affected by T1D, improvements and innovations to our current treatments must continue.

II. Continuous Subcutaneous Insulin Infusion (CSII)

PEDIATRICS

David Maahs, MD, PhD, and H. Peter Chase, MD

Standard of Care

A consensus statement on the use of insulin pump therapy, CSII, in youth with type 1 diabetes (T1D) is available, and will be referred to intermittently.[1]

Who Should Use a Pump?

Pump therapy has been successfully used in pediatric patients of all ages, including preschoolers.[2-5] The decision to initiate insulin pump therapy is made by parents, youth (referring to children or adolescents), and their diabetes care providers. In very young children, parents work with the medical team to make the decision. Important factors to consider are outlined in the Table 12.II.1.[6] Fortunately, most health insurance companies require proof of a minimum of four blood glucose (BG) values per day in order to help fund CSII therapy. Subjects who do not routinely meet this criterion cannot safely use an insulin pump. In addition to the items in Table 12.II.1, many centers require knowledge of carbohydrate counting prior to initiating pump therapy. Only experienced pediatric diabetes care providers should treat youth initiating pump therapy.

Table 12.II.1 Factors to Consider in Initiating Insulin Pump Therapy[6]

Self-monitoring of blood sugar levels

Motivation

Compliance

Family involvement and support

Knowledge

Adequate diabetes knowledge

Adequate communication with the diabetes team

Realistic expectations

Problem solving skills

Manual dexterity

Health insurance

Literacy

Parameters Associated with Insulin Pump Use in Pediatrics

Youth (and parents of infants) usually state that the main reason for wanting to use a pump is to reduce the number of insulin injections per day.[7] Clinical parameters to consider include:

1. Reduction of A1C Levels: As with a meta-analysis of primarily adult studies, a reduction of 0.5% in A1C levels compared to prepump values is common, assuming proper patient selection for pump use and adequate follow-up.[8-12] Other real-life data collected in the T1D Exchange Registry in the U.S. found a significant reduction (P <0.001) in A1C levels for all age-groups in 10,065 pump users, compared to 8,051 subjects using insulin injections.[10] In a clinical trial of 485 people with T1D (STAR 3), youth and adults were randomized to remain on injections and BG checking or to use an insulin pump and a continuous glucose monitor (CGM).[11] The latter group (for all ages) had statistically lower A1C levels by 0.5% (P <0.001) after one year. Youth who do more frequent BG checks and more frequent insulin boluses tend to have lower A1C levels.[8-12]
2. Severe Hypoglycemia (SH): As with a meta-analysis of primarily adult studies, studies of youth using insulin pumps have shown a significant reduction in SH.[9-13] In other real-life data, the T1D Exchange Registry has reported a lower incidence of SH in subjects using insulin pumps versus injections for people <50 years old.[10] In contrast, the incidence of SH in the closely monitored STAR 3 trial was 13 episodes/100 person years in both the control and the pump/CGM groups.[11]
3. Exercise is the number one factor associated with SH in children (particularly delayed hypoglycemia at night following heavy daytime exercise).[14] A major advantage of CSII in youth is the ability to reduce or discontinue insulin during and following exercise to prevent hypoglycemia.[15-16]
4. Diabetic Ketoacidosis (DKA): The incidence of DKA (6.2/100 person years) was similar to that of SH (6.6/100 person years) in 1,041 youth from 17 countries who used an insulin pump.[13] In a study of 291 youth with T1D, the incidence of DKA was 1.4/100 person years in the year prior to initiation.[9] After initiation of CSII therapy the incidence of DKA was 4.0/100 person years in the subsequent 1–9 years (mean 3.8 years; P = 0.08). The incidence in the same entire pediatric diabetes clinic (youth using and not using CSII) was 8/100 person years (with an incidence of 10/100 person years for youth not using CSII).[17] Youth and families were screened and chosen to begin CSII therapy, resulting in the lesser likelihood of DKA. In the same pediatric diabetes clinic, 80% of cases of DKA occurred in 20% of the population.[17] As DKA is the greatest cause of mortality in people under age 30 years, it is important to be selective in choosing youth for CSII therapy.[18-19] For example, if rapid-acting insulin delivery is interrupted, hyperglycemia and ketonemia can develop within 3 h.[20] In the absence of basal insulin, it is imperative that people using CSII routinely check their BG and, if elevated, blood or urine ketones. According preventative measures can then be taken. In other real-life data, the incidence of DKA in the first year of

monitoring in the T1D Exchange Registry showed the highest rates in the 12–17 and the 18–25-year-old age groups using CSII therapy.[10] The main cause of DKA in youth using insulin pumps is insertion-set occlusion with loss of available insulin.[21] The use of a CGM to warn youth of high glucose levels essentially eliminated DKA in the STAR 3 trial.[11] In summary, DKA may be slightly increased in youth after initiating CSII therapy; however, it is likely lower than in a general pediatric diabetes clinic population.[9–17]

5. Psychosocial Parameters: Many youths who do not elect to use CSII report that they "do not want to be continually attached to something."[6] There have been many studies of patient satisfaction in youth before and after using CSII and the results are usually "improved" or "no changes."[4,22] A meta-analysis of the psychosocial impact of CSII (including five pediatric studies) found no consistent differences in anxiety, depression, quality of life, self-esteem, or family functioning.[23] Further references to psychosocial issues can be found in the pediatric pump consensus statement.[1]

New Advances in Pump Therapy

Technologies will continue to advance for all people using insulin pumps. Patch pumps with no tubing between the pump and the infusion set have been popular with youth and will continue to improve. Incorporation of pump intelligence into a cell phone is already feasible but will require FDA approval for eventual use. The discontinuation of CSII with a low glucose level (Low Glucose Suspend) detected with CGM is already available in many countries and has been shown to result in less time spent in hypoglycemia.[24–26]

The use of CGM with a pump has been referred to above in the STAR 3 trial.[11] The JDRF-CGM study demonstrated that use of a CGM in youth is only helpful when used 6 or more days/week.[27] Unfortunately, 75% of youth do not succeed in this endeavor.[10] The development of smaller, more comfortable, user-friendly, and more accurate sensors may help to encourage consistent CGM use. These technological advances will make CGM/insulin pump use, and life without SH and DKA, more likely for youth with T1D.

ADULTS

Howard Wolpert, MD

There are several published meta-analyses comparing insulin pumps and multiple daily injections (MDIs) as tools for intensifying glycemic control in adults with type 1 diabetes (T1D). These analyses of the randomized controlled trials in the literature indicate that adults using pump therapy have a 0.4–0.5% lower A1C than with MDI, without an increase in hypoglycemia and with lower insulin requirements. Several national and international clinical guidelines recommend continuous subcutaneous insulin infusion (CSII) as a therapeutic option for adults with T1D with hypoglycemia unawareness and severe hypoglycemia or poor glycemic control. However, because of methodologic issues, the different meta-analyses regarding reduction of hypoglycemia with pump therapy have been conflicting. The meta-analysis conducted by Pickup, which was restricted to studies with a baseline rate of severe hypoglycemia of more than 10/100 episodes/patient years, showed that pump therapy was associated with a 2.9-fold reduction in severe hypoglycemia. Another meta-analysis, commissioned by the Endocrine Society, reached different conclusions that CSII is not associated with a significant reduction in either severe or nocturnal hypoglycemia. The validity of these conclusions is limited by the inclusion of short duration studies with low severe hypoglycemia incidence rates that would bias against detection of any treatment-related differences. In addition, the studies examined in this analysis predominantly involved use of older pumps that did not have bolus calculator software that can limit hypoglycemia from insulin stacking.

The potential complications of pump therapy such as device malfunction, infusion site problems, and ketoacidosis are often not reported in the clinical trials. Patient education about infusion site care and troubleshooting for unexplained hyperglycemia are crucial in decreasing the risk for ketoacidosis in pump users.

CLINICAL INDICATIONS AND PRACTICAL BENEFITS

As in the pediatric population, the adults wishing to start on pump therapy need to be motivated and adherent with the requirements of intensive diabetes self-management and have an adequate diabetes knowledge base. In addition to the benefits of CSII as a tool to intensify glycemic control and minimize hypoglycemia, pump therapy can be advantageous in certain individual circumstances. These include preconception and pregnancy (see chapter 17), diurnal variation in basal insulin requirements (e.g., dawn phenomenon or steroid therapy) or low insulin requirements (better dosing accuracy and precision than injection therapy), and optimization of bolus coverage for gastroparesis and higher fat/complex carbohydrate meals that are more slowly absorbed. The published literature suggests that pump therapy is associated with improved quality of life; however, this has not been confirmed in all studies. This may relate to individual differences in perception about the trade-offs between potential benefits (such as increased lifestyle flexibility and reduced fear for hypoglycemia) relative to some of the negatives associated with wearing a pump (including body image concerns). In practice, ease of bolusing with the pump can be helpful to facilitate interprandial correction bolusing, coverage of snacks, and eating out at restaurants. Unrealistic notions, including the expectation that use of technology reduces need for attentiveness to self-care, need to be dispelled before patients start on pump therapy (see Table 12.II.2).

Relative contraindications to initiation of pump therapy include infrequent self-blood glucose monitoring (with related failure to detect and promptly treat unexplained hyperglycemia, and associated risk for ketoacidosis) and eating disorders with insulin omission and chronically elevated glucoses (with related failure to recognize hyperglycemia from insulin nondelivery). The development of cognitive impairment with compromised judgment, psychiatric problems with inattentiveness to self-care, and visual impairment (unless close family members can assist with pump/infusion set troubleshooting) can be grounds for discontinuing pump therapy in adults.

INSULIN DOSES

Considerations in calculating starting insulin doses for patients changing from MDI to pump therapy and optimizing both basal and bolus doses are covered in several publications, and therefore, will not be discussed here.

TROUBLESHOOTING ERRATIC GLUCOSE CONTROL IN THE PUMP PATIENT

There are several pump-specific issues the clinician should consider in the pump patient presenting with erratic glucoses:

1. Routine history should include questions about frequency of catheter kinking or dislodgement and frequency of catheter and reservoir replacement.

Table 12.II.2 Factors That Predict Success with CSII

Pediatrics and Adults

Minimum of 4–6 home blood glucose tests/day (if not using CGM)

Knowing the carbohydrate counts of the most commonly consumed foods

Understanding the risk for rapid rise in blood glucose levels and progression to DKA, within 6–8 h, if any interruption in insulin infusion occurs and is not recognized and corrected

Having insurance that will pay for pump and supplies

CSII (vs. MDI) is preferred in the following situations:

    Significant dawn phenomenon

    Changes in daily schedule (e.g., shift work, erratic school activities)

    Gastroparesis (adults)

    Frequently changing basal requirements (e.g., exercise)

2. Routine examination should include evaluation of pump infusion sites for scarring and lipohypertrophy, which are not uncommon causes of erratic glucoses, especially in the long-term pump patient.
3. Review of blood glucose data should include evaluation to determine if erratic or elevated glucoses are more common in the period preceding set changes.
4. Review of pump downloads can be informative:
   a. Priming history to determine frequency of reservoir change.
   b. Bolus history to detect missed boluses.
   c. Percent basal to bolus insulin. Basal > bolus in the patient with frequent hyperglycemia may indicate that bolus doses are being missed, whereas in the patient with frequent hypoglycemia this may indicate that high basal rates are contributing to hypoglycemia and would point to need to reevaluate basal settings.
   d. Pump suspension or inappropriate basal rate reduction to determine if this is contributing to hyperglycemia.

PUMP USE IN THE HOSPITALIZED PATIENT

To date only a few hospital facilities have introduced formal policies and procedures regarding the continued use of CSII pumps in patients with diabetes, however with more widespread use of pumps this is an issue that will need attention from hospital oversight bodies. Since most hospital staff do not have expertise with pump use, the patient needs to be alert and orientated and able to self-manage his or her pump (including administering boluses and changing reservoirs and infusion sets) in order to safely continue with pump therapy during hospitalization. Continued use of CSII pumps is contraindicated in patients who are critically ill or metabolically unstable. Because of the risk for overdelivery by insulin pumps that are in proximity to magnetic resonance imaging (MRI), it is critically important for hospitals and radiology facilities to have protocols to ensure that patients remove their pumps before entry into MRI suites.

GAPS IN CURRENT KNOWLEDGE

There are always questions about whether information obtained from well-done randomized research studies vs. collection of real-life clinical data is more useful. The answer is, of course, that both are useful. It will be important to verify the lower A1C levels found in the STAR 3 Study in real-life situations.[1] The T1D Exchange Registry, with large T1D patient numbers (~26,000 subjects), is now starting to fill this gap in the U.S.[2] Funded by the Helmsley Charitable Trust, this registry plans to continue to provide longitudinal data to assist care providers and families of youth with T1D to select the best treatments available.

New Advances in Pump Technology

The next decade promises several technical improvements in pumps (including the introduction of smaller patch pumps with larger and prefilled insulin reservoirs) and infusion catheters that lead to more rapid insulin absorption, as well as advances of the insulin dosing software incorporated into insulin pumps. Current software incorporated into insulin pumps can be helpful in assisting patients with calculation of bolus doses to cover carbohydrates and correct hyperglycemia, and can be very important tools for reducing risk for hypoglycemia from stacking of insulin boluses. The insulin duration of action programmed into the pump software is a key factor in individualizing this function of the bolus calculator; if the duration of action is set too short (i.e., less than actual action time of the insulin bolus) the pump will indicate that there is less insulin on board than is the case, leading to dose stacking and hypoglycemia. In this regard it is important for the clinician setting the duration of action in the pump software to consider the pharmacodynamics, not the pharmacokinetics, of insulin boluses. The pumps currently in use apply different rules for this calculation; for example, the Insulet pump does not consider insulin from meal boluses when compensating for insulin on board. In addition to refinements of this function, future developments in pump software will include the incorporation of preprogrammable boluses to cover more complex meals and adaptive algorithms to refine basal insulin infusion rates.

CONCLUSION

The pharmacologic treatment tools and general approaches for T1D management have quickly and dramatically changed. In spite of this, the current treatment paradigm is still imperfect. The fundamental challenge, which separates T1D for all age groups from other chronic conditions, is the fact that for success, self-management will be required. Specific attention to diet and to the timing of insulin and vast attention to detail about all factors that impact blood glucose need to be appreciated by both patients and their families. The good news is many patients today can take advantage of these advances, especially in insulin and its delivery systems, and the burden of diabetes-related complications has dramatically lessened. The result is a new phenomenon, which we are just starting to appreciate: geriatric T1D. It is difficult to predict the public health magnitude this issue will be in 20 years, but it will likely be a major focus of public policy for organizations such as the American Diabetes Association. The already-developed tools described in this chapter are now allowing children and adults with T1D to be successful in all aspects of their life, an accomplishment never imagined just a few years ago.

REFERENCES

Insulin

1. Diabetes Control and Complications Trial Research Group: The effect of intensive treatment of diabetes on the development and progression of long-term complications in insulin-dependent diabetes mellitus. *N Engl J Med* 329:977–986, 1993
2. Hirsch IB, Skyler JS: Management of type 1 diabetes. In *Atlas of Diabetes.* Skyler JS, Ed. New York, Springer Science + Business Media, LLC, 2012, p. 95–113

3. Garber AJ, King AB, Del Prato S, Sreenan S, Balci MK, Muñoz-Torres M, Rosenstock J, Endahl LA, Francisco AM, Hollander P: NN1250-3582 (BEGIN BB T2D) Trial Investigators: Insulin degludec, an ultra-longacting basal insulin, versus insulin glargine in basal-bolus treatment with meal-time insulin aspart in type 2 diabetes (BEGIN Basal-Bolus Type 2): a phase 3, randomised, open-label, treat-to-target non-inferiority trial. *Lancet* 379:1498–1507, 2012

4. Heller S, Buse J, Fisher M, Garg S, Marre M, Merker L, Renard E, Russell-Jones D, Philotheou A, Francisco AM, Pei H, Bode B: BEGIN Basal-Bolus Type 1 Trial Investigators: Insulin degludec, an ultra-longacting basal insulin, versus insulin glargine in basal-bolus treatment with mealtime insulin aspart in type 1 diabetes (BEGIN Basal-Bolus Type 1): a phase 3, randomised, open-label, treat-to-target non-inferiority trial. *Lancet* 379:1489–1497, 2012

5. American Diabetes Association: *Medical Management of Type 1 Diabetes*. 5th ed. Kaufman, FR, Ed. Alexandria, VA, American Diabetes Association, 2008: 51–82; table on 58

6. Hirsch, IB: Insulin Analogues. *N Engl J Med* 352:174–183; table on 177, 2005

7. Hirsch LJ, Gibney MA, Albanese J, Qu S, Kassler-Taub K, Klaff LJ, Bailey TS: Comparative glycemic control, safety and patient ratings for a new 4mm×32G insulin pen needle in adults with diabetes. *Curr Med Res Opin* 26:1531–1541, 2010

8. McKay M, Compion G, Lytzen L: A comparison of insulin injection needles on patients' perceptions of pain, handling, and acceptability: a randomized, open-label, crossover study in subjects with diabetes. *Diabetes Technol Ther* 11:195–201, 2009

9. Siegmund T, Blankenfield H, Schumm-Drager P: Comparison of usability and patient preference for insulin pen needles produced with different production techniques. *Diabetes Technol Ther* 11:523–528, 2009

10. Marino MT, Costello D, Baughman R, et al. Pharmacokinetics and pharmacodynamics of inhaled GLP-1 (MKC253): proof of concept studies in healthy normal volunteers and in patients with type 2 diabetes. *Clinical Pharmacology & Therapeutics* 88:243–250, 2010

11. Marino MT, Cassidy JR, Baughman RA, et al.: A new C-peptide correction model used to assess bioavailability of regular human insulin. *Biopharmaceutics & Drug Disposition* 31:428–435, 2010

12. www.clinicaltrials.gov. Accessed 4 October 2012

13. Miles HL, Acerini CL: Insulin analog preparations and their use in children and adolescents with type 1 diabetes mellitus. *Paediatr Drugs* 10:163–176, 2008

ADDITIONAL REFERENCES: INSULIN

American Diabetes Association: Clinical practice recommendations. *Diabetes Care* 35 (Suppl. 1), 2012

Maahs DM, Nadeau K, Snell-Bergeon JK, Schauer I, Bergman B, West NA, Rewers M, Daniels SR, Ogden LG, Hamman RF, Dabelea D: Association of insulin sensitivity to lipids across the lifespan in people with type 1 diabetes. *Diabet Med* 28:148–155, 2011. doi: 10.1111/j.1464-5491.2010.03143.x

Marino MT, Cassidy JR, Baughman RA, et al.: A new c-peptide correction model used to assess bioavailability of regular human insulin. *Biopharmaceuticals & Drug Disposition* 31:428–435, 2010.

Nadeau KJ, Regensteiner JG, Bauer TA, Brown MS, Dorosz JL, Hull A, Zeitler P, Draznin B, Reusch JE: Insulin resistance in adolescents with type 1 diabetes and its relationship to cardiovascular function. *J Clin Endocrinol Metab* 95:513–521, 2010. Epub 13 November 2009

O'Riordan SMP, Robinson PD, Donaghue KC, Moran A.: Management of cystic fibrosis-related diabetes. *Pediatr Diabetes* 10 (Suppl. 12):43–50, 2009

Paris CA, Imperatore G, Klingensmith G, et al.: Predictors of insulin regimens and impact on outcomes in youth with type 1 diabetes: the SEARCH for Diabetes in Youth Study. *J Pediatr* 155:161–162, 2009

Pickup JC, Renard E: Long-acting insulin analogs versus insulin pump therapy for the treatment of type 1 and type 2 diabetes. *Diabetes Care* 31 (Suppl. 2): S140–S145, 2008

Weinzimer SA, Ternand C, Howard C, Chang CT, Becker DJ, Laffel LM: Insulin Aspart Pediatric Pump Study Group: A randomized trial comparing continuous subcutaneous insulin infusion of insulin aspart versus insulin lispro in children and adolescents with type 1 diabetes. *Diabetes Care* 31:210–215, 2008. Epub 5 November 2007

REFERENCES

Continuous Subcutaneous Insulin Infusion (CSII): Pediatrics

1. Phillip M, Danne T, Battelino T, Kaufman F, Rodriguez H: Use of insulin pump therapy in the pediatric age-group. *Diabetes Care* 30:1653–1662, 2007

2. Weinzimer SA, Ahern JH, Doyle EA, Vincent MR, Dziura J, Steffen AT, Tamborlane WV: Persistence of benefits of continuous subcutaneous insulin infusion in very young children with type 1 diabetes: a follow-up report. *Pediatrics* 114:1601–1605, 2004

3. Wilson DM, Buckingham BA, Kunselman EL, Sullivan MM, Paguntalan HU, Gitelman SE: A two-center randomized controlled feasibility trial of insulin pump therapy in young children with diabetes. *Diabetes Care* 28:15–19, 2005

4. Fox LA, Buckloh LM, Smith SD, Wysocki T, Mauras N: A randomized controlled trial of insulin pump therapy in young children with type 1 diabetes. *Diabetes Care* 28:1277–1281, 2005

5. Oprpari-Arrigan L, Fredericks EM, Burkart N, Dale L, Hodge M, Foster C: Continuous subcutaneous insulin infusion benefits quality of life in preschool-age children with type 1 diabetes mellitus. *Pediatr Diabetes* 8:377–383, 2007

6. Chase HP, Messer L: *Understanding Insulin Pumps and Continuous Glucose Monitors.* 2nd ed. Denver, Children's Diabetes Foundation at Denver, 2010

7. Maahs DM, Horten LA, Chase HP: The use of insulin pumps in youth with type 1 diabetes. *Diabetes Tech Ther* 12:S59–S65, 2010

8. Pickup J, Mattock M, Kerry S: Glycaemic control with continuous subcutaneous insulin infusion compared with intensive insulin injection in patients with type 1 diabetes: meta-analysis of randomized controlled trials. *BMJ* 324:1–6, 2002

9. Scrimgeour L, Cobry E, McFann K, Burdick P, Weimer C, Slover R, Chase HP: Improved glycaemic control after long-term insulin pump use in pediatric patients with type 1 diabetes. *Diabetes Technol and Ther* 9:421–428, 2007

10. T1D Exchange Registry Symposium: Advanced Technologies and Treatments for Diabetes, February 2012. Barcelona, Spain

11. Bergenstal R, Tamborlane W, Ahmann A, Buse JB, Dailey G, Davis SN, Joyce C, Peoples T, Perkins BA, Welsh JB, Willi SM, Wood MA; STAR 3 Study Group: Effectiveness of sensor-augmented insulin-pump therapy in type 1 diabetes. *N Engl J Med* 363:311–320, 2010

12. Danne T, Battelino T, Jarosz-Chobor P, Pankowska E, Ludvigsson J, et al: Establishing glycaemic control with continuous subcutaneous insulin infusion in children and adolescents with type 1 diabetes: experience of the PedPump study in 17 countries. *Diabetologia* 51:1594–1601, 2008

13. Pickup JC, Sutton AJ: Severe hypoglycemia and glycaemic control in type 1 diabetes: meta-analysis of multiple daily injections compared with subcutaneous insulin infusion. *Diabet Med* 25:765–774, 2008

14. Bhatia V, Wolfsdorf JI: Severe hypoglycemia in youth with insulin dependent diabetes mellitus: frequency and causative factors. *Pediatrics* 88:1187–1189, 1991

15. Tsalikian E, Mauras N, Beck RW, Tamborlane WV, Janz KF, Chase HP, et al: Diabetes Research In Children Network Direcnet Study Group: Impact of exercise on overnight glycemic control in children with type 1 diabetes mellitus. *J Pediatr* 147:528–523, 2005

16. Taplin CE, Cobry E, Messer L, McFann K, Chase HP, Fiallo-Scharer R: Preventing post-exercise nocturnal hypoglycemia in children with type 1 diabetes. *J Pediatr* 157:784–788, 2010

17. Rewers A, Chase HP, Mackenzie T, Walravens P, Roback M, Rewers M, Hamman RF, Klingensmith G: Predictors of acute complications in children with type 1 diabetes. *JAMA* 287:2511–2518, 2002

18. Patterson CC, Dahlquist G, Harjutsalo V, Joner G, Feltbower RG, Svensson J, Schober E, Gyürüs E, Castell C, Urbonaité B, Rosenbauer J, Iotova V, Thorsson AV, Soltész G: Early mortality in EURODIAB population-based cohorts of type 1 diabetes diagnosed in childhood since 1989. *Diabetologia* 50:2439–2442, 2007

19. Dalhquist G, Kallen B: Mortality in childhood-onset type 1 diabetes. *Diabetes Care* 28:2384–2387, 2005

20. Orsini-Federici M, Akwi JA, Canonico V, Celleno R, Ferolla P, Pippi R, Tassi C, Timi A, Benedetti MM: Early detection of insulin deprivation in continuous subcutaneous insulin infusion-treated patients with type 1 diabetes. *Diabetes Technol Ther* 8:67–75, 2006

21. Hannas R, Lindgren F, Lindblad B: A 2-year national population study of pediatric ketoacidosis in Sweden: predisposing conditions and insulin pump use. *Pediatr Diabetes* 10:33–37, 2009

22. McMahon SK, Airey FL, Marangou DA, McElwee KJ, Carne CL, Clarey AJ, Davis EA, Jones TW: Insulin pump therapy in children and adolescents: improvements in key parameters of diabetes management including quality of life. *Diabet Med* 22:92–96, 2005
23. Weissberg-Benchell J, Antisdel-Lomaglio J, Seshadri R: Insulin pump therapy: a meta-analysis. *Diabetes Care* 26:1079–1087, 2003
24. Danne T, Kordonouri O, Holder M, Haberland H, Golembowski S, Remus K, Bläsig S, Wadien T, Zierow S, Hartmann R, Thomas A: Prevention of hypoglycemia by using low glucose suspend function in sensor-augmented pump therapy. *Diabetes Technol Ther* 13:1129–1134, 2011
25. Choudhary P, Shin J, Evans ML, Hammond PJ, Kerr D, Shaw JA, Pickup JC, Amiel SA: Insulin pump therapy with automated insulin suspension in response to hypoglycemia. *Diabetes Care* 34:2023–2025, 2011
26. Agrawal P, Welsh JB, Kannard B, Askari S, Yang Q, Kaufman FR.: Usage and effectiveness of the low glucose suspend feature of the Medtronic Paradigm Veo insulin pump. *J Diabetes Sci Technol* 5:1137–1141, 2011
27. Chase HP, Beck RW, Xing D, Tamborlane WV, Coffey J, Fox LA, Ives B, Keady J, Kollman C, Laffel L, Ruedy KJ: Continuous glucose monitoring in youth with type 1 diabetes: 12-month follow-up of the Juvenile Diabetes Research Foundation continuous glucose monitoring randomized trial. *Diabetes Technol Ther* 12:507–515, 2010

REFERENCES

Continuous Subcutaneous Insulin Infusion (CSII): Adults

American Diabetes Association: Continuous subcutaneous insulin infusion. *Diabetes Care* 27 (Suppl. 1):S110, 2004
Barnard KD, Lloyd CE, Skinner TC: Systematic literature review: quality of life associated with insulin pump use in type 1 diabetes. *Diabet Med* 24:607–617, 2007
Barnard KD, Skinner TC: Cross-sectional study into quality of life issues surrounding insulin pump use in type 1 diabetes. *Practical Diabetes International* 25, 2008
Fatourechi MM, Kudva YC, Murad MH, Elamin MB, Tabini CC, Montori VM: Hypoglycemia with intensive insulin therapy: a systematic review and meta-analyses of randomized trials of continuous subcutaneous insulin infusion versus multiple daily injections. *J Clin Endocrinol Metab* 94:729–740, 2009
Hammond P, Boardman S, Greenwood R: ABCD position paper on insulin pumps. *Practical Diabetes International* 23:395–400, 2006
Heinemann L: Insulin pump therapy: what is the evidence for using different types of boluses for coverage of prandial insulin requirements? *J Diabetes Sci Technol* 3:1490–1500, 2009
Jeitler K, Horvath K, Berghold A, Gratzer TW, Neeser K, Pieber TR, Siebenhofer A: Continuous subcutaneous insulin infusion versus multiple daily insulin injections in patients with diabetes mellitus: systematic review and meta-analysis. *Diabetologia* 51:941–951, 2008

Kerr D, Morton J, Whately-Smith C, Everett J, Begley JP: Laboratory-based non-clinical comparison of occlusion rates using three rapid-acting insulin analogs in continuous subcutaneous insulin infusion catheters using low flow rates. *J Diabetes Sci Technol* 2:450–455, 2008

Linkeschova R, Raoul M, Bott U, Berger M, Spraul M: Less severe hypoglycae-mia, better metabolic control, and improved quality of life in type 1 diabetes mellitus with continuous subcutaneous insulin infusion (CSII) therapy; an observational study of 100 consecutive patients followed for a mean of 2 years. *Diabet Med* 19:746–751, 2002

Mecklenburg RS, Benson EA, Benson JW Jr, Fredlund PN, Guinn T, Metz RJ, Nielsen RL, Sanner CA: Acute complications associated with insulin infusion ther-apy. Report of experience with 161 patients. *JAMA* 252:3265–3269, 1984

Perriello G, De Feo P, Torlone E, Fanelli C, Santeusanio F, Brunetti P, Bolli GB: The dawn phenomenon in type 1 (insulin-dependent) diabetes mellitus: mag-nitude, frequency, variability, and dependency on glucose counterregulation and insulin sensitivity. *Diabetologia* 34:21–28, 1991

Pickup J, Mattock M, Kerry S: Glycaemic control with continuous subcutaneous insulin infusion compared with intensive insulin injections in patients with type 1 diabetes: meta-analysis of randomised controlled trials. *BMJ* 324:705, 2002

Pickup JC, Hammond P: NICE guidance on continuous subcutaneous insulin infusion 2008: review of the technology appraisal guidance. *Diabet Med* 26: 1–4, 2009

Pickup JC, Sutton AJ: Severe hypoglycaemia and glycaemic control in type 1 diabetes: meta-analysis of multiple daily insulin injections compared with continuous subcutaneous insulin infusion. *Diabet Med* 25:765–774, 2008

Retnakaran R, Hochman J, DeVries JH, Hanaire-Broutin H, Heine RJ, Melki V, Zinman B: Continuous subcutaneous insulin infusion versus multiple daily injections: the impact of baseline A1C. *Diabetes Care* 27:2590–2596, 2004

Ritholz MD, Smaldone A, Lee J, Castillo A, Wolpert H, Weinger K: Perceptions of psychosocial factors and the insulin pump. *Diabetes Care* 30:549–554, 2007

Swan KL, Dziura JD, Steil GM, Voskanyan GR, Sikes KA, Steffen AT, Martin ML, Tamborlane WV, Weinzimer SA: Effect of age of infusion site and type of rapid-acting analog on pharmacodynamic parameters of insulin boluses in youth with type 1 diabetes receiving insulin pump therapy. *Diabetes Care* 32:240–244, 2009

Weissberg-Benchell J, Antisdel-Lomaglio J, Seshadri R: Insulin pump therapy: a meta-analysis. *Diabetes Care* 26:1079–1087, 2003

Wolpert H: *Smart Pumping: A Practical Approach to Mastering the Insulin Pump.* Alexandria, VA, American Diabetes Association, 2002

Zisser H, Robinson L, Bevier W, Dassau E, Ellingsen C, Doyle FJ, Jovanovic L: Bolus calculator: a review of four "smart" insulin pumps. *J Diabetes Technol Ther* 10:441–444, 2008

REFERENCES

Gaps in Current Knowledge

1. Bergenstal R, Tamborlane W, Ahmann A, Buse JB, Dailey G, Davis SN, Joyce C, Peoples T, Perkins BA, Welsh JB, Willi SM, Wood MA; STAR 3 Study Group: Effectiveness of sensor-augmented insulin-pump therapy in type 1 diabetes. *N Engl J Med* 363:311–320, 2010
2. T1D Exchange Registry Symposium: Advanced Technologies and Treatments for Diabetes, February 2012. Barcelona, Spain

13

Adjunctive Therapies

Jeremy Hodson Pettus, MD, and Steven Edelman, MD

INTRODUCTION

T he discovery of insulin over 90 years ago remains one of the greatest success stories in the history of medicine. Although insulin remains the mainstay of therapy for patients with type 1 diabetes (T1D), the greatest deterrents to the use of intensive insulin regimens are hypoglycemia, weight gain, and the need for frequent fine-tuning of insulin doses on a day-to-day basis. Furthermore, despite advances in diabetic technologies and new insulin formulations, the majority of T1D patients do not reach an A1C of less than 7%, putting them at higher risk for developing diabetic complications over time. There exists a very real need to explore other therapeutic agents that may assist T1D patients to reach therapeutic goals, reduce hypoglycemia, minimize glucose variability, and offset weight gain. While we have seen an explosion of therapeutic agents available for type 2 diabetes (T2D), only one other medication, pramlintide, has been approved by the FDA (Food and Drug Administration) for use in T1D. In this chapter we will review the use of pramlintide in T1D as well as discuss other medications that may have clinical benefits in T1D.

AMYLIN, THE HORMONE

Amylin is a 37 amino acid β-cell hormone that is packaged together and cosecreted with insulin during times of nutrient intake. In healthy individuals, amylin is secreted in a similar manner to insulin, whereby low baseline plasma concentrations are followed by surges at mealtimes (see Figure 13.1).[1-5] However, in T1D, there is an absolute deficiency in amylin. Experiments in rodents have demonstrated that amylin exerts its effects as a neuroendocrine hormone, activating specific amylin receptors in the area postrema and nucleus accumbens, components of the central nervous system.[6] Via this central binding, amylin acts to slow the appearance of glucose in the circulation through three different mechanisms: glucagon suppression, slowing of gastric emptying, and promotion of early satiety.[7-12] Together, these actions complement insulin's effects on postprandial glucose regulation, help to reduce glycemic fluctuations, and maintain glucose homeostasis (see Figure 13.2).[13]

PRAMLINTIDE

Pramlintide aggregates into amyloid when injected subcutaneously, making the physiological hormone itself unsuitable for therapeutic use. Pramlintide, an

DOI: 10.2337/9781580404785ch13

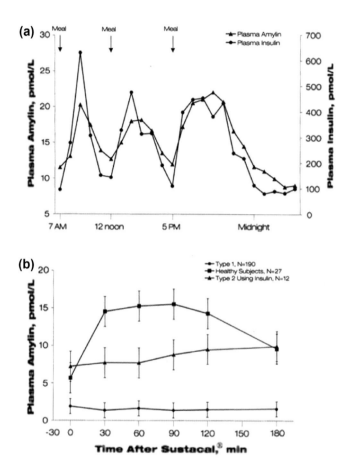

Figure 13.1 (a) Amylin is colocated and cosecreted with insulin and T1D patients have an absolute deficiency of amylin.

Source: Original work: (a) Koda JE, Fineman MS, Kolterman OG, et al.: 24 hour plasma amylin profiles are elevated in IGT subjects vs. normal controls [abstract 876]. *Diabetes* 44 (Suppl. 1):A238, 1995. (b) Fineman MS, Giotta MP, Thompson RG, et al.: Amylin response following Sustacal ingestion is diminished in type II diabetic patients treated with insulin. *Diabetologia* 39 (Suppl.1):A149, 1996. Taken from: Kruger DF, Gatcomb PM, Owen SK: Clinical implications of amylin and amylin deficiency. *Diabetes Educ* 25:389–397; quiz 398, 1999. Reprinted with permission from the publisher.

amylin analogue, was therefore developed as a pharmaceutical agent via manipulation of three of the amino acids, allowing the hormone to be injected subcutaneously and exert its physiological effects without aggregating. Peak concentrations of pramlintide are achieved 20 min after the injection, regardless of the dose. Pramlintide has a half-life of approximately 50 min, and is cleared by the kidneys.

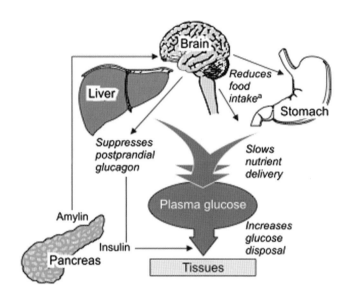

Figure 13.2 Collective mechanisms by which amylin and insulin act to maintain glucose homeostasis.

Source: Edelman SV, Weyer C: Unresolved challenges with insulin therapy in type 1 and type 2 diabetes: potential benefit of replacing amylin, a second beta-cell hormone. *Diabetes Technol Ther* 4:175–189, 2002. Reprinted with permission from the publisher.

Slowing of Gastric Emptying

In healthy individuals, pramlintide acts via the vagus nerve to modulate the rate of gastric emptying. Slowing of gastric emptying acts to modulate the inflow of nutrients to the small intestine, which in turn aids in reducing the postprandial rise in glucose. The rate of gastric emptying is accelerated in patients with T1D, with increases in postprandial glucose directly proportional to the rate of gastric emptying.[14] When pramlintide is administered, the rate of gastric emptying is slowed or normalized and postprandial hyperglycemia is mitigated. Studies in patients with T1D have found that pramlintide prolonged the half-gastric emptying time of meals by 60 to 90 min without influencing emptying rates of subsequent meals.[15,16]

Postprandial Glucagon Suppression

Glucagon is produced by the α-cells in the islets of the pancreas and acts to increase glucose production in the liver. It has a central role in maintaining appropriate levels of glucose in the circulation during times of fasting and is normally suppressed during and after meals. Patients with T1D not only fail to suppress glucagon in the postprandial period but often have a paradoxical increase in glucagon release. Pramlintide administration inhibits this inappropriate increase in postprandial glucagon, thereby lowering postprandial blood glucose levels.[17,18]

It is important to note that in the setting of hypoglycemia, glucagon release is not inhibited by pramlintide.[19,20]

Regulation of Food Intake

Pramlintide has also been shown to promote early satiety via its action on the central nervous system, specifically the area postrema.[21] A study specifically designed to assess this effect of pramlintide showed that pramlintide administered as a single preprandial injection increased levels of satiety, leading to reduced food intake.[22] In addition, the satiety effect appears to be independent of the nausea that can accompany pramlintide treatment. The effect of early satiety leading to reduced nutrient intake appears to be the mechanism that leads to the weight loss seen in multiple clinical trials as described below.

Postprandial Glucose Control

The collective mechanisms of action of pramlintide described above complement insulin in the postprandial period by slowing the appearance of glucose in the circulation, thereby reducing postprandial hyperglycemia (Figure 13.2). The ability of pramlintide to control postprandial glucose has been evaluated in multiple randomized, placebo-controlled trials. Specifically, when administered prior to a standardized meal, pramlintide was shown to reduce postprandial glucose excursions compared to insulin therapy alone (see Figure 13.3).[23]

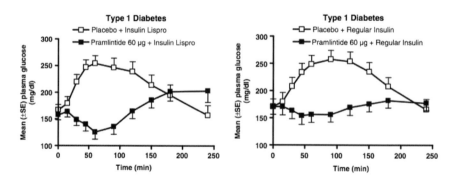

Figure 13.3 Pramlintide's effect on postprandial glucose control when added to insulin.

Source: Chart taken from: Edelman SV, Darsow T, Frias JP: Pramlintide in the treatment of diabetes. *Int J Clin Pract* 60:1647–1653, 2006. Original work: Weyer C, Gottlieb A, Kim DD, Lutz K, Schwartz S, Gutierrez M, Wang Y, Ruggles JA, Kolterman OG, Maggs DG: Pramlintide reduces postprandial glucose excursions when added to regular insulin or insulin lispro in subjects with type 1 diabetes: a dose-timing study. *Diabetes Care* 26:3074–3079, 2003. Reprinted with permission from the publisher.

This effect was seen with both regular and a rapid-acting insulin analog. In a separate study using continuous glucose monitoring, pramlintide therapy led to significantly less glucose variability during the 4 weeks of treatment compared to baseline readings.[24] Finally, in both T1D and T2D patients, 6 months of open-label pramlintide reduced postprandial glucose values and resulted in smoother self-monitored glucose profiles when compared to baseline (see Figure 13.4).[25–27]

Long-Term Placebo-Controlled Trials

The long-term effects of pramlintide treatment in patients with T2D and T1D were investigated in four separate randomized, placebo-controlled, 52-week trials.[28–31] The studies consistently demonstrated that adding pramlintide to existing insulin therapy improved long-term glycemic and weight control.

Specifically in T1D, two 52-week trials (n = 480 and n = 651) showed an A1C reduction of –0.39% and –0.34% with pramlintide at 30 or 60 mcg doses 4 times daily, respectively. In patients with T1D who completed 2 years of pramlintide treatment, these A1C reductions were sustained over the treatment period. Furthermore, a statistically significant increase in the number of patients reaching an A1C goal of <7% was reported in both studies. In the initial trial, a three-fold greater proportion of patients achieved this goal, and in the second trial, more than twice the proportion of patients in the pramlintide arm reached an

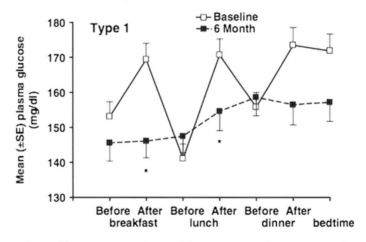

Figure 13.4 Glucose excursions with and without pramlintide therapy at baseline and 6 months.

Source: Original work: Guthrie R, Karl DM, Wang Y et al: In an open-label clinical study pramlintide lowered A1C, body weight, and insulin use in patients with type 1 diabetes failing to achieve glycemic targets with insulin therapy. *Diabetes* 54 (Suppl. 1): A118, 2005. Chart taken from: Pullman J, Darsow, Frias JP: Pramlintide in the management of insulin-using patients with type 2 and type 1 diabetes. *Vasc Health and Risk Management* 2:203–212, 2006. Reprinted with permission from the publisher.

A1C <7%. This improved glycemic profile was achieved while mitigating the usual increase in insulin dose seen over time. Over a 1-year period, insulin dose increased by 2.3% in the pramlintide group and 10.3% in the control arm during one study. Changes in insulin dose were typically in the mealtime insulin rather than basal rates (see Figure 13.5).[26,28,31]

Weight Loss

Weight gain is associated with intensive insulin regimens. During the first year of the DCCT, subjects assigned to intensive insulin therapy gained twice as much weight as those given conventional therapy.[32] This increased weight is concerning in diabetes as it can lead to and exacerbate factors such as hypertension and hyperlipidemia that place patients at even higher risk for cardiovascular complications. Fortunately, improved glycemic control in pramlintide-treated patients in long-term, placebo-controlled studies was not accompanied by weight gain, but instead was associated with a sustained and significant reduction in body weight. Following 6 months of pramlintide treatment, patients with T1D lost an average of approximately 1 kg compared with an average gain of 0.6 kg in placebo-treated patients (see Figure 13.5).[28,31] Weight reductions were sustained up to 1 year, however, in an open-label extension trial, patients who continued on pramlintide tended to begin to regain weight. Stratification of patients based on baseline body mass index demonstrated that body weight reductions were greatest in patients who were overweight or obese, and that pramlintide did not change weight in lean patients.

Dose Titration Study

Hypoglycemia was a concern highlighted by the early pivotal trials. This side effect was typically noticed in the initiation of the medication (first 4 weeks) without any proactive reduction in insulin dosing and no titration of the dose, both of which led to an FDA black box warning. To address initiation strategies,

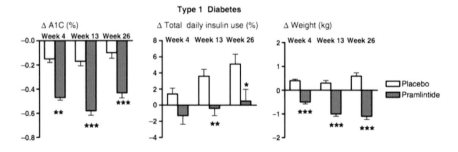

Figure 13.5 Effects from combined placebo-controlled trials on A1C, insulin dose, and weight.

Source: Taken from: Edelman SV, Darsow T, Frias JP: Pramlintide in the treatment of diabetes. *Int J Clin Pract* 60:1647–1653, 2006. Reprinted with permission from the publisher.

a 29-week, placebo-controlled dose titration study was conducted in which pramlintide was initiated at 15 mcg with a 30–50% proactive reduction in mealtime insulin dosing. Pramlintide was then increased to a goal dose of 60 mcg before meals as tolerated with insulin doses adjusted to blood glucose values. Using this strategy, hypoglycemic events during initiation of pramlintide were reduced and not statistically different from placebo. Consistent with previous studies, significant reductions in postprandial glucose, insulin dose, and weight were observed.[33]

Side Effects

Hypoglycemia. Pramlintide does not cause hypoglycemia when administered alone. However, the addition of an antihyperglycemic agent to a patient's insulin therapy has the potential to increase the risk of insulin-induced hypoglycemia, particularly at the start of therapy. As mentioned above, hypoglycemia was observed more frequently in the initial trials when insulin doses were not prophylactively reduced and pramlintide was initiated at the highest recommended dose of 60 mcg. It has since been demonstrated that this risk was short-term and manageable with adequate glucose monitoring, a 30–50% reduction of preprandial insulin doses at initiation of pramlintide, and gradual upward titration of the pramlintide dose during its initiation.[33]

Gastrointestinal. Beyond hypoglycemia, the most common side effects seen with pramlintide are nausea followed by anorexia and vomiting.[28,31] Nausea is particularly an issue in the T1D population, with rates as high as 48% in the initiation period. Practitioners and patients need to be aware of this common phenomenon and address it specifically at the time of initiation. It seems as though, based on the authors extensive clinical experience, the longer the duration of T1D, the more susceptible the individual is to nausea. With diligent slow up-titration, the effect can be minimized. Furthermore, it should be emphasized to the patient that the gastrointestinal side effects are typically mild to moderate in intensity and transient. However, given that pramlintide slows the rate of gastric emptying, this can lead to more severe symptoms in patients with established gastroparesis.

Clinical Use

Pramlintide is an appropriate adjunct to mealtime insulin to consider for any patient with T1D that is not meeting their desired A1C goal. However, there are some basic concepts to keep in mind prior to initiation. Patients should begin with reasonable blood glucose control with an A1C <9% indicating a somewhat stable insulin regimen and compliance with their insulin therapy. Patients should monitor their blood glucose frequently (or use a continuous glucose monitor) and have frequent contact with a health care provider skilled in insulin use. Pramlintide should be avoided in patients with hypoglycemia unawareness or with episodes of severe hypoglycemia in the preceding 6 months. Patients with severe gastroparesis should not use pramlintide as its effect on slowing gastric emptying can exacerbate these symptoms. In patients with mild gastroparesis the effects of pramlintide can actually improve symptoms because it helps to prevent over eating, which makes the stomach wall atonic. The pramlintide dose should be gradually titrated upwards with an initial 50% decrease in mealtime insulin. In the clinical trials the final reduction in mealtime insulin was ~30% so a discussion with the patient telling them that the 50% may be too much and to expect higher blood glucose values upon initiation. Doses of both pramlintide and insulin should be adjusted according to the patient based on symptoms and home or continuous glucose monitoring. Figure 13.6 details dose titration when initiating pramlintide.

The timing of the mealtime insulin bolus should also be taken into consideration. Pramlintide reduces the postprandial glucose concentrations via the mechanisms described above. Dosing a rapid-acting insulin analog before a meal in a typical fashion may result in an initial reduction in postprandial glucose, but can also result in a late, gradual increase in glucose concentrations after peak mealtime insulin action (see Figure 13.3). Experimenting with dosing the rapid-acting analog insulin after the meal or using an extended wave bolus via an insulin pump may help to further fine-tune the overall postprandial glucose profile in patients using pramlintide and provide a better matching of the pharmacokinetics of rapid-acting insulin.

Pramlintide in the Pediatric Population

Pramlintide is currently FDA-approved for adults but not in the pediatric population; however, several small trials have evaluated its use in children and

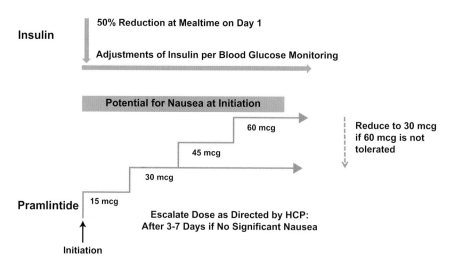

Figure 13.6 Stepwise approach to initiating pramlintide therapy.
Adapted from: Pramlintide Acetate Prescribing Information [package insert], 2005

adolescents.[34–37] Overall, these trials have demonstrated similar effects as seen in the adult population in regard to decreasing postprandial hyperglycemia, reducing insulin dose, and improving body weight profiles—an overall proof of concept. The aim of these trials has largely been to establish a safe dose that can be administered without undue side effects. Pramlintide is frequently used in the adolescent population; however, this is an off-label indication. A 4-month trial comparing pramlintide with insulin vs. exenatide and insulin in 12–21 year olds is currently underway and may help answer some of these questions.

Future Roles of Pramlintide in Insulin Pumps and the Artificial Pancreas

With the improvement in continuous glucose monitors, insulin pumps, and insulin formulations, the artificial pancreas has become an increasingly possible technology. Studies have commenced testing prototype models for at home use in real-world situations.[38] However, the lag time between insulin infusion in the subcutaneous tissue and its onset of metabolic action remains a significant barrier to perfecting the insulin delivery algorithms. This lag can result in unacceptable postprandial glucose spikes with potential late hypoglycemic reactions. To solve this problem, one could imagine multiple possible solutions. One solution would be to add pramlintide into the infusion device itself along with insulin to help mitigate postprandial hyperglycemia. This addition, however, would mean a separate chamber for pramlintide in the device with a separate infusion site since the two medications are currently believed to be incompatible. Furthermore, the larger clinical trials above only assessed pramlintide as an adjunct in a mealtime fashion. Therefore, it remains to be seen if infusion of the medication in a basal-bolus fashion would confer any additional benefits beyond mealtime delivery alone.

Several small trials have begun to address these issues. A 16-week open-label study of 11 patients with long-standing T1D used pramlintide in a basal-bolus fashion administered via an insulin pump. A continuous infusion was maintained at 9 mcg/hr with boluses at mealtime titrated up to 60 mcg. Over the study period, patients had lower A1C values, and lower fasting glucoses, and lost weight.[39] However, there was no control group that used pramlintide in a bolus fashion only, making it impossible to determine the benefit of a continuous infusion. A similar study was done in adolescents where 13 patients were observed on insulin monotherapy and then crossed over to insulin along with pramlintide in a basal-bolus fashion.[40] Improvement in glucose variability, reduction in insulin dose, and decreased glucagon response were all observed with the addition of pramlintide. Together these trials show that it is technically possible and safe to administer pramlintide in a continuous fashion along with insulin therapy. However, larger studies need to be done with an appropriate control group.

The need for separate infusions of pramlintide and insulin is cumbersome. To address this issue, one randomized, placebo-controlled study of 51 patients evaluated the effects of mixing various insulin formulations with pramlintide and ultimately found that this had no effect on the area under the concentration-vs.-time curve and the maximum concentration of serum-free insulin.[41] However, it remains unknown if the two can be mixed in a pump.

Pramlintide has been shown to be a useful addition to insulin in the treatment of T1D. Not only has it been shown to reduce A1C in the adult population but it does so while reducing overall insulin dose and weight. Furthermore, with proper dose titration at initiation, side effects can be effectively reduced, making the medication safe and tolerable. Going forward, the medication will need to be evaluated in the pediatric population, and if deemed safe and effective, would add a long-awaited adjunct in this group. Finally, with the advent of the artificial pancreas looming in the near future, the role of pramlintide in a continuous infusion setting along with insulin needs to be evaluated. The beneficial postprandial glucose profile provided by pramlintide could potentially help to close the loop sooner.

GLP-1 AGONISTS

The incretin effect was discovered after experiments found that administration of oral glucose resulted in an increased insulin secretion compared to the same amount of intravenous glucose in healthy controls.[42] This effect was eventually ascribed to two hormones produced in the gut, glucagon-like-peptide-1 (GLP-1) and glucose-dependent insulinotropic peptide (GIP). Both hormones have roles in controlling glucose appearance similar to that of amylin. GLP-1 has been shown to suppress glucagon production, augment glucose-dependent insulin secretion, promote early satiety, and delay gastric emptying.[43] Given this physiological abnormality and the beneficial clinical effects, the first GLP-1 analog, exenatide, was approved by the FDA in 2005 for use in T2D.

The incretin effect is somewhat different in T1D patients when compared to T2D. The incretin effect was originally measured by noting the increased release of insulin from an oral glucose load as compared to an IV load. As T1D patients typically do not make insulin, this same effect cannot be demonstrated. However, studies have been done in T1D patients in which levels of GIP and GLP-1 were directly measured after an oral glucose load. These studies have shown that T1D patients seem to make a normal amount of the incretin hormones when compared to controls. However, it was shown that T1D patients had an increased glucagon response to an oral compared to IV load.[44] Taken together, these findings make the argument that while T1D patients produce a normal amount of these gut hormones, there still appears to be a dysregulation between the gut and pancreas in which glucagon is not effectively suppressed (see Figure 13.7). This phenomenon raises the possibility that therapeutic intervention with GLP-1 agonists may have beneficial effects in T1D.

Several studies have begun to look specifically at the clinical benefits of GLP-1 agonists in T1D. One such study took 30 patients with T1D and gave them liraglutide once daily over a 4-week period.[45] This study broke patients into C-peptide–positive and C-peptide–negative subgroups and compared the effect of the liraglutide with insulin vs. insulin therapy alone. In both C-peptide negative (<0.03 nmol/l) and C-peptide–positive groups (>0.06 nmol/l), the addition of once daily liraglutide showed a trend toward lowered A1C (–0.2% and –0.5%, respectively) at 4 weeks but was not statistically significant. Liraglutide did lead to significantly lower total insulin dose (approximately –0.2 U/kg) and weight

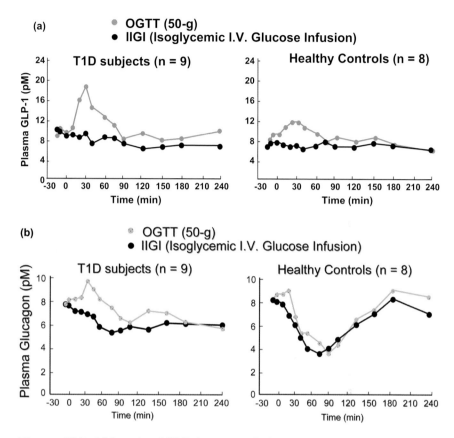

Figure 13.7 (a) Levels of GLP-1 are not diminished in T1D. (b) Paradoxical increased glucagon levels in response to oral glucose load compared to IV load in T1D.

Source: Hare KJ, Vilsbøll T, Holst JJ, Knop FK: Inappropriate glucagon response after oral compared with isoglycemic intravenous glucose administration in patients with type 1 diabetes. *Am J Physiol Endocrinol Metab* 298:E832–E837, 2010. Reprinted with permission from the publisher.

loss (–2.3 kg). Hypoglycemia was not increased with liraglutide but mild and transient nausea was noted at initiation. The degree of insulin dose reduction was found to correlate with underlying β-cell function in that the C-peptide–positive group was able to reduce insulin usage more than the C-peptide–negative group. This study highlights that the clinical benefits of GLP-1 agonists may go beyond glucose dependent insulin secretion as both C-peptide–positive and C-peptide–negative patients trended toward improved glycemic control (see Figure 13.8).[45]

Change in insulin dose, mean BG, HbA$_{1c}$ and stimulated C-peptide in T1D patients with (C-peptide positive) and without (C-peptide negative) residual ϖ-cell function before (week 0) and during (week 4) 4 weeks of treatment with liraglutide or insulin alone

Treatment	C-peptide positive Liraglutide + insulin		C-peptide negative Liraglutide + insulin		C-peptide negative Insulin only	
	Week 0	Week 4	Week 0	Week 4	Week 0	Week 4
Insulin dose (units/kg per day)	0.50 ± 0.06	0.31 ± 0.08*	0.72 ± 0.08	0.59 ± 0.06†	0.62 ± 0.04	0.64 ± 0.05 (NS)
Mean blood glucose (mmol/l)	6.0 ± 0.2	6.3 ± 0.3 (NS)	7.5 ± 0.4	7.7 ± 0.4(NS)	7.5 ± 0.4	7.5 ± 0.6 (NS)
HbA$_{1c}$ (%)	6.6 ± 0.3	6.4 ± 0.2†	7.5 ± 0.2	7.0 ± 0.1†	7.1 ± 0.3	6.9 ± 0.2 (NS)
C-peptide (pmol/L)‡	520 ± 106	457 ± 79(NS)	—	—	—	—

Data are means ± SE. Mean blood glucose levels are derived from continuous glucose montitoring as mean values during 3 days with identical food intake and physical activity in week 0 and week 4. NS, nonsignificant vs. week 4. *P < 0.001 and † p < 0.05 vs. week 0 in the same group. ‡ n = 8.

Figure 13.8 Four weeks of liraglutide reduced A1C while reducing insulin dose in C-peptide positive and negative patients. *Source:* Kielgast U, Krarup T, Holst JJ, Madsbad S: Four weeks of treatment with liraglutide reduces insulin dose without loss of glycemic control in type 1 diabetic patients with and without residual beta-cell function. *Diabetes Care* 34:1463–1468, 2011. Reprinted with permission from the publisher.

In the above-mentioned study, the trial duration of only 4 weeks makes improvements in A1C difficult to detect. In a longer running trial, 14 C-peptide–negative patients were given once-daily liraglutide for one week in addition to insulin therapy. Eight patients then continued on to receive the intervention for 6 months. Over the 6-month period, fasting glucose was reduced, the mean A1C fell (6.5 to 6.1%), total insulin dose was reduced (0.65 to 0.47 U/kg), and there was substantial weight loss (4.5 +/– 1.5 kg) without an increase in hypoglycemia (see Figure 13.9).[46]

Effects of liraglutide treatment for a mean duration of 24 weeks in eight patients

Parameters	Before treatment (1 week)	On liraglutide (24 weeks)	P Value
Weight (kg)	68 ± 5	63.5 ± 4	0.02
HBA1c (%)	6.5 ± 0.5	6.1 ± 0.4	0.02
Insulin dose (U/day)			
Basal	26.5 ± 7	13.5 ± 5	< 0.01
Bolus	25.5 ± 6	14 ± 4	< 0.01
Mean blood glucose (mg/d)			
Fasting	128 ± 10	108 ± 8	< 0.01
Weekly	134 ± 20	111 ± 12	< 0.01
Time spent in hyperglycemia (% time)			
>150 mg/dl	27.5 ± 6	21 ± 5	0.02
>200 mg/dl	17.5 ± 5	6.5 ± 2	< 0.01
>250 Mg/dl	8.0 ± 2	2.0 ⊥ 1	< 0.01
Time spent in hypoglycemia (% time)			
<70 mg/dl	2.1 ± 2	2.3 ± 2	0.08
<40 mg/dl	0.11 ± 0.2	0.12 ± 0.3	0.12
Mean S.D. Weekly (mg/dl)	53.10	27 ± 6	< 0.01
Coefficient of variation weekly (%)	39.5 ± 10	24.3 ± 8	< 0.01

Figure 13.9 Six months of liraglutide lowered A1C and fasting blood glucose while reducing weight, insulin dose, duration of hyperglycemia, and glucose variability.

Source: Varanasi A, Bellini N, Rawal D, Vora M, Makdissi A, Dhindsa S, Chaudhuri A, Dandona P: Liraglutide as additional treatment for type 1 diabetes. *Eur J Endocrinol* 165:77–84, 2011. Reprinted with permission from the publisher.

In summary, GLP-1 agonists have a potential therapeutic role in T1D both in long-standing and new-onset disease. In general, the medication has similar effects as pramlintide by reducing postprandial hyperglycemia while reducing insulin usage and promoting weight loss. An additional advantage of the GLP-1 agonists is the longer dosing intervals. Once-weekly exenatide has recently been FDA approved for use in T2D patients and even longer formulation including once-monthly and even once/year-infusion devices are being studied. If such formulations could be approved for T1D, the fear of multiple injections would be somewhat alleviated. In the adult patients, longer duration trials and head-to-head comparisons with pramlintide are in process.

DPP-4 INHIBITORS

Both GLP-1 and GIP are rapidly degraded by the enzyme dipeptidyl peptidase-4 (DPP-4) with circulating half-lives of only several minutes. Therefore, effectively inhibiting this enzyme results in prolonged duration of endogenous GLP-1. Sitagliptin, the first DPP-4 inhibitor, was approved for use in T2D in 2006 and has proven to be a valuable addition in the armamentarium of treating T2D. Like GLP-1 agonists, DPP-4 inhibitors have shown to reduce postprandial hyperglycemia without increased incidence of hypoglycemia.[47] They do not show the weight loss that GLP-1 agonists do but carry the benefit of being an oral medication while GLP-1 agonists are exclusively injectables.

One randomized, double-blind trial evaluated the effect of sitagliptin 100 mg/day in 20 patients with T1D. Patients were given sitagliptin 100 mg/day or placebo for 4 weeks and then crossed over. Compared to placebo, sitagliptin was shown to reduce A1C at 4 weeks (–0.27%), reduce postprandial hyperglycemia, and reduce total insulin dose (–0.051 U/kg). No change in weight or hypoglycemic episodes was observed. Limitations were a small sample size, a short trial interval of only 4 weeks, and large placebo effect (see Figure 13.10).[48]

As with the GLP-1 agonists, larger studies are needed to define the clinical effect of DPP-4 inhibitors in T1D. Additionally, as this class of medication has shown immune modulatory effects, its role in early onset disease is being evaluated. A study funded by the JDRF is underway in which new-onset T1D with disease duration of less than 6 months will be randomized to sitagliptin and lansoprazole (thought to aid β-cell survival by increasing endogenous gastrin levels) vs. placebo with a primary outcome of C-peptide response to a mixed meal tolerance test at baseline compared to at 1 year.

METFORMIN

Metformin is an established oral agent that is widely used as a first line agent in the treatment of T2D.[49] Its mechanism of action centers around decreasing hepatic glucose production and improving insulin sensitivity. Administration is associated with A1C reduction, weight loss, an improved lipid profile, and decreased levels of inflammation represented by C-reactive protein in T2D. These beneficial effects have led to multiple trials evaluating its use in T1D. Two large reviews have compiled the clinical evidence to date.

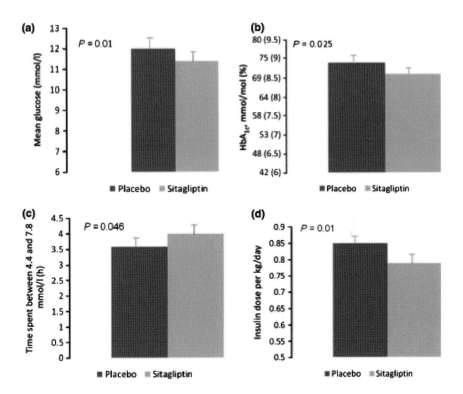

Figure 13.10 Sitagliptin reduced mean glucose, A1C, and insulin dose while increasing time spent in eucglycemia.

Source: Ellis SL, Moser EG, Snell-Bergeon JK, Rodionova AS, Hazenfield RM, Garg SK: Effect of sitagliptin on glucose control in adult patients with type 1 diabetes: a pilot, double-blind, randomized, crossover trial. *Diabet Med* 28:1176–1181, 2011. Reprinted with permission from the publisher.

In 2009, a Cochrane review was published on the addition of metformin to insulin in adolescents with T1D.[50] After searching for any randomized control trial of at least 3-months duration, only two studies could be included. Both trials were 3 months in length and included 30 poorly controlled adolescents (average baseline A1C of around 9%) randomized to placebo vs. metformin up to 2 g/day in addition to insulin. Both studies suggested that metformin therapy led to a reduction in A1C values. There were no comments about lipid profiles or insulin sensitivity although one study noted a 10% reduction in total insulin dosage. Given these findings, the authors conclude that there is some evidence that metformin can improve glycemic control in adolescents but larger studies of longer duration are needed.

A second review was published in 2010 that evaluated the effect of adding metformin to insulin therapy in any patient with T1D.[51] The authors ultimately found nine studies that met their search criteria, two of which were also in the Cochrane review noted above. Due to heterogeneity between studies, only five could be included into a formal meta-analysis. In these five studies, metformin had no statistically significant change in A1C but was found to lower insulin dosage by 6.6 U/day. Of note, the largest and longest trial included was of 100 patients randomized to metformin 1g BID vs. placebo and followed for 1 year. In this study, there again was no statistically significant change in A1C, however total daily insulin dose was reduced (–5.7 U/day) and weight loss was observed (–1.74 kg).[52]

Taking all the data together, metformin appears to have a beneficial effect on insulin sensitivity with reduction in overall insulin requirements and weight. The effect on overall glycemic control is somewhat less clear. As a result, metformin is not currently advocated as an adjunctive therapy for any subgroup of patients with T1D. Clinical data makes it difficult to firmly recommend or refute the use of metformin in an off-label fashion as some patients may benefit from the medication. The group of patients that would theoretically show the most benefit would be poorly controlled diabetics who are overweight and requiring large amounts of insulin.

A large trial entitled "REducing With MetfOrmin Vascular Adverse Lesions in Type 1 Diabetes (REMOVAL)" is currently underway to evaluate the effects of metformin on cardiovascular and metabolic outcomes in T1D. The trial will enroll 500 patients, randomize them to 1g BID of metformin vs. placebo and then follow them for 3 years. The primary outcome will be change in averaged mean common carotid artery intima-media thickness. Multiple other secondary outcomes including A1C and lipid profiles will be evaluated. This study will be the largest and longest running study to date and will hopefully provide a clear answer to the role of metformin in T1D. It is estimated to reach completion in 2016.

LEPTIN

Leptin is a 167 amino acid neurohormone produced by adipocytes that plays a key role in the central regulation of appetite, fat and glucose metabolism, and weight. Recombinant leptin (metrelpetin) therapy has shown to have beneficial metabolic effects in patients with lipodystrophy.[53] In T1D, mouse studies have shown that administration of leptin alone can restore the health of insulin-deficient animals by eliminating ketoacidosis, effectively making it the only hormone other than insulin with this ability.[54,55] Leptin inhibits glucagon production and serves to offset the anabolic effects of insulin on lipids by inhibiting lipogenesis and cholesterol biosynthesis. A pilot study is underway evaluating the use of adjunctive leptin therapy in T1D. Fifteen patients will be treated with recombinant human leptin and will serve as their own controls. The endpoints will include A1C, energy intake, glucose variability, insulin dose, and others. The study is expected to reach completion in early 2013.

C-PEPTIDE

Following cleavage of proinsulin in the islet cells, C-peptide is released along with insulin in equimolar amounts into the portal circulation. C-peptide has long been viewed as an inert byproduct of insulin production, but a recent surge in research has revealed that the peptide has biological activity as its own hormone. Research involving the therapeutic replacement of C-peptide has revealed conflicting results in the T1D and T2D populations. In T2D patients, C-peptide was found to accumulate in carotid artery walls and may promote athrogenic lesions.[56] T1D studies, however, have shown more promising results.

A growing amount of evidence in the T1D population has shown that C-peptide replacement can prevent or even reverse diabetic complications in rats, namely neuropathy and nephropathy.[57-60] Several human trials have gone on to demonstrate that therapeutic administration has positive effects on diabetic neuropathy as evidenced by improving nerve conduction velocities.[61,62] These findings represent a paradigm shift in how we view C-peptide. The protein has long been useful as a surrogate marker for insulin production, and it is well known that preservation of C-peptide status leads to a lower incidence of diabetic complications.[32] With evidence of its utility as a therapeutic, it may be the peptide itself that is leading to favorable outcomes. Development of a longer acting subcutaneous injection of C-peptide is underway, which will assist in furthering clinical trials.[63]

OTHERS

In addition to the therapeutic agents described above, studies have looked into α-glucosidase inhibitors, colesevelam, thiazolidinediones (TZDs), and others.[64-66] In general, these studies enrolled very few patients and showed, at best, mild clinical benefits. Therefore, the benefit of these medications is unknown and thus they are not recommended at this time.

CONCLUSIONS

Since the discovery of insulin, therapies for T1D have focused on different insulin formulations, meal planning around dosing, correction doses, and other interventions that could be described as insulin-centric. However, with the relatively recent discovery of amylin deficiency in T1D, a newfound interest in investigating other potential pathways to treat this patient population has emerged. Furthermore, the proven clinical benefits and FDA approval of pramlintide has shown that adjunctive therapies in T1D can be effectively implemented into clinical practice. This fact has opened the door for an expanded investigation into other therapies. Currently, the incretin-based therapies may have the most promise, as more evidence is accumulating regarding their clinical benefits. Furthermore, with oral administration of the DPP-4 inhibitors and longer acting GLP-1 agonists, patient compliance may increase. Going forward, more clinical trials with larger patient numbers and study durations will need to be done. With some of these already underway, practitioners can expect that the repertoire of medications used to treat patients with T1D will expand in the near future.

REFERENCES

1. Koda JE, Fineman M, Rink TJ, Dailey GE, Muchmore DB, Linarelli LG: Amylin concentrations and glucose control. *Lancet* 339:1179–1180, 1992
2. Weyer C, Maggs DG, Young AA, Kolterman OG: Amylin replacement with pramlintide as an adjunct to insulin therapy in type 1 and type 2 diabetes mellitus: a physiological approach toward improved metabolic control. *Curr Pharm Des* 7:1353–1373, 2001
3. Kruger DF, Gatcomb PM, Owen SK: Clinical implications of amylin and amylin deficiency. *Diabetes Educ* 25:389–397; quiz 398, 1999
4. Koda JE, Fineman MS, Kolterman OG, et al.: 24 hour plasma amylin profiles are elevated in IGT subjects vs. normal controls [abstract 876]. *Diabetes* 44 (Suppl. 1):A238, 1995
5. Fineman MS, Giotta MP, Thompson RG, et al.: Amylin response following Sustacal ingestion is diminished in type II diabetic patients treated with insulin. *Diabetologia* 39 (Suppl. 1):A149, 1996
6. Beaumont K, Kenney MA, Young AA, Rink TJ: High affinity amylin binding sites in rat brain. *Mol Pharmacol* 44:493–497, 1993
7. Gedulin BR, Rink TJ, Young AA: Dose-response for glucagonostatic effect of amylin in rats. *Metabolism* 46:67–70, 1997
8. Silvestre RA, Rodríguez-Gallardo J, Jodka C, Parkes DG, Pittner RA, Young AA, Marco J: Selective amylin inhibition of the glucagon response to arginine is extrinsic to the pancreas. *Am J Physiol Endocrinol Metab* 280:E443–E449, 2001
9. Young AA, Gedulin B, Vine W, Percy A, Rink TJ: Gastric emptying is accelerated in diabetic BB rats and is slowed by subcutaneous injections of amylin. *Diabetologia* 38:642–648, 1995
10. Young AA, Gedulin BR, Rink TJ: Dose-responses for the slowing of gastric emptying in a rodent model by glucagon-like peptide (7-36) NH2, amylin, cholecystokinin, and other possible regulators of nutrient uptake. *Metabolism* 45:1–3, 1996
11. Rushing PA, Hagan MM, Seeley RJ, Lutz TA, Woods SC: Amylin: a novel action in the brain to reduce body weight. *Endocrinology* 141:850–853, 2000
12. Rushing PA:,Central amylin signaling and the regulation of energy homeostasis. *Curr Pharm Des* 9:819–825, 2003
13. Edelman SV, Weyer C: Unresolved challenges with insulin therapy in type 1 and type 2 diabetes: potential benefit of replacing amylin, a second beta-cell hormone. *Diabetes Technol Ther* 4:175–189, 2002
14. Rayner CK, Samsom M, Jones KL, Horowitz M: Relationships of upper gastrointestinal motor and sensory function with glycemic control. *Diabetes Care* 24:371–381, 2001
15. Kong MF, King P, Macdonald IA, Stubbs TA, Perkins AC, Blackshaw PE, Moyses C, Tattersall RB: Infusion of pramlintide, a human amylin analogue, delays gastric emptying in men with IDDM. *Diabetologia* 40:82–88, 1997
16. Kong MF, Stubbs TA, King P, Macdonald IA, Lambourne JE, Blackshaw PE, Perkins AC, Tattersall RB: The effect of single doses of pramlintide on gastric emptying of two meals in men with IDDM. *Diabetologia* 41:577–583, 1998

17. Fineman M, Weyer C, Maggs DG, Strobel S, Kolterman OG: The human amylin analog, pramlintide, reduces postprandial hyperglucagonemia in patients with type 2 diabetes mellitus. *Horm Metab Res* 34:504–508, 2002

18. Fineman MS, Koda JE, Shen LZ, Strobel SA, Maggs DG, Weyer C, Kolterman OG: The human amylin analog, pramlintide, corrects postprandial hyperglucagonemia in patients with type 1 diabetes. *Metabolism* 51:636–641, 2002

19. Amiel SA, Heller SR, Macdonald IA, Schwartz SL, Klaff LJ, Ruggles JA, Weyer C, Kolterman OG, Maggs DG: The effect of pramlintide on hormonal, metabolic or symptomatic responses to insulin-induced hypoglycaemia in patients with type 1 diabetes. *Diabetes Obes Metab* 7:504–516, 2005

20. Nyholm B, Møller N, Gravholt CH, Orskov L, Mengel A, Bryan G, Moyses C, Alberti KG, Schmitz O: Acute effects of the human amylin analog AC137 on basal and insulin-stimulated euglycemic and hypoglycemic fuel metabolism in patients with insulin-dependent diabetes mellitus. *J Clin Endocrinol Metab* 81:1083–1089, 1996

21. Potes CS, Turek VF, Cole RL, Vu C, Roland BL, Roth JD, Riediger T, Lutz TA: Noradrenergic neurons of the area postrema mediate amylin's hypophagic action. *Am J Physiol Regul Integr Comp Physiol* 299:R623–R631, 2010

22. Chapman I, Parker B, Doran S, Feinle-Bisset C, Wishart J, Strobel S, Wang Y, Burns C, Lush C, Weyer C, Horowitz M: Effect of pramlintide on satiety and food intake in obese subjects and subjects with type 2 diabetes. *Diabetologia* 48:838–848, 2005

23. Weyer C, Gottlieb A, Kim DD, Lutz K, Schwartz S, Gutierrez M, Wang Y, Ruggles JA, Kolterman OG, Maggs DG: Pramlintide reduces postprandial glucose excursions when added to regular insulin or insulin lispro in subjects with type 1 diabetes: a dose-timing study. *Diabetes Care* 26:3074–3079, 2003

24. Levetan C, Want LL, Weyer C, Strobel SA, Crean J, Wang Y, Maggs DG, Kolterman OG, Chandran M, Mudaliar SR, Henry RR: Impact of pramlintide on glucose fluctuations and postprandial glucose, glucagon, and triglyceride excursions among patients with type 1 diabetes intensively treated with insulin pumps. *Diabetes Care* 26:1–8, 2003

25. Karl D, Philis-Tsimikas A, Darsow T, Lorenzi G, Kellmeyer T, Lutz K, Wang Y, Frias JP: Pramlintide as an adjunct to insulin in patients with type 2 diabetes in a clinical practice setting reduced A1C, postprandial glucose excursions, and weight. *Diabetes Technol Ther* 9:191–199, 2007

26. Edelman SV, Darsow T, Frias JP: Pramlintide in the treatment of diabetes. *Int J Clin Pract* 60:1647–1653, 2006

27. Maggs DG, Fineman M, Kornstein J, Burrell T, Schwartz S, Wang Y, Ruggles JA, Kolterman OG, Weyer C: Pramlintide reduces postprandial glucose excursions when added to insulin lispro in subjects with type 2 diabetes: a dose-timing study. *Diabetes Metab Res Rev* 20:55–60, 2004

28. Whitehouse F, Kruger DF, Fineman M, Shen L, Ruggles JA, Maggs DG, Weyer C, Kolterman OG: A randomized study and open-label extension evaluating the long-term efficacy of pramlintide as an adjunct to insulin therapy in type 1 diabetes. *Diabetes Care* 25:724–730, 2002

29. Ratner RE, Want LL, Fineman MS, Velte MJ, Ruggles JA, Gottlieb A, Weyer C, Kolterman OG: Adjunctive therapy with the amylin analogue pramlintide leads to a combined improvement in glycemic and weight control in insulin-treated subjects with type 2 diabetes. *Diabetes Technol Ther* 4:51–61, 2002
30. Hollander PA, Levy P, Fineman MS, Maggs DG, Shen LZ, Strobel SA, Weyer C, Kolterman OG: Pramlintide as an adjunct to insulin therapy improves long-term glycemic and weight control in patients with type 2 diabetes: a 1-year randomized controlled trial. *Diabetes Care* 26:784–790, 2003
31. Ratner RE, Dickey R, Fineman M, Maggs DG, Shen L, Strobel SA, Weyer C, Kolterman OG: Amylin replacement with pramlintide as an adjunct to insulin therapy improves long-term glycaemic and weight control in type 1 diabetes mellitus: a 1-year, randomized controlled trial. *Diabet Med* 21:1204–1212, 2004
32. Diabetes Control and Complications Trial Research Group: The effect of intensive treatment of diabetes on the development and progression of long-term complications in insulin-dependent diabetes mellitus. *N Engl J Med* 329:977–986, 1993
33. Edelman S, Garg S, Frias J, Maggs D, Wang Y, Zhang B, Strobel S, Lutz K, Kolterman O: A double-blind, placebo-controlled trial assessing pramlintide treatment in the setting of intensive insulin therapy in type 1 diabetes. *Diabetes Care* 29:2189–2195, 2006
34. Kishiyama CM, Burdick PL, Cobry EC, Gage VL, Messer LH, McFann K, Chase HP: A pilot trial of pramlintide home usage in adolescents with type 1 diabetes. *Pediatrics* 124:1344–1347, 2009
35. Chase HP, Lutz K, Pencek R, Zhang B, Porter L: Pramlintide lowered glucose excursions and was well-tolerated in adolescents with type 1 diabetes: results from a randomized, single-blind, placebo-controlled, crossover study. *J Pediatr* 155:369–373, 2009
36. Hassan K, Heptulla RA: Reducing postprandial hyperglycemia with adjuvant premeal pramlintide and postmeal insulin in children with type 1 diabetes mellitus. *Pediatr Diabetes* 10:264–268, 2009
37. Raman VS, Mason KJ, Rodriguez LM, Hassan K, Yu X, Bomgaars L, Heptulla RA: The role of adjunctive exenatide therapy in pediatric type 1 diabetes. *Diabetes Care* 33:1294–1296, 2010
38. Hovorka R, Kumareswaran K, Harris J, Allen JM, Elleri D, Xing D, Kollman C, Nodale M, Murphy HR, Dunger DB, Amiel SA, Heller SR, Wilinska ME, Evans ML: Overnight closed loop insulin delivery (artificial pancreas) in adults with type 1 diabetes: crossover randomised controlled studies. *BMJ* 342:d1855, 2011
39. Huffman DM, McLean GW, Seagrove MA: Continuous subcutaneous pramlintide infusion therapy in patients with type 1 diabetes: observations from a pilot study. *Endocr Pract* 15:689–695, 2009
40. Heptulla RA, Rodriguez LM, Mason KJ, Haymond MW: Twenty-four-hour simultaneous subcutaneous Basal-bolus administration of insulin and amylin in adolescents with type 1 diabetes decreases postprandial hyperglycemia. *J Clin Endocrinol Metab* 94:1608–1611, 2009

41. Weyer C, Fineman MS, Strobel S, Shen L, Data J, Kolterman OG, Sylvestri MF: Properties of pramlintide and insulin upon mixing. *Am J Health Syst Pharm* 62:816–822, 2005

42. Nauck MA, Homberger E, Siegel EG, Allen RC, Eaton RP, Ebert R, Creutzfeldt W: Incretin effects of increasing glucose loads in man calculated from venous insulin and C-peptide responses. *J Clin Endocrinol Metab* 63:492–498, 1986

43. Hare KJ, Knop FK: Incretin-based therapy and type 2 diabetes. *Vitam Horm* 84:389–413, 2010

44. Hare KJ, Vilsbøll T, Holst JJ, Knop FK: Inappropriate glucagon response after oral compared with isoglycemic intravenous glucose administration in patients with type 1 diabetes. *Am J Physiol Endocrinol Metab* 298:E832–E837, 2010

45. Kielgast U, Krarup T, Holst JJ, Madsbad S: Four weeks of treatment with liraglutide reduces insulin dose without loss of glycemic control in type 1 diabetic patients with and without residual beta-cell function. *Diabetes Care* 34:1463–1468, 2011

46. Varanasi A, Bellini N, Rawal D, Vora M, Makdissi A, Dhindsa S, Chaudhuri A, Dandona P: Liraglutide as additional treatment for type 1 diabetes. *Eur J Endocrinol* 165:77–84, 2011

47. Nauck MA: Incretin-based therapies for type 2 diabetes mellitus: properties, functions, and clinical implications. *Am J Med* 124 (Suppl. 1):S3–S18, 2011

48. Ellis SL, Moser EG, Snell-Bergeon JK, Rodionova AS, Hazenfield RM, Garg SK: Effect of sitagliptin on glucose control in adult patients with type 1 diabetes: a pilot, double-blind, randomized, crossover trial. *Diabet Med* 28:1176–1181, 2011

49. Standards of medical care in diabetes: 2012. *Diabetes Care* 35 (Suppl. 1):S11–S63, 2012

50. Abdelghaffar S, Attia AM: Metformin added to insulin therapy for type 1 diabetes mellitus in adolescents. *Cochrane Database Syst Rev* CD006691, 2009

51. Vella S, Buetow L, Royle P, Livingstone S, Colhoun HM, Petrie JR: The use of metformin in type 1 diabetes: a systematic review of efficacy. *Diabetologia* 53:809–820, 2010

52. Lund SS, Tarnow L, Astrup AS, Hovind P, Jacobsen PK, Alibegovic AC, Parving I, Pietraszek L, Frandsen M, Rossing P, Parving HH, Vaag AA: Effect of adjunct metformin treatment in patients with type-1 diabetes and persistent inadequate glycaemic control. A randomized study. *PLoS One* 3:e3363, 2008

53. Oral EA, Chan JL: Rationale for leptin-replacement therapy for severe lipodystrophy. *Endocr Pract* 16:324–333, 2010

54. Fujikawa T, Chuang JC, Sakata I, Ramadori G, Coppari R: Leptin therapy improves insulin-deficient type 1 diabetes by CNS-dependent mechanisms in mice. *Proc Natl Acad Sci U S A* 107:17391–17396, 2010

55. Wang MY, Chen L, Clark GO, Lee Y, Stevens RD, Ilkayeva OR, Wenner BR, Bain JR, Charron MJ, Newgard CB, Unger RH: Leptin therapy in insulin-deficient type I diabetes. *Proc Natl Acad Sci U S A* 107:4813–4819, 2010

56. Marx N, Walcher D, Raichle C, Aleksic M, Bach H, Grüb M, Hombach V, Libby P, Zieske A, Homma S, Strong J: C-peptide colocalizes with macrophages in early arteriosclerotic lesions of diabetic subjects and induces monocyte chemotaxis in vitro. *Arterioscler Thromb Vasc Biol* 24:540–545, 2004
57. Zhang W, Kamiya H, Ekberg K, Wahren J, Sima AA: C-peptide improves neuropathy in type 1 diabetic BB/Wor-rats. *Diabetes Metab Res Rev* 23:63–70, 2007
58. Sima AA, Zhang W, Sugimoto K, Henry D, Li Z, Wahren J, Grunberger G: C-peptide prevents and improves chronic type I diabetic polyneuropathy in the BB/Wor rat. *Diabetologia* 44:889–897, 2001
59. Samnegard B, Jacobson SH, Jaremko G, Johansson BL, Ekberg K, Isaksson B, Eriksson L, Wahren J, Sjöquist M: C-peptide prevents glomerular hypertrophy and mesangial matrix expansion in diabetic rats. *Nephrol Dial Transplant* 20:532–538, 2005
60. Maezawa Y, Yokote K, Sonezaki K, Fujimoto M, Kobayashi K, Kawamura H, Tokuyama T, Takemoto M, Ueda S, Kuwaki T, Mori S, Wahren J, Saito Y: Influence of C-peptide on early glomerular changes in diabetic mice. *Diabetes Metab Res Rev* 22:313–322, 2006
61. Ekberg K, Brismar T, Johansson BL, Lindström P, Juntti-Berggren L, Norrby A, Berne C, Arnqvist HJ, Bolinder J, Wahren J: C-peptide replacement therapy and sensory nerve function in type 1 diabetic neuropathy. *Diabetes Care* 30:71–76, 2007
62. Ekberg K, Brismar T, Johansson BL, Jonsson B, Lindström P, Wahren J: Amelioration of sensory nerve dysfunction by C-Peptide in patients with type 1 diabetes. *Diabetes* 52:536–541, 2003
63. Wahren J, Kallas A, Sima AA: The clinical potential of C-Peptide replacement in type 1 diabetes. *Diabetes* 61:761–772, 2012
64. Garg SK, Ritchie PJ, Moser EG, Snell-Bergeon JK, Freson BJ, Hazenfield RM: Effects of colesevelam on LDL-C, A1c and GLP-1 levels in patients with type 1 diabetes: a pilot randomized double-blind trial. *Diabetes Obes Metab* 13:137–143, 2011
65. Rabasa-Lhoret R, Burelle Y, Ducros F, Bourque J, Lavoie C, Massicotte D, Péronnet F, Chiasson JL: Use of an alpha-glucosidase inhibitor to maintain glucose homoeostasis during postprandial exercise in intensively treated type 1 diabetic subjects. *Diabet Med* 18:739–744, 2001
66. Kawano Y, Irie J, Nakatani H, Yamada S: Pioglitazone might prevent the progression of slowly progressive type 1 diabetes. *Intern Med* 48:1037–1039, 2009

14

Hypoglycemia

Elizabeth R. Seaquist, MD, and William L. Clarke, MD

INTRODUCTION

People of all ages with type 1 diabetes (T1D) are at risk for hypoglycemia. The severity of hypoglycemia varies from the generation of classic symptoms to a loss of consciousness. Hypoglycemic symptoms differ within and across individuals and are influenced by therapeutic, biologic, and behavioral factors. Hypoglycemia unawareness may occur at any age. Infants and toddlers are unable to express the early symptoms of low blood glucose (BG) they may be experiencing. Older individuals who are attempting to achieve near-normal glycemic control are also at increased risk of hypoglycemia and often develop hypoglycemia unawareness. Hypoglycemia has been considered the limiting factor to the achievement of normal BG and A1C levels even with currently available designer insulins and advanced diabetes technologies. This chapter reviews the physiology of glucose counterregulation and its impairment in T1D and advanced type 2 diabetes that requires insulin for treatment. We will review the following aspects of hypoglycemia: counterregulation, causes, approaches to treatment, complications associated with its occurrence, and prevention in both the pediatric and adult populations with T1D, distinguishing between the different age groups. This chapter concludes with future directions for clinical research.

DEFINITION

Hypoglycemia is defined by the ADA Workgroup on Hypoglycemia as BG <70 mg/dl and severe hypoglycemia (SH) as loss of consciousness or inability to self-treat to raise BG.[1]

COUNTERREGULATION

In response to falling BG, humans have developed a redundant series of compensatory responses that serve to restore BG to normal.[2] When BG falls below ~85 mg/dl, a reduction in insulin secretion from the β-cell occurs to maintain normoglycemia (Fig. 14.1). If BG continues to fall to <70 mg/dl, hypoglycemia-induced glucagon secretion from the pancreatic α-cell secretion ensues. In patients with T1D, neither of these two lines of defense is operative. First, a reduction in insulin secretion cannot occur because the β-cells have been destroyed by the autoimmune process that led to the disease. Second, hypoglycemia-induced glucagon secretion also fails to occur, most likely because a reduction in the insulin concentration released in a paracrine fashion from the β-cell, which does not occur in T1D, is required to trigger this response.[3]

DOI: 10.2337/9781580404785ch14

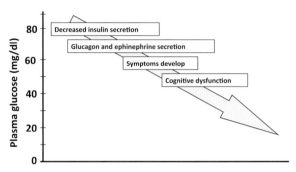

Figure 14.1 Neuroendocrine responses to hypoglycemia

NEUROGENIC AND NEUROGLYCOPENIC SYMPTOMS

Because hypoglycemia-induced glucagon secretion fails to occur, patients with T1D must depend on an increase in adrenomedullary epinephrine secretion and activation of the sympathetic nervous system to detect a fall in BG.[3,4] This counter-regulatory response produces neurogenic symptoms, such as pounding heart, trembling, sweating, tingling, nervousness, and anxiety. Neuroglycopenia occurs when the brain has inadequate fuel to maintain normal function and results in symptoms, such a blurred vision, difficulty concentrating, confused thinking, slurred speech, numbness, drowsiness, seizures, coma, and death.[2] Commonly occurring neurogenic and neuroglycopenic symptoms are listed in Table 14.1.

The BG threshold for neurogenic and neuroglycopenic symptoms may differ between children and adults.[5] Children with T1D may counterregulate at a higher BG than adults,[6] and thus their low BG symptoms may occur with normal BG. It has been shown, however, that epinephrine responses to hypoglycemia occurring during the night while asleep are blunted in both adolescents with T1D and adolescents who are control subjects, thereby increasing the risk for SH.[7] Symptoms of low BG in children have been difficult to assess with confidence, but behavioral disturbances appear to be more significant signals of low BG in children than in adults.[8] The frequency of occurrence of SH in both children and adults is shown in Table 14.2.

It has been estimated that that the average person with T1D will experience two symptomatic hypoglycemic events each week and that asymptomatic or nocturnal hypoglycemia may be much more common.[9] Indeed continuous glucose monitoring of children with T1D has identified low BG (<50 mg/dl) occurring up to 35% of nights with durations of up to 2 h.[10–12] Most of these events were asymptomatic.

CAUSES OF HYPOGLYCEMIA

All hypoglycemia is the result of a mismatch between insulin, food, and physical activity. This mismatch can be the result of therapeutic, biologic, and behavioral factors (Table 14.3). Effective diabetes treatment results from the right balance of insulin, diet, and exercise. Prospective field studies of adults

Table 14.1 Hypoglycemic Symptoms

Adrenergic Symptoms	Neuroglycopenic Symptoms
Trembling or Shaking	Slow Thinking
Sweating	Blurred Vision
Pounding Heart	Slurred Speech
Rapid Pulse	Incoordination
Changes in Temperature	Numbness
Tingling in Extremities	Difficulty Concentrating
Heavy Breathing	Dizziness
	Fatigue or Sleepiness
	Loss of Consciousness
	Seizure
	Death

Unknown Etiology

Hunger

Weakness

Headache

Nausea

Mood Changes

Feeling of Something Not Right

with T1D have confirmed that the occurrence of low BG can be predicted by regression models that utilize the variables of more insulin, less food, and more exercise.[13] Insulin analogs, including lispro, glargine, and detemir have each been shown to be associated with significant reductions in the frequency of low BG when compared with NPH-based insulin regimens.[14–17] This may be because near physiological insulin replacement is possible with insulin analogs, or it may be due to intrinsic differences between insulins. These results have been demonstrated for both adults and children with T1D. The route of insulin administration also is associated with differences in the frequency of hypoglycemia. Continuous subcutaneous insulin infusion systems (insulin pumps) reduce the risk of hypoglycemia for adults and for children,[18,19] and intraperitoneal insulin delivery reduces the occurrence of SH compared to continuous subcutaneous insulin infusion.[20]

Exercise has both immediate and long-term effects on glycemia. Studies in children with T1D have shown that as little as one hour of afternoon exercise led the to occurrence of nocturnal hypoglycemia in nearly half of the children studied.[21] Antecedent low BG reduces the counterregulatory response to

Table 14.2 Event Rates for SH in Patients with T1D (Episodes/100 patient years)

Study (author)	Year	N	Rate	Reference
PEDIATRICS				
Rewers	2002	1243	19	22
Hvidoere	2007	2100	27	—
O'Connell	2011	1683	5.6	24
Katz	2012	255	37.6	25
PEDIATRICS/ADULTS				
DCCT	1993	711	62	26
EDIC Conventional	2005	606	39.6	27
EDIC Intensive	2005	620	48.4	27
JDRF CGM	2011	436	17.9	28
ADULTS				
UK Hypoglycemia	2007	57	320	29
Donnelly	2005	94	115	30

Notes: DCCT = Diabetes Control and Complications Trial; EDIC = Epidemiology of Diabetes Interventions and Complications; CGM = continuous glucose monitoring

subsequent euglycemic exercise, and exercise itself reduces glucose counter-regulation for at least 24 h regardless of its effect on BG.[31,32] (See chapter 11, Exercise.)

Biologic factors that may be precursors to low BG include insulin sensitivity, low BG itself, and comorbid conditions and their treatments. In addition, the presence of residual C-peptide is associated with reduced risk of SH. Sensitivity to the glucose-lowering effects of subcutaneous insulin varies between individuals based not only on weight but also on age and duration of disease. Comorbid conditions such as celiac disease, gastroparesis, inflammatory bowel disorders, or thyroid disease can affect the absorption of carbohydrates and other nutrients from the gastrointestinal tract and predispose individuals to variable glucose levels. Diseases that impair glucose counterregulation like adrenal and growth hormone insufficiency or that disrupt gluconeogenesis and glycogenolysis like liver and kidney failure may rarely present as hypoglycemia. Medications such as metaclopramide or acarbose may also affect nutrient absorption, the threshold for glucose counterregulation, or the perception or ability to effectively respond to low BG symptoms. The elderly may have biologic risk factors, such as irregular eating habits, dementia, and changes in drug

Table 14.3 Causes of SH

Therapy Associated

Insulin – types and routes of delivery (e.g., giving wrong insulin type [glargine instead of lispro] or intramuscular injection)

Food – carbohydrates versus fats, liquids versus solids

Exercise – intensity, duration, time of day

Mismatch of insulin, food, and exercise

Biologic Factors

Insulin sensitivity

Low BG – altered physiologic responses and symptom intensity

Failure of glucose counterregulation – disease duration, time of day, recurrent hypoglycemia

Comorbidities and the drugs used to treat them

Gastrointestinal illness

Behavioral Factors

Reduced awareness of low BG

Symptom awareness

Low BG detection

Judgment to treat

Treatment choices

---

absorption, distribution, metabolism, and clearance, which are different from those of younger adults.[33,34] In addition, age and duration of insulin use have been shown to be predictors of SH in this group, as have potentially nondiabetes-related comorbidities, such as reduced glomerular filtration rate (GFR) and peripheral neuropathies.[34]

Behavioral factors, such as symptom awareness, low BG detection, judgment to treat, and treatment choices themselves, can be causes of SH. Symptom awareness is usually idiosyncratic and can be influenced by a variety of factors, including competing circumstances, illness, fatigue, and the use of alcohol, caffeine, or medications, such as β-blockers.[35] Even when low BG symptoms are perceived, a significant number of individuals with T1D fail to detect or recognize that their BG is low.[36] The causes of this failure to detect low BG include misattribution of symptoms, lack of knowledge about symptoms, inaccurate symptom beliefs, and denial. Deciding whether to immediately treat a detected low BG involves an assessment of the current risk associated with low BG as well as previous experience tolerating different degrees of low BG.[35] The decision not to treat a detected low BG may be based on the conclusion that immediate treatment might prove either embarrassing or inconvenient.

TREATMENT

Low BG should be treated at the first sign or symptom with rapid-acting carbohydrates (Table 14.4). A good rule of thumb is that 1 g of glucose will raise the BG level by 3 mg/dl. To avoid overcorrecting low BG and becoming hyperglycemic, patients should correct their BG with enough grams of glucose to raise their BG to 100 mg/dl. In practical terms, it may be easier to advise patients and their caregivers to administer 15 g of carbohydrate for a BG <70 mg/dl with symptoms of hypoglycemia and then wait 15 min before rechecking the BG to determine whether another 15 g of carbohydrate should be given. Complex carbohydrates and foods that contain fats along with glucose should be discouraged because fats often slow the absorption of carbohydrates from the gastrointestinal tract (Table 14.5). In field studies of subjects with and without a history of recurrent SH, it has been shown that subjects with recurrent SH are less likely to treat their low BG with a rapid-acting carbohydrate and are more likely to use foods that do not raise BG quickly.[37]

Table 14.4(a) Treatment of Mild to Moderate Hypoglycemia (15–20 grams of rapid-acting carbohydrate)

Source	Quantity
Glucose Tablets	3–4
Lifesavers	8–10
Airheads	10
Brach's Hard Candies	8–10
Raisins	2 tbsp
Regular Soft Drinks	4–6 oz
Fruit Juice	4–6oz
No- or Low-Fat Milk	8 oz

Table 14.4(b) Treatment of SH (loss of consciousness, seizure, coma, inability to consume oral agents)

Glucagon Emergency Kit –

	10–30 mcg/kg body weight intramuscularly or
	0.5 mg for ages <12 years
	1.0 mg for age >12 years

Table 14.5 Poor Choices for Emergency Treatment of Low BG

Ice Cream	Milkshake	Pizza
Doughnuts	Candy Bars	Nuts
Pies, Cakes	Cheese	Potatoes
French Fries	Cookie Dough	Chips
Meats		

Persons experiencing SH should always be treated with intramuscular glucagon or, when located in a medical setting, a bolus of intravenous (IV) glucose (Table 14.4). During SH, a person will be unable to treat themselves, so their care providers must be instructed on how and when to give glucagon. Glucagon should be available for trained support individuals (e.g., family member, roommate, coworker) to administer during SH events. In addition, care providers should always carry a glucagon kit with them or have ready access to this medication. Low-dose glucagon administration using the rather simple algorithm shown in Table 14.6 has been used successfully in children who are ill or unable to consume sufficient amounts of rapid-acting carbohydrates to raise and maintain their BG in a euglycemic range.[38] (See chapter 18.II for glucose safety at school.)

COMPLICATIONS

One of the most feared complications of hypoglycemia is that it will impair an individual's ability to detect a subsequent episode of hypoglycemia. It has been well documented that the occurrence of a single BG <70mg/dl will shift the glucose level at which the counterregulatory response is triggered to a lower

Table 14.6 Minidose Glucagon Treatment of Mild to Moderate Hypoglycemia

1) Mix glucagon vial as per printed instructions
2) Determine dose based on age
3) Administer glucagon dose subcutaneously
4) Measure BG every 30 min for 1 h, and then every hour
5) If in 30 min, BG has not risen, administer a double dose and recheck BG in 30 min

Age	Units on Insulin Syringe
<2 years	2 units
2–15 years	1 unit per year of age
>15 years	15 units (maximum dose)

glucose level for many days.[4,39] As a result, a patient must drop to a lower glucose level before the counterregulatory response is activated. Unfortunately, the glucose level at which neuroglycopenia develops during subsequent hypoglycemia is not affected by a single episode of low BG, meaning that patients with frequent hypoglycemia may find that their first symptoms of hypoglycemia are those associated with neuroglycopenia. The magnitude of the hormonal counterregulatory response is also reduced by a previous episode of hypoglycemia. Interestingly, patients with T1D and hypoglycemia unawareness appear to have different patterns of cerebral activation during hypoglycemia than do patients with T1D who develop symptoms with hypoglycemia, suggesting that recurrent hypoglycemia leads to an alteration in the way the brain detects and responds to hypoglycemia.[40] Fortunately, hypoglycemia unawareness can be ameliorated by the strict avoidance of hypoglycemia for several weeks.[41]

COGNITIVE DYSFUNCTION

During acute hypoglycemia, many patients experience the temporary disruption of cognitive functioning.[42,43] Whether or not there is a long-lasting association between hypoglycemia and cognitive function remains unclear. Recent studies of adults with a long history of T1D have shown a slowing of mental speed, motor speed, and flexibility. A meta-analysis of 33 studies comparing cognition in adults with and without T1D has shown significantly lower intelligence, speed of information processing, psychomotor efficiency, visual and sustained attention, cognitive flexibility, and visual perception in the T1D subjects.[44] These findings were associated with the presence of microvascular complications and an indirect measure of persistent hyperglycemia, but not with the occurrence of SH episodes or poor metabolic control. The 18-year follow-up of the Diabetes Control and Complications Trial cohort also failed to show an association between decrements in learning, memory, spatial information processing, and psychomotor efficiency and SH.[45] Another study of adults with T1D with and without exposure to SH as young children (<10 years old) has shown decreased problem solving, verbal function, and psychomotor efficiency in those with the history of SH.[46] Exposure to SH has been associated with increased hippocampal volumes in children with T1D, which has been hypothesized to represent a pathological response to recurrent hypoglycemia.[47] Thus, the impact of hypoglycemia on long-term cognitive function is probably small and dependent in part on the patient's age at the time of the hypoglycemia. Nevertheless, it does have the potential to influence the performance of everyday activities, including treatment decisions that could increase the frequency of hypoglycemia.

FEAR OF HYPOGLYCEMIA

Fear of hypoglycemia is common among adults and children with T1D and not unsurprisingly among parents of children with T1D.[48,49] Fear of hypoglycemia is most commonly assessed using the Hypoglycemia Fear Survey (HFS), an instrument that has been well validated and shown to have test–retest reliability and internal consistency.[50] The HFS has two subscales: Worry and Behavior. Worry scores are associated with a history of SH and with the number of symptoms associated with mild hypoglycemia and Behavior scores are associated with elevated BG levels and poorer glucose control. The HFS has been shown to be reliable for adults, adolescents, and children as young as 6 to 8 years of age.[51] Detection of low BG by children (ages 6 to 11 years) and their parents is poor, with both groups making clinically significant errors as frequently as clinically accurate assessments. Thus, it is not surprising that parents and children have higher levels of fear of hypoglycemia than adults with T1D.[48,49,52] Fear is related to both trait and state anxiety, and significant evidence demonstrates its impact on diabetes management, metabolic control, and health outcomes.[48,49,51]

PREVENTING HYPOGLYCEMIA

Because a variety of causes or pathways can lead to SH, individuals also have a variety of different ways to reduce the risk of its occurrence (Table 14.7).

Clearly, avoiding low BG (<70mg/dl) is critical to preventing SH and to restoring the adrenomedullary response to hypoglycemia in persons with hypoglycemia-associated autonomic failure (HAAF). But this syndrome is one of several pathways to SH. Preventing hypoglycemia involves patient education, self-examination of the treatment regimen, and the courage to alter usual self-management practices or lifestyle. Health care professionals need to listen carefully to their patients' description of their hypoglycemic episodes and to ask questions about events preceding and surrounding the episode to identify the causes of the episode. They also need to educate their patients as to how future episodes might be prevented and encourage them to take steps to reduce their

---

Table 14.7 Preventing Recurrent Hypoglycemia

Assess Problems with Hypoglycemia by Patient Interview

Review Comorbid Conditions and Medications

Review SBGM and CGM Data

Review Treatment Regimen

    Assess Insulin Peaks – Timing, Delivery System

    Assess Meal-Related BG Peaks

    Assess Timing, Duration, and Intensity of Exercise

Identify Personal Symptoms of Low BG

Identify Factors Competing for Low BG Detection

Identify Barriers to Immediate Treatment of Low BG

Review Low-BG Treatment Choices

Negotiate Changes Identified to Reduce Risk

vulnerability to SH. Each and every occurrence of low BG has the potential to be a learning experience.

Preventing nocturnal hypoglycemia, particularly after a day of exercise, has been the focus of much research. The fat content of a bedtime snack does not seem to alter overnight glycemia in active children with T1D.[53] Some studies have demonstrated that the addition of uncooked cornstarch to a bedtime snack can significantly reduce nighttime and morning hypoglycemia in this population.[54] The response of nonexercising adults with T1D to a bedtime snack containing uncooked cornstarch may be different. In a controlled laboratory setting, overnight glycemia after ingestion of a bedtime snack containing uncooked cornstarch was the same as it was after having no snack in such adults.[55] Future investigation will be necessary to see whether uncooked cornstarch as part of a bedtime snack prevents nocturnal hypoglycemia only after exercise or only in children.

Bedtime administration of the β-agonist terbutaline has been found to prevent nocturnal hypoglycemia in patients with diabetes, but at the cost of morning hyperglycemia.[55] Although this effect may be dose dependent,[56] a large trial demonstrating efficacy has not yet been done.

GLUCOSE MONITORING

Glucose monitoring, using either traditional self-BG-monitoring (SBGM) systems or newer continuous glucose sensor technology is an essential tool for the prevention of low BG. Studies have shown that the frequency of SBGM testing is inversely related to the occurrence of low BG and SH in individuals with T1D.[57] Patients need to be encouraged to measure their BG not just when they feel poorly but at other times of the day, including before and after meals; before, after, and during prolonged intense exercise; before retiring for sleep; and in the middle of the night during a day in which vigorous exercise occurred. Frequent BG should also accompany any change in routine, including changes in insulin delivery systems or insulin doses, meal times, activity level, work schedules, or travel across time zones. Such carefully collected BG data forms the basis for beginning to assist the patient in preventing SH.

Continuous glucose monitoring has been shown to be a valuable addition to SBGM in identifying times of day when low BG is most likely to occur. Although these systems are less accurate in the hypoglycemic range (<70mg/dl) than in either the euglycemic or hyperglycemic range, their use has been associated with a reduction in time spent with low BG, even in the absence of specific instructions as to how to modify insulin, food, or exercise in response to the information displayed.[58] Of particular importance has been the documentation that a significant number of children with T1D experience prolonged periods of unrecognized low BG during the night and that the suspension of insulin delivered by continuous subcutaneous infusion pumps for up to 2 h at the first sign of impending hypoglycemia can reduce the frequency of low BG without precipitating serious hyperglycemia.[59]

Armed with BG information, health care professionals and their patients can work together to review how the individual's insulin regimen and meal choices affect their risk for SH. (See chapters 12 and 10 for in-depth discussions of insulin and nutrition, respectively.) Such information also can be used to direct adjustments in insulin delivery and food choices for anticipated or unplanned exercise. Specific algorithms based on the timing, duration, intensity, and pre-exercise BG level have been developed to assist with these decisions (see chapter 11, Exercise).

Preventing SH involves more than educating the patient about how the treatment regimen affects his or her BG levels. Psychobehavioral factors, such as symptom awareness, low BG detection, judgment to treat, and self-treatment behaviors are critical to preventing SH, especially when unanticipated low BG occurs. Blood Glucose Awareness Training (BGAT) is an eight-week biobehavioral intervention designed to improve the accuracy of BG detection and includes group sessions on insulin, diet, exercise, moods, low and high BG–associated symptoms, and symptom perception as well as daily self-monitoring exercises.[60] BGAT has been shown to improve the accuracy of BG detection, reduce the frequency of low BG, and reduce nocturnal hypoglycemia without causing an increase in overall glucose control as measured by A1C. BGAT has been shown to be effective for subjects with T1D who have reduced awareness of hypoglycemia as well as those who have normal awareness and those with defective glucose counterregulation. But BGAT is effective only when it includes both treatment and psychobehavioral content.[61] Neither alone are sufficient to produce the results described earlier. This suggests that in addition to educating patients regarding the importance of balancing insulin, food, and exercise to reduce the risk of SH, they need to be guided to identify their personal symptoms (warning cues) of low BG, to recognize and affirm when those symptoms are occurring, to treat symptoms immediately regardless of any potential personal embarrassment or inconvenience, and to treat each occurrence with rapid-acting carbohydrates. An Internet version of BGAT has been pilot tested but is not as yet available for dissemination.[62]

FUTURE CLINICAL RESEARCH: FILLING THE GAPS

Hypoglycemia will continue to be a barrier to euglycemia in people with T1D as long as mismatches in insulin, diet, and exercise occur and there is inability to preserve residual β-cell function following the onset of T1D. Thus, research is being directed toward ways to better detect, predict, and alert patients regarding their immediate and future risk of hypoglycemia. Manufacturers of SBGM systems have been improving the accuracy of these devices especially in the low BG (<70mg/dl) range. Continuous glucose-monitoring systems currently include alarms that are activated when the glucose level has reached a preset threshold or is rapidly falling into the low range. Unfortunately, studies have shown that these alarms are often ignored or not recognized during sleep.[63]

The rapid development of the artificial pancreas,[64] in which continuous glucose monitoring is coupled with an insulin pump, has been the focus of much research (see chapter 9, Monitoring). Initial studies with closed-loop systems have demonstrated their superiority over open-loop systems in reducing the occurrence of nocturnal hypoglycemia and maintaining BG levels overnight in a euglycemic range.[65] Further progress has demonstrated that these systems can maintain euglycemia during afternoon ergometer exercise and throughout the following night.[65,66] One manufacturer has developed a product in which the continuous glucose monitoring is programmed to tell the pump to suspend insulin infusion when the interstitial glucose level is either at a preset low threshold or when low BG is predicted,[67] but this product is not available in all countries. At the time of this writing, studies are planned around the world to test the ability of such coupled systems to manage both fasting and postprandial glycemia.

As work on the artificial pancreas continues to evolve, it is probable that it will stimulate research and development in other areas of diabetes treatment. A specific example is the development of insulin analogs that are more rapidly absorbed than current rapid-acting insulins and whose peak action more closely coincides with that of postprandial glycemia. Such an improvement in matching may prevent postprandial hypoglycemia in some individuals. Closed-loop research with a bihormonal pump that can infuse both insulin and glucagon may encourage the development of a more stable and user-friendly glucagon product. Research efforts are focused on understanding why and how an episode of hypoglycemia leads to hypoglycemia unawareness, with the hope that new therapies will come from the insights gained from this work. Current research is focused on the role of the central nervous system in the detection of hypoglycemia and the coordination the hormone response that restores BG to normal following an episode of hypoglycemia..[22,68,69] Recent work, including experiments that have demonstrated that the defective counterregulation associated with HAAF can be prevented by opioid receptor blockade and that a six-week administration of a serotonin reuptake inhibitor can increase epinephrine and norepinephrine secretion to hypoglycemia[70,71] raise the possibility that new therapies will be developed to prevent and treat HAAF.

Until new therapies become available, health care professionals and their patients at risk for hypoglycemia must continue to focus on perfecting the balance between insulin, diet, and exercise and on identifying personal behavioral factors that may increase the risk of SH.

GAPS ACCORDING TO THE EDITORS

1. There are ongoing needs to prevent or reduce SH.
2. There is an ongoing need to preserve residual β-cell function.
3. There is a need for improved continuous glucose-monitoring systems with improved accuracy and effective alarms.
4. Ongoing research is needed to provide a closed-loop, artificial pancreas that will avoid SH.
5. Studies are needed to identify patients at greatest risk for SH and autonomic failure with approaches to reverse or prevent the defects.
6. There is a need to better understand "dead in bed" phenomenon.

REFERENCES

1. American Diabetes Association Workgroup on Hypoglycemia: Defining and reporting hypoglycemia in diabetes. *Diabetes Care* 28:1245–1249, 2005
2. Tesfaye N, Seaquist E: Neuroendocrine responses to hypoglycemia. *Ann N.Y. Acad Sci* 1212:12–28, 2010
3. Cooperberg B, Cryer P: Insulin reciprocally regulates glucagon secretion in humans. *Diabetes* 59:2936–2940, 2010
4. Cryer P: Hypoglycemia in type 1 diabetes mellitus. *Endocrinol Metab Clin N Am* 39:641–654, 2010
5. Clarke W, Gonder-Frederick L, Richards F, Cryer P: Multifactorial origin of hypoglycemic symptom unawareness in IDDM. *Diabetes* 40:680–685, 1991
6. Jones T, Boulware S, Kraemer D, Caprio S, Sherwin R, Tamborlane W: Independent effects of youth and poor diabetes control on responses to hypoglycemia in children. *Diabetes* 40:358–363, 1991
7. Jones T, Porter P, Sherwin R, Davis E, O'Leary P, Frazer F, Byrne G, Stick S, Tamborlane W: Decreased epinephrine responses to hypoglycemia during sleep. *New Engl J Med* 338:1657–1662, 1998
8. McCrimmon R, Gold A, Deary I, Kelnar C, Frier B: Symptoms of hypoglycemia in children with IDDM. *Diabetes Care* 18:858–861, 1995
9. Cryer P, Axelrod L, Grossman A, Heller S, Montori V, Seaquist E, Service F: Evaluation and management of adult hypoglycemic disorders: an endocrine society clinical practice guideline. *J Clin Endocrinol Metab* 94:709–728, 2009
10. Kaufman F, Austin J, Neinstein A, Jeng L, Halvorson M, Devoe D, Pitukcheewanont P: Nocturnal hypoglycemia detected with the continuous glucose monitoring system in pediatric patients with type 1 diabetes. *J Pediatr* 141:625–630, 2002
11. Amin R, Ross K, Acerini C, Edge J, Warner J, Dunger D: Hypoglycemia prevalence in prepubertal children with type 1 diabetes on standard insulin regimen: use of continuous glucose monitoring system. *Diabetes Care* 26:662–667, 2003
12. Juvenile Diabetes Research Foundation Continuous Glucose Monitoring Study Group 2010: Prolonged nocturnal hypoglycemia is common during 12 months of continuous glucose monitoring in children and adults with type 1 diabetes. *Diabetes Care* 33:1004–1008, 2010
13. Clarke W, Cox D, Gonder-Frederick L, Julian D, Kovatchev B, Young-Hyman D: Biopsychobehavioral model of risk of severe hypoglycemia-self-management behaviors. *Diabetes Care* 22:580–584, 1999
14. Pfutzner A, Kustner E, Forst B, Schulze-Schleppinghoff B, Trautmann M, Haslbeck M, Schatz H, Beyer J: Intensive insulin therapy with insulin lispro in patients with type 1 diabetes reduces the frequency of hypoglycemic episodes. *Exp Clin Endocrinol* 104:25–30, 1996
15. Standl E, Lang H, Roberts A: The 12-month efficacy and safety of insulin detemir and NPH insulin in basal-bolus therapy for the treatment of type 1 diabetes. *Diab Technol Ther* 6:579–588, 2004
16. Rosenstock J, Dailey G, Mass-Benedetti M, Fritsche A, Lin Z, Salzman A: Reduced hypoglycemia risk with insulin glargine. *Diabetes Care* 28:950–955, 2005

17. Alemzadeh R, Berhe T, Wyatt D: Flexible insulin therapy with glargine insulin improved glycemic control and reduced severe hypoglycemia among preschool-aged children with type 1 diabetes mellitus. *Pediatrics* 115:1320–1324, 2005
18. Fatourechi M, Kudva Y, Hassan Murad M, Elamin M, Tabini C, Montori V: Hypoglycemia with intensive insulin therapy: a systematic review and meta-analyses of randomized trials of continuous subcutaneous insulin infusion versus multiple daily injections. *J Clin Endocrinol Metab* 94:729–740, 2009
19. Bode B, Steed R, Davidson P: Reduction in severe hypoglycemia with long-term continuous subcutaneous insulin infusion in type 1 diabetes. *Diabetes Care* 19:324–327, 1996
20. Liebl A, Hoogma R, Renard E, Geelhoed-Duijvestijn P, Klein E, Diglas J, Kessler L, Melki V, Diem P, Brun J, Schaepelynck-Bélicar P, Frei T: A reduction in severe hypoglycaemia in type 1 diabetes in a randomized crossover study of continuous intraperitoneal compared with subcutaneous insulin infusion. *Diab, Obes and Metab* 11:1001–1008, 2009
21. The Diabetes Research in Children Network (DirecNet) Study Group: Impact of exercise on overnight glycemic control in children with type 1 diabetes mellitus. *J Pediatr* 147:528–534, 2005
22. Rewers A, Chase H, Mackenzie T, Walravens P, Roback M, Rewers M, Hamman R, Klingensmith G: Predictors of acute complications in children with type 1 diabetes. *JAMA* 287:2511–2518, 2002
23. De Beaufort C, Swift P, Skinner C, et al.: Continuing stability of center differences in pediatric diabetes care: do advances in diabetes treatment improve outcome? *Diabetes Care* 30:2245–2250, 2007
24. O'Connell S, Cooper M, Bulsara M, Davis E, Jones T: Reducing rates of severe hypoglycemia in a population-based cohort of children and adolescents with type 1 diabetes over the decade 2000–2009. *Diabetes Care* 34:2379–2380, 2011
25. Katz M, Volkening L, Anderson B, Laffel L: Contemporary rates of severe hypoglycemia in youth with type 1 diabetes: variability by insulin regimen. *Diabet Med* doi:10.1111/j.1464-5491, 2012
26. Diabetes Control and Complications Trial Research Group: The effect of intensive treatment of diabetes on the development and progression of long-term complications in insulin-dependent diabetes mellitus. *N Engl J Med* 329:977–986, 1993
27. Diabetes Control and Complications Trial/Epidemiology of Diabetes Interventions and Complications (DCCT/EDIC) Research Group: Modern day clinical course of type 1 diabetes mellitus after 30 years' duration. *Arch Intern Med* 169:1307–1316, 2009
28. Juvenile Diabetes Research Foundation: Continuous glucose monitoring study group. Factors predictive of severe hypoglycemia in type 1 diabetes. *Diabetes Care* 34:586–590, 2011
29. UK Hypoglycemia Study Group: Risk of hypoglycemia in types 1 and 2 diabetes; effects of treatment modalities and their duration. *Diabetologia* 50:1140–1147, 2007
30. Donnelly L, Morris A, Frier B, Ellis J, Donnan P, Durrant T, Band M, Reekie G, Leese G: Frequency and predictors of hypoglycaemia in type 1 and insulin-treated type 2 diabetes: a population-based study. *Diabet Med* 22:749–755, 2005

31. Galassetti P, Tate D, Neill R, Morrey S, Wasserman D, Davis S: Effect of antecedent hypoglycemia on counterregulatory responses to subsequent euglycemic exercise in type 1 diabetes. *Diabetes* 52:1761–1769, 2003

32. Cryer, P: Exercise-related hypoglycemia-associated autonomic failure in diabetes. *Diabetes* 58:1951–1952, 2009

33. Amiel S, Dixon T, Mann R, Jameson K: Hypoglycaemia in type 2 diabetes. *Diab Med* 25:245–254, 2008

34. Davis S, Mann S, Briscoe V, Ertl A, Tate D: Effects of intensive therapy and antecedent hypoglycemia on counterregulatory responses to hypoglycemia in type 2 diabetes. *Diabetes* 58:701–709, 2009

35. Gonder-Frederick L, Cox D, Kovatchev B, Schlundt D, Clarke W: A biopsychobehavioral model of risk of severe hypoglycemia. *Diabetes Care* 20:661–669, 1997

36. Cox D, Clarke W, Gonder-Frederick L, Pohl S, Hoover C, Snyder A, Zimbelman L, Carter W: Accuracy of perceiving blood glucose in IDDM patients. *Diabetes Care* 8:529–536, 1985

37. Cox D, Gonder-Frederick L, Kovatchev B, Young-Hyman D, Donner T, Julian D, Clarke W: Biopsychobehavioral model of severe hypoglycemia. II. Understanding the risk of severe hypoglycemia. *Diabetes Care* 22:2018–2025, 1999

38. Haymond M, Schreiner B: Mini-dose glucagon rescue for hypoglycemia in children with type 1 diabetes. *Diabetes Care* 24:643–645, 2001

39. Cryer, P: The barrier of hypoglycemia in diabetes. *Diabetes* 57:3169–3176, 2008

40. Dunn J, Cranston I, Marsden P, Amiel S, Reed L: Attenuation of amygdala and frontal cortical responses to low blood glucose concentration in symptomatic hypoglycemia in type 1 diabetes: a new player in hypoglycemia unawareness? *Diabetes* 56:2766–2773, 2007

41. Fanelli C, Pampanelli S, Epifano L, Rambotti A, DiVincenzo A, Modarelli F, Ciolfetta M, Lepore M, Annibale B, Torlone E, et al.: Long-term recovery from unawareness, deficient counterregulation and lack of cognitive dysfunction during hypoglycemia following institution of rational, intensive therapy in IDDM. *Diabetologia* 37:1265–1276, 1994

42. Gonder-Frederick L, Zrebiec J, Bauchowitz A, Ritterband L, Magee J, Cox D, Clarke W: Cognitive function is disrupted by both hypo-and hyperglycemia in school-aged children with type 1 diabetes: a field study. *Diabetes Care* 32:1001–1006, 2009

43. Strachan M, Deary I, Ewing F, Frier B: Recovery of cognitive function and mood after severe hypoglycemia in adults with insulin-treated diabetes. *Diabetes Care* 23:305–311, 2000

44. Brands A, Biessels G, de Haan E, Kappelle L, Kessels R: The effects of type 1 diabetes on cognitive performance. *Diabetes Care* 28:726–735, 2005

45. Jacobson A, Ryan C, Cleary P, Waberski B, Weinger K, Musen G, Dahms W, DCCT/EDIC Research Group: Biomedical risk factors for decreased cognitive functioning in type 1 diabetes: an 18 year follow-up of the Diabetes Control and Complications Trial (DCCT) cohort. *Diabetologia* 29:1883–1889, 2010

46. Asvold B, Sand T, Hestad K, Bjorgaas M: Cognitive function in type 1 diabetic adults with early exposure to severe hypoglycemia. *Diabetes Care* 33:1945–1947, 2010

47. Hershey T, Perantie D, Wu J, Weaver P, Black K, White N: Hippocampal volumes in youth with type 1 diabetes. *Diabetes* 59:236–241, 2010
48. Gonder-Frederick L, Fisher C, Ritterband L, Cox D, Hou L, DasGupta A, Clarke W: Predictors of fear of hypoglycemia in adolescents with type 1 diabetes and their parents. *Ped Diab* 7:215–222, 2006
49. Wild D, von Maltzah R, Brohan E, Christensen T, Clauson P, Gonder-Frederick L: A critical review of the literature on fear of hypoglycemia in diabetes: implications for diabetes management and patient education. *Patient Education and Counseling* 68:10–15, 2007
50. Gonder-Frederick L, Schmidt K, Vajda K, Greear M, Singh H, Shepard J, Cox D: Psychometric properties of the Hypoglycemia Fear Survey-II for adults with type 1 diabetes. *Diabetes Care* 34:801–806, 2011
51. Gonder-Frederick L, Nyer M, Shepard J, Vajda K, Clarke W: Assessing fear of hypoglycemia in children with type 1 diabetes and their parents. *Diabetes Manage* 1:627–639, 2011
52. Clarke W, Gonder-Frederick L, Snyder A, Cox D: Maternal fear of hypoglycemia in their children with insulin dependent diabetes mellitus. *J Ped Endocrinol & Metab* 11:189–194, 1998
53. Wilson D, Chase P, Kollman C, Xing D, Caswell K, Tansley M, Fox L, Weinzimer S, Beck R, Ruedy K, Tamborlane W: Low-fat vs high-fat bedtime snacks in children and adolescents with type 1 diabetes. *Pediatric Diabetes* 9:320–325, 2008
54. Kaufman F, Halvorson M, Kaufman N: A randomized, blinded trial of uncooked cornstarch to diminish nocturnal hypoglycemia at diabetes camp. *Diab Res Clin Prac* 30: 205–209, 1995
55. Raju B, Arbelaez A, Breckenridge S, Cryer P: Nocturnal hypoglycemia in type 1 diabetes: an assessment of preventive bedtime treatments. *J Clin Endocrinol Metab* 91:2087–2092, 2006
56. Cooperberg B, Breckennridge S, Arbelaez A, Cryer P: Terbutaline and the prevention of nocturnal hypoglycemia in type 1 diabetes. *Diabetes Care* 31:2271–2272, 2008
57. Silverstein J, Klingensmith G, Copeland K, Plotnick L, Kaufman F, Laffel L, Deeb L, Grey M, Anderson B, Holzmeister L, Clark N: Care of children and adolescents with type 1 diabetes. *Diabetes Care* 28:186–212, 2005
58. Ly T, Hewitt J, Davey R, Lim E, Davis E, Jones T: Improving epinephrine responses in hypoglycemia unawareness with real-time continuous glucose monitoring in adolescents with type 1 diabetes. *Diabetes Care* 34:50–52, 2011
59. Buckingham B, Chase H, Dassau E, Cobry E, Clinton P, Gage V, Caswell K, Wilkinson J, Cameron F, Lee H, Bequette B, Doyle F: Prevention of nocturnal hypoglycemia using predictive alarm algorithms and insulin pump suspension. *Diabetes Care* 33:1013–1017, 2010
60. Cox D, Gonder-Frederick L, Ritterband L, Patel K, Schachinger H, Ferhm-Wolfsdorf G, Hermanns N, Snoek F, Zrebiec J, Polonsky W, Schlundt D: Blood glucose awareness training: what is it, where is it, and where is it going? *Diabetes Spectrum* 19:43–49, 2006
61. Cox D, Gonder-Frederick L, Julian D, Cryer P, Lee J, Richards F, Clarke W: Intensive versus standard blood glucose awareness training (bgat) with insulin dependent diabetes: mechanism and ancillary effects. *Psychosomatic Medicine* 53:453–462, 1991

62. Cox D, Ritterband L, Magee J, Clarke W, Gonder-Frederick L: Blood glucose awareness training delivered over the Internet. *Diabetes Care* 31: 1527–1528, 2008

63. Buckingham B, Block J, Burdick J, Kalajian A, Kollman C, Choy M, Wilson D, Chase P: Response to nocturnal alarms using a real-time glucose sensor. *Diabetes Technol Ther* 7:440–447, 2005

64. Cobelli C, Renard E, Kovatchev B: Artificial pancreas: past, present, future. *Diabetes* 60:2672–2682, 2011

65. Kovatchev B, Cobelli C, Renard E, Anderson S, Breton M, Patek S, Clarke W, Bruttomesso D, Maran A, Costa S, Avogaro A, Man C, Facchinetti A, Magni L, De Nicolao G, Place J, Farret A: Multinational study of subcutaneous model-predictive closed-loop control in type 1 diabetes mellitus: summary of the results. *J Diabetes Sci Tech* 4:1374–1381, 2010

66. Castle J, Engle J, Youssef J, Massoud R, Yuen K, Ryland K, Ward W: Novel use of glucagon in a closed-loop system for prevention of hypoglycemia in type 1 diabetes. *Diabetes Care* 33:1282–1287, 2010

67. Garg S, Brazg L, Bailey T, Buckingham B, Slover R, Klonoff D, Shin J, Welsh J, Kaufman F: Reduction in duration of hypoglycemia by automatic suspension of insulin delivery: the In-clinic ASPIRE study. *Diabetes Thechnol Ther* 14:205–209, 2012

68. Cryer, P: Elimination of hypoglycemia from the lives of people affected by diabetes. *Diabetes* 60:24–27, 2011

69. McCrimmon R, Sherwin R: Hypoglycemia in type 1 diabetes. *Diabetes* 59:2333–2339, 2010

70. Leu J, Cui M, Shamoon H, Gabriely I: Hypoglycemia-associated autonomic failure is prevented by opioid receptor blockade. *J Clin Endocrinol Metab* 94:3372–3380, 2009

71. Briscoe V, Ertl A, Tate D, Davis S: Effects of the selective serotonin reuptake inhibitor fluoxetine on counterregulatory responses to hypoglycemia in individuals with type 1 diabetes. *Diabetes* 57:3315–3322, 2008

15

Diabetic Ketoacidosis
I. Pediatrics

Joseph I. Wolfsdorf, MB BCh

D iabetic ketoacidosis (DKA) is a clinical syndrome resulting from absolute or relative deficiency of circulating insulin and the combined effects of increased levels of the counterregulatory hormones and cytokines that impair insulin action.[1]

DEFINITION OF DKA

The biochemical criteria for the diagnosis of DKA include the following:[2]

- Hyperglycemia (blood glucose >11 mmol/L [≈200 mg/dL])
- Venous pH <7.3 or bicarbonate <15 mmol/L
- Ketonemia and ketonuria

Children who have been partially treated or who have consumed little or no carbohydrate may, occasionally, have only mild hyperglycemia ("euglycemic ketoacidosis").[3]

Type 2 diabetes (T2D) now accounts for up to one half of all newly diagnosed diabetes in children ages 10 to 21 years.[4] In the U.S., the SEARCH for Diabetes in Youth Study found that 29.4% of participants less than 20 years of age with type 1 diabetes (T1D) presented with DKA as compared to 9.7% of youth with T2D.[5] DKA has, rarely, been reported in patients with cystic fibrosis–related diabetes,[6-8] in patients receiving the calcineurin inhibitor tacrolimus after solid organ transplantation,[9] and during therapy for acute lymphoblastic leukemia.[10] The severity of DKA is categorized by the degree of acidosis:[2]

- Mild: venous pH <7.3 or bicarbonate <15 mmol/L
- Moderate: pH <7.2, bicarbonate <10 mmol/L
- Severe: pH <7.1, bicarbonate <5 mmol/L

Hyperglycemic Hyperosmolar State

Hyperglycemic hyperosmolar state (HHS), characterized by extreme elevations in serum glucose concentrations and hyperosmolality without significant ketosis may occur in young patients with T2D. Recent reports suggest an increasing incidence of this disorder in children and adolescents.[11-18] Criteria for the diagnosis of HHS include the following:[16]

- Serum glucose concentration >600 mg/dL (33 mmol/L)
- Serum osmolality >330 mOsm/Kg

DOI: 10.2337/9781580404785ch15s1

■ No significant ketosis and acidosis (serum bicarbonate >15 mmol/L, urine ketone [acetoacetate] concentration <15 mg/dL [1.5 mmol/L]; negative or trace ketonuria)

Overlap between HHS and DKA may occur, and some patients with HHS—especially when there is severe dehydration—experience mild or moderate acidosis. Conversely, some children with T1D may have severe hyperglycemia if high–carbohydrate-containing beverages have been used to quench thirst before diagnosis.[19] Therapy must be appropriately modified to address the pathophysiology and unique biochemical disturbances of each patient.

EPIDEMIOLOGY

At Disease Onset

Worldwide incidence rates inversely correlate with the regional incidence of T1D. Frequencies range from ~15 to 67% in Europe and North America[5,20–25] and even higher rates of DKA at presentation have been reported from Africa.[26,27] DKA is more common and frequently more severe in children less than 5 years of age, which may be related to a delay in diagnosis and more aggressive β-cell destruction, and in children who do not have ready access to medical care for social or economic reasons.[5,24,25,28–33] Despite an increasing incidence of diabetes in children, large series reported from major pediatric diabetes centers in Austria, Germany, and Brazil have shown no reduction in the frequency of DKA at presentation over the past 10 to 20 years.[24,30,34]

In Children with Established Diabetes

The risk of DKA in established T1D is 1.4–10 per 100 patient-years.[23,35–37]

Risk is increased in the following:[38]

■ Children with poor metabolic control or previous episodes of DKA
■ Peripubertal and adolescent girls
■ Children with psychiatric disorders, including those with eating disorders
■ Children with dysfunctional or unstable family circumstances (e.g., parental abuse)
■ Children of immigrant families[37]
■ Children who omit insulin[36,39]
■ Children with limited access to medical services
■ Patients who use insulin pump therapy (as only rapid- or short-acting insulin is used in pumps, interruption of insulin delivery for any reason rapidly leads to insulin deficiency)[40]

Despite their long duration of action, patients using long-acting insulin analogs (glargine, detemir) have a higher incidence of DKA than those who use intermediate-acting insulin (neutral protamine Hagedorn [NPH]).[41] An intercurrent infection is seldom the cause when the patient or family is properly educated in diabetes management and is receiving appropriate follow-up care by a diabetes care team that is available to provide 24 h telephone advice.[42–45]

PATHOPHYSIOLOGY

Absolute insulin deficiency occurs in previously undiagnosed T1D and when established patients deliberately or inadvertently do not take insulin, especially the long-acting component of a basal-bolus regimen.[41] Patients who use an insulin pump can rapidly develop DKA when insulin delivery fails for any reason.[40] Relative insulin deficiency occurs when the concentrations of counterregulatory hormones increase in response to stress caused by sepsis, trauma, or gastrointestinal illness with diarrhea and vomiting.

The pathophysiology of DKA in children is shown in Fig. 15.I.1. Absolute or relative insulin deficiency and excess counterregulatory hormones cause increased glucose production from glycogenolysis and gluconeogenesis while limiting glucose utilization, resulting in hyperglycemia, osmotic diuresis, electrolyte loss, dehydration, decreased glomerular filtration, and hyperosmolarity. Lipolysis increases free fatty acid levels and β-oxidation in the liver facilitates gluconeogenesis and generates acetoacetic and β-hydroxybutyric acids (ketones), which overwhelm the buffering capacity and results in metabolic acidosis. Poor tissue perfusion or sepsis may cause lactic acidosis. Progressive dehydration, hyperosmolarity, acidosis, and electrolyte disturbances further stimulate stress hormone secretion, which leads to progressive metabolic decompensation.

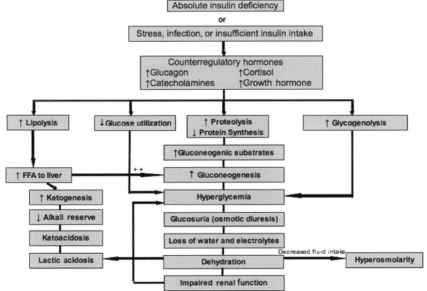

Figure 15.I.1 Pathophysiology of DKA.

CLINICAL MANIFESTATIONS OF DKA

The clinical manifestations are polyuria, polydipsia, signs of dehydration, "Kussmaul breathing" (rapid, deep respirations to reduce carbon dioxide partial pressure [PCO2]), and progressive obtundation, leading to coma. Water and electrolytes are lost from both the intra- and extracellular fluid compartments; the range of losses is shown in Table 15.I.1. Despite dehydration, patients maintain normal blood pressure and children with severe DKA may have mild hypertension.[46] Urine output occurs until extreme volume depletion leads to a critical decrease in renal blood flow and glomerular filtration. The magnitude of specific deficits in an individual patient varies depending on the duration and severity of illness, the extent to which the patient was able to maintain intake of fluid and electrolytes, and the content of food and fluids consumed before coming to medical attention. For example, consumption of juices or sugar-containing soft drinks exacerbate the hyperglycemia and patients may present with extreme hyperglycemia and hyperosmolality.[19]

Patients with DKA have an extracellular fluid (ECF) volume deficit usually in the range from 4 to 10%.[47-50] The severity of dehydration may be more severe in patients with mixed DKA and HHS.[16] Children ≤2 years of age are often more dehydrated than older children.[51] Shock is rare in pediatric DKA. Clinical estimates of the volume deficit are subjective and inaccurate[49,52,53] and the magnitude of dehydration cannot be assessed accurately by either clinical or biochemical parameters. Unless the patient is hemodynamically unstable, a relatively restrictive regimen of fluid administration is associated with timely correction of DKA.[50]

Table 15.I.1 Usual Losses of Fluids and Electrolytes in DKA and Maintenance Requirements in Children

	Average (range) Losses (per kg)	Maintenance Requirements (24 h)
Water	70 mL (30–100)	≤10 kg 100 mL/kg/24 h
		11–20 kg 1000 mL + 50 mL/kg/24 h for each kg from 11–20
		>20 kg 1500 mL + 20 mL/kg/24 h for each kg >20
Sodium	6 mmol (5–13)	2–4 mmol[†]
Potassium	5 mmol (3–6)	2–3 mmol
Chloride	4 mmol (3–9)	2–3 mmol
Phosphate	0.5–2.5 mmol	1–2 mmol[*]

Note: Data are from measurements in only a few children and adolescents.[47,48,54-56] In any individual patient, actual losses may be less or greater than the ranges shown in the table.

[†] per 100 mL of maintenance fluid.
[*] Data are from 57.

The effective osmolality (= 2x(Na + K) + glucose mOsm/kg) is frequently in the range of 300–350 mmol/Kg.

Increased serum urea nitrogen and hematocrit are useful indicators of the severity of ECF contraction,[58,59] whereas serum sodium concentration is an unreliable measure of ECF contraction because glucose causes osmotic movement of water into the extracellular space and dilutional hyponatremia.[60,61] It is important to calculate the corrected sodium concentration and monitor its changes throughout the course of therapy.

Corrected sodium = measured Na + 0.02 ([plasma glucose - 100]) mg/dL.[60,61]

As the plasma glucose concentration decreases after administering fluid and insulin, the measured serum sodium concentration should increase, but this does not indicate a worsening of the hypertonic state. A failure of measured serum sodium levels to rise or a decrease in serum sodium levels with therapy is a potentially ominous sign of impending cerebral edema.[62–64]

Total body *potassium* deficits are on the order of 3 to ≥6 mmol/kg.[47,48,54–56] Intracellular potassium is depleted because of transcellular shifts caused by hypertonicity (increased plasma osmolality causes solvent drag in which water and potassium are drawn out of cells). In addition, glycogenolysis and proteolysis cause potassium efflux from cells. Potassium is also lost because of vomiting and osmotic diuresis, and volume depletion causes secondary hyperaldosteronism, which promotes urinary potassium excretion. At presentation, serum potassium levels may be normal, increased or decreased.[65]

Phosphate is lost as a result of osmotic diuresis leading to intracellular phosphate depletion.[47,48,54]

PRESENTATION: DIFFERENTIAL DIAGNOSIS

Starvation ketosis and alcoholic ketoacidosis are distinguished by clinical history and plasma glucose concentrations ranging from hypoglycemia in the former to mildly elevated (but rarely >200 mg/dL) in the latter condition.[66] DKA must also be distinguished from other causes of increased anion gap metabolic acidosis, including lactic acidosis and ingestion of such drugs as salicylate, methanol, ethylene glycol, and paraldehyde. These low–molecular-weight organic compounds can produce an osmolar gap in addition to the anion gap acidosis.[67] In infancy, rare inborn errors of metabolism, such as propionic acidemia,[68] the chronic intermittent form of isovaleric acidemia,[69] and defects of ketolysis (succinyl-CoA 3-oxoacid CoA transferase deficiency and mitochondrial acetoacetyl-CoA thiolase deficiency) present with recurrent episodes of ketoacidosis and usually are accompanied by normoglycemia or hypoglycemia, but rarely by hyperglycemia in older children, that mimics DKA.[70,71]

Following are the clinical manifestations of DKA:

- Dehydration
- Rapid, deep, sighing (Kussmaul respiration); air hunger

- Nausea, vomiting, and abdominal pain mimicking an acute abdomen
- Progressive obtundation and loss of consciousness
- Increased leukocyte count with left shift
- Nonspecific elevation of serum amylase[73-76]
- Fever only when infection is present[42]

EMERGENCY ASSESSMENT

An emergency assessment for DKA includes the following:

- Perform a clinical evaluation to confirm the diagnosis and determine its cause (look for evidence of infection; in recurrent DKA, insulin omission or failure to follow sick day or pump failure management guidelines accounts for most episodes).
- Weigh the patient.* This weight should be used for calculations and not the weight from a previous office visit or hospital record.

  - Look for acanthosis nigricans, suggesting insulin resistance and T2D.

- Clinical assessment of dehydration is inaccurate and generally shows only fair to moderate agreement among examiners. The three most useful individual signs for assessing dehydration in young children and predicting at least 5% dehydration and acidosis are as follows:

  - Prolonged capillary refill time (normal is ≤1.5–2 s)
  - Abnormal skin turgor (tenting or inelastic skin)
  - Hyperpnea[77]

- Other useful signs include dry mucus membranes, sunken eyes, absent tears, weak pulses, and cool extremities. More signs of dehydration tend to be associated with more severe dehydration.[77]

  - ≥10% dehydration is suggested by weak or impalpable peripheral pulses, hypotension, and oliguria.

- Assess level of consciousness (Glasgow coma scale†).[78,79]
- Obtain a blood sample for measurement of plasma glucose, electrolytes (including bicarbonate or total carbon dioxide [TCO2]), urea nitrogen, creatinine, osmolality, venous (arterial only in critically ill patient) pH, PCO2, PO2, hemoglobin and hematocrit or complete blood count,‡ calcium, phosphorus, and magnesium concentrations, blood β-hydroxybutyrate concentration,[80,81] A1C.
- Perform a urinalysis for ketones.
- If there is evidence of infection, obtain appropriate specimens for culture (blood, urine, throat).
- If laboratory measurement of serum potassium is delayed, perform an electrocardiogram for baseline evaluation of potassium status.[82,83]

---

*If body surface area is used for fluid therapy calculations, measure height or length to determine surface area.

†See Appendix 15.I.A for details.

‡An increased white blood cell count in response to stress is characteristic of DKA and is not indicative of infection.

SUPPORTIVE MEASURES

The following supportive measures should be taken:

- In the unconscious or severely obtunded patient, secure the airway and empty the stomach by continuous nasogastric suction to prevent pulmonary aspiration.
- A peripheral intravenous (IV) catheter should be placed for blood sampling.
- Use continuous electrocardiographic monitoring to assess T-waves for evidence of hyper- or hypokalemia and monitor for arrhythmias.[82,83]
- Give oxygen to patients with circulatory impairment or shock.
- Give antibiotics to febrile patients after obtaining cultures of body fluids.
- Bladder catheterization is usually not necessary, but if the child is unconscious or unable to void on demand (infants and very ill young children), the bladder should be catheterized.
- Central venous pressure monitoring rarely may be required to guide fluid management in the critically ill or neurologically compromised patient.[§]

WHERE SHOULD THE CHILD BE MANAGED?

The child should receive care in a unit that has the following:

- Experienced nursing staff trained in monitoring and management
- Access to a laboratory that can provide frequent and timely evaluation of biochemical variables
- Specialist with expertise in the management of DKA should direct management.
- Children with severe DKA (long duration of symptoms, compromised circulation, or depressed level of consciousness) or those who are at increased risk for cerebral edema (e.g., <5 years of age, low PCO_2, high urea nitrogen) should be treated in a pediatric intensive care unit.[2]

CLINICAL AND BIOCHEMICAL MONITORING

Management of DKA and HHS requires meticulous monitoring of the clinical and biochemical response to treatment so that timely adjustments in treatment can be made when indicated.

Monitoring and documentation on a flow chart should include the following:

- Hourly (or more frequently as indicated) vital signs (heart rate, respiratory rate, blood pressure).
- Hourly (or more frequently as indicated) neurological observations for warning signs and symptoms of cerebral edema (see below signs and symptoms suggestive of cerebral edema).
- Noninvasive end-tidal CO_2 monitoring (capnography) is a valuable and reliable tool to continuously monitor acidosis in pediatric patients with

---

[§]Central lines in children with DKA are frequently associated with thrombosis and should be resorted to only when absolutely necessary.

DKA. Continuous end-tidal CO_2 monitoring supplements data obtained from intermittent blood gas determinations and provides early warning of unexpected changes in acidosis.[84]

- Amount of administered insulin.
- Hourly (or more frequently as indicated) fluid input and output.
- Capillary blood glucose should be measured hourly (but must be cross-checked against laboratory venous glucose because capillary methods may be inaccurate in the presence of poor peripheral circulation and acidosis).
- Laboratory tests: serum electrolytes, glucose, calcium, magnesium, phosphorus, and blood gases should be repeated every 2–4 h, or more frequently, as clinically indicated, in more severe cases. BUN, creatinine, and hematocrit should be repeated at 6–8 h intervals until they are normal.
- Urine ketones until cleared.
- If the laboratory cannot provide timely results, a portable biochemical analyzer that measures plasma glucose, serum electrolytes, and blood ketones on fingerstick blood samples at the bedside is a useful adjunct to laboratory-based determinations.
- Calculations:

    - Anion gap = Na – (Cl + HCO_3): normal is 12 ± 2 mmol/L
    - Corrected sodium = measured Na + 0.02([plasma glucose - 100]) mg/dL.
    - Effective osmolality = 2x(Na + K) + glucose mmol/L (mg/dL ÷ 18)

Following are the goals of therapy:

- Correct dehydration
- Correct acidosis and reverse ketosis
- Restore blood glucose to near normal
- Avoid complications of therapy
- Identify and treat any precipitating event

MANAGEMENT

Volume Expansion; Water and Salt Replacement

Fluid replacement alone will reverse many of the clinical and biochemical derangements seen in DKA.[85] The principles described in this section were developed after a comprehensive review of the literature and were accepted and endorsed by a panel of expert physicians representing the Lawson Wilkins Pediatric Endocrine Society (LWPES), the European Society for Paediatric Endocrinology (ESPE), and the International Society for Pediatric and Adolescent Diabetes (ISPAD).[2,86]

Begin fluid replacement before starting insulin therapy. If needed to restore peripheral circulation, volume expansion (resuscitation) should begin immediately with 0.9% saline. The volume and rate of fluid administration depends on circulatory status. The volume administered typically is 10–20 mL/kg over 1–2 h and may be repeated if necessary. Because of the increased risk of thromboembolism, femoral and central vein catheters should be avoided if possible.[87] Subsequent fluid administration should aim to rehydrate evenly over 48 h at a rate seldom more than 1.5 to 2 times the usual daily maintenance requirement beginning with 0.9% saline for at least 4–6 h.[58,62,88–90] Thereafter, deficit replacement should be with a solution that has a tonicity at least equal to or greater than 0.45% saline with added potassium (see the subsection Potassium).[58,62,88,91,92] See Tables 15.I.2 and 15.I.3 for examples of calculations.

Calculation of effective osmolality is a valuable guide to fluid and electrolyte therapy. Urinary losses should not routinely be added to the calculation of replacement fluid, but, rarely, it may be necessary in the profoundly dehydrated patient with mixed DKA and HHS. The sodium content of the fluid may need to be increased if the measured serum sodium concentration is low and does not rise appropriately as the plasma glucose concentration falls.[62,93] Hyperchloremic metabolic acidosis from large volumes of 0.9% saline is a frequent complication of treatment.[94,95]

Insulin

Although rehydration alone causes a significant decrease in blood glucose concentration,[85,96] insulin therapy is essential to normalize blood glucose, suppress lipolysis and ketogenesis, and reverse acidosis.[97] Several factors, in addition to the rate of insulin infusion,[98] influence the rate of decline in serum glucose concentration. These include the initial degree of compromise of renal function caused by dehydration, rate of IV fluid, and the timing and amount of dextrose administration. Prospective data from randomized trials in pediatric DKA are almost nonexistent;[99] however, extensive evidence indicates that low-dose IV insulin administration should be the standard of care.[100]

IV insulin infusion should commence 1–2 h after starting fluid replacement therapy—that is, after the patient has received initial volume expansion.[72] The starting dose is 0.1 unit/kg per hour (dilute 50 units of regular [soluble] insulin in 50 mL normal saline, 1 unit = 1 mL).[98,100] An IV priming dose or bolus is unnecessary,[101,102] may increase the risk of cerebral edema,[72] and should *not* be used at the start of therapy. The dose of insulin should usually remain at 0.1 unit/kg per hour

---

Table 15.I.2 Fluid and Electrolyte Losses Based on Assumed 10% Dehydration in a Child (weight 30 kg, surface area 1 m²) with DKA

Fluid and Electrolyte	Approximate Losses with 10% Dehydration	Approximate Requirements for Maintenance (48 h)	Working Total (48 h)
Water mL	3000	3000	6000
Sodium mEq	180	90	270
Potassium mEq	150	70	220
Chloride mEq	120	60	180
Phosphate mmol	75	20	95

until resolution of DKA (pH >7.30, anion gap normal, bicarbonate >15 mmol/L, β-OHB <0.6 mmol/L), which invariably takes longer than normalization of blood glucose concentrations.[103] If, however, the patient appears to be sensitive to insulin (e.g., some young children, patients with HHS, and some older children with established diabetes) or there is difficulty maintaining normal serum potassium concentrations, the dose may be decreased to 0.05 unit/kg per hour, or less, provided that metabolic acidosis continues to resolve.

Recent nonrandomized, observational[104] and retrospective[105] studies have shown that low-dose (0.05 unit/kg per hour) is as effective as standard-dose (0.1 units/kg per hour) IV insulin infusion in the initial treatment (less than 6 h)[104] or 12 h[105] of DKA in children.

During initial volume expansion, the plasma glucose concentration falls steeply.[85] Thereafter, and after commencing insulin therapy, the plasma glucose concentration typically decreases at a rate of 40 to 90 mg/dL per hour, depending on the timing and amount of glucose administration.[106] Adding dextrose to the IV fluid infusion modulates the rate of decline in glucose concentrations.[107] To prevent an unduly rapid decrease in plasma glucose concentration and hypoglycemia, 5% glucose should be added to the IV fluid when the plasma glucose is 250–300 mg/dL, or sooner if the rate of fall is precipitous. It may be necessary to use 10% or even 12.5% dextrose to prevent hypoglycemia while continuing to infuse the amount of insulin necessary to correct the metabolic acidosis.

If biochemical parameters of DKA (pH, anion gap, β-OHB) do not improve, consider possible causes of impaired response to insulin—for example, infection or errors in insulin preparation.

When continuous IV administration is not possible and in patients with uncomplicated DKA, hourly or two hourly subcutaneous (SC) or intramuscular (IM) administration of a rapid-acting insulin analog (insulin lispro or insulin aspart) is safe and may be as effective as IV regular insulin infusion,[108–110] but it should not be used in subjects whose peripheral circulation is impaired. A recommended SC regimen for treatment of DKA consists of an initial SC dose of 0.3 unit/kg, followed 1 h later by SC insulin (lispro or aspart) at 0.1 unit/kg every hour or 0.15–0.20 units/kg every 2 h. If blood glucose falls to ≤250 mg/dL before DKA has resolved, reduce the dose of SC insulin to 0.05 unit/kg per hour to keep BG ≈200 mg/dL until DKA resolves.

Potassium

At the time of presentation, serum potassium levels may be normal, increased, or decreased.[65] Renal dysfunction, by enhancing hyperglycemia and reducing potassium excretion, contributes to hyperkalemia.[65] Administration of insulin and the correction of acidosis drive potassium back into the cells, decreasing serum levels.[111] The serum potassium concentration may decrease abruptly, predisposing the patient to cardiac arrhythmias.

Potassium replacement therapy is required regardless of the serum potassium concentration.[112,113] If the patient's serum potassium concentration is low at presentation, assume that total body potassium depletion is severe and start potassium replacement *at the time of* initial volume expansion and *before* starting insulin therapy. If potassium is given with the initial rapid volume expansion, a concentration of 20–40 mmol/L should be used. If the patient has hyperkalemia, *defer* potassium replacement therapy until urine output is documented. Otherwise, start replacing potassium *after* initial volume expansion and concurrent with starting insulin therapy.

If immediate serum potassium measurements are unavailable, an electrocardiogram (ECG) may help to determine whether the child has hyper- or hypokalemia.[82] Flattening of the T wave, widening of the QT interval, and the appearance of U waves indicate hypokalemia. Tall, peaked, symmetrical, T waves and shortening of the QT interval are signs of hyperkalemia. Prolonged QTc of unclear significance frequently occurs during DKA and is correlated with ketosis.[114]

The starting potassium concentration in the infusate should be 40 mmol/L. Potassium phosphate may be used together with potassium chloride or acetate—for example, 20 mmol/L potassium chloride and 20 mmol/L potassium phosphate or 20 mmol/L potassium phosphate and 20 mmol/L potassium acetate. Subsequent potassium replacement therapy should be based on serum potassium measurements and continue throughout IV fluid therapy. The maximum recommended rate of IV potassium replacement is 0.5 mmol/kg per hour. If hypokalemia persists despite a maximum rate of potassium replacement, the rate of insulin infusion should be reduced.

Phosphate

Phosphate is lost as a result of osmotic diuresis,[47,48,54] resulting in intracellular phosphate depletion. Insulin promotes phosphate entry into cells[115,116] and plasma phosphate levels fall after starting treatment. Total body phosphate depletion has been associated with a variety of metabolic disturbances.[117–119] Prospective studies have not shown clinical benefit from phosphate replacement, however.[120–125] Nonetheless, severe hypophosphatemia (<1 mg/dL), which may manifest as weakness, should be treated even in the absence of symptoms.[126,127] Potassium phosphate may be administered safely provided that careful monitoring of serum calcium is performed to avoid hypocalcemia.[128,129]

Acidosis and Bicarbonate

Insulin stops further ketoacid production and allows ketoacids to be metabolized, which generates bicarbonate. Treatment of hypovolemia improves tissue perfusion and renal function, thereby decreasing lactic acid production and increasing organic acid excretion. Controlled trials have shown no clinical benefit from bicarbonate administration.[130–133] Bicarbonate therapy may cause paradoxical central nervous system acidosis,[134,135] and rapid correction of acidosis with bicarbonate causes hypokalemia.[134,136,137] In general, there is no evidence that bicarbonate is necessary, and its administration is not recommended routinely; however, selected patients may benefit from cautious alkali therapy. These include patients with severe acidemia (arterial pH <6.9) in whom decreased cardiac contractility and peripheral vasodilatation can further impair tissue perfusion, and patients with life-threatening hyperkalemia.[138] If bicarbonate is considered necessary, cautiously give 1–2 mmol/kg over 60 min.

Table 15.I.2 Fluid and Electrolyte Replacement for a Child (30 kg, 1 m²) with DKA Estimated to be 10% Dehydrated

Approximate Duration and Rate	Fluid Composition and Volume	Sodium mEq	Potassium mEq	Chloride mEq	Phos-phate mmol
Hour 1 (300 mL/h)	300 mL 0.9% NaCl (normal saline)	46	–	46	–
Hour 2–4 (125 mL/h) Start regular insulin at 0.1 unit/kg per hour	375 mL normal saline + 20 mEq K acetate/L + 20 mEq K phosphate/L	58	15	58	5.1
Hours 5–48 (125 mL/h) Continue regular insulin (0.1 unit/kg per hour until pH ≥7.3, anion gap 12±2, or HCO₃ ≥15 mEq/L)	5,500 mL 1/2 normal saline + dextrose +20 mEq K acetate/L + 20 mEq K phosphate/L	424	220	424	75
Total in 48 h	**6,175 mL fluid**	**528**	**235**	**528**	**80**

Note: Normal saline 10 mL/kg is given over 1 h for initial volume expansion; thereafter, the child is rehydrated over 48 h at an even rate at two times the maintenance rate of fluid requirement. Potassium phosphate: 4.4 mEq potassium and 3 mmol phosphate (1 mEq K and 0.68 mmol phosphate).

COMPLICATIONS OF TREATMENT

In national population studies, the mortality rate from DKA in children is 0.15 to 0.30%,[139,140] and cerebral edema accounts for 60 to 90% of all DKA deaths.[64,141] From 10 to 25% of survivors of cerebral edema have significant residual morbidity.[64,141,142]

Cerebral Edema

The incidence of cerebral edema in national population studies is 0.5 to 0.9% and the mortality rate is 21 to 24%.[64,141,142] The pathogenesis of cerebral edema is incompletely understood. Evidence for disruption of the blood–brain barrier has been found in cases of fatal cerebral edema associated with DKA.[143] The degree of edema formation during DKA in children correlates with the degree of dehydration and hyperventilation at presentation, but it does not correlate with factors related to initial osmolality or osmotic changes during treatment. There is no convincing evidence of an association between the rate of fluid or sodium administration used to treat DKA and the development of cerebral edema.[144] Although not definitively proven, recent data suggest that the pathophysiology of cerebral edema is not the result of acute changes in serum osmolality, but it may be a consequence of cerebral ischemia from hypoperfusion and reperfusion leading to vasogenic edema.[145–148]

Demographic factors associated with an increased risk of cerebral edema include the following:

■ Younger age[149]
■ New onset diabetes[140,149]
■ Longer duration of symptoms[150]

These risk associations may reflect more severe DKA.
Epidemiological studies have identified several potential risk factors at diagnosis or during treatment of DKA:

■ More severe hypocapnia at presentation after adjusting for degree of acidosis[64,146,151]
■ Increased serum urea nitrogen at presentation[64,146]
■ More severe acidosis at presentation[152,153]
■ Bicarbonate treatment[64,154]
■ An attenuated rise in measured serum sodium concentrations during therapy[62-64]
■ Greater volumes of fluid given in the first 4 h[153]
■ Administration of insulin in the first hour of fluid treatment[153]

Following are signs and symptoms suggestive of cerebral edema:

■ Headache
■ Slowing of heart rate
■ Recurrence of vomiting
■ Change in neurological status (restlessness, irritability, increased drowsiness, age-inappropriate incontinence)
■ Specific neurological signs (e.g., cranial nerve palsies, abnormal pupillary responses)
■ Rising blood pressure
■ Decreased oxygen saturation

Clinically significant cerebral edema usually develops 4–12 h after treatment has started, but it can occur even before treatment has begun,[64,142,155-158] or, rarely, it may develop as late as 24–48 h after the start of treatment.[64,149,159] Following is a method of clinical diagnosis based on bedside evaluation of neurological state:[160]

Diagnostic criteria.

■ Abnormal motor or verbal response to pain
■ Decorticate or decerebrate posturing
■ Cranial nerve palsy (especially III, IV, and VI)
■ Abnormal neurogenic respiratory pattern (e.g., grunting, tachypnea, Cheyne–Stokes respiration, apneusis)

Major criteria.

■ Altered mentation or fluctuating level of consciousness
■ Sustained heart rate deceleration (decrease more than 20 beats per minute) not attributable to improved intravascular volume or sleep state
■ Age-inappropriate incontinence

Minor criteria.

- Vomiting
- Headache
- Lethargy or not easily aroused
- Diastolic blood pressure >90 mm Hg
- Age <5 years

One diagnostic criterion, two major criteria, or one major and two minor criteria have a sensitivity of 92% and a false positive rate of only 4%.[160] A chart with the reference ranges for blood pressure and heart rate, which vary depending on height, weight, and gender, should be readily available at the bedside.

Treatment of cerebral edema.

- Initiate treatment as soon as the condition is suspected.
- Give mannitol 0.5-1 g/kg IV over 20 min and repeat if there is no initial response in 30 min.[161–163]
- Reduce fluid administration rate by one-third.
- Hypertonic saline (3%), 5–10 mL/kg over 30 min, may be an alternative to mannitol, especially if there is no initial response to mannitol.[164,165] Mannitol or hypertonic saline should be available at the bedside.
- Elevate the head of the bed.
- Intubation may be necessary for the patient with impending respiratory failure, but aggressive hyperventilation (to a PCO2 <22 mm Hg [2.9 kPa]) has been associated with poor outcome and is not recommended.[166]
- *After* treatment for cerebral edema has been started, a cranial CT scan should be obtained to rule out other possible intracerebral causes of neurologic deterioration (≈10% of cases), especially thrombosis and cerebral infarction,[167–171] or intracerebral haemorrhage,[172–174] or dural sinus thrombosis,[169,175] which may benefit from specific therapy.

Other Causes of Morbidity and Mortality

The following are other causes of morbidity and mortality:

- Hypoglycemia
- Hyperchloremic metabolic acidosis
- Prothrombotic tendency and peripheral venous thrombosis
- Sepsis
- Rhino-orbital-cerebral, auricular, or pulmonary mucormycosis
- Aspiration pneumonia
- Pulmonary edema
- Adult respiratory distress syndrome (ARDS)
- Pneumothorax, pneumomediastinum, and subcutaneous emphysema
- Rhabdomyolysis
- Acute renal failure
- Acute pancreatitis

WHEN HAS DKA RESOLVED?

Serial measurements of point-of-care capillary blood β-hydroxybutyrate (β-OHB) concentrations have been used to monitor biochemical resolution of DKA and to determine when IV insulin infusion should be stopped. Blood β-OHB levels decrease to <1 mmol/L many hours before the urine becomes ketone free.[176] Absence of ketonuria should *not* be used as an endpoint for determining resolution of DKA.

Introduction of Oral Fluids and Transition to SC Insulin Injections

Oral fluids should be introduced after ketoacidosis has resolved (venous pH >7.3, closure of the anion gap, serum bicarbonate ≥15 mEq/L, β-OHB <0.6 mmol/L) and plasma glucose <200 mg/dL. Note that the anion gap normalizes earlier than the bicarbonate concentration in children treated with normal saline.[177] The most convenient time to change to SC insulin is just before a mealtime. To prevent rebound hyperglycemia, the first SC injection should be given 15–30 min (with rapid-acting analog insulin) or 1 h (with short-acting, regular insulin) before stopping the insulin infusion, depending on the plasma glucose concentration, to allow sufficient time for the injected insulin to be absorbed. For patients on a basal-bolus insulin regimen, the first dose of basal insulin (glargine or detemir) may be administered in the evening and the insulin infusion is stopped the next morning.

In patients with established diabetes, the patient's usual insulin regimen may be resumed. See chapter 12 (Insulin Therapy) for details about starting an SC insulin regimen after resolution of DKA in newly diagnosed patients. After transitioning to SC insulin, frequent blood glucose monitoring is required to avoid marked hyperglycemia and hypoglycemia. Supplemental rapid-acting insulin is given at ~3 to 4 h intervals to correct blood glucose levels that exceed 200 mg/dL.

PREVENTION OF DKA

Primary Prevention in Undiagnosed Patients

Programs to raise awareness of school personnel and primary care physicians. Progression of metabolic deterioration to DKA generally is related to a long duration of ignored or misdiagnosed hyperglycemia-related symptoms. In the Parma area of Italy, Vanelli and colleagues implemented a highly successful DKA prevention program in children ages 6 to 14 years.[178,179] A poster showing the classic symptoms of diabetes (and highlighting the special significance of nocturnal enuresis in a previously dry child) was displayed in 177 primary and secondary public schools. Pediatricians working in the area were given equipment to measure glucosuria and blood glucose levels, as well as cards listing guidelines for the early diagnosis of diabetes to be given to patients. A toll-free number provided free access to health providers experienced in diabetes diagnosis. This intervention resulted in a decrease in the cumulative frequency of DKA in new-onset diabetes from 78% during the 4-year period before initiation to 12.5% during the subsequent 8 years after the information about diabetes was introduced to teachers, students, parents, and pediatricians. The campaign to prevent DKA was still effective 8 years after it was promoted and confirmed that enuresis is the most important symptom for the early diagnosis of T1D. To maintain its effectiveness, the campaign should be periodically renewed (possibly every 5 years).[180]

Screening in High-Risk Individuals

When children at increased risk of developing T1D (e.g., family history of T1D, positive pancreatic autoantibodies, or expression of diabetes-associated human leukocyte antigen [HLA] genotypes) are regularly screened and followed prospectively, many are asymptomatic and have a normal A1C concentration at the time of diagnosis.[181] DKA is infrequent, the onset of diabetes is less severe, A1C is lower at diagnosis, fewer patients are hospitalized, and patients have a milder clinical course in the first year after diagnosis.[181–184] In one study, however, no substantial benefit with respect to A1C and insulin dose was observed during the first 5 years after diagnosis.[183]

Secondary Prevention in Established Patients

Prevention of recurrent DKA. Insulin omission, either inadvertently or deliberately, is the cause of DKA, in most cases, and management of an episode of DKA should not be considered complete until its cause has been identified and an attempt made to address it. A psychiatric social worker or clinical psychologist should be consulted to identify possible psychosocial reasons that may be contributing to DKA. Reasons for insulin omission include the following: an attempt to lose weight in an adolescent girl with an eating disorder, a means of escaping an intolerable or abusive home situation, or clinical depression causing inability of the patient to manage diabetes unassisted. An infection that is not associated with vomiting and diarrhea is seldom the cause when the patient or family is properly educated in diabetes management and is receiving appropriate follow-up care by a diabetes team with a 24-h telephone helpline that patients access for assistance when ketosis develops.[185]

Insulin omission can be prevented by education, psychosocial evaluation, and treatment combined with adult supervision of insulin administration.[186] When a responsible adult administers insulin, there may be as much as a tenfold reduction in frequency of recurrent DKA,[186] and a more recent study has shown that intensive behavioral intervention reduces admissions for DKA and related costs in high-risk youth with poorly controlled diabetes.[187]

The most common cause of DKA in patients who use insulin pumps is failure to take extra insulin with a pen or syringe when hyperglycemia and hyperketonemia or ketonuria occur. Home measurement of blood 3-β-OHB concentrations, when compared to urine ketone testing, decreases diabetes-related hospital visits thanks to the early identification and treatment of ketosis.[188] Blood β-OHB measurements may be especially valuable to prevent DKA in patients who use a pump because interrupted insulin delivery rapidly leads to ketosis,[189,190] and serum β-OHB concentrations may be increased to levels consistent with DKA when urine is still ketone negative or shows only trace or small ketonuria.[191]

Parents and patients should learn how to recognize and treat impending DKA with additional rapid- or short-acting insulin and oral fluids, and patients should have access to a 24-h telephone helpline for emergency advice and treatment.[43]

Sick-Day Management

Illness and stress are common and can trigger counterregulation and subsequent metabolic deterioration. Sick-day management requires increased monitoring of blood glucose levels and measurement of blood or urine ketones. Urine testing for ketones had been the standard approach to sick-day management until the advent of self-monitoring of blood 3-β-hydroxybutyrate levels.[191,192]

As the majority of patients presenting with DKA have established diabetes, outpatient education directed at sick-day management and the early identification and treatment of impending DKA are important elements of a comprehensive diabetes education program. Teaching and reinforcement of sick-day "rules" and, especially, the vital importance of frequent self-monitoring of blood glucose and ketone levels and timely administration of supplemental rapid-acting insulin and oral salt and water reduce episodes of DKA in patients with established T1D.

HYPERGLYCEMIC HYPEROSMOLAR STATE

Hyperglycemic hyperosmolar state (HHS) is a syndrome characterized by extreme elevations in serum glucose concentrations and hyperosmolality without significant ketosis.[16] Although the incidence of HHS is increasing,[13,14,18] it is less frequent in children than DKA.

Unlike the usual symptoms of DKA (hyperventilation, vomiting, and abdominal pain), which typically bring children to medical attention, the gradually increasing polyuria and polydipsia of HHS may go unrecognized resulting in profound dehydration and electrolyte losses at the time of presentation. In adults, fluid losses in HHS have been estimated to be twice those of DKA; furthermore, obesity and hyperosmolality can make the clinical assessment of dehydration challenging. Despite severe volume depletion and electrolyte losses, hypertonicity preserves intravascular volume and signs of dehydration may be less evident.

During therapy, decreasing serum osmolality (from enhanced glucosuria and insulin-mediated glucose uptake) results in movement of water out of the intravascular space resulting in decreased intravascular volume, and osmotic diuresis may continue for hours in patients with extremely increased plasma glucose concentrations. Early in the course of treatment, urinary fluid losses may be considerable. Because intravascular volume may decrease rapidly during treatment in patients with HHS, more aggressive replacement of intravascular volume (as compared to treatment of children with DKA) is required to avoid vascular collapse.

Treatment of HHS

There are no prospective data to guide treatment of children and adolescents with HHS. The following recommendations are based on extensive experience in adults and an appreciation of the pathophysiological differences between HHS and DKA (see Fig. 15.I.2).[16] Patients should be admitted to an intensive care unit or comparable setting where expert medical, nursing, and laboratory services are available.

Fluid therapy. The goal of initial fluid therapy is to expand the intra- and extravascular volume and restore normal renal perfusion. The rate of fluid replacement should be more rapid than is recommended for DKA. The initial bolus should be ≥20 mL/kg of isotonic saline (0.9% NaCl) and a fluid deficit of ~12 to 15% of body weight should be assumed. Additional fluid boluses should be given, if necessary, to restore peripheral perfusion; thereafter, 0.45 to 0.75% NaCl should be administered to replace the deficit over 24 to 48 h. The goal is to promote a gradual decline in serum sodium concentration and osmolality. Because isotonic fluids are more effective in maintaining circulatory volume, isotonic saline should be restarted if perfusion and hemodynamic status appear inadequate as serum osmolality declines. Serum sodium concentrations should be frequently measured and the sodium concentration in fluids adjusted to promote a gradual decline in corrected serum sodium concentration. A rate of 0.5 mmol/L per hour has been recommended for hypernatremic dehydration. With adequate rehydration, serum glucose concentrations should decrease by 75 to 100 mg/dL per hour. A more rapid rate of decline in serum glucose concentration is typical during the first several hours of treatment when an expanded vascular volume leads to improved renal perfusion. Failure of the expected decrease of plasma glucose concentration should prompt reassessment and evaluation of renal function. Unlike treatment of DKA,

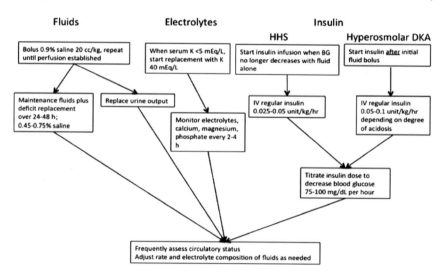

Figure 15.1.2 Treatment of HHS.

Reprinted from Zeitler et al.,[16] with permission from the publisher.

replacement of urinary losses is recommended.[193] The typical urine sodium concentration during an osmotic diuresis approximates 0.45% saline; however, when there is concern about the adequacy of circulatory volume, urinary losses may be replaced with a fluid containing a higher sodium concentration.

Insulin therapy. Whereas tissue hypoperfusion in HHS commonly causes lactic acidosis, ketosis usually is minimal. Early insulin administration is unnecessary in nonketotic HHS. Fluid administration alone causes a marked decline in serum glucose concentration as a result of dilution, improved renal perfusion leading to glucosuria, and increased tissue uptake with improved circulation. The osmotic pressure that glucose exerts within the vascular space contributes to the maintenance of blood volume. A rapid fall in serum glucose concentration and osmolality after insulin administration may lead to circulatory compromise and thrombosis unless fluid replacement is adequate. Patients with HHS also have extreme potassium deficits, and a rapid insulin-induced shift of potassium to the intracellular space can trigger arrhythmia.

Insulin administration should be initiated when serum glucose concentration is no longer declining at a rate of at least 50 mg/dL per hour with fluid administration alone. In patients with more severe ketosis and acidosis, however, insulin administration should be initiated earlier. Continuous administration of 0.025 to 0.05 units per kg per hour can be used initially, with the dosage titrated to achieve a decrease in glucose concentration of 50 to 75 mg/dL per hour. Insulin boluses are not recommended.

Electrolytes. In general, deficits of potassium, phosphate, and magnesium are greater in HHS than DKA. Potassium replacement (40 mmol/L of replacement fluid) should begin as soon serum potassium concentration is within the normal range and adequate renal function has been established. Higher rates of administration may be necessary after starting an insulin infusion and serum potassium concentrations should be monitored every 2–3 h along with ECG monitoring. Hourly potassium measurements may be necessary if the patient has hypokalemia. Bicarbonate therapy is not indicated; it increases the risk of hypokalemia and may adversely affect tissue oxygen delivery.

Severe hypophosphatemia may lead to rhabdomyolysis, hemolytic uremia, muscle weakness, and paralysis. Although administration of phosphate is associated with a risk of hypocalcemia, an IV solution that contains a 50:50 mixture of potassium phosphate and another suitable potassium salt (potassium chloride or potassium acetate) generally permits adequate phosphate replacement while avoiding clinically significant hypocalcemia. Serum phosphate concentrations should be measured every 3 to 4 h.

Patients with HHS frequently have large magnesium deficits, but there are no data to determine whether replacement of magnesium is beneficial. Replacement of magnesium should be considered in the occasional patient who experiences severe hypomagnesemia and hypocalcemia during therapy. The recommended dose is 25 to 50 mg/kg per dose for 3 to 4 doses given every 4 to 6 h with a maximum infusion rate of 150 mg/min and 2 g/h.

Complications. Venous thrombosis associated with use of central venous catheters is a common hazard in HHS.[87] Prophylactic use of low-dose heparin has been suggested in adults, but there are no data to indicate benefit from this practice. Heparin treatment should be reserved for children who require central venous catheters for physiologic monitoring or venous access and are immobile for more than 24 to 48 h.[16]

Rhabdomyolysis may occur in children with HHS resulting in acute kidney failure, severe hyperkalemia, hypocalcemia, and muscle swelling causing compartment syndrome.[194] The classic symptom triad of rhabdomyolysis includes myalgia, weakness, and dark urine, and monitoring creatine kinase concentrations every 2 to 3 h is recommended for early detection.

For unknown reasons, several children with HHS have had clinical manifestations consistent with malignant hyperthermia.[11,15,195,196] Patients who have a fever associated with a rise in creatine kinase concentrations should be treated with dantrolene, which reduces release of calcium from the sarcoplasmic reticulum and stabilizes calcium metabolism within muscle cells.

Altered mental status is common in adults whose serum osmolality exceeds 330 mOsm/kg; however, cerebral edema is rare. A decline in mental status after hyperosmolality has improved with treatment is unusual and should be promptly investigated.

MIXED HHS AND DKA

Treatment must take into account potential complications of both DKA and HHS. Mental status must be closely monitored and frequent reassessment of circulatory status and fluid balance is necessary to guide therapy. To maintain an adequate circulatory volume, the rate of fluid and electrolyte administration usually exceeds that required for the typical case of DKA. Insulin is necessary to resolve ketosis and arrest hepatic gluconeogenesis; however, insulin infusion should be deferred until after the patient has received an initial fluid bolus and the circulation has been stabilized. Serum potassium and phosphate concentrations should be carefully monitored as described above for DKA.

APPENDIX 15.I.A

Glasgow Coma Scale or Score

The Glasgow Coma Scale (GCS)[78,79] consists of three parameters and is scored between 3 and 15, with 3 being the worst and 15 the best. One of the components of the GCS is the best verbal response, which cannot be assessed in nonverbal young children. A modification of the GCS was created for children too young to talk.

Table 15.I.A.1 Glasgow Coma Scale

Best Eye Response	Best Verbal Response	Best Verbal Response (nonverbal children)	Best Motor Response
No eye opening	No verbal response	No response	No motor response
Eyes open to pain	No words, only incomprehensible sounds; moaning and groaning	Inconsolable, irritable, restless, cries	Extension to pain (decerebrate posture)
Eyes open to verbal command		Inconsistently consolable and moans; makes vocal sounds	
Eyes open spontaneously	Words, but incoherent*		Flexion to pain (decorticate posture)
	Confused, disoriented conversation**	Consolable when crying and interacts inappropriately	Withdrawal from pain
	Orientated, normal conversation	Smiles, oriented to sound, follows objects and interacts	Localizes pain
			Obeys commands

Note:

* Inappropriate words, no sustained conversational exchange
** Attention can be held; responds in a conversational manner, but shows some disorientation.

REFERENCES

1. Kitabchi AE, Umpierrez GE, Murphy MB, Kreisberg RA: Hyperglycemic crises in adult patients with diabetes: a consensus statement from the American Diabetes Association. *Diabetes Care* 29(12):2739–2748, 2006
2. Dunger DB, Sperling MA, Acerini CL, Bohn DJ, Daneman D, Danne TP, et al.: ESPE/LWPES consensus statement on diabetic ketoacidosis in children and adolescents. *Arch Dis Child* 89(2):188–194, 2004
3. Pinkey JH, Bingley PJ, Sawtell PA, Dunger DB, Gale EA: Presentation and progress of childhood diabetes mellitus: a prospective population-based study. Bart's-Oxford Study Group. *Diabetologia* 37(1):70–74, 1994
4. American Diabetes Association: Type 2 diabetes in children and adolescents (consensus statement). *Diabetes Care* 23(3):381–389, 2000
5. Rewers A, Klingensmith G, Davis C, Petitti DB, Pihoker C, Rodriguez B, et al.: Presence of diabetic ketoacidosis at diagnosis of diabetes mellitus in youth: the Search for Diabetes in Youth study. *Pediatrics* 121(5):e1258–e1266, 2008
6. Atlas AB, Finegold DN, Becker D, Trucco M, Kurland G.: Diabetic ketoacidosis in cystic fibrosis. *Am J Dis Child* 146(12):1457–1458, 1992
7. Swartz LM, Laffel LM: A teenage girl with cystic fibrosis–related diabetes, diabetic ketoacidosis, and cerebral edema. *Pediatric Diabetes* [Case Reports] 9(4 Pt 2):426–430, 2008
8. Eenkhoorn V, Van den Driessche A, Van Gaal L, Desager K, De Block C: Diabetic keto-acidosis as a presentation of cystic fibrosis-related diabetes: a case report. *J Diabetes Complications* [Case Reports] 25(2):137–141, 2011
9. Dehghani SM, Nikeghbalian S, Eshraghian A, Haghighat M, Imanieh MH, Bahador A, et al.: New-onset diabetes mellitus presenting with diabetic ketoacidosis after pediatric liver transplantation. *Pediatr Transplant* [Case Reports] 13(5):536–539, 2009
10. Roberson JR, Raju S, Shelso J, Pui CH, Howard SC: Diabetic ketoacidosis during therapy for pediatric acute lymphoblastic leukemia. *Pediatr Blood Cancer* [Research Support, N.I.H., Extramural Research Support, Non-U.S. Gov't] 50(6):1207–1212, 2008
11. Morales AE, Rosenbloom AL: Death caused by hyperglycemic hyperosmolar state at the onset of type 2 diabetes. *J Pediatr* 144(2):270–273, 2004
12. Kershaw MJ, Newton T, Barrett TG, Berry K, Kirk J: Childhood diabetes presenting with hyperosmolar dehydration but without ketoacidosis: a report of three cases. *Diabet Med* 22(5):645–647, 2005
13. Canarie MF, Bogue CW, Banasiak KJ, Weinzimer SA, Tamborlane WV: Decompensated hyperglycemic hyperosmolarity without significant ketoacidosis in the adolescent and young adult population. *J Pediatr Endocrinol Metab* 20(10):1115–1124, 2007
14. Fourtner SH, Weinzimer SA, Levitt Katz LE: Hyperglycemic hyperosmolar non-ketotic syndrome in children with type 2 diabetes. *Pediatr Diabetes* 6(3):129–135, 2005
15. Hollander AS, Olney RC, Blackett PR, Marshall BA: Fatal malignant hyperthermia-like syndrome with rhabdomyolysis complicating the presentation of diabetes mellitus in adolescent males. *Pediatrics* 111(6 Pt 1):1447–1452, 2003

16. Zeitler P, Haqq A, Rosenbloom A, Glaser N: Hyperglycemic hyperosmolar syndrome in children: pathophysiological considerations and suggested guidelines for treatment. *J Pediatr* [Review] 158(1):9–14, e1–e2, 2011
17. Rosenbloom AL: Hyperglycemic crises and their complications in children. *J Pediatr Endocrinol Metab* 20(1):5–18, 2007
18. Rosenbloom AL: Hyperglycemic hyperosmolar state: an emerging pediatric problem. *J Pediatr* 156(2):180–184, 2010
19. McDonnell CM, Pedreira CC, Vadamalayan B, Cameron FJ, Werther GA: Diabetic ketoacidosis, hyperosmolarity and hypernatremia: are high-carbohydrate drinks worsening initial presentation? *Pediatr Diabetes* 6(2): 90–94, 2005
20. Levy-Marchal C, Papoz L, de Beaufort C, Doutreix J, Froment V, Voirin J, et al.: Clinical and laboratory features of type 1 diabetic children at the time of diagnosis. *Diabet Med* (3):279–284, 1992
21. Komulainen J, Lounamaa R, Knip M, Kaprio EA, Akerblom HK: Keto-acidosis at the diagnosis of type 1 (insulin dependent) diabetes mellitus is related to poor residual beta cell function. Childhood Diabetes in Finland Study Group. *Arch Dis Child* 75(5):410–415, 1996
22. Levy-Marchal C, Patterson CC, Green A: Geographical variation of presentation at diagnosis of type I diabetes in children: the EURODIAB study. *Diabetologia* 44(Suppl. 3):B75–B80, 2001
23. Hanas R, Lindgren F, Lindblad B: Diabetic ketoacidosis and cerebral oedema in Sweden—a 2-year paediatric population study. *Diabet Med* 24(10):1080–1085, 2007
24. Rodacki M, Pereira JR, Nabuco de Oliveira AM, Barone B, Mac Dowell R, Perricelli P, et al.: Ethnicity and young age influence the frequency of diabetic ketoacidosis at the onset of type 1 diabetes. *Diabetes Res Clin Pract* 78(2):259–262, 2007
25. Hekkala A, Knip M, Veijola R: Ketoacidosis at diagnosis of type 1 diabetes in children in northern Finland: temporal changes over 20 years. *Diabetes Care* 30(4):861–866, 2007
26. Majaliwa ES, Munubhi E, Ramaiya K, Mpembeni R, Sanyiwa A, Mohn A, et al.: Survey on acute and chronic complications in children and adolescents with type 1 diabetes at Muhimbili National Hospital in Dar es Salaam, Tanzania. *Diabetes Care* 30(9):2187–2192, 2007
27. Elamin A, Altahir H, Ismail B, Tuvemo T: Clinical pattern of childhood type 1 (insulin-dependent) diabetes mellitus in the Sudan. *Diabetologia* [Research Support, Non-U.S. Gov't] 35(7):645–648, 1992
28. Quinn M, Fleischman A, Rosner B, Nigrin DJ, Wolfsdorf JI: Characteristics at diagnosis of type 1 diabetes in children younger than 6 years. *J Pediatr* 148(3):366–371, 2006
29. Szypowska A, Skorka A: The risk factors of ketoacidosis in children with newly diagnosed type 1 diabetes mellitus. *Pediatric Diabetes* 12(4 Pt 1):302–306, 2011
30. Schober E, Rami B, Waldhoer T: Diabetic ketoacidosis at diagnosis in Austrian children in 1989–2008: a population-based analysis. *Diabetologia* [Research Support, Non-U.S. Gov't] 53(6):1057–1061, 2010
31. Bui H, To T, Stein R, Fung K, Daneman D: Is diabetic ketoacidosis at disease onset a result of missed diagnosis? *J Pediatr* 156(3):472–477, 2010

32. Abdul-Rasoul M, Al-Mahdi M, Al-Qattan H, Al-Tarkait N, Alkhouly M, Al-Safi R, et al.: Ketoacidosis at presentation of type 1 diabetes in children in Kuwait: frequency and clinical characteristics. *Pediatric Diabetes* 11(5):351–356, 2010

33. Pawlowicz M, Birkholz D, Niedzwiecki M, Balcerska A: Difficulties or mistakes in diagnosing type 1 diabetes in children?—demographic factors influencing delayed diagnosis. *Pediatric Diabetes* 10(8):542–549, 2009

34. Neu A, Hofer SE, Karges B, Oeverink R, Rosenbauer J, Holl RW: Ketoacidosis at diabetes onset is still frequent in children and adolescents: a multicenter analysis of 14,664 patients from 106 institutions. *Diabetes Care* 32(9):1647–1648, 2009

35. Rosilio M, Cotton JB, Wieliczko MC, Gendrault B, Carel JC, Couvaras O, et al.: Factors associated with glycemic control. A cross-sectional nationwide study in 2,579 French children with type 1 diabetes. French Pediatric Diabetes Group [see comments]. *Diabetes Care* 21(7):1146–1153, 1998

36. Smith CP, Firth D, Bennett S, Howard C, Chisholm P: Ketoacidosis occurring in newly diagnosed and established diabetic children. *Acta Pediatr* 87(5):537–541, 1998

37. Fritsch M, Rosenbauer J, Schober E, Neu A, Placzek K, Holl RW: Predictors of diabetic ketoacidosis in children and adolescents with type 1 diabetes. Experience from a large multicentre database. *Pediatric Diabetes* [Research Support, Non-U.S. Gov't] 12(4 Pt 1):307–312, 2011

38. Rewers A, Chase HP, Mackenzie T, Walravens P, Roback M, Rewers M, et al.: Predictors of acute complications in children with type 1 diabetes. *JAMA* 287(19):2511–2518, 2002

39. Morris AD, Boyle DI, McMahon AD, Greene SA, MacDonald TM, Newton RW: Adherence to insulin treatment, glycaemic control, and ketoacidosis in insulin-dependent diabetes mellitus. DARTS/MEMO Collaboration. Diabetes Audit and Research in Tayside Scotland. Medicines Monitoring Unit. *Lancet* 350(9090):1505–1510, 1997

40. Hanas R, Lindgren F, Lindblad B: A 2-yr national population study of pediatric ketoacidosis in Sweden: predisposing conditions and insulin pump use. *Pediatr Diabetes* 10(1):33–37, 2009

41. Karges B, Kapellen T, Neu A, Hofer SE, Rohrer T, Rosenbauer J, et al.: Long-acting insulin analogs and the risk of diabetic ketoacidosis in children and adolescents with type 1 diabetes A prospective study of 10,682 patients from 271 institutions. *Diabetes Care* 33:1031–1033, 2010

42. Flood RG, Chiang VW: Rate and prediction of infection in children with diabetic ketoacidosis. *Am J Emerg Med* 19(4):270–273, 2001

43. Hoffman WH, O'Neill P, Khoury C, Bernstein SS: Service and education for the insulin-dependent child. *Diabetes Care* 1(5):285–288, 1978

44. Drozda DJ, Dawson VA, Long DJ, Freson LS, Sperling MA: Assessment of the effect of a comprehensive diabetes management program on hospital admission rates of children with diabetes mellitus. *Diabetes Educ* 16(5):389–393, 1990

45. Grey M, Boland EA, Davidson M, Li J, Tamborlane WV: Coping skills training for youth with diabetes mellitus has long-lasting effects on metabolic control and quality of life. *J Pediatr* 137(1):107–113, 2000

46. Deeter KH, Roberts JS, Bradford H, Richards T, Shaw D, Marro K, et al.: Hypertension despite dehydration during severe pediatric diabetic ketoacidosis. *Pediatric Diabetes* 12(4 Pt 1):295–301, 2011

47. Atchley D, Loeb R, Richards D, Jr., Benedict E, Driscoll M: On diabetic ketoacidosis: a detailed study of electrolyte balances following the withdrawal and reestablishment of insulin therapy. *J Clin Invest* 12:297–326, 1933

48. Nabarro J, Spencer A, Stowers J: Metabolic studies in severe diabetic ketosis. *Q J Med* 82:225–248, 1952

49. Fagan MJ, Avner J, Khine H: Initial fluid resuscitation for patients with diabetic ketoacidosis: how dry are they? *Clin Pediatr* 47(9):851–855, 2008

50. Sottosanti M, Morrison GC, Singh RN, Sharma AP, Fraser DD, Alawi K, et al.: Dehydration in children with diabetic ketoacidosis: a prospective study. *Arch Dis Child* [Research Support, Non-U.S. Gov't] 97(2):96–100, 2012

51. Yanovski JA, Sobel DO, Abbassi V: The differing presentation of insulin-dependent diabetes mellitus in infants and children. *Clin Pediatr* [Comparative Study] 33(9):556–560, 1994

52. Mackenzie A, Barnes G, Shann F: Clinical signs of dehydration in children. *Lancet* 2(8663):605–607, 1989

53. Koves IH, Neutze J, Donath S, Lee W, Werther GA, Barnett P, et al.: The accuracy of clinical assessment of dehydration during diabetic ketoacidosis in childhood. *Diabetes Care* 27(10):2485–2487, 2004

54. Butler A, Talbot N, Burnett C, Stanbury J, MacLachlan E: Metabolic studies in diabetic coma. *Tans Assoc Am Physicians* 60:102–109, 1947

55. Danowski T, Peters J, Rathbun J, Quashnock J, Greenman L: Studies in diabetic acidosis and coma, with particular emphasis on the retention of administered potassium. *J Clin Invest* 28:1–9, 1949

56. Darrow D, Pratt E: Retention of water and electrolyte during recovery in a patient with diabetic acidosis. *J Pediatr* 41:688–696, 1952

57. Taketomo C, Hodding J, Kraus D: *Pediatric Dosage Handbook.* 12th ed. Hudson, OH, Lexi-Comp, 2005

58. Harris GD, Fiordalisi I: Physiologic management of diabetic ketoacidemia. A 5-year prospective pediatric experience in 231 episodes. *Arch Pediatr Adolesc Med* 148(10):1046–1052, 1994

59. Linares MY, Schunk JE, Lindsay R: Laboratory presentation in diabetic ketoacidosis and duration of therapy. *Pediatr Emerg Care* 12(5):347–351, 1996

60. Katz MA: Hyperglycemia-induced hyponatremia—calculation of expected serum sodium depression. *N Engl J Med* 289(16):843–844, 1973

61. Hillier TA, Abbott RD, Barrett EJ: Hyponatremia: evaluating the correction factor for hyperglycemia. *Am J Med* 106(4):399–403, 1999

62. Harris GD, Fiordalisi I, Harris WL, Mosovich LL, Finberg L: Minimizing the risk of brain herniation during treatment of diabetic ketoacidemia: a retrospective and prospective study. *J Pediatr* 117:22–31, 1990

63. Hale PM, Rezvani I, Braunstein AW, Lipman TH, Martinez N, Garibaldi L: Factors predicting cerebral edema in young children with diabetic ketoacidosis and new onset type I diabetes. *Acta Pediatr* 86(6):626–631, 1997

64. Glaser N, Barnett P, McCaslin I, Nelson D, Trainor J, Louie J, et al.: Risk factors for cerebral edema in children with diabetic ketoacidosis. Pediatric Emergency Medicine Collaborative Research Committee of the American Academy of Pediatrics. *N Engl J Med* 344(4):264–269, 2001

65. Adrogue HJ, Lederer ED, Suki WN, Eknoyan G: Determinants of plasma potassium levels in diabetic ketoacidosis. *Medicine* 65(3):163–172, 1986

66. Umpierrez GE, DiGirolamo M, Tuvlin JA, Isaacs SD, Bhoola SM, Kokko JP: Differences in metabolic and hormonal milieu in diabetic- and alcohol-induced ketoacidosis. *J Crit Care* [Comparative Study Research Support, Non-U.S. Gov't] 15(2):52–59, 2000

67. DeFronzo RA, Matsuda M, Barrett EJ: Diabetic ketoacidosis: a combined metabolic-nephrologic approach to therapy. *Diabetes Reviews* 2:209–238, 1994

68. Dweikat IM, Naser EN, Abu Libdeh AI, Naser OJ, Abu Gharbieh NN, Maraqa NF, et al.: Propionic acidemia mimicking diabetic ketoacidosis. *Brain Dev* [Case Reports] 33(5):428–431, 2011

69. Erdem E, Cayonu N, Uysalol E, Yildirmak ZY: Chronic intermittent form of isovaleric acidemia mimicking diabetic ketoacidosis. *JPEM* [Case Reports] 23(5):503–505, 2010

70. Saudubray JM, Specola N, Middleton B, Lombes A, Bonnefont JP, Jakobs C, et al.: Hyperketotic states due to inherited defects of ketolysis. *Enzyme* [Review] 38(1–4):80–90, 1987

71. Fukao T, Scriver CR, Kondo N: The clinical phenotype and outcome of mitochondrial acetoacetyl-CoA thiolase deficiency (beta-ketothiolase or T2 deficiency) in 26 enzymatically proved and mutation-defined patients. *Mol Genet Metab* 72(2):109–114, 2001

72. Edge JA, Jakes RW, Roy Y, Hawkins M, Winter D, Ford-Adams ME, et al.: The UK case-control study of cerebral oedema complicating diabetic keto-acidosis in children. *Diabetologia* 49(9):2002–2009, 2006

73. Haddad NG, Croffie JM, Eugster EA: Pancreatic enzyme elevations in children with diabetic ketoacidosis. *J Pediatr* 145(1):122–124, 2004

74. Quiros JA, Marcin JP, Kuppermann N, Nasrollahzadeh F, Rewers A, DiCarlo J, et al.: Elevated serum amylase and lipase in pediatric diabetic ketoacidosis. *Pediatr Crit Care Med* 9(4):418–422, 2008

75. Vinicor F, Lehrner LM, Karn RC, Merritt AD: Hyperamylasemia in diabetic ketoacidosis: sources and significance. *Ann Intern Med* 91(2):200–204, 1979

76. Warshaw AL, Feller ER, Lee K-H: On the cause of raised serum amylase in diabetic ketoacidosis. *Lancet* 1:929–931, 1977

77. Steiner MJ, DeWalt DA, Byerley JS: Is this child dehydrated? *JAMA* 291(22):2746–2754, 2004

78. Teasdale G, Jennett B: Assessment of coma and impaired consciousness. A practical scale. *Lancet* 2(7872):81–84, 1974

79. Reilly PL, Simpson DA, Sprod R, Thomas L: Assessing the conscious level in infants and young children: a paediatric version of the Glasgow Coma Scale. *Childs Nerv Syst* 4(1):30–33, 1988

80. Wiggam MI, O'Kane MJ, Harper R, Atkinson AB, Hadden DR, Trimble ER, et al.: Treatment of diabetic ketoacidosis using normalization of blood

3-hydroxybutyrate concentration as the endpoint of emergency management. A randomized controlled study. *Diabetes Care* 20(9):1347–1352, 1997
81. Rewers A, McFann K, Chase HP: Bedside monitoring of blood beta-hydroxybutyrate levels in the management of diabetic ketoacidosis in children. *Diabetes Technol Ther* 8(6):671–676, 2006
82. Malone JI, Brodsky SJ: The value of electrocardiogram monitoring in diabetic ketoacidosis. *Diabetes Care* 3(4):543–547, 1980
83. Soler NG, Bennett MA, Fitzgerald MG, Malins JM: Electrocardiogram as a guide to potassium replacement in diabetic ketoacidosis. *Diabetes* 23(7):610–615, 1974
84. Agus MS, Alexander JL, Mantell PA: Continuous non-invasive end-tidal CO2 monitoring in pediatric inpatients with diabetic ketoacidosis. *Pediatric Diabetes* 7(4):196–200, 2006
85. Waldhausl W, Kleinberger G, Korn A, Dudczak R, Bratusch-Marrain P, Nowotny P: Severe hyperglycemia: effects of rehydration on endocrine derangements and blood glucose concentration. *Diabetes* 28(6):577–584, 1979
86. Dunger DB, Sperling MA, Acerini CL, Bohn DJ, Daneman D, Danne TP, et al.: European Society for Paediatric Endocrinology/Lawson Wilkins Pediatric Endocrine Society consensus statement on diabetic ketoacidosis in children and adolescents. *Pediatrics* 113(2):e133–e140, 2004
87. Gutierrez JA, Bagatell R, Samson MP, Theodorou AA, Berg RA: Femoral central venous catheter-associated deep venous thrombosis in children with diabetic ketoacidosis. *Crit Care Med* 31(1):80–83, 2003
88. Adrogue HJ, Barrero J, Eknoyan G: Salutary effects of modest fluid replacement in the treatment of adults with diabetic ketoacidosis. Use in patients without extreme volume deficit. *JAMA* 262(15):2108–2113, 1989
89. Mel JM, Werther GA: Incidence and outcome of diabetic cerebral oedema in childhood: are there predictors? *J Pediatr Child Health* 31(1):17–20, 1995
90. Wagner A, Risse A, Brill HL, Wienhausen-Wilke V, Rottmann M, Sondern K, et al.: Therapy of severe diabetic ketoacidosis. Zero-mortality under very-low-dose insulin application. *Diabetes Care* 22(5):674–677, 1999
91. Rother KI, Schwenk WF, 2nd: Effect of rehydration fluid with 75 mmol/L of sodium on serum sodium concentration and serum osmolality in young patients with diabetic ketoacidosis. *Mayo Clin Proc* 69(12):1149–1153, 1994
92. Felner EI, White PC: Improving management of diabetic ketoacidosis in children. *Pediatrics* 108(3):735–740, 2001
93. Duck SC, Wyatt DT: Factors associated with brain herniation in the treatment of diabetic ketoacidosis. *J Pediatr* 113:10–14, 1988
94. Adrogue HJ, Eknoyan G, Suki WK: Diabetic ketoacidosis: role of the kidney in the acid-base homeostasis re-evaluated. *Kidney Int* 25(4):591–598, 1984
95. Oh MS, Carroll HJ, Uribarri J: Mechanism of normochloremic and hyperchloremic acidosis in diabetic ketoacidosis. *Nephron* 54(1):1–6, 1990
96. Owen OE, Licht JH, Sapir DG: Renal function and effects of partial rehydration during diabetic ketoacidosis. *Diabetes* 30(6):510–518, 1981
97. Luzi L, Barrett EJ, Groop LC, Ferrannini E, DeFronzo RA: Metabolic effects of low-dose insulin therapy on glucose metabolism in diabetic ketoacidosis. *Diabetes* 37(11):1470–1477, 1988

98. Schade DS, Eaton RP: Dose response to insulin in man: differential effects on glucose and ketone body regulation. *J Clin Endocrinol Metab* 44(6):1038–1053, 1977

99. Marcin JP, Kuppermann N, Tancredi DJ, Glaser NS: Insulin administration for treatment of pediatric diabetic ketoacidosis: are lower rates of infusion beneficial? *Pediatr Crit Care Med* [Comment Editorial] 12(2):217–219, 2011

100. Kitabchi AE: Low-dose insulin therapy in diabetic ketoacidosis: fact or fiction? *Diabetes Metab Rev* 5(4):337–363, 1989

101. Lindsay R, Bolte RG: The use of an insulin bolus in low-dose insulin infusion for pediatric diabetic ketoacidosis. *Pediatr Emerg Care* 5(2):77–79, 1989

102. Kitabchi AE, Murphy MB, Spencer J, Matteri R, Karas J: Is a priming dose of insulin necessary in a low-dose insulin protocol for the treatment of diabetic ketoacidosis? *Diabetes Care* [Randomized Controlled Trial Research Support, N.I.H., Extramural] 31(11):2081–2085, 2008

103. Soler NG, FitzGerald MG, Wright AD, Malins JM: Comparative study of different insulin regimens in management of diabetic ketoacidosis. *Lancet* 2(7947):1221–1224, 1975

104. Puttha R, Cooke D, Subbarayan A, Odeka E, Ariyawansa I, Bone M, et al.: Low dose (0.05 units/kg/h) is comparable with standard dose (0.1 units/kg/h) intravenous insulin infusion for the initial treatment of diabetic ketoacidosis in children with type 1 diabetes—an observational study. *Pediatr Diabetes* 11:12–17, 2010

105. Al Hanshi S, Shann F: Insulin infused at 0.05 versus 0.1 units/kg/hr in children admitted to intensive care with diabetic ketoacidosis. *Pediatr Crit Care Med* [Comparative Study] 12(2):137–140, 2011

106. Burghen GA, Etteldorf JN, Fisher JN, Kitabchi AQ: Comparison of high-dose and low-dose insulin by continuous intravenous infusion in the treatment of diabetic ketoacidosis in children. *Diabetes Care* 3(1):15–20, 1980

107. Grimberg A, Cerri RW, Satin-Smith M, Cohen P: The "two bag system" for variable intravenous dextrose and fluid administration: benefits in diabetic ketoacidosis management. *J Pediatr* [Comparative Study Research Support, Non-U.S. Gov't] 134(3):376–378, 1999

108. Umpierrez GE, Latif K, Stoever J, Cuervo R, Park L, Freire AX, et al.: Efficacy of subcutaneous insulin lispro versus continuous intravenous regular insulin for the treatment of patients with diabetic ketoacidosis. *Am J Med* 117(5):291–296, 2004

109. Umpierrez GE, Cuervo R, Karabell A, Latif K, Freire AX, Kitabchi AE: Treatment of diabetic ketoacidosis with subcutaneous insulin aspart. *Diabetes Care* 27(8):1873–1878, 2004

110. Della Manna T, Steinmetz L, Campos PR, Farhat SC, Schvartsman C, Kuperman H, et al.: Subcutaneous use of a fast-acting insulin analog: an alternative treatment for pediatric patients with diabetic ketoacidosis. *Diabetes Care* 28(8):1856–1861, 2005

111. DeFronzo RA, Felig P, Ferrannini E, Wahren J: Effect of graded doses of insulin on splanchnic and peripheral potassium metabolism in man. *Am J Physiol* 238(5):E421–E427, 1980

112. Tattersall RB: A paper which changed clinical practice (slowly). Jacob Holler on potassium deficiency in diabetic acidosis (1946). *Diabet Med* 16(12):978–984, 1999

113. Nabarro JD, Spencer AG, Stowers JM: Treatment of diabetic ketosis. *Lancet* 1(20):983–989, 1952

114. Kuppermann N, Park J, Glatter K, Marcin JP, Glaser NS: Prolonged QT interval corrected for heart rate during diabetic ketoacidosis in children. *Arch Pediatr Adolesc Med* 162(6):544–549, 2008

115. Guest G, Rapoport S: Electrolytes of blood plasma and cells in diabetic acidosis and during recovery. *Proc Am Diabetes Assoc* 7:95–115, 1947

116. Riley MS, Schade DS, Eaton RP: Effects of insulin infusion on plasma phosphate in diabetic patients. *Metabolism* 28(3):191–194, 1979

117. Alberti KG, Emerson PM, Darley JH, Hockaday TD: 2,3-Diphosphoglycerate and tissue oxygenation in uncontrolled diabetes mellitus. *Lancet* 2(7774):391–395, 1972

118. Knochel JP: The pathophysiology and clinical characteristics of severe hypophosphatemia. *Arch Intern Med* 137(2):203–220, 1977

119. O'Connor LR, Wheeler WS, Bethune JE: Effect of hypophosphatemia on myocardial performance in man. *N Engl J Med* 297(17):901–903, 1977

120. Gibby OM, Veale KE, Hayes TM, Jones JG, Wardrop CA: Oxygen availability from the blood and the effect of phosphate replacement on erythrocyte 2,3-diphosphoglycerate and haemoglobin-oxygen affinity in diabetic ketoacidosis. *Diabetologia* 15(5):381–385, 1978

121. Keller U, Berger W: Prevention of hypophosphatemia by phosphate infusion during treatment of diabetic ketoacidosis and hyperosmolar coma. *Diabetes* 29(2):87–95, 1980

122. Wilson HK, Keuer SP, Lea AS, Boyd AE, III, Eknoyan G: Phosphate therapy in diabetic ketoacidosis. *Arch Intern Med* 142(3):517–520, 1982

123. Becker DJ, Brown DR, Steranka BH, Drash AL: Phosphate replacement during treatment of diabetic ketosis. Effects on calcium and phosphorus homeostasis. *Am J Dis Child* 137(3):241–246, 1983

124. Fisher JN, Kitabchi AE: A randomized study of phosphate therapy in the treatment of diabetic ketoacidosis. *J Clin Endocrinol Metab* 57(1):177–180, 1983

125. Clerbaux T, Reynaert M, Willems E, Frans A: Effect of phosphate on oxygen-hemoglobin affinity, diphosphoglycerate and blood gases during recovery from diabetic ketoacidosis. *Intensive Care Med* 15(8):495–498, 1989

126. Bohannon NJ: Large phosphate shifts with treatment for hyperglycemia. *Arch Intern Med* 149(6):1423–1425, 1989

127. de Oliveira Iglesias SB, Pons Leite H, de Carvalho WB: Hypophosphatemia-induced seizure in a child with diabetic ketoacidosis. *Pediatr Emerg Care* [Case Reports] 25(12):859–861, 2009

128. Zipf WB, Bacon GE, Spencer ML, Kelch RP, Hopwood NJ, Hawker CD: Hypocalcemia, hypomagnesemia, and transient hypoparathyroidism during therapy with potassium phosphate in diabetic ketoacidosis. *Diabetes Care* 2(3):265–268, 1979

129. Winter RJ, Harris CJ, Phillips LS, Green OC: Diabetic ketoacidosis. Induction of hypocalcemia and hypomagnesemia by phosphate therapy. *Am J Med* 67(5):897–900, 1979
130. Hale PJ, Crase J, Nattrass M: Metabolic effects of bicarbonate in the treatment of diabetic ketoacidosis. *Br Med J (Clin Res Ed)* 289(6451):1035–1038, 1984
131. Morris LR, Murphy MB, Kitabchi AE: Bicarbonate therapy in severe diabetic ketoacidosis. *Ann Intern Med* 105(6):836–840, 1986
132. Okuda Y, Adrogue HJ, Field JB, Nohara H, Yamashita K: Counterproductive effects of sodium bicarbonate in diabetic ketoacidosis. *J Clin Endocrinol Metab* 81(1):314–320, 1996
133. Green SM, Rothrock SG, Ho JD, Gallant RD, Borger R, Thomas TL, et al.: Failure of adjunctive bicarbonate to improve outcome in severe pediatric diabetic ketoacidosis. *Ann Emerg Med* 31(1):41–48, 1998.
134. Assal JP, Aoki TT, Manzano FM, Kozak GP: Metabolic effects of sodium bicarbonate in management of diabetic ketoacidosis. *Diabetes* 23(5):405–411, 1974
135. Ohman JL, Jr., Marliss EB, Aoki TT, Munichoodappa CS, Khanna VV, Kozak GP: The cerebrospinal fluid in diabetic ketoacidosis. *N Engl J Med* 284(6):283–290, 1971
136. Soler NG, Bennett MA, Dixon K, FitzGerald MG, Malins JM: Potassium balance during treatment of diabetic ketoacidosis with special reference to the use of bicarbonate. *Lancet* 2(7779):665–667, 1972
137. Lever E, Jaspan JB: Sodium bicarbonate therapy in severe diabetic ketoacidosis. *Am J Med* 75(2):263–268, 1983
138. Narins RG, Cohen JJ: Bicarbonate therapy for organic acidosis: the case for its continued use. *Ann Intern Med* 106(4):615–618, 1987
139. Curtis JR, To T, Muirhead S, Cummings E, Daneman D: Recent trends in hospitalization for diabetic ketoacidosis in Ontario children. *Diabetes Care* 25(9):1591–1596, 2002
140. Edge JA, Ford-Adams ME, Dunger DB: Causes of death in children with insulin dependent diabetes 1990–96. *Arch Dis Child* 81(4):318–323, 1999
141. Edge JA, Hawkins MM, Winter DL, Dunger DB: The risk and outcome of cerebral oedema developing during diabetic ketoacidosis. *Arch Dis Child* 85(1):16–22, 2001
142. Lawrence SE, Cummings EA, Gaboury I, Daneman D: Population-based study of incidence and risk factors for cerebral edema in pediatric diabetic ketoacidosis. *J Pediatr* 146(5):688–692, 2005
143. Hoffman WH, Stamatovic SM, Andjelkovic AV: Inflammatory mediators and blood brain barrier disruption in fatal brain edema of diabetic ketoacidosis. *Brain Res* 1254:138–148, 2009
144. Brown TB: Cerebral oedema in childhood diabetic ketoacidosis: is treatment a factor? *J Emerg Med* 21(2):141–144, 2004
145. Yuen N, Anderson SE, Glaser N, Tancredi DJ, O'Donnell ME: Cerebral blood flow and cerebral edema in rats with diabetic ketoacidosis. *Diabetes* 57(10):2588–2594, 2008
146. Glaser NS, Marcin JP, Wootton-Gorges SL, Buonocore MH, Rewers A, Strain J, et al.: Correlation of clinical and biochemical findings with diabetic

ketoacidosis-related cerebral edema in children using magnetic resonance diffusion-weighted imaging. *J Pediatr* 153(4):541–546, 2008

147. Glaser N: Cerebral injury and cerebral edema in children with diabetic ketoacidosis: could cerebral ischemia and reperfusion injury be involved? *Pediatr Diabetes* 10(8):534–541, 2009

148. Glaser N, Yuen N, Anderson SE, Tancredi DJ, O'Donnell ME: Cerebral metabolic alterations in rats with diabetic ketoacidosis: effects of treatment with insulin and intravenous fluids and effects of bumetanide. *Diabetes* [Research Support, N.I.H., Extramural Research Support, U.S. Gov't, Non-P.H.S.] 59(3):702–709, 2010.

149. Rosenbloom AL: Intracerebral crises during treatment of diabetic ketoacidosis. *Diabetes Care* 13(1):22–33, 1990

150. Bello FA, Sotos JF: Cerebral oedema in diabetic ketoacidosis in children [letter]. *Lancet* 336(8706):64, 1990

151. Mahoney CP, Vlcek BW, DelAguila M: Risk factors for developing brain herniation during diabetic ketoacidosis. *Pediatr Neurol* 21(4):721–727, 1999

152. Durr JA, Hoffman WH, Sklar AH, el Gammal T, Steinhart CM: Correlates of brain edema in uncontrolled IDDM. *Diabetes* 41(5):627–632, 1992

153. Edge JA, Jakes RW, Roy Y, Hawkins M, Winter D, Ford-Adams ME, et al: The UK case-control study of cerebral oedema complicating diabetic ketoacidosis in children. *Diabetologia* 49:2002–2009, 2006

154. Bureau MA, Begin R, Berthiaume Y, Shapcott D, Khoury K, Gagnon N: Cerebral hypoxia from bicarbonate infusion in diabetic acidosis. *J Pediatr* 96(6):968–973, 1980

155. Deeb L: Development of fatal cerebral edema during outpatient therapy for diabetic ketoacidosis. *Pract Diab* 6:212–213, 1989

156. Glasgow AM: Devastating cerebral edema in diabetic ketoacidosis before therapy [letter]. *Diabetes Care* 14(1):77–78, 1991

157. Couch RM, Acott PD, Wong GW: Early onset fatal cerebral edema in diabetic ketoacidosis. *Diabetes Care* 14(1):78–79, 1991

158. Fiordalisi I, Harris GD, Gilliland MG: Prehospital cardiac arrest in diabetic ketoacidemia: why brain swelling may lead to death before treatment. *J Diabetes Complications* 16(3):214–219, 2002

159. Edge JA: Cerebral oedema during treatment of diabetic ketoacidosis: are we any nearer finding a cause? *Diabetes Metab Res Rev* 16(5):316–324, 2000

160. Muir AB, Quisling RG, Yang MC, Rosenbloom AL. Cerebral edema in childhood diabetic ketoacidosis: natural history, radiographic findings, and early identification. *Diabetes Care* 27(7):1541–1546, 2004

161. Franklin B, Liu J, Ginsberg-Fellner F: Cerebral edema and ophthalmoplegia reversed by mannitol in a new case of insulin-dependent diabetes mellitus. *Pediatrics* 69(1):87–90, 1982

162. Shabbir N, Oberfield SE, Corrales R, Kairam R, Levine LS: Recovery from symptomatic brain swelling in diabetic ketoacidosis. *Clin Pediatr* 31(9):570–573, 1992

163. Roberts MD, Slover RH, Chase HP: Diabetic ketoacidosis with intracerebral complications. *Pediatric Diabetes* 2:109–114, 2001

164. Curtis JR, Bohn D, Daneman D: Use of hypertonic saline in the treatment of cerebral edema in diabetic ketoacidosis (DKA). *Pediatr Diabetes* 2(4):191–194, 2001

165. Kamat P, Vats A, Gross M, Checchia PA: Use of hypertonic saline for the treatment of altered mental status associated with diabetic ketoacidosis. *Pediatr Crit Care Med* 4(2):239–242, 2003

166. Marcin JP, Glaser N, Barnett P, McCaslin I, Nelson D, Trainor J, et al.: Factors associated with adverse outcomes in children with diabetic ketoacidosis-related cerebral edema. *J Pediatr* 141(6):793–797, 2002

167. Kanter RK, Oliphant M, Zimmerman JJ, Stuart MJ: Arterial thrombosis causing cerebral edema in association with diabetic ketoacidosis. *Crit Care Med* 15(2):175–176, 1987

168. Roe TF, Crawford TO, Huff KR, Costin G, Kaufman FR, Nelson MD, Jr.: Brain infarction in children with diabetic ketoacidosis. *J Diabetes Complications* 10(2):100–108, 1996

169. Keane S, Gallagher A, Ackroyd S, McShane MA, Edge JA: Cerebral venous thrombosis during diabetic ketoacidosis. *Arch Dis Child* 86(3):204–205, 2002

170. Rosenbloom AL: Fatal cerebral infarctions in diabetic ketoacidosis in a child with previously unknown heterozygosity for factor V Leiden deficiency. *J Pediatr* 145(4):561–562, 2004

171. Lee HS, Hwang JS: Cerebral infarction associated with transient visual loss in child with diabetic ketoacidosis. *Diabet Med* [Case Reports] 28(5):516–518, 2011

172. Lin JJ, Lin KL, Wang HS, Wong AM, Hsia SH: Occult infarct with acute hemorrhagic stroke in juvenile diabetic ketoacidosis. *Brain Dev* [Case Reports] 30(1):91–93, 2008

173. Foster JR, Morrison G, Fraser DD: Diabetic ketoacidosis-associated stroke in children and youth. *Stroke Research and Treatment* 2011:219706, 2011. doi:10.4061/2011/219706

174. Mahmud FH, Ramsay DA, Levin SD, Singh RN, Kotylak T, Fraser DD: Coma with diffuse white matter hemorrhages in juvenile diabetic ketoacidosis. *Pediatrics* [Case Reports Research Support, Non-U.S. Gov't] 120(6):e1540–e1546, 2007

175. Zerah M, Patterson R, Hansen I, Briones M, Dion J, Renfroe B: Resolution of severe sinus vein thrombosis with super selective thrombolysis in a pre-adolescent with diabetic ketoacidosis and a prothrombin gene mutation. *JPEM* [Case Reports] 20(6):725–731, 2007

176. Noyes KJ, Crofton P, Bath LE, Holmes A, Stark L, Oxley CD, et al.: Hydroxybutyrate near-patient testing to evaluate a new end-point for intravenous insulin therapy in the treatment of diabetic ketoacidosis in children. *Pediatr Diabetes* 8(3):150–156, 2007

177. Mrozik LT, Yung M: Hyperchloraemic metabolic acidosis slows recovery in children with diabetic ketoacidosis: a retrospective audit. *Aust Crit Care* 22(4):172–177, 2009

178. Vanelli M, Chiari G, Ghizzoni L, Costi G, Giacalone T, Chiarelli F: Effectiveness of a prevention program for diabetic ketoacidosis in children. An 8-year study in schools and private practices. *Diabetes Care* 22(1):7–9, 1999

179. Vanelli M, Scarabello C, Fainardi V: Available tools for primary ketoacidosis prevention at diabetes diagnosis in children and adolescents. "The Parma campaign." *Acta Biomed* 79(1):73–78, 2008
180. Vanelli M, Chiari G, Lacava S, Iovane B: Campaign for diabetic ketoacidosis prevention still effective 8 years later [letter]. *Diabetes Care* 30(4):e12, 2007
181. Triolo TM, Chase HP, Barker JM: Diabetic subjects diagnosed through the Diabetes Prevention Trial-Type 1 (DPT-1) are often asymptomatic with normal A1C at diabetes onset. *Diabetes Care* 32(5):769–773, 2009
182. Barker JM, Goehrig SH, Barriga K, Hoffman M, Slover R, Eisenbarth GS, et al.: Clinical characteristics of children diagnosed with type 1 diabetes through intensive screening and follow-up. *Diabetes Care* 27(6):1399–1404, 2004
183. Winkler C, Schober E, Ziegler AG, Holl RW: Markedly reduced rate of diabetic ketoacidosis at onset of type 1 diabetes in relatives screened for islet autoantibodies. *Pediatric Diabetes* 13:308–313, 2012
184. Elding Larsson H, Vehik K, Bell R, Dabelea D, Dolan L, Pihoker C, et al.: Reduced prevalence of diabetic ketoacidosis at diagnosis of type 1 diabetes in young children participating in longitudinal follow-up. *Diabetes Care* [Research Support, N.I.H., Extramural Research Support, U.S. Gov't, P.H.S.] 34(11):2347–2352, 2011
185. Farrell K, Holmes-Walker DJ: Mobile phone support is associated with reduced ketoacidosis in young adults. *Diabet Med* [Evaluation Studies] 28(8):1001–1004, 2011
186. Golden MP, Herrold AJ, Orr DP: An approach to prevention of recurrent diabetic ketoacidosis in the pediatric population. *J Pediatr* 107:195–200, 1985
187. Ellis D, Naar-King S, Templin T, Frey M, Cunningham P, Sheidow A, et al.: Multisystemic therapy for adolescents with poorly controlled type 1 diabetes: reduced diabetic ketoacidosis admissions and related costs over 24 months. *Diabetes Care* 31(9):1746–1747, 2008
188. Laffel LM, Wentzell K, Loughlin C, Tovar A, Moltz K, Brink S: Sick day management using blood 3-hydroxybutyrate (3-OHB) compared with urine ketone monitoring reduces hospital visits in young people with T1DM: a randomized clinical trial. *Diabet Med* 23(3):278–284, 2006
189. Attia N, Jones TW, Holcombe J, Tamborlane WV: Comparison of human regular and lispro insulins after interruption of continuous subcutaneous insulin infusion and in the treatment of acutely decompensated IDDM. *Diabetes Care* 21(5):817–821, 1998
190. Guerci B, Meyer L, Salle A, Charrie A, Dousset B, Ziegler O, et al.: Comparison of metabolic deterioration between insulin analog and regular insulin after a 5-hour interruption of a continuous subcutaneous insulin infusion in type 1 diabetic patients. *J Clin Endocrinol Metab* 84(8):2673–2678, 1999
191. Laffel L. Sick-day management in type 1 diabetes. *Endocrinol Metab Clin North Am* 29(4):707–723, 2000
192. Bismuth E, Laffel L: Can we prevent diabetic ketoacidosis in children? *Pediatr Diabetes* 8(Suppl. 6):S24–S33, 2007
193. Kitabchi AE, Umpierrez GE, Fisher JN, Murphy MB, Stentz FB: Thirty years of personal experience in hyperglycemic crises: diabetic ketoacidosis

and hyperglycemic hyperosmolar state. *J Clin Endocrinol Metab* [Research Support, N.I.H., Extramural Research Support, Non-U.S. Gov't Review] 93(5):1541–1552, 2008

194. Mannix R, Tan ML, Wright R, Baskin M: Acute pediatric rhabdomyolysis: causes and rates of renal failure. *Pediatrics* 118(5):2119–2125, 2006

195. Carcillo JA, Tasker RC: Fluid resuscitation of hypovolemic shock: acute medicine's great triumph for children. *Intensive Care Med* 32(7):958–961, 2006

196. Kilbane BJ, Mehta S, Backeljauw PF, Shanley TP, Crimmins NA: Approach to management of malignant hyperthermia-like syndrome in pediatric diabetes mellitus. *Pediatr Crit Care Med.* 7(2):169–173, 2006

II. Adults

Guillermo E. Umpierrez, MD

INTRODUCTION

Diabetic ketoacidosis (DKA) is the most serious hyperglycemic emergency in patients with type 1 (T1D) and type 2 diabetes (T2D).[1,2] In the U.S., the annual number of cases between 1995 and 2005 has increased by 30%, and currently more than 130,000 people are admitted for DKA per year.[3] Treatment of DKA utilizes many resources, accounting for an estimated annual total cost of U.S. $2.4 billion.[4] In adult patients, recent controlled studies have reported a mortality rate less than 2%; mortality is increased in the elderly and in patients with concomitant life-threatening illnesses. Successful treatment of DKA requires frequent monitoring, replacement of fluid and electrolyte deficits to restore circulatory volume and tissue perfusion, correction of hyperglycemia, and a careful search for the precipitating cause.

EPIDEMIOLOGY

Observational studies have reported that DKA accounts for 4–9% of hospital discharges among patients admitted with a primary diagnosis of diabetes.[5,6] In a Danish study, the incidence was 8.5 per 100,000 total population in the years 1975–1979.[7] A higher figure was reported by the EURODIAB study where 8.6% of 3,250 subjects with T1D throughout Europe had been admitted with DKA in the previous 12 months.[8] Recent epidemiological studies indicate that hospitalizations for DKA during the past two decades are increasing, with the majority of cases occurring as recurrent cases in the same subjects.[5,9,10]

Most patients with DKA have autoimmune T1D; however, patients with T2D are also at risk during the catabolic stress of acute illness, such as trauma, surgery, or infections. In contrast to popular belief, DKA is more common in adults than in children.[11] In community-based studies, more than 40% of patients with DKA are older than 40 years and more than 20% are older than 55 years.[12] More than half of obese African Americans with newly diagnosed diabetes presenting with DKA have no apparent precipitating cause.[9,13] At presentation, they have markedly impaired insulin secretion and insulin action.[6,14] Intensified diabetic management results in significant improvement in β-cell function and insulin sensitivity sufficient to allow discontinuation of insulin therapy within a few months of follow-up.[15] This clinical presentation has been reported primarily in African Americans, but also in other minority ethnic groups, and has been referred to as idiopathic T1D, atypical diabetes, type 1.5 diabetes, and more recently as ketosis-prone T2D.[16–19] Despite their presentation in DKA, the presence of obesity, a strong family history of diabetes, measurable insulin secretion, and a low prevalence of autoimmune markers of β-cell destruction, these patients appear to have T2D.[15]

In adult subjects with DKA, the overall mortality is less than 1%;[20] however, a mortality rate higher than 5% has been reported in the elderly and in patients with concomitant life-threatening illnesses.[11,21] Death in these conditions is rarely due to the metabolic complications of hyperglycemia or ketoacidosis but relates to the underlying precipitating illness.[1,9] The prognosis of both conditions is substantially worsened at the extremes of age in the presence of coma, hypotension, and severe comorbidities.[1,22]

PRECIPITATING CAUSES

In patients with known diabetes, precipitating factors for DKA include infections, intercurrent illnesses, psychological stress, and noncompliance with therapy. Worldwide, infection remains the most common underlying cause, occurring in 30–50% of cases.[8,23] Urinary tract infection and pneumonia account for the majority of infections.[9,12] Other acute conditions that may precipitate DKA include cerebrovascular accident, alcohol abuse, pancreatitis, pulmonary embolism, myocardial infarction, and trauma. Drugs that affect carbohydrate metabolism, such as corticosteroids, sympathomimetic agents, and pentamidine, also may precipitate DKA. Recently, a number of case reports indicate that the conventional antipsychotic as well as atypical antipsychotic drugs produce diabetes.[24–26]

In adult patients with T1D, poor adherence to insulin therapy is reported as the major precipitating cause of DKA in inner-city populations.[10,27,28] A recent study determined clinical, socioeconomic, and psychological factors associated with recurrence of DKA in inner-city minority patients.[10] Discontinuation of insulin therapy accounted for more than two-thirds of all DKA admissions. Several behavioral, socioeconomic, and psychosocial factors contributed to poor treatment adherence. Among patients with poor compliance with insulin therapy, one-third of patients "just stopped" (gave no clear reason for stopping insulin), one-third reported financial troubles, and most of the rest reported being away from supply or did not know how to handle insulin on sick days. Other studies have reported that psychological risk factors, including eating disorders, in up to 20% of recurrent episodes of ketoacidosis in young women.[29] Recently, it was estimated that up to one-third of young women with T1D have eating disturbances.[30]

PATHOPHYSIOLOGY

DKA is a state of severe metabolic decompensation characterized by hyperglycemia, metabolic acidosis, and increased total ketone bodies or ketoacids. Ketoacidosis results from insulin deficiency and excess counterregulatory hormones, including glucagon, catecholamines, cortisol, and growth hormone.

The insulin deficiency of DKA can be absolute in T1D or relative as in T2D in the presence of stress or intercurrent illness, which causes sudden worsening of insulin resistance and impairment of insulin secretion.[1,2] In DKA, reduced effective insulin concentrations and increased concentrations of counterregulatory hormones (catecholamines, cortisol, glucagon, and growth hormone) lead to hyperglycemia and ketosis. Hyperglycemia develops as a result of three processes: increased gluconeogenesis, accelerated glycogenolysis, and impaired glucose utilization by peripheral tissues.[31-35] This is magnified by transient insulin resistance resulting from the hormone imbalance as well as the elevated free fatty acid (FFA) concentrations.[4,18] The combination of insulin deficiency and increased counterregulatory hormones in DKA also leads to the release of FFAs into the circulation from adipose tissue (lipolysis) and to unrestrained hepatic fatty acid oxidation in the liver to ketone bodies (β-hydroxybutyrate [β-OHB] and acetoacetate),[36] with resulting ketonemia and metabolic acidosis.

Increasing evidence indicates that hyperglycemia in patients with DKA is associated with a severe inflammatory state characterized by an elevation of proinflammatory cytokines, reactive oxygen species, and cardiovascular risk factors in the absence of obvious infection or cardiovascular pathology.[37] Circulating levels of tumor necrosis factor-α, interleukin (IL)-6, IL-1β, and IL-8, C-reactive protein, plasminogen activator inhibitor-1, FFAs, cortisol, and growth hormone are significantly increased two- to fourfold on admission in patients with hyperglycemic crises compared with control subjects, and levels returned to normal levels after insulin treatment and resolution of hyperglycemic crises.

DIAGNOSIS

Symptoms and Signs

Clinical features of DKA at presentation can be nonspecific, but in general, patients complain of polydypsia and polyuria for several days before the development of DKA. Generalized weakness, weight loss, and gastrointestinal symptoms, including nausea, vomiting, and abdominal pain, are frequently present on admission.[38] A prospective study of 189 consecutive patients with DKA reported that abdominal pain was present in 46% of patients with DKA, and its presence related to the severity of metabolic acidosis and not to the severity of hyperglycemia or dehydration.[38] In DKA subjects with abdominal pain, the mean serum bicarbonate (9 $\pm$ 1 mmol/L) and blood pH (7.12 $\pm$ 0.02) were lower than in patients without pain (15 $\pm$ 1 mmol/L and 7.24 $\pm$ 0.09), respectively. Delayed gastric emptying and ileus induced by electrolyte disturbance and metabolic acidosis have been implicated as possible causes of abdominal pain in DKA.[39] In the majority of patients, the abdominal pain spontaneously resolves after correction of metabolic disturbance; thus, in the absence of an overt cause for abdominal pain, allowing several hours to treat the underlying acidosis constitutes the best diagnostic tool to elucidate the etiology of abdominal pain in DKA.

Physical examination reveals signs of dehydration, including loss of skin turgor, dry mucous membranes, tachycardia, and hypotension. Most patients are normothermic or even hypothermic at presentation. Acetone on breath and labored Kussmaul respiration may also be present on admission, particularly in patients with severe metabolic acidosis. Mental status can vary from full alertness to profound lethargy; however, fewer than 20% of patients are hospitalized with loss of consciousness.[40,41] Abnormalities in mental status correlated better with increased serum osmolality than with the severity of metabolic acidosis, patient's age, or duration of diabetes.

Laboratory Findings

DKA consists of the biochemical triad of hyperglycemia, ketonemia, and metabolic acidosis. Until recently, the most widely used diagnostic criteria for DKA are blood glucose greater than 250 mg/dL, serum bicarbonate lower than 15 mEq/L, arterial pH lower than 7.3, an increased anion gap metabolic acidosis, and a moderate degree of ketonemia. The severity of DKA is now classified as mild, moderate, or severe based primarily on the severity of metabolic acidosis (blood pH, bicarbonate, ketones) and the presence of altered mental status (Table 15.II.1). The key diagnostic feature is the elevation in circulating total blood ketone concentration.

Assessment of ketonemia is usually performed by the nitroprusside reaction, which provides a semiquantitative estimation of acetoacetate and acetone levels. Although, the nitroprusside test (both in urine and in serum) is highly sensitive, it can underestimate the severity of ketoacidosis because this assay does not recognize the presence of β-hydroxybutyrate, the main metabolic product in

Table 15.II.1 Diagnostic Criteria for DKA

	Mild	Moderate	Severe
Plasma glucose (mg/dl)	>250	>250	>250
Arterial pH	7.25–7.30	7.00–7.24	<7.0
Serum bicarbonate (mEq/l)	15–18	10–<15	<10
Urine ketones*	Positive	Positive	Positive
Serum ketones*	Positive	Positive	Positive
Effective serum osmolality (mOsm/kg)†	Variable	Variable	Variable
Anion gap‡	>10	>12	>12
Alteration in sensoria or mental obtundation	Alert	Alert/drowsy	Stupor/coma

Note:
* Nitroprusside reaction method
† Effective serum osmolality = $2[Na^+ (mEq/l)] + [glucose (mg/dl)/18]$
‡ Anion gap = $[Na^+] - [Cl^- + HCO_3^-]$

Source: Adapted from Kitabchi AE, Umpierrez GE, Miles JM, Fisher JN: Hyperglycemic crises in adult patients with diabetes. *Diabetes Care* 32:1335–1343, 2009.

ketoacidosis.[32,42] If available, measurement of serum β-hydroxybutyrate may be useful for diagnosis.[43] Accumulation of ketoacids results in an increased anion gap metabolic acidosis. The anion gap is calculated by subtracting the sum of chloride and bicarbonate concentration from the sodium concentration:

$$\text{Anion gap} = [Na - (Cl + HCO_3)]$$

A normal anion gap is between 7 and 9 mEq/l, and an anion gap >10–12 mEq/l indicates the presence of increased anion gap metabolic acidosis.[1]

Differential Diagnosis

Not all patients who present with anion gap acidosis or ketoacidosis have DKA. Patients with chronic ethanol abuse with a recent binge culminating in nausea, vomiting, and acute starvation may present with alcoholic ketoacidosis (AKA).[44] In most cases, making a distinction between DKA and AKA is straightforward. Most patients with DKA have a known history of T1D and present with severe hyperglycemia, whereas patients with AKA have a history of chronic ethanol abuse and decreased food intake and present with normal or low blood glucose concentration.[44] The absence of hyperglycemia in AKA results from the combination of prolonged starvation with glycogen depletion[45] and impaired gluconeogenesis because of decreased nicotinamide adenosine dinucleotide (NAD), a cofactor critical for the utilization of gluconeogenic precursors.[46]

Some patients with decreased food intake (lower than 500 calories/day) for several days may present with starvation ketosis.[38,47,48] Because of the progressive accumulation of ketone bodies during fasting, a healthy subject is able to adapt by enhancing the kidney's ability to excrete large amount of ammonia to compensate for the increased acid production.[49] Therefore, a patient with starvation ketosis rarely presents with a serum bicarbonate concentration less than 18 mEq/L.[50]

DKA must also be distinguished from other causes of high anion gap metabolic acidosis, including lactic acidosis, advanced chronic renal failure, and ingestion of such drugs as salicylate, methanol, ethylene glycol, and paraldehyde.[17]

TREATMENT

The therapeutic goals in DKA management are as follows:

■ Improve circulatory volume and tissue perfusion
■ Decrease serum glucose
■ Clear serum ketoacids
■ Correct electrolyte imbalances

Successful therapy of DKA depends on frequent monitoring, replacement of fluid losses, correction of the hyperglycemia and metabolic acidosis, replacement of electrolytes losses, and careful scrutiny for precipitating factors for metabolic decompensation (Table 15.II.2).

There are no guidelines determining the safety and cost effectiveness of treating adult patients with DKA in an intensive care unit (ICU) or in non-ICU

Table 15.II.2 Treatment Protocol for the Management of DKA

1. **Intravenous (IV) fluids:**
   1. 0.9% saline at 500–1,000 mL/h for 2 h
   2. 0.45% saline at 250–500 mL/h until blood glucose <250 mg/dL
   3. Dextrose 5% in 0.45% saline at 150–250 ml/h until resolution of DKA

2. **Potassium replacement:**
   1. If serum K^+ >5.5 mmol/L, do not give K^+ but check serum K^+ every 2 h
   2. K^+ = 4–5.5 mmol/L, add 20 mmol of KCl to each liter of IV fluid
   3. K^+ = 3–<4 mmol/L, add 40 mmol of KCl to each liter of IV fluid
   4. K^+ = <3 mmol/L, give 10–20 mmol of KCl per hour until serum K^+ >3 mmol/L, then add 20–40 mmol of KCl of each liter of IV fluid

3. **Insulin therapy:**

   A. IV regular insulin:
   1. Initial IV bolus: 0.1 unit/kg body weight, followed by
   2. Continuous insulin infusion at 0.1 U/kg per hour
   3. When blood glucose <200 mg/dL, change IV fluids to D5% 0.45% saline and reduce insulin infusion rate to 0.05 unit/kg/hr to keep glucose ~200 mg/dl until resolution of DKA.

   B. Subcutaneous (SC) rapid-acting insulin analog (lispro, aspart, glulisine) every 1 h:
   1. Initial dose SC: 0.2U/kg of body weight, followed by
   2. SC lispro/aspart/glulisine insulin at 0.1 unit/kg every hour
   3. When blood glucose <200 mg/dL, change IV fluids to D5% 0.45% saline and reduce SC lispro/aspart insulin to 0.05 unit/kg per hour to keep glucose ~200 mg/dL until resolution of DKA.

   C. SC rapid-acting insulin analog (lispro, aspart, glulisine) every 2 h:
   1. Initial dose SC: 0.3 U/kg of body weight, followed by
   2. SC lispro/aspart/glulisine insulin at 0.2 units 1 h later and every 2 h
   3. When blood glucose <200 mg/dL, change IV fluids to D5% 0.45% saline and reduce SC lispro/aspart to 0.1 unit/kg every 2 h to keep glucose ~200 mg/dL until resolution of DKA.

4. **Bicarbonate**

   Arterial pH <6.9, administer 44.6 mEq in 200 ml 0.45% saline over 1 h until pH increases to ≥6.9–7.0. Do not give bicarbonate if pH ≥7.0.

5. **Phosphate**

   Not routinely recommended: if indicated (<1 mg/dl), 20–30 mmol of potassium phosphate can be added to replacement fluids. Monitor serum calcium level.

6. **Glucose monitoring and laboratory**

   During therapy, capillary blood glucose should be determined every 1–2 h at the bedside using a glucose oxidase reagent strip. Blood should be drawn every 4 h for determination of serum electrolytes, glucose, blood urea nitrogen, creatinine, phosphorus, and venous pH.

7. Transition to SC insulin therapy

Insulin infusion should be continued until resolution of ketoacidosis (glucose <200 mg/dL, bicarbonate ≥18 mEq/L, pH ≥7.30, anion gap <12 mEq/L). When this occurs, start SC insulin regimen. In patients with known diabetes who were receiving insulin prior to admission, restart previous insulin regimen. In patients with newly diagnosed diabetes, start insulin at 0.6 units/kg/day. Consider basal bolus regimen with basal insulin (glargine once daily or detemir once or twice daily) and rapid-acting insulin analogs (lispro, aspart, glulisine) before meals. To prevent recurrence of DKA during the transition period to SC insulin, IV insulin should be continued for 1–2 h after SC insulin is given.

settings. Several observational and prospective studies have indicated no clear benefits resulting from treating DKA patients in the ICU compared to step-down units or general medicine wards.[51–53] The mortality rate, length of hospital stay, or time to resolve ketoacidosis are similar between patients treated in ICU and non-ICU settings. In addition, ICU admission has been shown to be associated with more testing and significantly higher hospitalization cost in patients with DKA.[47,51] Thus, the majority of patients with mild to moderate DKA can be safely managed in the emergency department or in step-down units,[54,55] and only patients with severe DKA or those with a critical illness as precipitating cause (i.e., myocardial infarction, gastrointestinal bleeding, sepsis) should be treated in the ICU.

Fluid Replacement

Patients with DKA are invariably volume depleted with an estimated water deficit of ~100 ml/kg of body weight.[41] Expansion of extracellular fluid with intravenous (IV) fluids results in significant improvement of hyperglycemia, hypertonicity, and metabolic acidosis because of a decline in counterregulatory hormones levels.[37,56] The volume expansion also improves renal perfusion, which subsequently leads to increased urinary clearance of glucose.[57] The severity of dehydration and volume depletion can be estimated by clinical examination (orthostasis) and by calculating plasma osmolality.[58,59] An effective plasma osmolality >320 mOsm/kg H_2O is associated with large fluid deficits. The water deficit can be estimated, based on corrected serum sodium concentration, using the following equation:

$$\text{Water deficit} = (0.6)(\text{body weight in kilograms}) \times ([\text{corrected sodium} / 140] - 1)^{60}$$

The initial fluid of choice is isotonic saline (0.9% NaCl). Generally 1 or 2 L of saline at a rate of 500–1000 mL/h are sufficient to restore blood pressure and renal perfusion. Subsequent choice and rate of fluid replacement depends on hemodynamics, the state of hydration, serum electrolyte levels, and urinary output. In general, 0.45% NaCl infused at 250–500 ml/h is appropriate if the corrected serum sodium is normal or elevated; 0.9% NaCl at a similar rate is appropriate if the corrected serum sodium is low.

During treatment of DKA, hyperglycemia is corrected faster than ketoacidosis. The mean duration of treatment until blood glucose reaches <250 mg/dl and ketoacidosis is corrected (pH >7.30, bicarbonate >18 mmol/l) is 6 and 12 h, respectively.[9,61] Once the plasma glucose is ~250 mg/dL, 5–10% dextrose should be added to replacement fluids to allow continued insulin administration until ketonemia is controlled, while at the same time avoiding hypoglycemia. An additional important aspect of fluid management is to replace the volume of urinary losses, especially in those subjects with excessive polyuria. Failure to adjust fluid replacement for urinary losses may delay correction of water deficit.

Insulin Therapy

The cornerstone of DKA management after initial hydration is insulin administration. Insulin increases peripheral glucose utilization and decreases hepatic glucose production, thereby lowering blood glucose concentration.[31] In addition, insulin therapy inhibits the release of FFA from adipose tissue and decreases ketogenesis, both of which lead to the reversal of ketogenesis.[62] Randomized controlled studies in patients with DKA have shown that insulin therapy is effective regardless of the route of administration.[63,64] The administration of continuous IV infusion of regular insulin is the preferred route because of its short half-life and easy titration.[63,64] Recent evidence indicates that rapid-acting insulin analogs (aspart, lispro, glulisine) given by intramuscular or subcutaneous (SC) route may represent alternatives to the use of IV regular insulin in the treatment of DKA. Treatment of patients with mild and moderate DKA with SC aspart insulin every 1 or 2 h in non-ICU settings was shown to be as safe and effective as the treatment with IV regular insulin in the ICU.[53,65]

A common and effective practice includes an initial IV bolus of regular insulin of 0.1 units/kg of body weight, followed by a continuous infusion of regular insulin at a dose of 0.1 units/kg per hour.[4] Low dose insulin infusion decreases glucose concentration at a rate of 50–75 mg/dl per hour.[4,64] Once the serum glucose has declined to ~250 mg/dL an infusion of glucose (D5% 0.45% normal saline) should be started at 150–200 ml/h, and the insulin infusion rate should be reduced to 0.05 units/kg per hour. Thereafter, the rate of insulin administration may need to be adjusted to maintain glucose levels at ~200 mg/dL and continued until ketoacidosis is resolved.

Potassium

Despite a total body potassium deficit of ~3–5 mEq/kg of body weight, most patients with DKA have a serum potassium level at or above the upper limits of normal.[66–68] With initiation of therapy, the extracellular potassium concentration invariably falls. Rehydration lowers the serum potassium level by exerting a dilutional effect and by increasing urinary potassium excretion.[31] Both insulin therapy and correction of acidosis decrease serum potassium levels by stimulating cellular potassium uptake in peripheral tissues.[69] Therefore to prevent hypokalemia, most patients require IV potassium during the course of DKA therapy. The treatment goal is to maintain serum potassium levels within the normal range of 4 to 5 mEq/L. Generally, 20–30 mEq potassium in each liter of infusion fluid is sufficient to maintain a serum potassium concentration within the normal range. In some hyperglycemic patients admitted with severe potassium deficiency, insulin administration may precipitate profound hypokalemia, which can induce life-threatening arrhythmias and respiratory muscle weakness.[31,70,71] Thus, if the initial serum potassium is ≤3.0 mEq/L, potassium replacement should begin immediately by an infusion at a rate of 10–20 mEq per hour. One should consider withholding insulin therapy for 1–2 h until sufficient potassium replacement is given.

Bicarbonate

Severe metabolic acidosis can lead to impaired myocardial contractility, cerebral vasodilatation and coma, and several gastrointestinal complications;[72–74] however, several studies have reported that bicarbonate therapy for DKA offers no advantage in improving cardiac and neurologic functions or in the rate of recovery of hyperglycemia and ketoacidosis.[75–77] Nine small studies have evaluated the effect of alkalinization in a total of 434 patients with KDA, 217 treated with bicarbonate, and 178 patients without alkali therapy.[45,46,48–50,75,78–80] Moreover, several deleterious effects of bicarbonate therapy have been reported, such as increased risk of hypokalemia,[78] decreased tissue oxygen uptake,[81] and cerebral edema.[82] Despite that lack of evidence in support of the use of bicarbonate therapy in patients with DKA, clinical guidelines recommend that in patients with severe metabolic acidosis (pH <6.9), 50–100 mmol of sodium bicarbonate should be given as isotonic solution (in 200 ml of water) every 2 h until pH rises to ~6.9–7.0. In patients with arterial pH >7.0, no bicarbonate therapy is necessary.

Phosphate

The serum phosphate level in patients with DKA is usually normal or elevated, but the admission serum phosphate does not reflect the actual body deficit. This is possibly due to an extracellular shift that may exist, similar to the shift seen with potassium.[83] During insulin therapy and fluid replacement, phosphate reenters the intracellular compartment, leading to mild to moderate reductions in serum phosphate concentrations. Prospective randomized studies have failed to show any beneficial effect of phosphate replacement on the clinical outcome in DKA,[83] and overzealous phosphate therapy can cause severe hypocalcemia.[84] In the presence of severe hypophosphatemia, 20–30 mEq/l of potassium phosphate can be added to replacement fluids.[85]

Transition to Subcutaneous Insulin

Patients with DKA should be treated with continuous IV insulin until ketoacidosis is resolved. Criteria for resolution of ketoacidosis include the following:

- Blood glucose lower than 200 mg/dL
- Serum bicarbonate level equal to or greater than 18 mEq/L

■ Venous pH greater than 7.3
■ Calculated anion gap equal to or lower than 14 mEq/L[4]

When this occurs, SC insulin therapy can be started. The American Diabetes Association (ADA) position statement recommends a transition to a split-mixed insulin regimen with neutral protamine Hagedorn (NPH) and regular insulin twice daily or to a multidose regimen of short- or rapid-acting and intermediate- or long-acting insulins.[1,86] Several studies have reported hospital rates of hypoglycemic events up to 30% with the use of NPH and regular insulin after discontinuation of IV insulin.[6,9,87] The inadequate duration of action of NPH insulin and an undesirable peak activity at 4–6 h after injection,[88] as well as the high day-to-day variability in absorption,[89] partially explain the high rate of hypoglycemic events. A recent randomized study compared the safety and efficacy of insulin analogs and human insulins during the transition from intravenous to SC insulin in patients with DKA. During the transition to SC insulin, there were no differences in mean daily glucose levels, but 41% patients treated with NPH and regular insulin had higher rates of hypoglycemia compared to 15% of patients treated with glargine once daily and glulisine before meals. Thus, a basal bolus regimen with insulin analogs is safer and should be preferred over NPH and regular insulin following the resolution of DKA. In patients with newly diagnosed diabetes and initial insulin total insulin dose of 0.6 unit/kg per day, it is usually sufficient to achieve and maintain metabolic control.[47,87] To prevent recurrence of hyperglycemia or ketoacidosis during the transition period to SC insulin, it is important to allow an overlap of 1–2 h between discontinuation of IV insulin and the administration of SC insulin.

COMPLICATIONS

The two most common acute complications associated with the treatment of DKA in adult subjects are hypoglycemia and hypokalemia. Hypoglycemia is reported in 10–25% of patients during insulin therapy.[9,87] Hypoglycemic events most commonly occur after several hours of insulin infusion (between 8 and 16 h) or during the transition phase. The failure to reduce the insulin infusion rate or to use dextrose-containing solutions when glucose levels reach 250 mg/dL are the two most common causes of hypoglycemia during insulin therapy.[9] Frequent blood glucose monitoring (every 1–2 h) is mandatory to recognize hypoglycemia because many patients with DKA who develop hypoglycemia during treatment do not experience adrenergic manifestations of sweating, nervousness, fatigue, hunger, and tachycardia. Both insulin therapy and correction of acidosis decrease serum potassium levels by stimulating cellular potassium uptake in peripheral tissues and may lead to hypokalemia. Aggressive potassium replacement early in the management has been shown to minimize the risk of hypokalemia.[4,90] To prevent hypokalemia, initiate replacement with intravenous potassium as soon as the serum potassium concentration is <5.5 mEq/L. In addition, in patients who present with normal or reduced serum potassium, aggressive IV potassium replacement should begin immediately, and insulin therapy should be held until serum potassium is >3.3 mEq/L.[4,65]

Relapse of DKA may occur after sudden interruption of IV insulin therapy or in patients without concomitant use of SC insulin administration or lack of frequent monitoring. To prevent recurrence of ketoacidosis during the transition period to SC insulin, it is important to allow an overlap of 1–2 h between discontinuation of IV insulin and the administration of SC regular insulin. Other complications of diabetes include hyperchloremic acidosis with an excessive use of NaCl or KCl, resulting in a nonanionic gap metabolic acidosis.[44,62,91] This acidosis has no adverse clinical effects and is gradually corrected over the subsequent 24–48 h by enhanced renal acid excretion. The development of hyperchloremia can be prevented with the reduction of the chloride load by judicious use of hydration solutions.[91]

Cerebral Edema

Cerebral edema is a rare complications in adult patients with DKA.[4] Symptoms and signs of cerebral edema are variable and include onset of headache, gradual deterioration in level of consciousness, seizures, sphincter incontinence, pupillary changes, papilledema, bradycardia, elevation in blood pressure, and respiratory arrest.[92,93] Cerebral edema typically occurs 4–12 h after treatment is activated, but it can be present before treatment has begun or may develop any time during treatment for DKA.[93] Although, no single factor has been identified that can be used to predict the development of cerebral edema, a number of mechanisms have been proposed, including the role of cerebral ischemia and hypoxia, the generation of various inflammatory mediators,[94] increased cerebral blood flow, disruption of cell membrane ion transport, and rapid shift in extracellular and intracellular fluids resulting in changes in osmolality.[95–98]

PREVENTION

The most common precipitating causes of DKA include infection, intercurrent illness, psychological stress, and noncompliance with therapy. With improved outpatient treatment programs and better adherence to self-care, ~50 to 75% of DKA admissions may be preventable.[4,10,27] Outpatient management is more cost effective and can minimize missed days of school and work for patients with diabetes and their family members.[1,99] The frequency of hospitalizations for DKA have been reduced following diabetes education programs, improved follow-up care, and access to medical advice. Many patients with recurrent DKA are unaware of sick-day management or the consequences of skipping or discontinuing insulin therapy.[10,27] Thus, diabetes education and sick-day management should be reviewed periodically in patients with diabetes and should include specific information on when to contact the health care provider, blood glucose and A1C goals, use of supplemental short- or rapid-acting insulin during illness, and, most important, the importance of never discontinuing insulin and of seeking immediate medical attention in the case of severe hyperglycemia. A recent study in adolescents reported that an intensive home-based multidisciplinary intervention resulted in a significant decrease in DKA admissions over 2 years.[100] In that study, a multidisciplinary diabetes team met with study patients frequently and addressed barriers to communication, access to care, and medical adherence on the family, school, and health care levels. Despite the expense of providing such an intensive intervention, the multidisciplinary intervention incurred less cost to the health care system because of the decreased number of DKA admissions. In addition, patients with T1D should be instructed on the use of home blood ketone monitoring during illness and persistent hyperglycemia, which may allow for early recognition of impending ketoacidosis, and in turn may help to guide insulin therapy at home and, possibly, may prevent hospitalization for DKA. Finally, the alarming rise in insulin discontinuation because of economic reasons as the precipitating cause for DKA in urban patients illustrates the need for health care legislation to ensure reimbursement for medications to treat diabetes. Novel approaches to patient education incorporating a variety of health care beliefs and socioeconomic issues are critical to an effective prevention program.[10]

FUTURE CLINICAL RESEARCH—FILLING IN THE GAPS

The following are selected research topics and questions proposed to guide the management of patients with DKA in various hospital settings:

- What are optimal and safe glycemic targets during continuous insulin infusion until resolution of DKA? It is not known if we need to maintain a glucose concentration in the hyperglycemic range between ~200 mg/dl and 250 mg/dl until resolution of ketoacidosis. This recommendation precludes the use of insulin infusion protocols commonly used in critically ill patients with hyperglycemia (glucose target 140–180 mg/dl).
- Is the use of bicarbonate needed in patients with severe DKA? Available studies suggest that for pH >6.9–7.0, the use of bicarbonate does not provide any advantage. No prospective randomized studies are available to establish efficacy of the use of bicarbonate in DKA for pH <6.9.
- What education and support systems are required to effectively prevent recurrence of ketoacidosis? Insulin discontinuation is the precipitating cause in two-thirds of patients with recurrent DKA. Novel approaches to patient education incorporating a variety of health care beliefs and socioeconomic issues are critical to an effective prevention program in inner-city patients.
- What is the role of continuous glucose monitoring (CGM) systems in the acute and postdischarge management of patients with hyperglycemic crises? The Endocrine Society Clinical Practice Guideline Committee on the use of CGM recently recommended against the use of this technology in critically ill patients.[101] This recommendation was based on the limited available data related to accuracy and the concerns regarding potential danger in their use in guiding insulin administration in an acute-care setting. The use of CGM may have an advantage over bedside point-of-care (POC) testing in that it has the potential to reduce unknown hypoglycemic events that may occur between POC measurements; however, there is concern about the accuracy of CGM at low blood glucose levels and the limited correlation between CGM and capillary and arterial samples when the blood glucose is less than 81 mg/dl.[102]

ACKNOWLEDGMENTS

Dr. Umpierrez is supported in part by research grants from the American Diabetes Association (7-03-CR-35), Public Health Service Grant UL1 RR025008 from the Clinical and Translational Science Award program, National Institutes of Health, National Center for Research Resources.

REFERENCES

1. Kitabchi AE, Umpierrez GE, Murphy MB, Barrett EJ, Kreisberg RA, Malone JI, Wall BM: Management of hyperglycemic crises in patients with diabetes. *Diabetes Care* 24:131–153, 2001
2. White NH: Diabetic ketoacidosis in children. *Endocrinol Metab Clin North Am* 29:657–682, 2000
3. Division of Diabetes Translation NCfCDPaHP, CDC: Number (in thousands) of hospital discharges with diabetic ketoacidosis as first-listed diagnosis, United States, 1980-2005. Diabetes Data & Trends, 2005. Available from http://www.cdc.gov/diabetes/statistics/dkafirst/diabetes_complications/fig1.htm. Accessed 2 March 2011
4. Kitabchi AE, Umpierrez GE, Miles JM, Fisher JN: Hyperglycemic crises in adult patients with diabetes. *Diabetes Care* 32:1335–1343, 2009
5. Faich GA, Fishbein HA, Ellis SE: The epidemiology of diabetic acidosis: a population-based study. *Am J Epidemiol* 117:551–558, 1983
6. Umpierrez GE, Casals MM, Gebhart SP, Mixon PS, Clark WS, Phillips LS: Diabetic ketoacidosis in obese African-Americans. *Diabetes* 44:790–795, 1995
7. Geiss LS, Herman WH, Goldschmid MG, DeStefano F, Eberhardt MS, Ford ES, German RR, Newman JM, Olson DR, Sepe SJ, et al.: Surveillance for diabetes mellitus—United States, 1980–1989. *Mor Mortal Wkly Rep CDC Surveill Summ* 42:1–20, 1993
8. Ellemann K, Soerensen JN, Pedersen L, Edsberg B, Andersen OO: Epidemiology and treatment of diabetic ketoacidosis in a community population. *Diabetes Care* 7:528–532, 1984
9. Umpierrez GE, Kelly JP, Navarrete JE, Casals MM, Kitabchi AE: Hyperglycemic crises in urban blacks. *Arch Intern Med* 157:669–675, 1997
10. Randall L, Begovic J, Hudson M, Smiley D, Peng L, Pitre N, Umpierrez D, Umpierrez G: Recurrent diabetic ketoacidosis in inner-city minority patients: behavioral, socioeconomic, and psychosocial factors. *Diabetes Care* 34:1891–1896, 2011
11. Graves EJ, Gillium BS: Detailed diagnosis and procedures: National Discharge Survey, 1995. National Center for Health Statistics. *Vital Health Stat* 13, 1997
12. Johnson DD, Palumbo PJ, Chu CP: Diabetic ketoacidosis in a community-based population. *Mayo Clin Proc* 55:83–88, 1980
13. Low JC, Felner EI, Muir AB, Brown M, Dorcelet M, Peng L, Umpierrez GE: Do obese children with diabetic ketoacidosis have type 1 or type 2 diabetes? *Prim Care Diabetes* 6:61–65, 2012

14. Mauvais-Jarvis F, Sobngwi E, Porcher R, Riveline JP, Kevorkian JP, Vaisse C, Charpentier G, Guillausseau PJ, Vexiau P, Gautier JF: Ketosis-prone type 2 diabetes in patients of sub-Saharan African origin: clinical pathophysiology and natural history of beta-cell dysfunction and insulin resistance. *Diabetes* 53:645–653, 2004

15. Umpierrez GE, Smiley D, Kitabchi AE: Narrative review: ketosis-prone type 2 diabetes mellitus. *Ann Intern Med* 144:350–357, 2006

16. Sobngwi E, Mauvais-Jarvis F, Vexiau P, Mbanya JC, Gautier JF: Diabetes in Africans. Part 2: Ketosis-prone atypical diabetes mellitus. *Diabetes Metab* 28:5–12, 2002

17. Sobngwi E, Gautier JF: Adult-onset idiopathic Type I or ketosis-prone Type II diabetes: evidence to revisit diabetes classification. *Diabetologia* 45:283–285, 2002

18. Maldonado MR, Otiniano ME, Lee R, Rodriguez L, Balasubramanyam A: Ethnic differences in beta-cell functional reserve and clinical features in patients with ketosis-prone diabetes. *Diabetes Care* 26:2469, 2003

19. Kitabchi AE: Ketosis-prone diabetes—a new subgroup of patients with atypical type 1 and type 2 diabetes? *J Clin Endocrinol Metab* 88:5087–5089, 2003

20. Baldwin D, Villanueva G, McNutt R, Bhatnagar S: Eliminating inpatient sliding-scale insulin: a reeducation project with medical house staff. *Diabetes Care* 28:1008–1011, 2005

21. Malone ML, Gennis V, Goodwin JS: Characteristics of diabetic ketoacidosis in older versus younger adults. *J Am Geriatr Soc* 40:1100–1104, 1992

22. Kreisberg RA: Diabetic ketoacidosis: an update. *Crit Care Clin* 3:817–834, 1987

23. Microvascular and acute complications in IDDM patients: the EURODIAB IDDM Complications Study. *Diabetologia* 37:278–285, 1994

24. Ananth J, Parameswaran S, Gunatilake S: Side effects of atypical antipsychotic drugs. *Curr Pharm Des* 10:2219–2229, 2004

25. Tavakoli SA, Arguisola MS: Diabetic ketoacidosis in a patient treated with olanzapine, valproic acid, and venlafaxine. *South Med J* 96:729–730, 2003

26. Wilson DR, D'Souza L, Sarkar N, Newton M, Hammond C: New-onset diabetes and ketoacidosis with atypical antipsychotics. *Schizophr Res* 59:1–6, 2003

27. Musey VC, Lee JK, Crawford R, Klatka MA, McAdams D, Phillips LS: Diabetes in urban African-Americans. I. Cessation of insulin therapy is the major precipitating cause of diabetic ketoacidosis. *Diabetes Care* 18:483–489, 1995

28. Maldonado MR, Chong ER, Oehl MA, Balasubramanyam A: Economic impact of diabetic ketoacidosis in a multiethnic indigent population: analysis of costs based on the precipitating cause. *Diabetes Care* 26:1265–1269, 2003

29. Polonsky WH, Anderson BJ, Lohrer PA, Aponte JE, Jacobson AM, Cole CF: Insulin omission in women with IDDM. *Diabetes Care* 17:1178–1185, 1994

30. Rydall AC, Rodin GM, Olmsted MP, Devenyi RG, Daneman D: Disordered eating behavior and microvascular complications in young women with insulin-dependent diabetes mellitus. *N Engl J Med* 336:1849–1854, 1997

31. DeFronzo RA, Matzuda M, Barret E: Diabetic ketoacidosis: a combined metabolic-nephrologic approach to therapy. *Diabetes Rev* 2:209–238, 1994
32. Foster DW, McGarry JD: The metabolic derangements and treatment of diabetic ketoacidosis. *N Engl J Med* 309:159–169, 1983
33. Luzi L, Barrett EJ, Groop LC, Ferrannini E, DeFronzo RA: Metabolic effects of low-dose insulin therapy on glucose metabolism in diabetic keto-acidosis. *Diabetes* 37:1470–1477, 1988
34. van de Werve G, Jeanrenaud B: Liver glycogen metabolism: an overview. *Diabetes Metab Rev* 3:47–78, 1987
35. Felig P, Sherwin RS, Soman V, Wahren J, Hendler R, Sacca L, Eigler N, Goldberg D, Walesky M: Hormonal interactions in the regulation of blood glucose. *Recent Prog Horm Res* 35:501–532, 1979
36. Miles JM, Haymond MW, Nissen S, Gerich JE: Effects of free fatty acid availability, glucagon excess and insulin deficiency on ketone body production in postabsorptive man. *J Clin Invest* 71:1554–1561, 1983
37. Stentz FB, Umpierrez GE, Cuervo R, Kitabchi AE: Proinflammatory cytokines, markers of cardiovascular risks, oxidative stress, and lipid peroxidation in patients with hyperglycemic crises. *Diabetes* 53:2079–2086, 2004
38. Umpierrez G, Freire AX: Abdominal pain in patients with hyperglycemic crises. *J Crit Care* 17:63–67, 2002
39. Campbell IW, Duncan LJ, Innes JA, MacCuish AC, Munro JF: Abdominal pain in diabetic metabolic decompensation. Clinical significance. *JAMA* 233:166–168, 1975
40. Wachtel TJ, Silliman RA, Lamberton P: Prognostic factors in the diabetic hyperosmolar state. *J Am Geriatr Soc* 35:737–741, 1987
41. Kitabchi AE, Wall BM: Diabetic ketoacidosis. *Med Clin North Am* 79:9–37, 1995
42. Stephens JM, Sulway MJ, Watkins PJ: Relationship of blood acetoacetate and 3-hydroxybutyrate in diabetes. *Diabetes* 20:485–489, 1971
43. Sheikh-Ali M, Karon BS, Basu A, Kudva YC, Muller LA, Xu J, Schwenk WF, Miles JM: Can serum beta-hydroxybutyrate be used to diagnose diabetic ketoacidosis? *Diabetes Care* 31:643–647, 2008
44. Umpierrez GE, DiGirolamo M, Tuvlin JA, Isaacs SD, Bhoola SM, Kokko JP: Differences in metabolic and hormonal milieu in diabetic- and alcohol-induced ketoacidosis. *J Crit Care* 15:52–59, 2000
45. Assal JP, Aoki TT, Manzano FM, Kozak GP: Metabolic effects of sodium bicarbonate in management of diabetic ketoacidosis. *Diabetes* 23:405–411, 1974
46. Hale PJ, Crase J, Nattrass M: Metabolic effects of bicarbonate in the treatment of diabetic ketoacidosis. *Br Med J (Clin Res Ed)* 289:1035–1038, 1984
47. Javor KA, Kotsanos JG, McDonald RC, Baron AD, Kesterson JG, Tierney WM: Diabetic ketoacidosis charges relative to medical charges of adult patients with type I diabetes. *Diabetes Care* 20:349–354, 1997
48. Gamba G, Oseguera J, Castrejon M, Gomez-Perez FJ: Bicarbonate therapy in severe diabetic ketoacidosis. A double blind, randomized, placebo controlled trial. *Rev Invest Clin* 43:234–238, 1991
49. Morris LR, Murphy MB, Kitabchi AE: Bicarbonate therapy in severe diabetic ketoacidosis. *Ann Intern Med* 105:836–840, 1986

50. Okuda Y, Adrogue HJ, Field JB, Nohara H, Yamashita K: Counterproductive effects of sodium bicarbonate in diabetic ketoacidosis. *J Clin Endocrinol Metab* 81:314–320, 1996
51. May ME, Young C, King J: Resource utilization in treatment of diabetic ketoacidosis in adults. *Am J Med Sci* 306:287–294, 1993
52. Moss JM: Diabetic ketoacidosis: effective low-cost treatment in a community hospital. *South Med J* 80:875–881, 1987
53. Umpierrez GE, Cuervo R, Karabell A, Latif K, Freire AX, Kitabchi AE: Treatment of diabetic ketoacidosis with subcutaneous insulin aspart. *Diabetes Care* 27:1873–1378, 2004
54. Umpierrez GE, Cuervo R, Karabell A, Latif K, Freire AX, Kitabchi AE: Treatment of diabetic ketoacidosis with subcutaneous insulin aspart. *Diabetes Care* 27:1873–1878, 2004
55. Freire AX, Umpierrez GE, Afessa B, Latif KA, Bridges L, Kitabchi AE: Predictors of intensive care unit and hospital length of stay in diabetic ketoacidosis. *J Crit Care* 17:207–211, 2002
56. Waldhausl W, Kleinberger G, Korn A, Dudczak R, Bratusch-Marrain P, Nowotny P: Severe hyperglycemia: effects of rehydration on endocrine derangements and blood glucose concentration. *Diabetes* 28:577–584, 1979
57. Owen OE, Licht JH, Sapir DG: Renal function and effects of partial rehydration during diabetic ketoacidosis. *Diabetes* 30:510–518, 1981
58. Hillman K: Fluid resuscitation in diabetic emergencies—a reappraisal. *Intensive Care Med* 13:4–8, 1987
59. Pinies JA, Cairo G, Gaztambide S, Vazquez JA: Course and prognosis of 132 patients with diabetic non ketotic hyperosmolar state. *Diabete Metab* 20:43–48, 1994
60. Feig PU, McCurdy DK: The hypertonic state. *N Engl J Med* 297:1444–1454, 1977
61. Umpierrez GE, Khajavi M, Kitabchi AE: Review: diabetic ketoacidosis and hyperglycemic hyperosmolar nonketotic syndrome. *Am J Med Sci* 311:225–233, 1996
62. Kitabchi AE, Fisher JN, Murphy MB, Rumbak MJ: Diabetic ketoacidosis and the hyperglycemic hyperosmolar nonketotic state. In *Joslin's Diabetes Mellitus*. 13th ed. Kahn CR, Weir GC, Eds. Philadelphia, PA, Lea & Febiger, 1994, p. 738–770.
63. Fisher JN, Shahshahani MN, Kitabchi AE: Diabetic ketoacidosis: low-dose insulin therapy by various routes. *N Engl J Med* 297:238–241, 1977
64. Kitabchi AE, Umpierrez GE, Fisher JN, Murphy MB, Stentz FB: Thirty years of personal experience in hyperglycemic crises: diabetic ketoacidosis and hyperglycemic hyperosmolar state. *J Clin Endocrinol Metab* 93:1541–1552, 2008
65. Umpierrez GE, Latif K, Stoever J, Cuervo R, Park L, Freire AX, Kitabchi EK: Efficacy of subcutaneous insulin lispro versus continuous intravenous regular insulin for the treatment of patients with diabetic ketoacidosis. *Am J Med* 117:291–296, 2004
66. Adrogue HJ, Lederer ED, Suki WN, Eknoyan G: Determinants of plasma potassium levels in diabetic ketoacidosis. *Medicine* 65:163–172, 1986

67. Adrogue HJ, Eknoyan G, Suki WK: Diabetic ketoacidosis: role of the kidney in the acid-base homeostasis re-evaluated. *Kidney Int* 25:591–598, 1984
68. Beigelman PM: Severe diabetic ketoacidosis (diabetic "coma"). 482 episodes in 257 patients; experience of three years. *Diabetes* 20:490–500, 1971
69. DeFronzo RA, Felig P, Ferrannini E, Wahren J: Effect of graded doses of insulin on splanchnic and peripheral potassium metabolism in man. *Am J Physiol* 238:E421–427, 1980
70. Kitabchi AE, Umpierrez GE, Murphy MB, Barrett EJ, Kreisberg RA, Malone JI, Wall BM: Hyperglycemic crises in patients with diabetes mellitus. *Diabetes Care* 26(Suppl. 1):S109–S117, 2003
71. Abramson E, Arky R: Diabetic acidosis with initial hypokalemia. Therapeutic implications. *JAMA* 196:401–403, 1966
72. Lebovitz HE: Diabetic ketoacidosis. *Lancet* 345:767–772, 1995
73. Mitchell JH, Wildenthal K, Johnson RL, Jr.: The effects of acid-base disturbances on cardiovascular and pulmonary function. *Kidney Int* 1:375–389, 1972
74. Housley E, Clarke SW, Hedworth-Whitty RB, Bishop JM: Effect of acute and chronic acidaemia and associated hypoxia on the pulmonary circulation of patients with chronic bronchitis. *Cardiovasc Res* 4:482–489, 1970
75. Latif KA, Freire AX, Kitabchi AE, Umpierrez GE, Qureshi N: The use of alkali therapy in severe diabetic ketoacidosis. *Diabetes Care* 25:2113–2114, 2002
76. Hale PJ, Crase J, Nattrass M: Metabolic effects of bicarbonate in the treatment of diabetic ketoacidosis. *Br Med J (Clin Res Ed)* 289:1035–1038, 1984
77. Morris LR, Murphy MB, Kitabchi AE: Bicarbonate therapy in severe diabetic ketoacidosis. *Ann Intern Med* 105:836–840, 1986
78. Lever E, Jaspan JB: Sodium bicarbonate therapy in severe diabetic ketoacidosis. *Am J Med* 75:263–268, 1983
79. Green SM, Rothrock SG, Ho JD, Gallant RD, Borger R, Thomas TL, Zimmerman GJ: Failure of adjunctive bicarbonate to improve outcome in severe pediatric diabetic ketoacidosis. *Ann Emerg Med* 31:41–48, 1998
80. Viallon A, Zeni F, Lafond P, Venet C, Tardy B, Page Y, Bertrand JC: Does bicarbonate therapy improve the management of severe diabetic ketoacidosis? *Crit Care Med* 27:2690–2693, 1999
81. Graf H, Leach W, Arieff AI: Evidence for a detrimental effect of bicarbonate therapy in hypoxic lactic acidosis. *Science* 227:754–756, 1985
82. Glaser N, Barnett P, McCaslin I, Nelson D, Trainor J, Louie J, Kaufman F, Quayle K, Roback M, Malley R, Kuppermann N: Risk factors for cerebral edema in children with diabetic ketoacidosis. The Pediatric Emergency Medicine Collaborative Research Committee of the American Academy of Pediatrics. *N Engl J Med* 344:264–269, 2001
83. Fisher JN, Kitabchi AE: A randomized study of phosphate therapy in the treatment of diabetic ketoacidosis. *J Clin Endocrinol Metab* 57:177–180, 1983
84. Winter RJ, Harris CJ, Phillips LS, Green OC: Diabetic ketoacidosis. Induction of hypocalcemia and hypomagnesemia by phosphate therapy. *Am J Med* 67:897–900, 1979
85. Miller DW, Slovis CM: Hypophosphatemia in the emergency department therapeutics. *Am J Emerg Med* 18:457–461, 2000

86. Kitabchi AE, Umpierrez GE, Murphy MB, Barrett EJ, Kreisberg RA, Malone JI, Wall BM: Hyperglycemic crises in diabetes. *Diabetes Care* 27(Suppl. 1):S94–S102, 2004

87. Umpierrez GE, Jones S, Smiley D, Mulligan P, Keyler T, Temponi A, Semakula C, Umpierrez D, Peng L, Ceron M, Robalino G: Insulin analogs versus human insulin in the treatment of patients with diabetic ketoacidosis: a randomized controlled trial. *Diabetes Care* 32:1164–1169, 2009

88. Owens DR, Coates PA, Luzio SD, Tinbergen JP, Kurzhals R: Pharmacokinetics of 125I-labeled insulin glargine (HOE 901) in healthy men: comparison with NPH insulin and the influence of different subcutaneous injection sites. *Diabetes Care* 23:813–819, 2000

89. Heinemann L: Variability of insulin absorption and insulin action. *Diabetes Technol Ther* 4:673–682, 2002

90. Sacks HS, Shahshahani M, Kitabchi AE, Fisher JN, Young RT: Similar responsiveness of diabetic ketoacidosis to low-dose insulin by intramuscular injection and albumin-free infusion. *Ann Intern Med* 90:36–42, 1979

91. Adrogue HJ, Wilson H, Boyd AE, 3rd, Suki WN, Eknoyan G: Plasma acid-base patterns in diabetic ketoacidosis. *N Engl J Med* 307:1603–1610, 1982

92. Rosenbloom AL: Intracerebral crises during treatment of diabetic ketoacidosis. *Diabetes Care* 13:22–33, 1990

93. Edge JA, Hawkins MM, Winter DL, Dunger DB: The risk and outcome of cerebral oedema developing during diabetic ketoacidosis. *Arch Dis Child* 85:16–22, 2001

94. Abbott NJ: Inflammatory mediators and modulation of blood-brain barrier permeability. *Cell Mol Neurobiol* 20:131–147, 2000

95. Silver SM, Clark EC, Schroeder BM, Sterns RH: Pathogenesis of cerebral edema after treatment of diabetic ketoacidosis. *Kidney Int* 51:1237–1244, 1997

96. Glaser N, Barnett P, McCaslin I, Nelson D, Trainor J, Louie J, Kaufman F, Quayle K, Roback M, Malley R, Kuppermann N: Risk factors for cerebral edema in children with diabetic ketoacidosis. The Pediatric Emergency Medicine Collaborative Research Committee of the American Academy of Pediatrics. *N Engl J Med* 344:264–269, 2001

97. Arieff AI, Kleeman CR: Cerebral edema in diabetic comas. II. Effects of hyperosmolality, hyperglycemia and insulin in diabetic rabbits. *J Clin Endocrinol Metab* 38:1057–1067, 1974

98. Dunger DB, Sperling MA, Acerini CL, Bohn DJ, Daneman D, Danne TP, Glaser NS, Hanas R, Hintz RL, Levitsky LL, Savage MO, Tasker RC, Wolfsdorf JI: ESPE/LWPES consensus statement on diabetic ketoacidosis in children and adolescents. *Arch Dis Child* 89:188–194, 2004

99. Laffel LM, Brackett J, Ho J, Anderson BJ: Changing the process of diabetes care improves metabolic outcomes and reduces hospitalizations. *Qual Manag Health Care* 6:53–62, 1998

100. Ellis D, Naar-King S, Templin T, Frey M, Cunningham P, Sheidow A, Cakan N, Idalski A: Multisystemic therapy for adolescents with poorly controlled type 1 diabetes: reduced diabetic ketoacidosis admissions and related costs over 24 months. *Diabetes Care* 31:1746–1747, 2008

101. Klonoff DC, Buckingham B, Christiansen JS, Montori VM, Tamborlane WV, Vigersky RA, Wolpert H: Continuous glucose monitoring: an Endocrine Society clinical practice guideline. *J Clin Endocrinol Metab* 96:2968–2979, 2011
102. Price GC, Stevenson K, Walsh TS: Evaluation of a continuous glucose monitor in an unselected general intensive care population. *Crit Care Resusc* 10:209–216, 2008

16

Complications: Detection and Management
I. Macrovascular Complications

Raynard Washington, PhD, MPH, and Trevor Orchard, MD, M Med Sci, FAHA, FACE

INTRODUCTION

Macrovascular complications in type 1 diabetes (T1D) include a group of cardiovascular diseases (CVD) caused predominantly by the development of atherosclerosis in blood vessels throughout the body. Atherosclerosis begins in childhood and adolescence.[1,2] Atheromatous plaques are formed in large part because of the accumulation of cholesterol resulting from the formation of foam cells, following low-density lipoproteins penetration into the arterial wall. Plaques lead to angina and may rupture and hemorrhage, leading to thrombotic occlusion and tissue infarction. Manifestation of atherosclerosis varies by location in the body. The three major types of CVD most often associated with T1D are coronary heart disease (CAD), peripheral vascular disease (PVD), and cerebrovascular disease.

CVD is the primary cause of premature death in people who have T1D for 20 or more years.[3] Young adults (ages 20–40 years) with childhood onset diabetes, in many cases T1D, have an estimated 8- to 41-fold increased risk of dying from ischemic heart disease compared to the general population.[4] It is thus critical to recognize that young adults (e.g., in their 30s) with longstanding (>20 years) T1D have CVD risk levels approaching those considered high risk (a 2% per year risk of major coronary event[5]). In contrast, a newly diagnosed T1D individual at the same age has a much lower risk that is close to normal, which has major management implications.[6,7]

Many children with T1D have subclinical evidence of atherosclerosis, with increased intimal medial thickness of the carotid arteries and aorta,[2] reduced endothelium-dependent arterial flow-mediated dilation, and increased arterial stiffness.[1,2,8–10] Young adults with childhood onset diabetes may have silent coronary atherosclerosis as measured by ultrasound.[11] In adults with T1D, macroangiopathy is a major cause of CAD, PVD, cerebrovascular disease and mortality.[12–14]

PATHOGENOSIS AND RISK FACTORS

Multiple potential mechanisms account for the increased risk of CVD outcomes in T1D, including gluco-oxidative damage, insulin resistance, inflammation, fibrosis, and autonomic dysfunction.[8] T1D historically has been strongly related to developing nephropathy, another T1D complication.[15] Decreased

DOI: 10.2337/9781580404785ch16s1

nitric oxide (NO) production, increased oxidative stress, and impaired function of endothelial progenitor cells have recently been implicated.[16] Histopathology studies have suggested differences in the histology of plaques in diabetes (especially in T1D), which has led to the suggestion of more extensive (but less vulnerable) plaques that may be less likely to rupture but more likely to be eroded by inflammatory processes.[6]

Many risk factors are thus associated with CVD in patients with T1D. Importantly, the well-established linkages between CVD and standard risk factors, including hypertension, dyslipidemia, insulin resistance, obesity, and smoking, are also operative in patients with T1D.[6,17–19] Studies of T1D in the young show that 25–75% of patients have at least one cardiovascular (CV) risk factor.[20,21] In the SEARCH study, the authors identified at least two CV risk factors in 14% of youth with T1D, as well as a clustering of risk factors.[22] Aggressive treatment of these standard risk factors is known to improve outcomes.[12] In addition, as discussed, diabetes-related risk factors also contribute to the increased risk.

Glycemic Control

The relationship between glycemia and CVD in T1D remains unclear. Although some studies have indicated that silent coronary atherosclerosis[11] and CV events[23–25] are associated with poor glycemic control, several large observational studies have shown little or no association in multivariable analyses between glycemic control and CVD.[17,26,27] Neither baseline nor cumulative glycemic control were predictors of CVD in the Pittsburgh Epidemiology of Diabetes Complications (EDC) study however, a follow-up analysis showed that change in A1C over time was directly related to CVD risk.[28] This finding would be consistent with results from the Diabetes Complications and Control Trial (DCCT), which showed that improved glycemic control for 6 years had a profound protection against >20-year CV risk.[24] There are many potential explanations for the contrast between the findings of these studies, including the level of control achieved (lower in the DCCT[24] and Swedish register),[23] duration (longer in observational cohorts[17,26,27]), and prevalence of renal disease (lower in the positive studies[24,25]). Finally, it is likely that intensive insulin therapy will have benefits beyond glycemia (e.g., on hypertension and dyslipidemia).[29,30] Unfortunately, the potential role of these factors in explaining the benefit of intensive therapy in the DCCT/EDIC has not been examined.

Nephropathy

It has been long recognized that the development of renal disease dramatically increases CVD risk in T1D.[6,15,17] The etiology of this increased risk is not clear, although renal disease worsens a number of the standard risk factors, particularly hypertension and dyslipidemia, and also is linked to insulin resistance.[6,31] Additionally, recent data from the Pittsburgh EDC study suggest that although the incidence of renal disease has declined remarkably over the past 30 years, CAD incidence has not.[32]

Insulin Resistance and Metabolic Syndrome

Even though usually associated with type 2 diabetes (T2D), the presence of insulin resistance (and central obesity) also increase CVD risk, reflecting a state called "double diabetes," wherein T1D and T2D coexist. Early suggestions of this state include the association of family history of T2D with CVD risk in T1D[33] and the association of family history of T2D with excess weight gain and dyslipidemia in the DCCT.[34] Closely related to insulin resistance is the metabolic syndrome, a clustering of abdominal obesity, dyslipidemia, hypertension, and glucose intolerance.[8,20] It affects 8–21% of young individuals with T1D depending on definitions.[22,35,36] Recent Australian and international studies indicate that the clinical combination of T1D and the metabolic syndrome portends a worse prognosis than T1D alone, providing further support that insulin resistance and its associated risk factors are major components of CVD risk in T1D.[35]

Genetic Factors

A number of genetic factors have been implicated in CVD risk in T1D. Predominant among these recently is the haptoglobin genotype (Hp) 2-2 association with CAD risk in T1D,[37] which is consistent with extensive T2D data.[38] The EDC study found more than a twofold increased risk of CAD among individuals carrying the Hp 2-2 genotype compared with those carrying the Hp 1-1 genotype in multivariable analyses in T1D, furthermore its remarkable specificity for diabetes has been confirmed in another T1D study, the CACTI study.[39]

CURRENT STANDARDS OF CARE

Standards of care for the macrovascular complications of patients with T1D should involve screening, prevention, and management of both CVD and its individual risk factors. The American Diabetes Association (ADA),[19] American Association of Clinical Endocrinologist (AACE),[40] American Heart Association (AHA),[12] National Heart, Lung, and Blood Institute,[41] National Cholesterol Education Program Adult Treatment Panel,[5] International Society for Pediatric and Adolescent Diabetes,[18] and American Academy of Pediatrics[42] have, among others, provided recommendations for either or both pediatric and adult management. This discussion focuses on these specific guidelines. A more detailed summary is given in Appendix 16.I.A. It should be noted that some standards are specific to T1D, whereas others are provided for all diabetes in general, which as discussed is a major problem.

Pediatric Screening

Risk factors. The ADA recommends obtaining a fasting lipid profile on children >2 years of age soon after diagnosis if there is a family history of hypercholesterolemia or CV events before age 55 years or if family history is unknown.

Otherwise, a fasting lipid profile should be obtained at puberty (>10 years of age).[19] Similar guidelines are also given in other recommendations.[12,41,42] Of note, the International Society for Pediatric and Adolescent Diabetes recommends lipid profile screening every 5 years after age 12, instead of age 10.[18] Most standards recommend measuring fasting lipid profiles annually in youth with abnormal baseline measurements. Current standards recommend routine blood pressure measurements in children with diabetes.[18,19] Recommendations for screening for glycemic control in youth are discussed elsewhere.

Macrovascular disease. Despite the capability to detect atherosclerosis in youth,[1,2,8] currently there are no recommendations available for screening for macrovascular disease in youth with T1D. The primary focus is screening for potential risk factors.[12,18,19,40]

Adult Screening

Risk factors. Current standards recommend measuring a fasting lipid profile in adults annually and blood pressure and body weight screening at all routine diabetes visits.[5,19,40] In addition, routine and thorough assessment of tobacco use is important to prevent smoking or encourage cessation.[19]

Macrovascular disease. Screening for macrovascular disease in adults with T1D involves taking a thorough history, with a detailed annual examination, and possibly a resting electrocardiogram as a baseline. In asymptomatic patients with T2D, routine screening for coronary artery disease is not recommended,[19,40] largely on the basis of the lack of benefit in one study.[43] AACE recommends measurement of coronary artery calcification or coronary imaging in long diabetes duration patients.[40] Again no specific guidelines were identified for T1D, although it is likely that similar recommendations apply, particularly in those with metabolic syndrome. The annual clinical assessment should include a history for new-onset symptoms of ischemic heart disease, including typical or atypical chest pain or unexplained dyspnea on exertion, and an examination for carotid bruits and lower limb pulses.[19] According to the ADA, candidates for cardiac stress testing include those with atypical cardiac symptoms and an abnormal ECG.[19]

Pediatric Management

Risk factors. The ADA recommends initial treatment of hypertension or dyslipidemia to include dietary intervention and exercise, aimed at improved weight management, increased physical activity, and reduced saturated fat intake.[19] If target blood pressure is not reached within 3–6 months, pharmacologic treatment should be considered, particularly angiotensin-converting-enzyme inhibitors (ACEIs).[19] For lipid lowering, pharmacologic options (preferably statins) can be used after age 10, as statin use is not generally recommended for use in those under the age of 10 years in the U.S.[18,19,42] Short-term trials have reported that simvastatin, lovastatin, and pravastatin are effective and safe in children and adolescents.[44–46] No significant side effects were observed in growth, pubertal Tanner staging, testicular volume, menarche, endocrine function parameters, or liver or muscle enzymes. Special attention should be paid to symptoms associated with muscles and connective tissues because there is an increased risk of rhabdomylysis.

Macrovascular disease. Currently, there are no separate standards for the medical management of macrovascular disease in youth with T1D, as CVD rarely manifests in children.

Adult Management

Risk factors. Numerous studies have shown the efficacy of controlling individual CVD risk factors in preventing or delaying the onset of CVD events in people with diabetes.[19] Large benefits are also seen when multiple risk factors are addressed globally.[47] Significantly, however, no direct evidence of benefit exists for T1D except for intensive glycemic therapy[24] and low-density lipoprotein (LDLc) lowering with simvastatin.[48] The first priority for most patients with diabetes is to decide an appropriate glycemic control goal. A recent consensus statement has reviewed the major controversy surrounding optimal glycemic control in T2D, including the negative results of three recent trials and current strategies.[49] The extent to which these trials affect T1D is unclear, especially given the positive benefits of intensive therapy seen in DCCT;[24] however, the concept of individualizing goals as the panel recommends for T2D would seem prudent at this point. This is particularly true as patients age when episodes of severe hypoglycemia appear to increase in frequency, which may necessitate raising glycemic control targets (see chapter 6, Targets).

Table 16.I.1 shows recommendations for glycemic, blood pressure, and lipid control for most adults with diabetes.[5,19,40]

LDL cholesterol management. The next priority would be to lower cholesterol to a target goal of <100 mg/dL.[5,19,40] Diabetes, in general (albeit primarily T2D), is recognized by the National Cholesterol Education Program Adult Treatment Panel III (NCEP ATP III) to be a CVD risk equivalent, thus justifying this cutpoint. Indeed, in a subsequent review, this panel designated the combination of CVD and diabetes to be the highest risk category and proposed a 70 mg/dl LDLc goal when feasible (again, primarily in individuals with T2D).[50] Although some patients might achieve their specific objective with lifestyle intervention (including medical nutrition therapy) alone, the majority will need medication, preferably a statin. Furthermore, in those with clinical CVD, or those who are over the age of 40 years with other CVD risk factors, the ADA recommends that treatment with statin medication should be added to lifestyle therapy, regardless of baseline LDL levels.[19] If targets are not reached, combination therapy with other statins or other lipid-lowering medications is a further possibility.[5,19,40]

Hypertension management. The Seventh Report of the Joint National Committee on Prevention, Detection, Evaluation, and Treatment of High Blood Pressure[51] reports that antihypertensive agents effectively lower blood pressure in T1D. Effects are similar to those seen in the general population.[52] Combinations of two or more drugs are often needed to achieve the target goal of <130/80 mmHg.[53] Thiazide diuretics, β-adrenergic blocking (BBs) agents, ACEIs, angiotensin II receptor blockers (ARBs), and calcium channel blockers (CCBs) reduce

Table 16.I.1 Summary of Recommendations for Glycemic, Blood Pressure, and Lipid Control for Most Adults with Diabetes Based on ADA,[19] AACE,[40] and NCEP[5] Guidelines

Measurement	Recommended Goal
A1C, %	<7.0%*
Systolic Blood Pressure, mmHg	<130†
Diastolic Blood Pressure, mmHg	<80
LDL Cholesterol, mg/dL	<100‡
HDL Cholesterol, mg/dL	>40 (males) >50 (females)
Triglycerides, mg/dL	<150

Note: *More or less stringent glycemic goals may be appropriate for individual patients. Goals should be individualized based on duration of diabetes, age/life expectancy, comorbid conditions, known CVD or advanced microvascular complications, hypoglycemia unawareness, and individual and patient considerations.[49]

†Based on patient characteristics and response to therapy, higher or lower SBP targets may be appropriate.

‡In individuals with overt CVD, a lower LDL cholesterol goal of <70 mg/dL (1.8 mmol/L), using a high dose of a statin, is an option.

Sources: ADA,[19] AACE,[40] and NCEP[5] Guidelines.

incidence of CVD and stroke in patients with diabetes.[53-55] Current standards recommend ACEIs and ARBs as first-line agents in adults with diabetes, without contraindication, based partially on their efficacy in suppression and microalbuminuria.[5,19,40] Recommendations for glycemic, blood pressure, and lipid control for most adults with diabetes are discussed in chapter 5.

Smoking cessation

A number of large, randomized clinical trials have demonstrated the efficacy and cost-effectiveness of brief counseling in smoking cessation, including the use of quit lines, in the reduction of tobacco use. For patients motivated to quit, adding pharmacological therapy to counseling is more effective than either treatment alone. Special considerations include assessment of the level of nicotine dependence, which is associated with difficulty in quitting and relapse.[56]

Macrovascular disease. Generally, in addition to the risk factor management noted early for blood pressure and LDL cholesterol, aspirin use is recommended for those with a history of major CV events, stroke, and limb revascularization.[5,19,40,51] The ADA notes that in patients with a previous myocardial infarction, β-blockers should be used for 2 years after the event.[19] There are few guidelines on specific surgical management of CVD in T1D, although the greater benefit of bypass over angioplasty[57] and more recently of early coronary artery bypass graft versus medical therapy alone in those with fairly severe CAD[58] in T2D are observations worthy of consideration in the management of T1D.

Prevention

Control of risk factors, particularly blood pressure, lipid profile, weight, and smoking are currently recommended as primary prevention of CVD in youth and adults with diabetes.[18,19,40] No specific pharmacologic prevention beyond addressing these factors is currently recommended apart from low-dose aspirin (and statin use for secondary prevention and high-risk primary prevention, irrespective of lipid profile) as primary and secondary prevention of CVD in high-risk adults with diabetes.[19,40]

GAPS IN CLINICAL RESEARCH AND HOW TO ADDRESS THEM

Although research has answered many questions regarding the risk for, and development of, CVD in patients with diabetes, in general, there is a dearth of specific evidence pertaining to risk factor intervention and clinical management in T1D. Although the different types of diabetes are similar in some aspects, there are distinct differences in the natural history of each, particularly as it relates to macrovascular complications.[6] Other important "diabetes-type" differences are the age of onset (much younger in T1D) and the influence of renal disease (historically much greater in T1D). These factors are important for they greatly render diabetes standard CVD risk engines (prediction equations) inappropriate,[59] necessitating specific models.[60,61] Furthermore, the lack of specific, duration-based T1D guidelines likely leads to inadequate intervention for some young adults. In this regard, recent models from the Swedish National Diabetes Register for 30- to 65-year-olds with T1D should be tested in other data sets and possibly refined to specific age- and duration-groups.[60] Risk factor control is far from satisfactory in the adult T1D population as recent data have shown.[62] Thus, separate clinical guidelines may be ideal.

Another issue is that there are several functioning sets of recommendations and guidelines for screening, management, and prevention of CVD in diabetes. Although in some regards these standards are consistent, there are inconsistencies and extensive gaps as indicated earlier and detailed in Appendix 16.I.A. The necessity for uniform recommendations is therefore a priority.

Recommendations

Recommendation 1. The convening of all key stakeholders to produce a single set of clinical recommendations based on available data would provide an initial solution to the two current problems identified namely as the following:

1. Lack of specific T1D guidelines especially for (a) the screening for subclinical CVD in young adults; (b) intensity of risk factor management in youth and young adults; and (c) the management of CVD in T1D.

2. Plethora of guidelines that impinge on the management of T1D from a CVD viewpoint but fail to provide a comprehensive plan.

Major gaps in the T1D evidence base that partially underlie these current guideline deficiencies include a lack of data that directly link CV risk factors in childhood T1D to CV events, and limited evidence of the preventive benefits of CVD intervention in adolescents and adults with T1D. Although the Adolescent Type 1 Diabetes Cardio-renal Intervention Trial (AdDIT)[63] will partially address this concern for adolescents with some surrogate CVD measures, the appropriate intensity and mode of CVD risk intervention in young adults with T1D with CVD event is unclear and thus a high priority. Current data sets have not been fully tapped to provide clinically helpful risk estimates.

Recommendation 2. A research program should be developed to address gaps in our evidence base for CVD prevention in T1D based on existing studies and potentially new trials. Specific gaps include *1)* duration specific estimates of CVD risk in youth and young adults, *2)* the linkage of risk factors and subclinical measures in youth to events in adulthood, and *3)* the benefit of intensive risk factor intervention in youth and young adults.

In addition, the linkage between some risk factors and CVD in T1D remains unclear, including glycemic control and renal disease, and merits further investigation—for example, from DCCT/EDC. It is disappointing to note that despite remarkable improvement in survival and renal disease, some studies do not show a comparable reduction in CAD events.[32]

Recommendation 3. A workshop should be convened to specifically address the roles of glycemic control and renal disease on CVD events in T1D and how these influences should affect management.

Finally, novel risk factors for CVD (e.g., insulin resistance and haptoglobin genotype) in T1D are emerging and require further study. Haptoglobin is particularly attractive as vitamin E therapy has shown potential for benefit in those with T2D and Hp2/2.[64]

Recommendation 4. A research program to evaluate one or more novel approaches to prevention of CVD in T1D should be developed with appropriate funding so that some of the considerable residual risk beyond standard risk factors and glycemic control can be addressed.

Although some shortfalls can be addressed by ongoing follow-up in major longitudinal studies, and consensus meetings on guidelines, others will, as suggested, require randomized controlled trials.

Recommendation 5. Thus, it is further recommended that a broad-based international standing committee or panel be convened to initially review and implement these recommendations, as appropriate, and thereafter periodically review and standardize existing guidelines and recommend future research priorities. This would help provide contemporaneous guidance to clinical practice and research and be of service to providers, payers, and, most important, patients.

EXISTING STANDARDS OF CARE FOR CVD AND RISK FACTORS IN T1D

Table 16.I.A.1 Summary of Existing Standards of Care for CVD in T1D

Guide-line	Pediatric Screening				Adult Screening				Pediatric Management				Adult Management			
	Lipids	Blood Pressure	Other Risk Factors	Disease	Lipids	Blood Pressure	Other Risk Factors	Disease	Lipids	Blood Pressure	Other Risk Factors	Disease	Lipids	Blood Pressure	Other Risk Factors	Disease
ADA	◆	◆	◆		◇	◇	◇	◇	◆	◆	◆		◇	◇	◇	◇
AACE					◇	◇	◇	◇					◇	◇	◇	
AHA	◆	◆	◆						◆	◆	◆					
NCEP					◆								◆			
ISPAD	◆	◆	◆						◆	◆	◆					
AAP	◇								◇							
NHLBI	◆	◆	◆						◆	◆	◆					
JNC 7						◇								◇		

◆ - Recommendation for patients with T1D

◇ - Recommendation for all patients with diabetes

AACE, American Association of Clinical Endocrinologists; AAP, American Academy of Pediatrics; ADA, American Diabetes Association; AHA, American Heart Association; ISPAD, International Society for Pediatric and Adolescent Diabetes; JNC 7, Seventh Report of the Joint National Committee on Prevention, Detection, Evaluation, and Treatment of High Blood Pressure; NCEP, National Cholesterol Education Program; NHLBI, National Heart, Lung, and Blood Institute.

Table 16.I.A.2 Existing Standards of Care for Pediatric CVD and Risk Factor Screening in T1D

Guideline	Pediatric Lipid Screening Recommendations
ADA	• If family history of hypercholesterolemia, CVD event before age 55, or unknown, obtain fasting lipid profile in children >2 years of age soon after diagnosis; or, obtain fasting lipid ≥10 years of age • If diagnosed after puberty (≥age 10), obtain fasting lipid soon after diagnosis • If abnormal, obtain fasting lipid annually; else repeat every 5 years
AHA	• Measure fasting lipid profile in patients with T1D.
ISPAD	• If family history of hypercholesterolemia, CVD event before age 55, or unknown, obtain fasting lipid profile in children >2 years of age soon after diagnosis; or, obtain fasting lipid ≥ 12 years of age • If diagnosed after age 12, obtain fasting lipid soon after diagnosis • If abnormal, obtain fasting lipid annually; else repeat every 5 years
AAP	• If family history of hypercholesterolemia, CVD event before age 55, or unknown, obtain fasting lipid profile in children >2 years of age; or, obtain fasting lipid ≥10 years of age • If diagnosed after puberty (age 10), obtain fasting lipid soon after diagnosis • If abnormal, obtain fasting lipid annually; or repeat every 3–5 years
NHLBI	• Obtain fasting lipid profile in patients with diabetes

Guideline	Pediatric Blood Pressure Screening Recommendations
ADA	• Blood pressure should be measured at all routine visits
AHA	• Blood pressure should be measured at all routine visits
ISPAD	• Blood pressure should be measured at least annually
NHLBI	• Blood pressure should be measured at all routine visits

Guideline	Pediatric Other Risk Factor Screening Recommendations
ADA	• Annual screening for microalbuminuria, with a random spot urine sample after 10 years old and diabetes for 5 years • Screen for smoking behavior routinely • Measure height, weight, and BMI
AHA	• Screen for family history of early CVD in expanded first-degree pedigree • Screen for smoking behavior routinely • Measure height, weight, and BMI
ISPAD	• Annual screening for microalbuminuria, after 11 years old with 2 years' diabetes duration and after 9 years old with 5 years' diabetes duration, and after 2 years' diabetes duration in adolescents • Screen for smoking behavior routinely • Measure height, weight, and BMI
NHLBI	• Screen for smoking behavior routinely • Measure height, weight, and BMI • Screen for diet, physical activity/exercise history

AAP, American Academy of Pediatrics; ADA, American Diabetes Association; AHA, American Heart Association; CVD, cardiovascular disease; ISPAD, International Society for Pediatric and Adolescent Diabetes; NCEP, National Cholesterol Education Program; NHLBI, National Heart, Lung, and Blood Institute.

Table 16.I.A.3 Existing Standards of Care for Adult CVD and Risk Factor Screening in T1D

Guideline	Adult Lipid Screening Recommendations
ADA	• Measure fasting lipids at least annually, except in low-risk patients (LDL <100 mg/dl, HDL >50 mg/dl, and triglycerides <150 mg/dl) measure every 2 years
AACE	• Measure fasting lipids at least annually, if not at target measure more frequently
NCEP	• Measure fasting lipids at least annually, if not at target measure more frequently

Guideline	Adult Blood Pressure Screening Recommendations
ADA	• Blood pressure should be measured at all routine visits
AACE	• Blood pressure should be measured at all routine visits
JNC 7	• Blood pressure should be measured at all routine visits

Guideline	Adult Other Risk Factor Screening Recommendations
ADA	• Perform A1C test at least two times a year in patients who meet goals and four times a year in patients not meeting goals • Screen for smoking behaviors at all routine visits • Test for urine albumin excretion annually in patients with diabetes duration ≥5 years, and measure serum creatinine annually in all patients
AACE	• Perform A1C test at least two times a year in patients who meet goals and four times a year in patients not meeting goals • Screen for smoking behaviors at all routine visits • Begin annual assessment of serum creatinine to estimate the GRF and urine albumin excretion 5 years after diagnosis

Guideline	Adult Disease Screening Recommendations
ADA	• No routine screening in asymptomatic patients • CVD risk factors should be assessed annually • Cardiac stress testing is appropriate for symptomatic patients and those with an abnormal ECG
AACE	• No routine screening in asymptomatic patients • CVD risk factors should be assessed annually • Measure coronary artery calcification or coronary imaging to determine if patient is a reasonable candidate for intensification of glycemic, lipid, and/or blood pressure control

AACE, American Association of Clinical Endocrinologists; ADA, American Diabetes Association; CVD, cardiovascular disease; ECG, electrocardiogram; JNC 7, Seventh Report of the Joint National Committee on Prevention, Detection, Evaluation, and Treatment of High Blood Pressure; NCEP, National Cholesterol Education Program.

Table 16.I.A.4 Existing Standards of Care for Pediatric CVD and Risk Factor Management in T1D

Guideline	Pediatric Lipid Management Recommendations
ADA	• Target: LDL <100 mg/dl • Initial therapy: optimize glucose control and MNT using step 2 AHA diet to decrease saturated fat intake • After age 10, add statin in patients who have LDL >160 mg/dl, or LDL >130 mg/dl and one or more CVD risk factor
AHA	• Target: LDL ≤100 mg/dl • Rigorous age-appropriate education in diet and physical activity • Initial therapy: optimize glucose control and lifestyle intervention (diet/physical activity) for up to 6 months • If age >10, add statin if goals are not achieved
ISPAD	• Target: LDL <100 mg/dl • Initial therapy: optimize glucose control and lifestyle intervention (diet/physical activity) • After age 10, add statin in patients who have LDL >130 mg/dl and one or more CVD risk factor
AAP	• Target: LDL <110–130 mg/dl • Initial therapy: optimize glucose control and lifestyle intervention (diet/physical activity) • If age ≥8, add statin in patients who have LDL >130 mg/dl and have not achieved goal with lifestyle intervention
NHLBI	• Target: LDL <100 mg/dl, triglyceride <90 mg/dl, non-HDL <120 mg/dl • Initial therapy: optimize glucose control and MNT using step 2 AHA diet to decrease saturated fat intake • After age 10, add statin in patients who have LDL >160 mg/dl, or LDL >130 mg/dl and one or more CVD risk factor
Guideline	Pediatric Blood Pressure Management Recommendations
ADA	• Target: <130/80 mmHg or below 90th percentile for age, sex, and height, whichever is lower • Initial therapy: dietary intervention and exercise • If target not reached in 3–6 months or if blood pressure exceeds 95th percentile or consistently >130/80 mmHg, pharmacologic treatment should be considered • ACEIs should be considered for initial treatment, after appropriate reproductive counselin
AHA	• Target: ≤90th percentile for age, sex, and height • Initial therapy : dietary intervention (including, no added salt) and exercise (6 months) • If target not reached or if blood pressure exceeds 95th percentile, pharmacologic treatment should be considered • ACEIs should be considered for first line therapy, target <90th percentile or <130/80 mmHg, whichever is lower

ISPAD	• Target: ≤90th percentile for age, sex, and height • Initial therapy : dietary intervention and exercise • If target not reached or if blood pressure exceeds 95th percentile, pharmacologic treatment should be considered • ACEIs should be considered for first line therapy
NHLBI	• Target: ≤90th percentile for age, sex, and height • Initial therapy: dietary intervention (including no added salt) and exercise (6 months) • If target not reached or if blood pressure exceeds 95th percentile, pharmacologic treatment should be considered • ACEIs should be considered for first line therapy
Guideline	Pediatric Other Risk Factor Management Recommendations
ADA	• Treat confirmed microalbuminuria (in 3 samples) with ACEIs • Smoking cessation should be offered to all patients
AHA	• Weight loss intervention, as needed; BMI ≤85th percentile for age and sex • Intensive glucose management • Smoking cessation should be offered to all patients
NHLBI	• Weight loss intervention, as needed; BMI ≤85th percentile for age and sex • Intensive glucose management • Smoking cessation should be offered to all patients

AAP, American Academy of Pediatrics; ACEI, angiotensin-converting-enzyme inhibitors; ADA, American Diabetes Association; AHA, American Heart Association; CVD, cardiovascular disease; HDL, high-density lipoprotein; ISPAD, International Society for Pediatric and Adolescent Diabetes; LDL, low-density lipoprotein; NHLBI, National Heart, Lung, and Blood Institute.

Table 16.I.A.5 Existing Standards of Care for Adult CVD and Risk Factor Management in T1D

Guideline	Adult Lipid Management Recommendations
ADA	• Target: LDL <100 mg/dl, <70 mg/dl (in patients with known CVD); HDL >40 mg/dl (males), >50 mg/dl (females); triglycerides <150 mg/dl • Initial therapy: lifestyle modification focusing on reduction of saturated fat, including weight loss intervention and physical activity • Statin therapy (if not contraindicated), regardless of baseline lipid levels, if known CVD or have one or more other CVD risk factor
AACE	• Target: LDL <100 mg/dl, <70 mg/dl (in patients with known CVD); HDL >40 mg/dl (males), >50 mg/dl (females); triglycerides <150 mg/dl • Initial therapy: lifestyle modification focusing on reduction of saturated fat, including weight loss intervention and physical activity; and consult with dietitian • If goal not met or known CVD statin therapy is preferred (if not contraindicated), may be combined with bile acid sequestrants, niacin, or cholesterol absorption inhibitors if targets not met
NCEP	• Target: LDL <130 mg/dl if at onset, LDL <100 mg/dl with increasing diabetes duration • Initial therapy: Lifestyle modification focusing on reduction of saturated fat, including weight loss intervention and physical activity • Statin therapy should be used if LDL ≥130 mg/dl (if not contraindicated)

Guideline	Adult Blood Pressure Management Recommendations
ADA	• Target: blood pressure <130/80 mmHg • If blood pressure <140/90, lifestyle therapy (DASH diet, physical activity) alone for a maximum of 3 months • If blood pressure ≥140/90, lifestyle therapy and pharmacologic therapy (diuretic, ACEI, ARB, combination)
AACE	• Target: blood pressure <130/80 mmHg • Lifestyle therapy (DASH diet, physical activity) and as needed consult with dietitian for all patients above target • Consider ACEIs or ARBs as first-line, combine with calcium channel antagonists, diuretics, and/or β-blockers to achieve goal
JNC 7	• Target: blood pressure <130/80 mmHg • Lifestyle therapy (DASH diet, physical activity, dietary sodium reduction, weight reduction, and moderation of alcohol consumption) • If goals not achieved, consider ACEIs, β-blockers, ARBs, and calcium antagonists as monotherapy or in combination to achieve goals

Guideline	Adult Other Risk Factor Management Recommendations
ADA	• Manage glycemic control and nephropathy (ACEI and/or ARB therapy) • Smoking cessation
AACE	• Manage glycemic control and nephropathy (ACEI and/or ARB therapy)

Guideline	Adult Disease Management Recommendations
ADA	• Patients with increased CHD risk should receive aspirin and a statin, and ACEI or ARB therapy (if hypertensive)
	• Patients with known CVD should receive aspirin and a statin, and ACEI to reduce risk of CVD event
	• In patients with MI, β-blockers should be used for at least 2 years after the event

AACE, American Association of Clinical Endocrinologists; ACEI, angiotensin-converting-enzyme inhibitors; ADA, American Diabetes Association; ARB, angiotensin II receptor blockers; CHD, coronary heart disease; CVD, cardiovascular disease; DASH, Dietary Approaches to Stop Hypertension; HDL, high-density lipoprotein; JNC 7, Seventh Report of the Joint National Committee on Prevention, Detection, Evaluation, and Treatment of High Blood Pressure; LDL, low-density lipoprotein; NCEP, National Cholesterol Education Program.

REFERENCES

1. Krantz JS, Mack WJ, Hodis HN, Liu CR, Liu CH, Kaufman FR: Early onset of subclinical atherosclerosis in young persons with type 1 diabetes. *J Pediatr* 145(4):452–457, 2004
2. Jarvisalo MJ, Putto-Laurila A, Jartti L, et al.: Carotid artery intima-media thickness in children with type 1 diabetes. *Diabetes* 51(2):493–498, 2005
3. Secrest AM, Becker DJ, Kelsey SF, Laporte RE, Orchard TJ: Cause-specific mortality trends in a large population-based cohort with long-standing childhood-onset type 1 diabetes. *Diabetes* 59(12):3216–3222, 2010
4. Laing SP, Swerdlow AJ, Slater SD, Burden AC, Morris A, Waugh NR, Bingley PH, Patterson CC: Mortality from heart disease in a cohort of 23,000 patients with insulin-treated diabetes. *Diabetologia* 46:760–765, 2004
5. National Cholesterol Education Program (NCEP) Expert Panel on Detection, Evaluation, and Treatment of High Blood Cholesterol in Adults (Adult Treatment Panel III): Third report of the National Cholesterol Education Program (NCEP) Expert Panel on Detection, Evaluation, and Treatment of High Blood Cholesterol in Adults (Adult Treatment Panel III) final report. *Circulation* 106(25):3143–3421, 2002
6. Orchard, T, Costacou T, Kretowski, A, Nesto R: Type 1 diabetes and coronary artery disease. *Diabetes Care* 29(11):2528–2538, 2006
7. Orchard TJ, Costacou T: When are type 1 diabetic patients at risk for cardiovascular disease? *Curr Diab Rep* 10(1):48–54, 2010
8. Nadeau KJ, Reusch JE: Cardiovascular function/dysfunction in adolescents with type 1 diabetes. *Curr Diab Rep* 11(3):185–192, 2011
9. Haller MJ, Samyn M, Nichols WW, et al.: Radial artery tonometry demonstrates arterial stiffness in children with type 1 diabetes. *Diabetes Care* 27(12):2911–2917, 2004
10. Llaurado G, Ceperuelo-Mallafre V, Vilardell C, et al.: Arterial stiffness is increased in patients with type 1 diabetes without cardiovascular disease: a potential role of low-grade inflammation. *Diabetes Care* 35:1083–1089, 2012
11. Larsen J, Brekke M, Sandvik L, Arnesen H, Hanssen KF, Dahl-Jorgensen K: Silent coronary atheromatosis in type 1 diabetic patients and its relation to long-term glycemic control. *Diabetes* 51(8):2637–2641, 2002

12. Kavey RE, Allada V, Daniels SR, et al.: Cardiovascular risk reduction in high-risk pediatric patients: a scientific statement from the American Heart Association Expert Panel on Population and Prevention Science; the Councils on Cardiovascular Disease in the Young, Epidemiology and Prevention, Nutrition, Physical Activity and Metabolism, High Blood Pressure Research, Cardiovascular Nursing, and the Kidney in Heart Disease; and the Interdisciplinary Working Group on Quality of Care and Outcomes Research: endorsed by the American Academy of Pediatrics. *Circulation* 114(24):2710–2738, 2006

13. Donahue RP, Orchard TJ: Diabetes mellitus and macrovascular complications. An epidemiological perspective. *Diabetes Care* 15(9):1141–1155, 1992

14. Laing SP, Swerdlow AJ, Slater SD, et al.: The British Diabetic Association cohort study, II: cause-specific mortality in patients with insulin-treated diabetes mellitus. *Diabet Med* 16(6):466–471, 1999

15. Jensen T, Borch-Johnsen K, Kofoed-Enevoldsen A, Deckert T: Coronary heart disease in young type 1 (insulin-dependent) diabetic patients with and without nephropathy: incidence and risk factors. *Diabetologia* 30:144–148, 1987

16. Tousoulis D, Kampoli AM, Stefanadis C: Diabetes mellitus and vascular endothelial dysfunction: current perspectives. *Curr Vasc Pharmacol* 10(1):19–32, 2012

17. Orchard TJ, Olson JC, Erbey JR, Williams K, Forrest KY-Z, Kinder LS, Ellis D, Becker DJ: Insulin resistance-related factors, but not glycemia, predict coronary artery disease in type 1 diabetes. *Diabetes Care* 26(5):1374–1379, 2003

18. International Diabetes Federation, International Society for Pediatric and Adolescent Diabetes: Global IDF/ISPAD guideline for diabetes in childhood and adolescence, 2011. Available at http://www.idf.org/sites/default/files/Diabetes%20in%20Childhood%20and%20Adolescence%20Guidelines_0.pdf. Accessed 28 February 2012

19. American Diabetes Association: Standards of medical care in diabetes—2012. *Diabetes Care* 35(Suppl. 1):S11–S63, 2012

20. Margeirsdottir HD, Larsen JR, Brunborg C, Overby NC, Dahl-Jorgensen K: High prevalence of cardiovascular risk factors in children and adolescents with type 1 diabetes: a population-based study. *Diabetologia* 51(4):554–561, 2008

21. Schwab KO, Doerfer J, Hecker W, et al.: Spectrum and prevalence of atherogenic risk factors in 27,358 children, adolescents, and young adults with type 1 diabetes: cross-sectional data from the German diabetes documentation and quality management system (DPV). *Diabetes Care* 29(2):218–225, 2006

22. Mayer-Davis EJ, Ma B, Lawson A, et al.: Cardiovascular disease risk factors in youth with type 1 and type 2 diabetes: implications of a factor analysis of clustering. *Metab Syndr Relat Disord* 7(2):89–95, 2009

23. Eeg-Olofsson K, Cederholm J, Nilsson PM, Zethelius B, Svensson AM, Gudbjörnsdóttir S, Eliasson B: Glycemic control and cardiovascular disease in 7,454 patients with type 1 diabetes: an observational study from the Swedish National Diabetes Register (NDR). *Diabetes Care* 33(7):1640–1646, 2010

24. Nathan DM, Cleary PA, Backlund JY, et al.: Intensive diabetes treatment and cardiovascular disease in patients with type 1 diabetes. *N Engl J Med* 353(25):2643–2653, 2005

25. Lehto S, Rönnemaa T, Pyörälä K, Laakso M: Poor glycaemic control predicts coronary heart disease events in patients with type 1 diabetes without nephropathy. *Arterioscler Thromb Vasc Biol* 19:1014–1019, 1999

26. Soedamah-Muthu SS, Chaturvedi N, Toeller M, Ferris, B, Reboldi, P, Michel G, Manes C, Fuller JH, The EURODIAB Prospective Complications Study Group: Risk factors for coronary heart disease in type 1 diabetic patients in Europe: the EURODIABE prospective cohort study. *Diabetes Care* 27:530–537, 2004

27. Klein BEK, Klein R, McBride PE, Cruickshanks KJ, Palta M, Knudtson ML, Moss SE, Reinke JO: Cardiovascular disease, mortality, and retinal microvascular characteristics in type 1 diabetes: Wisconsin epidemiologic study of diabetic retinopathy. *Arch Intern Med* 164:1917–1924, 2004

28. Prince CT, Becker DJ, Costacou T, Miller RG, Orchard TJ: Changes in glycaemic control and risk of coronary artery disease in type 1 diabetes mellitus: findings from the Pittsburgh EDC. *Diabetologia* 50:2280–2288, 2007

29. The DCCT Study Research Group: Effect of intensive diabetes management on macrovascular events and risk factors in the Diabetes Control and Complications Trial. *Am J Cardiol* 75(14):894–903, 1995

30. de Boer IH, Kestenbaum B, Rue TC, Steffes MW, Cleary PA, Molitch ME, Lachin JM, Weiss NS, Brunzell JD, Diabetes Control and Complications Trial (DCCT)/Epidemiology of Diabetes Interventions and Complications (EDIC) Study Research Group: Insulin therapy, hyperglycemia, and hypertension in type 1 diabetes mellitus. *Arch Intern Med* 168(17):1867–1873, 2008

31. Orchard TJ, Chang Y-F, Ferrell RE, Petro N, Ellis DE: Nephropathy in type 1 diabetes: a manifestation of insulin resistance and multiple genetic susceptibilities? Further evidence from the Pittsburgh Epidemiology of Diabetes Complication study. *Kidney Int* 62:963–970, 2002

32. Pambianco G, Costacou T, Ellis D, Becker DJ, Klein R, Orchard TJ: The 30-year natural history of type 1 diabetes complications: the Pittsburgh Epidemiology of Diabetes Complications study experience. *Diabetes* 55:1463–1469, 2006

33. Erbey JR, Kuller LH, Becker DJ, Orchard TJ: The association between a family history of type 2 diabetes and coronary artery disease in a type 1 diabetes population. *Diabetes Care* 21:610–614, 1998

34. Purnell JQ, Dev RK, Steffes MW, et al.: Relationship of family history of type 2 diabetes, hypoglycemia, and autoantibodies to weight gain and lipids with intensive and conventional therapy in the Diabetes Control and Complications Trial. *Diabetes* 52:2623–2629, 2003

35. McGill M, Molyneaux L, Twigg SM, Yue DK: The metabolic syndrome in type 1 diabetes: does it exist and does it matter? *J Diabetes Complications* 22(1):18–23, 2008

36. Pambianco G, Costacou T, Orchard TJ: The prediction of major outcomes of type 1 diabetes: a 12-year prospective evaluation of three sepa-

rate definitions of the metabolic syndrome and their components and estimated glucose disposal rate: the Pittsburgh Epidemiology of Diabetes Complications study experience. *Diabetes Care* 30(5):1248–1254, 2007

37. Costacou T, Ferrell RE, Orchard TJ: Haptoglobin genotype: a determinant of cardiovascular complication risk in type 1 diabetes. *Diabetes* 57(6):1702–1706, 2008

38. Levy AP, Hochberg I, Jablonski K, et al.: Haptoglobin genotype is an independent risk factor for cardiovascular disease in individuals with diabetes: the Strong Heart study. *J Am Coll Cardiol* 40:1984–1990, 2002

39. Simpson M, Snell-Bergeon JK, Kinney GL, et al.: Haptoglobin genotype predicts development of coronary artery calcification in a prospective cohort of patients with type 1 diabetes. *Cardiovasc Diabetol* 10:99–106, 2011.

40. Handelsman Y, Mechanick JI, Blonde L, et al., AACE Task Force for Developing Diabetes Comprehensive Care Plan: American Association of Clinical Endocrinologists medical guidelines for clinical practice for developing a diabetes mellitus comprehensive care plan. *Endocr Pract* 17(Suppl. 2):S1–S53, 2011

41. National Heart, Lung, and Blood Institute, National Institutes of Health: Expert Panel on Integrated Guidelines for Cardiovascular Health and Risk Reduction in Children and Adolescents: summary report, 2011. Available at http://www.nhlbi.nih.gov/guidelines/cvd_ped/summary.htm#chap11. Accessed 28 February 2011

42. Daniels SR, Greer FR, Committee on Nutrition: Lipid screening and cardiovascular health in childhood. *Pediatrics* 122(1):198–208, 2008

43. Scognamiglio R, Negut C, Ramondo A, Tiengo A, Avogaro A: Detection of coronary artery disease in asymptomatic patients with type 2 diabetes mellitus. *J Am Coll Cardiol* 47(1):65–71, 2006

44. de Jongh S, Ose L, Szamosi T, et al.: Efficacy and safety of statin therapy in children with familial hypercholesterolemia: a randomized, double-blind, placebo-controlled trial with simvastatin. *Circulation* 106(17):2231–2237, 2002

45. Stein EA, Illingworth DR, Kwiterovich PO, Jr., et al.: Efficacy and safety of lovastatin in adolescent males with heterozygous familial hypercholesterolemia: a randomized controlled trial. *JAMA* 281(2):137–144, 1999

46. Wiegman A, Hutten BA, de Groot E, et al.: Efficacy and safety of statin therapy in children with familial hypercholesterolemia: a randomized controlled trial. *JAMA* 292(3):331–337, 2004

47. Gaede P, Lund-Andersen H, Parving HH, Pedersen O: Effect of a multifactorial intervention on mortality in type 2 diabetes. *N Engl J Med* 358(6):580–591, 2008

48. Collins R, Armitage J, Parish S, Sleigh P, Peto R: MRC/BHF Heart Protection study of cholesterol-lowering with simvastatin in 5963 people with diabetes: a randomised placebo-controlled trial. *Lancet* 361(9374):2005–2016, 2003

49. Inzucchi SE, Bergenstal RM, Buse JB, et al.: Management of hyperglycaemia in type 2 diabetes: a patient-centered approach. Position statement of the American Diabetes Association (ADA) and the European Association for the Study of Diabetes (EASD). *Diabetologia* 55(6):1577–1596, 2012
50. Grundy SM, Cleeman JI, Merz CN, et al.: Implications of recent clinical trials for the National Cholesterol Education Program Adult Treatment Panel III guidelines. *Circulation* 110(2):227–239, 2004
51. U.S. Department of Health and Human Services: JNC 7 Express. The Seventh Report of the Joint National Committee on Prevention, Detection, Evaluation, and Treatment of High Blood Pressure, 2003. Available at http://www.nhlbi.nih.gov/guidelines/hypertension/jncintro.htm. Accessed 29 February 2012
52. Arauz-Pacheco C, Parrott MA, Raskin P: Treatment of hypertension in adults with diabetes. *Diabetes Care* 26(Suppl. 1):S80–S82, 2003
53. ALLHAT Officers and Coordinators for the ALLHAT Collaborative Research Group: Major outcomes in high-risk hypertensive patients randomized to angiotensin-converting enzyme inhibitor or calcium channel blocker vs diuretic: The Antihypertensive and Lipid-Lowering Treatment to Prevent Heart Attack Trial (ALLHAT). *JAMA* 288(23):2981–2997, 2002
54. UK Prospective Diabetes Study Group: Efficacy of atenolol and captopril in reducing risk of macrovascular and microvascular complications in type 2 diabetes: UKPDS 39. *BMJ* 317(7160):713–720, 1998
55. Lindholm LH, Ibsen H, Dahlof B, et al.: Cardiovascular morbidity and mortality in patients with diabetes in the Losartan Intervention For Endpoint reduction in hypertension study (LIFE): a randomised trial against atenolol. *Lancet* 359(9311):1004–1010, 2002
56. Ruger JP, Lazar CM: Economic evaluation of pharmaco- and behavioral therapies for smoking cessation: a critical and systematic review of empirical research. *Annu Rev Public Health* 33:279–305, 2012
57. Influence of diabetes on 5-year mortality and morbidity in a randomized trial comparing CABG and PTCA in patients with multivessel disease: the Bypass Angioplasty Revascularization Investigation (BARI). *Circulation* 96(6):1761–1769, 1997
58. Rutter MK, Nesto RW: The BARI 2D study: a randomised trial of therapies for type 2 diabetes and coronary artery disease. *Diab Vasc Dis Res* 7(1):69–72, 2010
59. Zgibor JC, Piatt GA, Ruppert K, et al.: Deficiencies of cardiovascular risk prediction models for type 1 diabetes. *Diabetes Care* 29:1860–1865, 2006
60. Zgibor JC, Ruppert K, Orchard TJ, et al.: Development of a coronary heart disease risk prediction model for type 1 diabetes: the Pittsburgh CHD in Type 1 Diabetes Risk Model. *Diabetes Res Clin Pract* 88(3):314–321, 2010
61. Cederholm J, Eeg-Olofsson K, Eliasson B, Zethelius B, Gudbjörnsdottir S, Swedish National Diabetes Register: A new model for 5-year risk of cardiovascular disease in type 1 diabetes; from the Swedish National Diabetes Register (NDR). *Diabet Med* 28(10):1213–1220, 2011

62 Snell-Bergeon JK, Nadeau K: Cardiovascular disease risk in young people with type 1 diabetes. *J Cardiovasc Transl Res* 5:446–462, 2012

63. Adolescent Type 1 Diabetes Cardio-renal Intervention Trial Research Group: Adolescent Type 1 Diabetes Cardio-renal Intervention Trial (AdDIT). *BMC Pediatr* 9:79, 2009

64. Milman U, Blum S, Shapira C, et al.: Vitamin E supplementation reduces cardiovascular events in a subgroup of middle-aged individuals with both type 2 diabetes mellitus and the haptoglobin 2-2 genotype: a prospective double-blinded clinical trial. *Arterioscler Thromb Vasc Biol* 28:341–347, 2008

II. Microvascular Complications

Bruce A. Perkins, MD, MPH, FRCP(C)

Damage to the microvascular and macrovascular components of the vascular system in type 1 diabetes (T1D) arise from many of the same etiologic factors and pathogenic mechanisms, and even share many common approaches to their treatment. The clinical presentations of retinopathy, nephropathy, and neuropathy, however, are conventionally classified as distinct "microvascular complications" to differentiate from the coronary heart disease (CAD), peripheral vascular disease (PVD), and cerebrovascular disease discussed as "macrovascular complications" in section I of this chapter. In view of their unique clinical presentations, substantial differences in the evidence base for their detection and management, and the consequent current research gaps, the three microvascular complications are discussed individually in this section.

NEUROPATHY

Background

Damage to the peripheral nervous system in people with diabetes is a complex process that involves etiologic factors other than the simple exposure to hyperglycemia.[1,2] The complexity begins with the diverse clinical presentation—in fact, the neuropathies associated with diabetes encompass two broad categories: focal and generalized neuropathies.[3,4] The former category includes the mononeuropathies, such as carpal tunnel syndrome, peroneal nerve palsy, third cranial nerve palsy, and proximal nerve conditions, such as diabetic amyotrophy. Carpal tunnel syndrome, in particular, is common in people with diabetes and can be difficult to diagnose.[5] Diabetic sensorimotor polyneuropathy is the most common generalized neuropathy, and by far is the most common among the neurological complications of diabetes. For this reason, but despite the many other presentations of neuropathy associated with diabetes, the simplified term "diabetic neuropathy" generally replaces "diabetic sensorimotor polyneuropathy" in the medical literature. Diabetic neuropathy is a *polyneuropathy*, given the diffuse damage to all peripheral nerve fibers—motor, sensory, and autonomic. Such damage occurs insidiously and progressively, usually beginning as a generalized and asymptomatic symmetrical peripheral nerve dysfunction, depending on the length of the involved nerves. At first, nerve damage is characterized by sensory symptoms and later motor function loss in a stocking-and-glove distribution, but it may progress to involve clinical autonomic dysfunction. Sensory manifestations include symptoms, such as numbness, tingling, or pain, and motor symptoms may involve loss of ankle reflexes, include weakness of the foot muscles, and contribute to imbalance. Autonomic neuropathy affects the nerves that regulate the heart, blood pressure, and the adrenergic response to hypoglycemia. Common manifestations

DOI: 10.2337/9781580404785ch16s2

include gastroparesis, neurogenic bladder, cardiac autonomic neuropathy (CAN), erectile dysfunction, and hypoglycemia unawareness.[4,6] CAN is generally considered to be a cardiovascular disease (CVD) risk factor.[6,7] Simple clinical tests, such as postural change in blood pressure or the measurement of heart rate variability, can be used to identify CAN.[8] Diabetic neuropathy is of profound importance because it potentiates severe sequelae, including lower limb skin ulceration, faulty healing, and gangrene.[4,9,10] Furthermore, peripheral neuropathy is sufficient to cause exquisite pain, imbalance, and Charcot joint deformity. Although not all patients with neuropathy have motor or sensory symptoms, the neuropathic pain associated with symptomatic disease is frequently bothersome and often limits physical activity, quality of life, and work productivity.[11] Additionally, patients with neuropathy use more health resources than those without this complication.[11] Beyond the fact that these sequelae dramatically affect quality of life, from a public health perspective, they also generate immense economic burden.[11,12]

Diabetic neuropathy has exceptionally high prevalence (and incidence) as it is observed in >50% of people with diabetes when evaluated using objective tests, such as nerve conduction studies even after only an average of 10 years of diabetes duration.[13] Remarkably, even up to one-half of children with T1D have evidence of asymptomatic nerve injury—but risk may rise even further with aging and longer duration of diabetes.[1,6] In the Diabetes Control and Complications Trial (DCCT) and its subsequent Epidemiology of Diabetes Interventions and Complications (EDIC) observation,[1,14] one-half of participants had subclinical evidence of neuropathy at the time of accrual, whereas after 6.5 years mean follow-up, one-half had clinical manifestations as symptoms of physical examination findings. This age and duration dependence has been corroborated in other studies such that it is generally believed that at least one-third of those 40 years or older will have clinical manifestations of neuropathy.[15] The other risk factors for neuropathy include elevated blood glucose levels, elevated triglycerides, high BMI, smoking, and hypertension.[2]

General Clinical Recommendations for Neuropathy Screening and Management in T1D

Screening for diabetic neuropathy. Screening recommendations are summarized in chapter 5. A variety of methods for screening exist, including physical examination of peripheral sensation, such as pinprick sensation, vibration perception (using a 128 Hz tuning fork), the later-stage motor involvement by ankle reflexes, or use of the 10 g Semmes–Weinstein monofilament to assess a combination of pressure and light-touch sensation.[7] Additionally, composite history and physical examination scores, such as the Michigan Neuropathy Screening Instrument, the Toronto Clinical Neuropathy Score, or the Utah Early Neuropathy Scale can be used for identification.[16–18] Simplified screening can be performed rapidly and fairly reliably using the 10 g Semmes–Weinstein monofilament or the 128 Hz tuning fork.[19–23] The methods for using the monofilament or tuning fork to detect diabetic neuropathy differ from those used for the prediction of foot complications, such as ulceration or amputation in patients known to have neuropathy.[19,20,23] In individuals with significant early progressive symptoms of neuropathy, or in whom a clinical suspicion of nondiabetic neuropathy exists, additional neurologic evaluation that may require referral is indicated, such as the search for causes other than diabetes. These include such conditions as chronic inflammatory demyelinating polyneuropathy, in which prominent motor manifestations are generally seen earlier than in diabetic neuropathy, or alcohol abuse, renal failure, thyroid disease, neurotoxic medications, a familial genetic cause, and vitamin B_{12} deficiency.[4,7]

Management of diabetic neuropathy. Intensive glycemic control is effective for the primary prevention and secondary intervention of neuropathy in people with T1D;[1,24–26] in fact, the benefits of intensive insulin treatment persist for more than a decade for the primary prevention of neuropathy.[14] No other disease-modifying treatments are currently available.

Foot care for those with neuropathy—for example, an annual comprehensive foot exam and general foot self-care education—is critical to prevent ulcers and nonhealing wounds; >60% of nontraumatic lower limb amputations occur in people with diabetes.[27] Although amputation and foot ulceration are common and major causes of morbidity and disability in people with diabetes, early recognition and management of risk factors can prevent or delay adverse outcomes.[7,9,10,13]

Multiple treatments are available for the management of neuropathic pain. Detailed evidence-based guidelines on the treatment of painful diabetic neuropathy have been demonstrated in systematic review,[28] and several drugs have been approved by the U.S. Food and Drug Administration (FDA) for the management of painful peripheral neuropathies.[7] The majority of evidence, however, does not arise from studies specific to patients with T1D. An important observation is that few patients have complete relief of painful symptoms with any treatment and that a 30–50% reduction in baseline pain is considered to be a clinically meaningful response in these trials. There are insufficient comparative studies to recommend which oral medication should be used first, although most practitioners advise against the use of opioids for painful diabetic neuropathy because of the potential for dependency, tolerance, dose escalation, and diversion.[28] Anticonvulsants[29–37] and antidepressants[38–47] are most often used as first-line therapy. Opioids are effective for painful diabetic neuropathy[48–52] and are used primarily when other treatments fail. Other effective therapeutic options include topical nitrate sprays,[53,54] topical capsaicin,[55–58] and the possible use of transcutaneous electrical nerve stimulation.[59,60] Effective treatment with capsaicin involves short-term pain that limits its acceptability and generalizability in clinical practice. The surgical release of distal lower limb nerves is not recommended because of lack of evidence supporting efficacy.[61]

Although subclinical autonomic neuropathic manifestations are common, symptomatic involvement is less frequent. The diagnosis of symptomatic autonomic neuropathy is based on the exclusion of specific cardiovascular, gastrointestinal, or genitourinary manifestations through an assessment by a specialist in the affected system. Dietary changes and prokinetic agents may improve gastroparesis symptoms associated with autonomic neuropathy.[7] Men with diabetes and erectile dysfunction should be investigated for hypogonadism,[62–65] and a 5-phosphodiesterase inhibitor, if there are no contraindications to its use, should be offered as first-line therapy to eugonadal men with diabetes and erectile dysfunction in either an on-demand[66–71] or scheduled-use[71,72] dosing regimen. Referral to a specialist should be considered for eugonadal men who do not respond to 5-phosphodiesterase inhibitors or for whom their use is contraindicated, or if ejaculatory dysfunction is present and fertility is desired.

Fundamental Future Research Needs for Diabetic Neuropathy

The need for clinical biomarkers of diabetic neuropathy. The fundamental shortfall in the area of diabetic neuropathy is the lack of an early objective clinical biomarker that overcomes issues inherent in the physical examination tests and the composite scores—in that they require subjective patient feedback, have limitations in reproducibility, and do not track changes in nerve integrity over time.[73] Consequently, the underdiagnosis of diabetic neuropathy that arises from these limitations further impedes the benefits of early identification, the emphasis on early management, and the prevention of neuropathy-related sequelae. Recommendations for screening—such as examination with the monofilament or vibration tuning fork—are not being systematically performed, which highlights the urgent need for a valid screening test in clinical practice that overcomes the limitations in their specificity as predictive markers for the future onset of neuropathy.[74] Rather than designing diagnostic studies intended to identify those with established diabetic neuropathy, we need studies that assess those without neuropathy to determine the biomarkers that predict its future onset, such as has been pursued with the monofilament examination.[20,23] Furthermore, the lack of such an early reliable clinical biomarker has truly hindered clinical research into the therapies for the prevention and treatment of diabetic neuropathy.

In view of the prevailing concept of the natural history of diabetic neuropathy—that the initiating injury to the peripheral nervous system occurs in the small, unmyelinated, and thinly myelinated Aδ and C-type nerve fibres[75,76]—there is an urgent research need to identify the most objective (morphological) small-fiber measures. Current candidate tests include examination of intraepidermal nerve fibers in skin biopsy samples or, as a noninvasive alternative, the small nerve fibers in the sub-basal nerve plexus adjacent to Bowman's layer of the cornea that can be directly visualized reliably and noninvasively by a technique of in vivo corneal confocal microscopy.[77–80] If shown to be efficacious, examination to identify those patients at risk of diabetic neuropathy could be harmonized with the annual eye specialist visits by the addition of a corneal confocal microscopy examination at the time of retinopathy screening.

The need to use novel biomarkers of early neuropathy (small-fiber morphology) in clinical trials of novel disease modifying therapies. Determination and testing of novel disease-modifying therapies is critical in light of the existing evidence that limits the clinician to intensification of glycemic control. Agents that have in the past decades failed in the clinical trials of diabetic neuropathy may have been limited by the design of those trials and the biomarkers used to assess the change in nerve integrity. At present, there is a major clinical trial focus on examining newer aldose-reductase-inhibitor agents, development of agents designed to counteract oxidative and nitrosative stress, and investigation of gene therapies that provide various forms of nerve growth factors.[81–83]

The need for better guidance on the treatment of painful diabetic neuropathy. For the management of painful neuropathy, there is a major need to *1)* determine the chronic effects and appropriate duration of drug therapies as existing studies are short term; *2)* determine the relative efficacy of agents through comparative studies and combination studies; *3)* standardize the measures of pain, physical function, and quality of life in clinical trials; and *4)* in view of the major public health burden of diabetic painful neuropathy, the determination of cost effectiveness of therapies is particularly essential.

The need for better guidance on wound-healing therapies in advanced diabetic neuropathy. For the management of late-stage diabetic neuropathy sequelae, such as therapy for diabetic foot ulcers, although the provision of a moist wound environment, debridement of nonviable tissue (nonischemic wounds), and offloading of pressure areas are evidence-based principles,[84] there is an urgent need to determine the role of specific dressing type or to support the routine use of adjunctive wound-healing therapies. Evaluation of such therapies include topical growth factors, granulocyte-colony stimulating factors, dermal substitutes, or hyperbaric oxygen therapy.[85–87]

NEPHROPATHY

Background

Chronic kidney disease (CKD) in diabetes—defined as abnormality in the urinary excretion of albumin or impairment in the level of glomerular filtration—is associated with significant reductions in both length and quality of life, and unfortunately, the lifetime risk of such diabetic nephropathy approaches 50%.[88] Diabetic nephropathy (in T1D and type 2 diabetes [T2D]) is the single leading cause of end-stage renal disease (ESRD).[7] Although progress has been made in slowing the progression of CKD to ESRD, the prevalence of CKD as a whole is rising.[89–91] In T1D, there is evidence that onset of ESRD has been shifted to older ages, which implies that glycemic intervention in itself is insufficient to curtail lifetime risk.[92,93] A variety of forms of kidney disease can be seen in people with diabetes, including diabetic nephropathy, ischemic damage related to vascular disease, and hypertension, as well as other renal diseases that are unrelated to diabetes.[94,95] Diabetic nephropathy has classically been described as a progressive increase in the level of urinary protein excretion in those with longstanding diabetes, followed by declining renal function that eventually can lead to ESRD.[88,96,97] Although the fundamental risk factor for developing nephropathy is greater glycemic exposure, long diabetes duration, hypertension, obesity, and cigarette smoking are important cofactors that exaggerate the effects of hyperglycemia.[1,98]

Although hyperfiltration has been described as a classical early manifestation of diabetic nephropathy, where the glomerular filtration rate is significantly higher than normal, its identification is not clinically useful because it is difficult to determine from standard clinical tests. Persistent albuminuria (abnormal levels of urinary albumin excretion) is considered to be the earliest clinical sign of diabetic nephropathy. Microalbuminuria, defined as low levels of albuminuria, has become the primary predictive marker of risk for eventual ESRD, as it was found in small studies to be associated with extraordinary risk of progression to high levels, termed "macroalbuminuria" and frequently referred to as "protein-uria."[99–103] Together with reports in cross-sectional clinical studies of association between renal function impairment with macroalbuminuria, observational studies gave plausibility to a simple model of diabetic nephropathy composed of three sequential stages. Microalbuminuria heralds macroalbuminuria, which after long-term exposure is associated with impaired renal function and leads to ESRD.[104] This model has become the paradigm for research on diabetic nephropathy and for the development of its preventive and therapeutic protocols.[105] Despite this prevailing model for diabetic nephropathy, the rate of progression of each of albuminuria and glomerular filtration rate (GFR) loss can vary between individuals. Furthermore, as discerned from studies in T2D, these measures may not correlate consistently well with one another or the severity of renal disease seen by renal biopsy.[106] For example, in T1D, microalbuminuria is a dynamic phenotype that may progress and subsequently regress, the initiation of GFR loss in many may begin early, even at the onset of microalbuminuria, and many individuals may develop impaired GFR without having developed albuminuria.[107,108]

CKD in adolescence. Although microalbuminuria is detected in 12–16% of adolescents with T1D, for many, it remits to normoalbuminuria, and if persistent or progressive, it generally does not lead to impaired renal function in childhood or adolescence.[109] In the 195 adolescents ages 13–17 years recruited into the DCCT, intensive therapy reduced the risk and progression of microalbuminuria by 54%. The difference in A1C was 8.1 vs. 9.8%. The benefits of intensive therapy persisted in the former adolescent cohort during the EDIC study; the intensively managed group had 48% less microalbuminuria and 85% less albuminuria.[110]

The prevalence of microalbuminuria is substantial in adolescence, although it is frequently transient and, when persistent, may remit to normoalbuminuria with time and without specific intervention.[111] Although renoprotection with agents that inhibit the renin-angiotensin-aldosterone system (RAAS) to prevent long-term complications is justified,[112] microalbuminuria is rarely treated with such agents before the age of 18 years. Rates of reversion of albumin excretion to normal at the end of puberty approach 50%, with only a smaller proportion (in the range of 15%) of patients progressing to macroalbuminura.[109] Risk for microalbuminuria can be predicted by higher levels of albumin excretion (although still within the normal range) as early as 1 year from diagnosis.[113] Moreover, normal-range albuminuria may not exclude risk of the loss of renal function in children with diabetes.[114]

CKD in adults. Adults with T1D and with microalbuminuria increasingly are being treated with angiotensin-converting-enzyme (ACE) inhibitors or angiotensin receptor blockers (ARBs), drugs that are known to reduce the risk of progression of microalbuminuria to macroalbuminuria.[109] In subjects with macroalbuminuria and impaired renal function, these drugs are known to reduce the risk of progressive renal function loss.[115] Despite significant improvements in the treatment of hyperglycemia and the development of new renal protective protocols, patients with T1D are still at high risk for progressive diabetic nephropathy and premature mortality.[93,116–118]

General Clinical Recommendations for Nephropathy Screening and Management in T1D

Screening and monitoring for diabetic nephropathy. Screening recommendations are briefly summarized in chapter 5. ADA guidelines[7] call for an annual test to assess albuminuria in T1D patients beginning 5 years after diagnosis, and measurement of serum creatinine at least annually in all adults with diabetes regardless of the degree of urine albumin excretion. For albuminuria, the test of choice is the random urine albumin-to-creatinine ratio (urinary ACR) as the 24-h collection—although considered a technical gold standard—is difficult to implement and subject to collection errors.[119–123] Owing to short-term variability and confounding factors, a diagnosis of albuminuria requires two out of three abnormal urine samples performed at approximately monthly intervals after an abnormal annual screen.[119–123] Furthermore, a finding of microalbuminuria requires urinalysis and urine microscopy to identify cellular or hemegranular casts that could indicate a cause of renal disease other than diabetes. Patients with microalbuminuria who progress to macroalbuminuria generally are considered to be at the highest risk for subsequent progression to ESRD, although many lose renal function without the development of macroalbuminuria.[108,124] Despite some problems with accuracy, serum creatinine should be used to calculate the estimated glomerular filtration rate (eGFR) and stage the level of CKD, if albuminuria is present, according to common GFR estimating equations, such as the four-variable modification of diet in renal disease (MDRD) equation.[120] CKD stage 1 is defined as a normal or increased GFR in the setting of albuminuria. Stage 2 is defined as having a mildly decreased GFR (60–89 mL/min/1.73m^2), and stage 3 is defined as a moderately decreased GFR (30–59 mL/min/1.73m^2).[117] The last two CKD stages are defined as a severely decreased GFR (15–29 mL/min/1.73m^2) or kidney failure as defined by GFR <15 or on dialysis. When eGFR is <60 ml/min/1.73m^2, potential complications of CKD should be evaluated and managed.[7] A diagnosis of CKD should be made in patients with a random urine albumin-to-creatinine concentration ratio >30 mg/g (or approximately >2.0 mg/mmol, both approximately equivalent to a 24-h urine collection demonstrating 30 mg/day or more of urinary albumin) on at least two out of three samples over a 3-month period or the presence of eGFR <60 mL/min/1.73m^2.

Consideration of an alternate cause of renal CKD should be considered particularly in the setting of extreme macroalbuminuria, persistent hematuria, or an active urinary sediment, a rapidly falling eGFR, impaired eGFR with little or no albuminuria, known duration of diabetes <5 years, lack of evidence of other complications, and a family history of nondiabetic renal disease.[125–128]

Management of Diabetic Nephropathy

Excellent control of blood pressure—through the use of ACE inhibitors or ARBs—and glycemia should be achieved in people with diabetes and normal urinary albumin excretion to prevent or delay the development of diabetic nephropathy and the long-term risk of impaired renal function.[88,94–96,129–134] In patients with CKD, cardiovascular events and progression to ESRD occur at unacceptably high rates, even with proven medical management.[7,115,135,136] Consequently, all patients with diabetes and CKD should receive a comprehensive, multifaceted approach to reduce cardiovascular risk based on the results of trials in patients with T2D.[102] Adults with diabetes and CKD with either hypertension or albuminuria should receive an ACE inhibitor or an ARB to delay progression of CKD.[105,115,137–141] The safe use of RAAS inhibitors warrants that people with diabetes on an ACE inhibitor or an ARB should have their serum creatinine and potassium levels checked within 1–2 weeks of initiation or titration of therapy, and during times of acute illness.[142,143] Patients must be educated about the fact that these medications may need to be held during times of acute illness, and women should be counseled to avoid pregnancy when receiving this therapy because use of medications that disrupt the RAAS has been associated with adverse fetal outcomes. Furthermore, oral antihyperglycemic and other medications may need to be discontinued or undergo dose adjustment in the setting of impaired GFR. Alternative drugs (e.g., diuretics, calcium channel blockers, β-blockers) also can be used to further lower blood pressure as needed or as an option for those who cannot tolerate RAAS inhibitors. Finally, from data in the T2D population, the use of a dual blockade of the RAAS achieved by combining an ACE inhibitor and an angiotensin-receptor antagonist, or by combining a direct renin inhibitor with either an ACE inhibitor or an angiotensin receptor antagonist should not be done as part of the routine management of patients with diabetes and CKD.[144,145] Referral to a nephrologist or internist with expertise in CKD should be considered in the setting of a suspected nondiabetic cause. Furthermore, this should be considered in the following cases: a chronic, progressive loss of kidney function; ACR persistently >60 mg/mmol (approximately equivalent to a 24-h urine collection demonstrating 1,000 mg/day or more or urinary albumin); eGFR <30 mL/min/1.73m^2; patient unable to remain on renal-protective therapies because of adverse effects, such as hyperkalemia or a >30% increase in serum creatinine within 3 months of starting an ACE inhibitor or ARB; or patient unable to achieve target blood pressure.

Fundamental Future Research Needs

The need for better predictive biomarkers of nephropathy onset and progression. As for diabetic neuropathy, a major gap in the management of diabetic neuropathy is the performance of existing clinical biomarkers. Although the discovery of microalbuminuria permitted the design of clinical trials and the discovery of RAAS inhibition as an important intervention for decreasing urinary albumin excretion, the predictive value of microalbuminuria on its own is poor (only one-third of patients with microalbuminuria subsequently lose renal function), and there is evidence that albuminuria may not represent the clinically relevant aspects of nephropathy. For example, RAAS inhibition does not consistently prevent progression to microalbuminuria or substantially affect the development of renal morphological lesions in those with normoalbuminuria and normotension.[146] Population data do not appear to show a decrease in the incidence of advanced kidney disease in T1D over the time period that RAAS inhibition became the standard of care,[93] and intensification of therapy to profoundly suppress albuminuria with dual RAAS blockade has not been shown to systematically decrease renal outcomes— and may even increase clinically important outcomes—in patients with T2D.[147] Furthermore, that microalbuminuria represents a dynamic functional abnormality that in the majority of T1D patients it remits to normoalbuminuria makes this a nonspecific marker of long-term impairment in renal function.[107,108,112,148–151] A promising approach that could ultimately serve as a clinical biomarker or lead to the development of valid biomarkers is the determination of "early GFR loss." As opposed to identifying impairment in GFR, when function is already reduced and the opportunity for prevention has passed, early GFR loss refers to the systematic downward trend (or slope) in GFR that occurs when renal function is still in the normal range. Creatinine-based estimates do not perform well to identify early GFR loss—rather, their performance is optimized for identifying those with stage 3 CKD (GFR <60 ml/min/1.73m^2). In observational study, the longitudinal course of GFR estimated by serum cystatin C, an endogenous marker of renal function that is better able than serum creatinine to detect changes in renal function within the normal range, leads to the finding that one-third of individuals with microalbuminuria initiate a process of renal function decline even as early as at the time of onset of microalbuminuria.[108,150,152–154] As such, sequential measurement of serum cystatin C in those with new-onset microalbuminuria potentially could identify the subset of patients who will have progressive renal function loss to ESRD. Alternatively, research could focus on the systemic and urinary factors—measured at one point in time—that are associated with early GFR loss. Unlike albuminuria, whose risk is strongly associated with glycemic exposure, the association of early GFR loss with glycemia is weak, whereas there is a strong relationship with levels of serum uric acid and markers of chronic inflammation such as soluble tumor necrosis factor (TNF) receptors. For example, a single determination of serum TNF receptor-α 1 or 2 is a strong predictor of the subsequent 12-year risk of early GFR loss and of stage 3 CKD, independent of albuminuria or of GFR. There is an urgent need to determine the role of such biomarkers—both systemic and urinary—for risk prediction of diabetic neuropathy, its progression, or as targets for therapy using uric acid lowering therapies, such as allopurinol or febuxostat, or anti-TNF monoclonal antibody therapies to prevent ESRD.[155–159] To improve risk prediction and elucidate new therapies to prevent ESRD, a major research need is to identify other biomarkers specific to early GFR loss, determine their potential applicability to clinical practice and clinical research, and also to determine their mechanistic roles that are specific to the initiation of GFR loss as opposed to those mechanisms that are specific to albuminuria. Subjects with levels of TNFR-1, for example, in the high-risk range for ESRD could be targeted in clinical trials for new interventions that despite additional costs, risks, and clinical complexity may be warranted in light of exaggerated ESRD risk.

The need to determine whether the profound efficacy of glycemic control observed for primary prevention could apply to secondary and tertiary ESRD prevention. Although it has been clarified through the DCCT/EDIC studies that glycemic interventions are effective for primary prevention of GFR loss in patients with normoalbuminuria, where one anticipates 5–10% long-term risk of GFR loss,[134,153] it has not been determined whether they will be equally effective at all stages, such as in micro- and macroalbuminuria, where such risk approximates 30 and 50%, respectively.[108,153] *Primary prevention* of GFR loss is defined as the maintenance of GFR in individuals with normoalbuminuria, whereas *secondary prevention of early GFR* loss is the maintenance of GFR in individuals who have declared risk of nephropathy according to the new onset of albuminuria. Finally, *tertiary prevention of late GFR* loss is defined as the maintenance of GFR—or perhaps its improvement—in individuals with advanced renal function impairment, defined by stage 3 CKD or worse. The absence of these systematic secondary and tertiary prevention clinical trials for prevention or reversal of GFR loss represents a major research gap. Design of these trials—as discussed—depends first on the development of novel, valid predictive biomarkers to target the individuals at highest risk for ESRD. Second, these trials must test both existing conventional strategies for A1C reduction such as insulin pump therapy and sensor-augmented pump therapy as well as more aggressive strategies, such as islet and whole-pancreas transplantation in which earlier interventions appear to be warranted.[160–162] Third, these studies will need to be long term—in the range of 5–10 years—and will need to determine the dynamic changes in GFR using sequential measures of the direct measures of GFR as well as to evaluate indirect measures that are more accurate in the normal and elevated renal function ranges, such as the use of serum cystatin C. The focus on renal function—the most clinically relevant end point proximal to ESRD—rather than the focus on urinary albumin excretion as the traditional renal end point of the past two decades is unquestionably of paramount importance.

The need to determine the efficacy of RAAS inhibition on long-term renal function outcomes, as opposed to its effect on albuminuria. The existing evidence for RAAS inhibition should be revisited in light of the evidence demonstrating divergence between albuminuria and renal function and concerns about effectiveness (the real-world benefit as opposed to efficacy in clinical trials). In view of the fact that the design of the DCCT/EDIC study required 16 years of follow-up to demonstrate the efficacy of 6.5 years of intensive glycemic control on the development of stage 3 CKD, these long-term clinical trials that evaluate the effect of RAAS inhibition on renal function will likely need to implement proxies, such as serum cystatin C or its biomarkers, to determine early GFR loss. Finally, in view of the risk of increased renal failure associated with high-dose or combination strategies using RAAS inhibition in T2D, aggressive RAAS inhibition strategies should be sufficiently studied in the setting of randomized controlled trials to determine safety and efficacy in T1D patients before such interventions become more common in clinical practice.

RETINOPATHY

Background

Although many classifications exist for the term diabetic retinopathy based on its forms and severity, it can be considered to encompass three distinct forms of disease: the spectrum of proliferative or nonproliferative diabetic retinopathy, macular edema, and retinal capillary closure.[163] The early spectrum of progressive development of morphological changes in the macula and posterior retina referred to as nonproliferative retinopathy includes microvascular abnormalities—such as microaneurysms, occlusions, and dilated and tortuous vessels—as well as retinal nerve fiber layer infarcts termed cotton-wool spots, intraretinal hemorrhage, and hard exudates. The advanced spectrum of proliferative diabetic retinopathy is marked by the presence of neovascularization of disc and retinal vessels, which can be complicated by preretinal and vitreous hemorrhage, fibrosis, and traction retinal detachment. Visual loss in this form of retinopathy may occur because of acute bleeding from these abnormal vessels into the vitreous, although the spontaneous resorption of this blood can fortunately lead to regain of vision. The permanent loss of vision may occur because of retinal detachment or macular ischemia. Regardless of stage in proliferative or nonproliferative retinopathy, visual loss can occur through the development of a distinct form of retinopathy termed diabetic macular edema (DME), a classification that includes diffuse or focal vascular leakage at the macula. It is termed clinically significant macular edema (CSME) if it is subjectively close to the fovea, the center of the macula responsible for high-acuity vision.[164] Finally, retinal capillary closure is a form of vascular change detected on fluorescein angiography that carries substantial risk of vision loss, but unlike the other two forms, it currently has no treatment options. Additionally, glaucoma, cataracts, and other disorders of the eye also occur earlier and more frequently than they do in the nondiabetic population.[7]

Together, the forms of damage referred to as diabetic retinopathy are the most common causes of new cases of legal blindness.[165] Population-based data have estimated a crude prevalence rate of retinopathy in the adult diabetic population of the U.S. in the range of 30–40%, for which the nonproliferative form is the most common.[166,167] For example, one-half of patients with T1D develop nonproliferative retinopathy after 7 years of duration, whereas the majority have at least one form of retinopathy after 20 years.[163] Sight-threatening forms of retinopathy (such as complicated proliferative retinopathy or macular edema) likely occur in ~5–8% of T1D patients.[15,163,165,167] For the more advanced and clinically meaningful stage of proliferative diabetic retinopathy, prevalence has been estimated to be ~25% in people T1D.[168] Macular edema in T1D has an estimated prevalence of ~10%.[169] Visual loss from any of the forms of diabetic retinopathy is associated with significant morbidity, including increased falls, hip fracture, and a fourfold increase in mortality.[170] In context, among individuals with T1D, limb amputation and visual loss because of diabetic retinopathy are the two strongest independent predictors of early death.[171]

Pediatrics

Traditionally, diabetic retinopathy has been thought to rarely develop in children with T1D <10 years of age regardless of the duration of diabetes.[172] Perhaps because of limitations in contemporary intensive glycemic management, however, diabetic retinopathy has its onset in a small subset of adolescents with T1D that may have a prevalence as high as 7%, even within 2–5 years of diabetes duration,[173] although it is almost uniformly characterized by non–sight-threatening disease during adolescence.[172,174] The prevalence rate increases sharply after 5 years' duration of diabetes in postpubertal children and young adults with T1D.[172,175–177] More recently, progression rates of diabetic retinopathy were prospectively evaluated.[178–180] In a mixed cohort of T1D and T2D, those with no diabetic retinopathy, background retinopathy, or mild preproliferative retinopathy had short-term (1-year) cumulative incidence of sight-threatening forms of retinopathy of 0.3%, 3.6%, and 13.5%, respectively.[178] Although the incidence of sight-threatening diabetic retinopathy in the group without baseline diabetic retinopathy was low, there have been no studies comparing various screening intervals in their effectiveness to reduce the risk of vision loss.[178–182]

Risk Factors

Risk factors for the onset and prevalence of CSME and nonproliferative or proliferative diabetic retinopathy include diabetes duration, presence of nephropathy, pregnancy, chronic hyperglycemia, hypertension, and dyslipidemia— and, to a lesser extent, a high BMI, a low level of physical activity, and insulin resistance.[7,12,183–186] Although the glycated hemoglobin level is fundamentally the strongest risk factor for predicting the development and progression of diabetic retinopathy, the disease appears to have a complex multifactorial pathogenesis.[187] For example, associations have been observed with sleep apnea,[188] nonalcoholic fatty liver disease,[189] and serum prolactin, adiponectin, and homocysteine levels.[183,190–192] Recent data have also identified an association between vitamin D deficiency and retinopathy in children and adolescents with T1D.[193] Genetic factors include mutations in the erythropoietin gene promoter,[193] and a relation between accelerated retinopathy and hereditary deficiency of a key regulatory enzyme in glucose metabolism, glucose-6-phosphate dehydrogenase (G6PD).[194]

General Clinical Recommendations for Retinopathy Screening and Management in T1D

Screening. Screening recommendations are briefly summarized in chapter 5. Because laser therapy for sight-threatening diabetic retinopathy reduces the risk of blindness,[164,174,195,196] ophthalmic screening strategies are intended primarily to detect disease treatable by this therapy. Patients with proliferative diabetic retinopathy or macular edema may be asymptomatic.[7] The goal is to detect clinically significant retinopathy before vision is threatened.[163] Screening recommendations call for annual screening and evaluation for retinopathy by an expert professional starting 5 years after the onset of diabetes.[7,163,172,175] A secondary purpose of the screening evaluation by an expert professional is to detect other common conditions, such as cataracts, glaucoma, and macular degeneration. The determination of 7-standard field, stereoscopic-color fundus photography with interpretation by a trained reader is considered the gold-standard screening examination, although direct ophthalmoscopy, indirect slit-lamp fundoscopy, or digital central fundus photography (all performed on a dilated pupil) are considered alternative screening methods when performed by eye specialists.[197] Pregnancy is a risk factor for progression of retinopathy.[163] Women with preexisting diabetes who are planning pregnancy or who have become pregnant should have a comprehensive eye examination and be counseled on the risk or development or progression of diabetic retinopathy. Eye examination should occur in the first trimester with close follow-up throughout pregnancy and for 1 year postpartum.[7]

Primary and Secondary Prevention

To prevent the onset and delay of the progression of diabetic retinopathy, people with diabetes should be treated to achieve optimal control of blood glucose[1,198] and blood pressure.[199] The DCCT demonstrated that intensive glycemic control reduced both the development and progression of retinopathy in T1D,[1,198,200] with the beneficial effects of intensive glycemic control persisting for up to 10 years after completion of the initial trials.[201,202] Although offset by long-term benefits, it is important to recognize that rapid improvement of glycemia in T1D may be associated with transient early worsening of retinopathy.[203] Blood pressure control is an important component of risk factor modification in diabetes and reduces the risk of retinopathy progression. The majority of evidence for this intervention, however, arises from studies in T2D.[199,204,205] Although a number of trials have examined the effect of RAAS inhibition on retinopathy progression or development among normotensive patients with diabetes, the results generally have been conflicting or inconclusive.[146,206,207] Although there may be justification for the use of the peroxisome-proliferator–activated receptor-α agonist fenofibrate in addition to statin therapy in patients with T2D to slow the progression of established retinopathy (although this agent is not indicated for CVD prevention or treatment), sufficient evidence to support its clinical use has not been established in T1D.[204] Furthermore, systematic review suggests that aspirin therapy neither decreases nor increases the incidence or progression of diabetic retinopathy.[208] Correspondingly, aspirin use does not appear to be associated with an increase in risk of vitreous hemorrhage or diabetic macular edema.[209,210]

Tertiary prevention of vision loss in patients with diabetic retinopathy: Laser therapy and local (intraocular) pharmacologic intervention. Patients with sight-threatening diabetic retinopathy should be assessed by a general ophthalmologist or retina specialist. Laser therapy and vitrectomy[164,195,211,212] or local intraocular pharmacologic intervention[213-217] should be considered. As determined in the Diabetic Retinopathy Study (DRS) and the Early Treatment Diabetic Retinopathy Study (ETDRS), laser therapy by panretinal photocoagulation to the retinal periphery reduces severe visual loss and reduces legal blindness by 90% in people with severe nonproliferative or proliferative retinopathy.[174,195,196] As determined by the ETDRS, focal or grid laser treatment to the macula for CSME reduces the incidence of moderate visual loss by half.[164] Long-term follow-up studies to the original laser photocoagulation trials confirm its benefit over several decades.[218] In the treatment of CSME, as defined by optical coherence tomography (OCT) or clinical examination, intraocular pharmacotherapy is an available therapeutic option. With the knowledge that the cytokine vascular endothelial growth factor (VEGF) plays a primary role in the development of DME, two anti-VEGF drugs are now widely used owing to the results of three masked phase III clinical trials that evaluated monthly Ranibizumab injection, and a humanized recombinant anti-VEGF antibody fragment, with or without prompt laser.[213,214] In these trials, use of Ranibizumab generally was associated with a twofold clinically important visual acuity gain from a comparable likelihood of 18% in the control arm over 1 or 2 years. Similar results were obtained by physician-based flexible treatment algorithms rather than a strict prescribed injection schedule.[219] Intraocular injection of Bevacizumab, a full-length antibody against VEGF, was associated with similar efficacy in comparison to macular laser therapy.[220] Unlike Ranibizumab, however, intraocular injection of Bevacizumab in diabetic retinopathy constitutes off-label use in many countries.

It is important to emphasize the controversial role of steroid administration in the treatment of DME. Intraocular injection of steroid combined with prompt macular laser was as effective as Ranibizumab in a single subgroup of patients characterized by previous cataract surgery.[219] Treatment with intraocular steroid, however, was associated with increased rates of glaucoma. Two phase III clinical trials investigating the implantation of a long-term drug delivery device containing Fluocinolone Acetonide met their primary and secondary outcomes (visual acuity and OCT), but it showed increased rates of glaucoma and cataract progression compared to sham.[215,216] The risk-to-benefit ratio was considered unacceptable and, as such, routine use is not universally recommended.[216]

Surgical intervention. The Diabetic Retinopathy Vitrectomy Study (DRVS) group evaluated the benefit of early vitrectomy in the treatment of severe vitreous hemorrhage[211] and severe proliferative diabetic retinopathy[212] for patients with persistent vitreous hemorrhage or significant vitreous scarring and debris.[217] People with T1D of <20 years' duration and severe vitreous hemorrhage were more likely to achieve good vision with early vitrectomy compared with conventional management.[211] Similarly, early vitrectomy was associated with a higher chance of visual recovery in people with either T1D or T2D with severe proliferative diabetic retinopathy.[212] Surgical advances in vitrectomy since the DRVS trials have demonstrated reduced side effects with more consistent favorable visual outcomes, thus supporting vitrectomy in advanced proliferative diabetic retinopathy.[221] Furthermore, these advances have expanded surgical indications to include vitrectomy for diffuse macular edema.[222] The use of perioperative acetylsalicylic acid (ASA)[210,223,224] and warfarin therapy[225] for those undergoing ophthalmic surgery does not appear to raise the risk of hemorrhagic complications.

Vision evaluation and rehabilitation. Visually disabled people should be referred for low-vision evaluation and rehabilitation. Despite the successes of tertiary intervention, it is important to encourage patients with even moderate visual loss to seek assistance from community services that provide spectacle correction, enhanced magnification, vision aids, and measures to encourage independence and ongoing quality of life.[226,227]

Fundamental Future Research Needs for Diabetic Retinopathy

The need to validate novel biomarkers of early retinopathy. Active research has implied that the standard measures to screen for and determine longitudinal change in the stages of diabetic retinopathy can be supplemented with extremely sensitive measures of retinal function and structure to determine the nature of the earliest stages of retinopathy.[183] For example, OCT detects thinning of the neuronal and synaptic layers, spectrophotometry can identify regional defects in mitochondrial metabolism, or electroretinography can indicate reduced cellular signal transmission.[183,228,229] Furthermore, methods have been developed to identify loss of contrast sensitivity, the presence of visual-field defects, or the morphology of vascular architecture, such as the caliber of retinal vessels or their fractal geometry.[230-232] These novel biomarkers could be used to predict subsequent microvascular lesions[233] and responses to improved metabolic control[234] and could be used to evaluate new therapies designed to target the earliest preclinical stages of diabetic retinopathy.

The need to use novel biomarkers in the evaluation of emerging therapies. Active investigation into the alternatives to photocoagulation and local (intraocular) pharmacological intervention[235] must evaluate the effect on earlier stages of diabetic retinopathy and incorporate the novel biomarkers for prediction of disease. Among the emerging therapies that require further research are the newer inhibitors of vascular endothelial growth factor, aptamer, and pegaptanib,[236] agents that may offer advantages over the existing inhibitors currently in clinical use. Inhibition of TNF-α[237] and the βIG-H3 protein,[238] targeted regulation of angiopoietin isoforms in the Ang/Tie system,[235] and therapies that modify pericyte-endothelial interaction present examples of novel targets for therapeutic intervention.[235] Recent data provide greater knowledge of the human vitreous proteome and reveal protein alterations that are possibly involved in the pathogenesis of diabetic retinopathy. Further investigation into the relationship of these proteins with established and novel biomarkers may provide new targets for prevention and treatment.[239]

The need to reconcile the efficacy of RAAS inhibition on diabetic retinopathy for primary and secondary prevention. Specifically for diabetic retinopathy, evidence does not demonstrate an unequivocal beneficial role of inhibition of the RAAS in patients with T1D who have established retinopathy, and it does not demonstrate a role in those with T2D regardless of retinopathy status. The normotensive patient with T1D and normoalbuminuria in whom retinopathy is minimal or absent, however, stands to benefit from reduction in retinopathy progression through inhibition of the RAAS. Despite this finding, there remains insufficient clinical trial evidence to recommend RAAS inhibition as primary or secondary prevention from retinopathy for all normotensive patients with diabetes.[146,203,204,240,241] For example, although the reduction in the risk of retinopathy observed in the RAAS study[146] paralleled that observed with intensive insulin therapy,[207] there is inconsistency in the literature in that the much larger Diabetic Retinopathy Candesartan Trial (DIRECT)–Prevent 1 trial of a different type of RAAS inhibitor reported a minor relative risk reduction (of borderline statistical insignificance, $P = 0.051$) for the advancement of retinal change.[206] In corresponding studies of candesartan therapy in subjects with both T1D and T2D who had retinopathy at baseline, the drug failed to mitigate retinopathy progression.[206,207] Differences in sample size and the drugs and doses administered might explain the inconsistencies among trials, which requires further work to reconcile. Finally, although preclinical studies suggest that inhibition of the renin–angiotensin system may ameliorate diabetic macular edema, a major cause of visual loss, this outcome has yet to be fully addressed.[242]

The need to reconcile the efficacy of fibrate therapy seen in T2D on diabetic retinopathy for primary and secondary prevention. Dyslipidemia is an independent risk factor for retinal hard exudates and clinically significant macular edema in T1D.[243,244] Although statin-based lipid-lowering therapies are an integral part of vascular protection in diabetes, the role of these agents in preventing the development or progression or retinopathy has not been established.[200,245] The role of the peroxisome-proliferator–activated receptor-α agonist fenofibrate has been assessed in two large-scale randomized controlled trials of patients with T2D. In the Fenofibrate Intervention and Event Lowering in Diabetes (FIELD) study, fenofibrate reduced both the requirement for laser therapy (a prespecified tertiary endpoint and mainly the result of a lower prevalence of macular edema) and retinopathy progression among patients with preexisting retinopathy.[240] In the ACCORD Eye study, the addition of fenofibrate to simvastatin was associated with a 40% reduction in the primary outcome of retinopathy progression over 4 years.[204] From the study's control and event rates, the number of patients needed to treat with combination statin and fenofibrate therapy to prevent one retinopathy progression event is estimated at 27 over the 4-year period. Thus, the addition of fenofibrate to statin therapy could be considered in patients with T2D to slow the progression of established retinopathy as an important pharmacological intervention that indicates an urgent need to determine potential efficacy in patients with T1D.

The need to establish an effective framework for clinical reporting of diabetic retinopathy. The potential future implementation into clinical practice of systemic antihypertensive and dyslipidemic therapies for the prevention of diabetic retinopathy will require a logistical framework for standardized, accurate, and timely reporting of retinal findings between eye specialists and diabetes care providers. Recommendations for such a clinical framework will require active research. For example, in the RAAS study, the majority of subjects had no evidence of retinopathy or earlier stages of nonproliferative retinopathy (corresponding to ETDRS scale values of 21 or less). This degree of detail in the quantitative reporting of diabetic retinopathy stage generally is not communicated between eye specialists in clinical practice to their diabetes care specialists. As such, generalizability of results that arise from a study such as the RAAS study would require innovations in the quantitative scoring of retinopathy as well as information sharing with those who would prescribe and monitor the safety of systemic therapies—these are not trivial tasks in clinical practice. Finally, the clinical assessment of retinopathy, such as through the fundus photography telemedicine programs that have been developed internationally for the identification and triage of patients with diabetic retinopathy, will need to be refined and harmonized with other aspects of clinical care, such as screening protocols for neuropathy, nephropathy, and CVD.[246]

REFERENCES

1. Diabetes Control and Complications Trial Research Group: The effect of intensive treatment of diabetes on the development and progression of long-term complications in insulin-dependent diabetes mellitus. *N Engl J Med* 329:977–986, 1993
2. Tesfaye S, Chaturvedi N, Eaton SE, et al.: Vascular risk factors and diabetic neuropathy. *N Engl J Med* 352:341–350, 2005
3. Vinik A, Mehrabyan A, Colen L, Boulton A: Focal entrapment neuropathies in diabetes. *Diabetes Care* 27:1783–1788, 2004
4. Tesfaye S, Boulton AJ, Dyck PJ, et al., Toronto Diabetic Neuropathy Expert Group: Diabetic neuropathies: update on definitions, diagnostic criteria, estimation of severity, and treatments. *Diabetes Care* 33:2285–2293, 2010
5. Perkins BA, Olaleye D, Bril V: Carpal tunnel syndrome in patients with diabetic polyneuropathy. *Diabetes Care* 25:565–569, 2002
6. Vinik AI, Ziegler D: Diabetic cardiovascular autonomic neuropathy. *Circulation* 115:387–397, 2007
7. American Diabetes Association: Standards of medical care in diabetes—2012. *Diabetes Care* 35(Suppl. 1):S11–S63, 2012
8. Pavy-Le Traon A, Fontaine S, Tap G, et al.: Cardiovascular autonomic neuropathy and other complications in type 1 diabetes. *Clin Auton Res* 20:153–160, 2010
9. Young MJ, Breddy JL, Veves A, et al.: The prediction of diabetic neuropathic foot ulceration using vibration perception thresholds: a prospective study. *Diabetes Care* 17:557–560, 1994
10. Reiber GE, Boyko EJ, Smith DG: Lower extremity foot ulcers and amputations in diabetes. In *Diabetes in America*. 2nd ed. Bethesda, MD, National Diabetes Data Group, National Institutes of Health, National Institute of Diabetes and Digestive and Kidney Diseases, 1995, p. 409–428
11. daCosta DiBonaventura M, Cappelleri JC, Joshi AV: A longitudinal assessment of painful diabetic peripheral neuropathy on health status, productivity, and health care utilization and cost. *Pain Med* 12:118–126, 2011
12. Dworkin RH, Malone DC, Panarites CJ, Armstrong EP, Pham SV: Impact of postherpetic neuralgia and painful diabetic peripheral neuropathy on health care costs. *J Pain* 11:360–368, 2010
13. Nelson D, Mah JK, Adams C, et al.: Comparison of conventional and noninvasive techniques for the early identification of diabetic neuropathy in children and adolescents with type 1 diabetes. *Pediatr Diabet* 7:305–310, 2006
14. Albers JW, Herman WH, Pop-Busui R, et al.: Effect of prior intensive insulin treatment during the Diabetes Control and Complications Trial (DCCT) on peripheral neuropathy in type 1 diabetes during the Epidemiology of Diabetes Interventions and Complications (EDIC) Study. *Diabetes Care* 33:1090–1096, 2010

15. Centers for Disease Control and Prevention: National Diabetes Fact Sheet: National Estimates and General Information on Diabetes and Prediabetes in the United States, 2011. Atlanta, GA, U.S. Department of Health and Human Services, Centers for Disease Control and Prevention, 2011

16. Herman WH, Pop-Busui R, Braffett BH, et al.: Use of the Michigan Neuropathy Screening Instrument as a measure of distal symmetrical peripheral neuropathy in type 1 diabetes: results from the Diabetes Control and Complications Trial/Epidemiology of Diabetes Interventions and Complications. *Diabet Med* 29:937–944, 2012

17. Bril V, Tomioka S, Buchanan RA, Perkins BA, mTCNS Study Group: Reliability and validity of the modified Toronto Clinical Neuropathy Score in diabetic sensorimotor polyneuropathy. *Diabet Med* 26:240–246, 2009

18. Singleton JR, Bixby B, Russell JW, Feldman EL, Peltier A, Goldstein J, Howard J, Smith AG: The Utah Early Neuropathy Scale: a sensitive clinical scale for early sensory predominant neuropathy. *J Peripher Nerv Syst* 13:218–227, 2008

19. Kanji JN, Anglin RE, Hunt DL, et al.: Does this patient with diabetes have large-fiber peripheral neuropathy? *JAMA* 303:1526–1532, 2010

20. Perkins BA, Olaleye D, Zinman B, et al.: Simple screening tests for peripheral neuropathy in the diabetes clinic. *Diabetes Care* 24:250–256, 2001

21. Rith-Najarian SJ, Stolusky T, Gohdes DM: Identifying diabetic patients at high risk for lower-extremity amputation in a primary health care setting: a prospective evaluation of simple screening criteria. *Diabetes Care* 15:1386–1389, 1992

22. Rahman M, Griffin SJ, Rathmann W, et al.: How should peripheral neuropathy be assessed in people with diabetes in primary care? A population-based comparison of four measures. *Diabet Med* 20:368–374, 2003

23. Perkins BA, Orszag A, Olaleye D, et al.: Prediction of incident diabetic neuropathy using the monofilament exam: a 4-year prospective study. *Diabetes Care* 33:1549–1554, 2010

24. Reichard P, Berglund B, Britz A, et al.: Intensified conventional insulin treatment retards the microvascular complications of insulin-dependent diabetes mellitus (IDDM): the Stockholm Diabetes Intervention Study (SDIS) after 5 years. *J Intern Med* 230:101–108, 1991

25. Diabetes Control and Complications Trial Research Group: The effect of intensive diabetes therapy on the development and progression of neuropathy. *Ann Intern Med* 122:561–568, 1995

26. Callaghan BC, Little AA, Feldman EL, Hughes RA: Enhanced glucose control for preventing and treating diabetic neuropathy. *Cochrane Database Syst Rev* CD007543, 2012

27. NDEP, U.S. Department of Health and Human Services, National Diabetes Education Program: The facts about diabetes: a leading cause of death in the U.S. Available at http://www.ndep.nih.gov/diabetes-facts/index.aspx. Accessed 13 April 2012

28. Bril V, England J, Franklin GM, et al.: Evidence-based guideline: treatment of painful diabetic neuropathy: report of the American Academy of Neurology, the American Association of Neuromuscular and Electrodiagnostic

Medicine, and the American Academy of Physical Medicine and Rehabilitation. *Neurology* 76:1758–1765, 2011

29. McQuay H, Carroll D, Jadad AR, Wiffen P, Moore A: Anticonvulsant drugs for management of pain: a systematic review. *BMJ* 311:1047–1052, 1995

30. Backonja M, Beydoun A, Edwards KR, et al.: Gabapentin for the symptomatic treatment of painful neuropathy in patients with diabetes mellitus: a randomized controlled trial. *JAMA* 280:1831–1836, 1998

31. Richter RW, Portenoy R, Sharma U, et al.: Relief of painful diabetic peripheral neuropathy with pregabalin: a randomized, placebo-controlled trial. *J Pain* 6:253–260, 2005

32. Lesser H, Sharma U, LaMoreaux L, et al.: Pregabalin relieves symptoms of painful diabetic neuropathy: a randomized controlled trial. *Neurology* 63:2104–2110, 2004

33. Rosenstock J, Tuchman M, LaMoreau L, et al.: Pregabalin for the treatment of painful diabetic peripheral neuropathy: a double-blind, placebo-controlled trial. *Pain* 110:628–638, 2004

34. Kochar DK, Jain N, Agarwal RP, et al.: Sodium valproate in the management of painful neuroapthy in type 2 diabetes: a randomized placebo controlled study. *Acta Neurol Scand* 106:248–252, 2002

35. Kochar DK, Rawat N, Agrawal RP, et al.: Sodium valproate for painful diabetic neuropathy: a randomized double-blind placebo-controlled study. *QJM* 97:33–38, 2004

36. Guan Y, Ding X, Cheng Y, et al.: Efficacy of pregabalin for peripheral neuropathic pain: results of an 8-week, flexible-dose, double-blind, placebo-controlled study conducted in China. *Clin Ther* 33:159–166, 2011

37. Satoh J, Yagihashi S, Baba M, et al.: Efficacy and safety of pregabalin for treating neuropathic pain associated with diabetic peripheral neuropathy: a 14 week, randomized, double-blind, placebo-controlled trial. *Diabet Med* 28:109–116, 2011

38. Max MB, Culnane M, Schafer SC, et al.: Amitriptyline relieves diabetic neuropathy pain in patients with normal or depressed mood. *Neurology* 37:589–596, 1987

39. Max MB, Lynch SA, Muir J, et al.: Effects of desipramine, amitriptyline, and fluoxetine on pain in diabetic neuropathy. *N Engl J Med* 326:1250–1256, 1992

40. Goldstein DJ, Lu Y, Detke MJ, et al.: Duloxetine vs. placebo in patients with painful diabetic neuropathy. *Pain* 116:109–118, 2005

41. Raskin J, Smith TR, Wong K, et al.: Duloxetine versus routine care in the long-term management of diabetic peripheral neuropathic pain. *J Palliat Med* 9:29–40, 2006

42. Raskin J, Wang F, Pritchett YL, et al.: A double-blind, randomized multicenter trial comparing duloxetine with placebo in the management of diabetic peripheral neuropathic pain. *Pain Med* 6:346–356, 2005

43. Wernicke JF, Pritchett YL, D'Souza DN, et al.: A randomized controlled trial of duloxetine in diabetic peripheral neuropathic pain. *Neurology* 67:1411–1420, 2006

452 *ADA/JDRF Type 1 Diabetes Sourcebook*

44. Rowbotham MC, Goli V, Kunz NR, et al.: Venlafaxine extended release in the treatment of painful diabetic neuropathy: a double-blind, placebo-controlled study. *Pain* 110:697–706, 2004
45. Kadiroglu AK, Sit D, Kayabasi H, et al.: The effect of venlafaxine HCl on painful peripheral diabetic neuropathy in patients with type 2 diabetes mellitus. *J Diabetes Complications* 22:241–245, 2008
46. Kaur H, Hota D, Bhansali A, et al.: A comparative evaluation of amitriptyline and duloxetine in painful diabetic neuropathy, a randomized, double-blind, cross-over clinical trial. *Diabetes Care* 34:818–822, 2011
47. Yasuda H, Hotta N, Nakao K, et al.: Superiority of duloxetine to placebo in improving diabetic neuropathic pain: results of a randomized controlled trial in Japan. *J Diab Inv* 2:132–139, 2011
48. Sang CN, Booher S, Gilron I, et al.: Dextromethorphan and memantine in painful diabetic neuropathy and postherpetic neuralgia: efficacy and dose-response trials. *Anesthesiology* 96:1053–1061, 2002
49. Nelson KA, Park KM, Robinovitz E, et al.: High-dose oral dextromethorphan versus placebo in painful diabetic neruopathy and postherpetic neuralgia. *Neurology* 48:1212–1218, 1997
50. Gimbel JS, Richards P, Portenoy RK: Controlled-release oxycodone for pain in diabetic neuropathy: a randomized controlled trial. *Neurology* 60:927–934, 2003
51. Harati Y, Gooch C, Swenson M, et al.: Double-blind randomized trial of tramadol for the treatment of the pain of diabetic neuropathy. *Neurology* 50:1842–1846, 1998
52. Schwartz S, Etropolski M, Shapiro DY, et al.: Safety and efficacy of tapentadol ER in patients with painful diabetic peripheral neuropathy: results of a randomized-withdrawal, placebo-controlled trial. *CMRO* 27:151–162, 2011
53. Yuen KC, Baker NR, Rayman G: Treatment of chronic painful diabetic neuropathy with isosorbidedinitrate spray: a double-blind placebo-controlled cross-over study. *Diabetes Care* 25:1699–1703, 2002
54. Agrawal RP, Choudhary R, Sharma P, et al.: Glyceryltrinitrate spray in the management of painful diabetic neuropathy: a randomized double blind placebo controlled cross-over study. *Diabetes Res Clin Pract* 77:161–167, 2007
55. Low PA, Opfer-Gehrking TL, Dyck PJ, et al.: Double-blind, placebo-controlled study of the application of capsaicin cream in chronic distal painful polyneuropathy. *Pain* 62:163–168, 1995
56. Capsaicin Study Group: Treatment of painful diabetic neuropathy with topical capsaicin: a multicenter, double-blind, vehicle-controlled study. *Arch Intern Med* 151:2225–2229, 1991
57. Tandan R, Lewis GA, Krusinski PB, et al.: Topical capsaicin in painful diabetic neuropathy: controlled study with long-term follow-up. *Diabetes Care* 15:8–14, 1992
58. Agrawal RP, Goswami J, Jain S, et al.: Management of diabetic neuropathy by sodium valproate and glyceryltrinitrate spray: a prospective double-blind randomized placebo-controlled study. *Diabetes Res Clin Pract* 83:371–378, 2009
59. Kumar D, Alvaro MS, Julka IS, et al.: Diabetic peripheral neuropathy: effectiveness of electrotherapy and amitriptyline for symptomatic relief. *Diabetes Care* 21:1322–1325, 1998

60. Bosi E, Conti M, Vermigli C, et al.: Effectiveness of frequency-modulated electromagnetic neural stimulation in the treatment of painful diabetic neuropathy. *Diabetologia* 48:817–823, 2005
61. Chaudhry V, Stevens JC, Kincaid J, et al.: Practice advisory: utility of surgical decompression for treatment of diabetic neuropathy: report of the Therapeutics and Technology Assessment Subcommittee of the American Academy of Neurology. *Neurology* 66:1805–1808, 2006
62. Alexopoulou O, Jamart J, Maiter D, Hermans MP, De Hertogh R, De Nayer P, Buysschaert M: Erectile dysfunction and lower androgenicity in type 1 diabetic patients. *Diabetes Metab* 27:329–336, 2001
63. Dhindsa S, Prabhakar S, Sethi M, Bandyopadhyay A, Chaudhuri A, Dandona P: Frequent occurrence of hypogonadotropic hypogonadism in type 2 diabetes. *J Clin Endocrinol Metab* 89:5462–5468, 2004
64. Boyanov MA, Boneva Z, Christov VG: Testosterone supplementation in men with type 2 diabetes, visceral obesity and partial androgen deficiency. *Aging Male* 6:1–7, 2003
65. Shabsigh R, Kaufman JM, Steidle C, Padma-Nathan H: Randomized study of testosterone gel as adjunctive therapy to sildenafil in hypogonadal men with erectile dysfunction who do not respond to sildenafil alone. *J Urol* 172:658–663, 2004
66. Fonseca V, Seftel A, Denne J, Fredlund P: Impact of diabetes mellitus on the severity of erectile dysfunction and response to treatment: analysis of data from tadalafil clinical trials. *Diabetologia* 47:1914–1923, 2004
67. Rendell MS, Rajfer J, Wicker PA, et al.: Sildenafil for treatment of erectile dysfunction in men with diabetes: a randomized controlled trial. *JAMA* 281:421–426, 1999
68. Boulton AJ, Selam JL, Sweeney M, Ziegler D: Sildenafil citrate for the treatment of erectile dysfunction in men with type II diabetes mellitus. *Diabetologia* 44:1296–1301, 2001
69. Goldstein I, Young JM, Fischer J, Bangerter K, Segerson T, Taylor T, Vardenafil Diabetes Study Group: Vardenafil, a new phosphodiesterase type 5 inhibitor, in the treatment of erectile dysfunction in men with diabetes: a multicenter double-blind placebo-controlled fixed-dose study. *Diabetes Care* 26:777–783, 2003
70. Monsod TP, Flanagan DE, Rife F, Saenz R, Caprio S, Sherwin RS, Tamborlane WV: Do sensor glucose levels accurately predict plasma glucose concentrations during hypoglycemia and hyperinsulinemia? *Diabetes Care* 25:889–893, 2002
71. Hatzichristou D, Gambla M, Rubio-Aurioles E, Buvat J, Brock GB, Spera G, Rose L, Lording D, Liang S: Efficacy of tadalafil once daily in men with diabetes mellitus and erectile dysfunction. *Diabet Med* 25:138–146, 2008
72. Buvat J, van Ahlen H, Schmitt H, Chan M, Kuepfer C, Varanese L: Efficacy and safety of two dosing regimens of tadalafil and patterns of sexual activity in men with diabetes mellitus and erectile dysfunction: Scheduled use vs. on-demand regimen evaluation (SURE) study in 14 European countries. *J Sex Med* 3:512–520, 2006

73. Ziegler D, Luft D: Clinical trials for drugs against diabetic neuropathy: can we combine scientific needs with clinical practicalities? *Int Rev Neurobiol* 50:431–463, 2002

74. Harris SB, Worall G, Macaulay A, Norton P, Webster-Bogaert S, Donner A, Murray A, Stewart M: Diabetes management in Canada: baseline results of the Group Practice Diabetes Management Study. *Can J Diabetes* 30:131–137, 2006

75. Smith AG, Singleton JR: Impaired glucose tolerance and neuropathy. *Neurologist* 14:23–29, 2008

76. Sumner CJ, Sheth S, Griffin JW, Cornblath DR, Polydefkis M: The spectrum of neuropathy in diabetes and impaired glucose tolerance. *Neurology* 60:108–111, 2003

77. England JD, Gronseth GS, Franklin G, Carter GT, Kinsella LJ, Cohen JA, Asbury AK, Szigeti K, Lupski JR, Latov N, Lewis RA, Low PA, Fisher MA, Herrmann DN, Howard JF Jr, Lauria G, Miller RG, Polydefkis M, Sumner AJ, American Academy of Neurology: Practice parameter: evaluation of distal symmetric polyneuropathy: role of autonomic testing, nerve biopsy, and skin biopsy (an evidence-based review): report of the American Academy of Neurology, American Association of Neuromuscular and Electrodiagnostic Medicine, and American Academy of Physical Medicine and Rehabilitation. *Neurology* 72:177–184, 2009

78. Malik RA, Kallinikos P, Abbott CA, van Schie CH, Morgan P, Efron N, Boulton AJ: Corneal confocal microscopy: a non-invasive surrogate of nerve fibre damage and repair in diabetic patients. *Diabetologia* 46:683–688, 2003

79. Tavakoli M, Quattrini C, Abbott C, Kallinikos P, Marshall A, Finnigan J, Morgan P, Efron N, Boulton AJ, Malik RA: Corneal confocal microscopy: a novel noninvasive test to diagnose and stratify the severity of human diabetic neuropathy. *Diabetes Care* 33:1792–1797, 2010

80. Ahmed A, Bril V, Orszag A, Paulson J, Yeung E, Ngo M, Orlov S, Perkins BA: Detection of diabetic sensorimotor polyneuropathy by corneal confocal microscopy in type 1 diabetes: a concurrent validity study. *Diabetes Care* 35:821–828, 2012. Epub 8 February 2012

81. Tahrani AA, Askwith T, Stevens MJ: Emerging drugs for diabetic neuropathy. *Expert Opin Emerg Drugs* 15:661–683, 2010

82. Salonia A, D'Addio F, Gremizzi C, et al.: Kidney-pancreas transplantation is associated with near-normal sexual function in uremic type 1 diabetic patients. *Transplantation* 92:802–808, 2011

83. Vincent AM, Callaghan BC, Smith AL, Feldman EL: Diabetic neuropathy: cellular mechanisms as therapeutic targets. *Nat Rev Neurol* 7:573–583, 2011

84. Steed DL, Donohoe D, Webster MW, Lindsley L: Effect of extensive debridement and treatment on the healing of diabetic foot ulcers: diabetic ulcer study group. *J Am Coll Surg* 183:61–64, 1996

85. Buchberger B, Follmann M, Freyer D, Huppertz H, Ehm A, Wasem J: The importance of growth factors for the treatment of chronic wounds in the case of diabetic foot ulcers. *GMS Health Technol Assess* 6:Doc12, 2010

86. Cruciani M, Lipsky BA, Mengoli C, de Lalla F: Granulocyte-colony stimulating factors as adjunctive therapy for diabetic foot infections. *Cochrane Database Syst Rev* CD006810, 2009

87. Löndahl M, Fagher K, Katzman P: What is the role of hyperbaric oxygen in the management of diabetic foot disease? *Curr Diab Rep* 11:285–293, 2011

88. Warram JH, Gearin G, Laffel L, et al.: Effect of duration of type I diabetes on the prevalence of stages of diabetic nephropathy defined by urinary albumin/creatinine ratio. *J Am Soc Nephrol* 7:930–937, 1996

89. Coresh J, Selvin E, Stevens LA, et al.: Prevalence of chronic kidney disease in the United States. *JAMA* 298:2038–2047, 2007

90. Rettig RA, Norris K, Nissenson AR: Chronic kidney disease in the United States: a public policy imperative. *Clin J Am Soc Nephrol* 3:1902–1910, 2008

91. Ruggenenti P, Remuzzi G: Kidney failure stabilizes after a two-decade increase: impact on global (renal and cardiovascular) health. *Clin J Am Soc Nephrol* 2:146–150, 2007

92. Perkins BA: Intensive therapy and GFR in type 1 diabetes. *N Engl J Med* 366:856; author reply 857–858, 2012

93. Rosolowsky ET, Skupien J, Smiles AM, et al.: Risk for ESRD in type 1 diabetes remains high despite renoprotection. *J Am Soc Nephrol* 22:545–553, 2011

94. Mazzucco G, Bertani T, Fortunato M, et al.: Different patterns of renal damage in type 2 diabetes mellitus: a multicentric study on 393 biopsies. *Am J Kidney Dis* 39:713–720, 2002

95. Gambara V, Mecca G, Remuzzi G, et al.: Heterogeneous nature of renal lesions in type II diabetes. *J Am Soc Nephrol* 3:1458–1466, 1993

96. Mathiesen ER, Ronn B, Storm B, et al.: The natural course of microalbuminuria in insulin-dependent diabetes: a 10-year prospective study. *Diabet Med* 12:482–487, 1995

97. Lemley KV, Abdullah I, Myers BD, et al.: Evolution of incipient nephropathy in type 2 diabetes mellitus. [erratum appears in *Kidney Int* 58:2257, 2000]. *Kidney Int* 58:1228–1237, 2000

98. Scott LJ, Warram JH, Hanna LS, Laffel LM, Ryan L, Krolewski AS: A nonlinear effect of hyperglycemia and current cigarette smoking are major determinants of the onset of microalbuminuria in type 1 diabetes. *Diabetes* 50:2842–2849, 2001

99. Viberti GC, Hill RD, Jarrett RJ, Argyropoulos A, et al.: Microalbuminuria as a predictor of clinical nephropathy in insulin-dependent diabetes mellitus. *Lancet* 1:1430–1432, 1982

100. Parving HH, Oxenboll B, Svendsen PA, et al.: Early detection of patients at risk of developing diabetic nephropathy: a longitudinal study of urinary albumin excretion. *Acta Endocrinol (Copenh)* 100:550–555, 1982

101. Mogensen CE, Christensen CK: Predicting diabetic nephropathy in insulin-dependent patients. *N Engl J Med* 311:89–93, 1984

102. Gall MA, Nielsen FS, Smidt UM, et al.: The course of kidney function in type 2 (non-insulin-dependent) diabetic patients with diabetic nephropathy. *Diabetologia* 36:1071–1078, 1993

103. Jacobsen P, Rossing K, Tarnow L, et al.: Progression of diabetic nephropathy in normotensive type 1 diabetic patients. *Kidney Int* 71(Suppl.): S101–S105, 1999

104. Williams ME: Diabetic nephropathy: the proteinuria hypothesis. *Am J Nephrol* 25:77–94, 2005
105. ACE Inhibitors in Diabetic Nephropathy Trialist Group: Should all patients with type 1 diabetes mellitus and microalbuminuria receive angiotensin-converting enzyme inhibitors? A meta-analysis of individual patient data. *Ann Intern Med* 134:370–379, 2001
106. Biesenbach G, Bodlaj G, Pieringer H, et al.: Clinical versus histological diagnosis of diabetic nephropathy—is renal biopsy required in type 2 diabetic patients with renal disease? *QJM* 104:771–774, 2011
107. Perkins BA, Ficociello LH, Silva KH, et al.: Regression of microalbuminuria in type 1 diabetes. *N Engl J Med* 348:2285–2293, 2003
108. Perkins BA, Ficociello LH, Roshan B, Warram JH, Krolewski AS: In patients with type 1 diabetes and new-onset microalbuminuria the development of advanced chronic kidney disease may not require progression to proteinuria. *Kidney Int* 77:57–64, 2010
109. Adolescent type 1 Diabetes Cardio-renal Intervention Trial Research Group: Adolescent Type 1 Diabetes Cardio-renal Intervention Trial (AdDIT). *BMC Pediatr* 9:79, 2009
110. DCCT/EDIC Research Group: Sustained effect of intensive treatment of type 1 diabetes mellitus on development and progression of diabetic nephropathy: the Epidemiology of Diabetes Interventions and Complications (EDIC) study. *JAMA* 290:2159–2167, 2003
111. Salgado PP, Silva IN, Vieira EC, Simoes e Silva AC: Risk factors for early onset of diabetic nephropathy in pediatric type 1 diabetes. *J Pediatr Endocrinol Metab* 23:1311–1320, 2010
112. Amin R, Widmer B, Prevost AT, et al.: Risk of microalbuminuria and progression to macroalbuminuria in a cohort with childhood onset type 1 diabetes: prospective observational study. *BMJ* 336:697–701, 2008
113. Schultz CJ, Neil HA, Dalton RN, Dunger DB. Risk of nephropathy can be detected before the onset of microalbuminuria during the early years after diagnosis of type 1 diabetes. *Diabetes Care* 23(12):1811–1815, 2000
114. Zachwieja J, Soltysiak J, Fichna P, et al.: Normal-range albuminuria does not exclude nephropathy in diabetic children. *Pediatr Nephrol* 25(8):1445–1451, 2010
115. Lewis EJ, Hunsicker LG, Bain RP, Rohde RD: The effect of angiotensin-converting-enzyme inhibition on diabetic nephropathy. The Collaborative Study Group. *N Engl J Med* 329(20):1456–1462, 1993
116. Krolewski A, Bonventre JV: New therapies are desperately needed to reduce risk of ESRD in type 1 diabetes, a call to action. *Semin Nephrol* 2012 (in press)
117. Pavlakis M: The timing of dialysis and kidney transplantation in type 1 diabetes. *Diabetes Obes Metab* 14:689–693, 2012
118. Forsblom C, Harjutsalo V, Thorn LM, et al.: Competing-risk analysis of ESRD and death among patients with type 1 diabetes and macroalbuminuria. *J Am Soc Nephrol* 22(3):537–544, 2011
119. Rodby RA, Rohde RD, Sharon Z, et al.: The urine protein to creatinine ratio as a predictor of 24-hour urine protein excretion in type 1 diabetic patients with nephropathy. The Collaborative Study Group. *Am J Kidney Dis* 26:904–909, 1995

120. Bakker AJ: Detection of microalbuminuria. Receiver operating characteristic curve analysis favors albumin-to-creatinine ratio over albumin concentration. *Diabetes Care* 22:307–313, 1999

121. Huttunen NP, Kaar M, Puukka R, et al.: Exercise-induced proteinuria in children and adolescents with type 1 (insulin dependent) diabetes. *Diabetologia* 21:495–497, 1981

122. Solling J, Solling K, Mogensen CE: Patterns of proteinuria and circulating immune complexes in febrile patients. *Acta Medica Scandinavica* 212:167–169, 1982

123. Wiseman M, Viberti G, Mackintosh D, et al.: Glycaemia, arterial pressure and micro-albuminuria in type 1 (insulin-dependent) diabetes mellitus. *Diabetologia* 26:401–405, 1984

124. Gall MA, Hougaard P, Borch-Johnsen K, Parving HH: Risk factors for development of incipient and overt diabetic nephropathy in patients with non-insulin dependent diabetes mellitus: prospective, observational study. *BMJ* 314(7083):783–788, 1997

125. Venkata Raman TV, Knickerbocker F, Sheldon CV: Unusual causes of renal failure in diabetics: two case studies. *Journal—Oklahoma State Medical Association* 83:164–168, 1990

126. Anonymous: Clinical path conference. Unusual renal complications in diabetes mellitus. *Minnesota Medicine* 50:387–393, 1967

127. Amoah E, Glickman JL, Malchoff CD, et al.: Clinical identification of non-diabetic renal disease in diabetic patients with type I and type II disease presenting with renal dysfunction. *Am J Nephrol* 8:204–211, 1988

128. El-Asrar AM, Al-Rubeaan KA, Al-Amro SA, et al.: Retinopathy as a predictor of other diabetic complications. *International Ophthalmology* 24:1–11, 2001

129. Reenders K, de Nobel E, van den Hoogen HJ, et al.: Diabetes and its long-term complications in general practice: a survey in a well-defined population. *Fam Pract* 10:169–172, 1993

130. Weir MR: Albuminuria predicting outcome in diabetes: incidence of microalbuminuria in Asia-Pacific Rim. *Kidney Int* 66:S38–S39, 2004

131. Canadian Institute for Health Information: Canadian Organ Replacement Register Annual Report: Treatment of End-Stage Organ Failure in Canada, 2000 to 2009. Ottawa, ON, Canada, 2011

132. Foley RN, Parfrey PS, Sarnak MJ: Clinical epidemiology of cardiovascular disease in chronic renal disease. *Am J Kidney Dis* 32:S112–119, 1998

133. Bell CM, Chapman RH, Stone PW, et al.: An off-the-shelf help list: a comprehensive catalog of preference scores from published cost-utility analyses. *Medical Decision Making* 21:288–294, 2001

134. de Boer IH, Sun W, Cleary PA, et al.: Intensive diabetes therapy and glomerular filtration rate in type 1 diabetes. *N Engl J Med* 365(25):2366–2376, 2011

135. Lewis EJ, Hunsicker LG, Clarke WR, et al.: Renoprotective effect of the angiotensin-receptor antagonist irbesartan in patients with nephropathy due to type 2 diabetes. *N Engl J Med* 345(12):851–860, 2001

136. KDOQI Clinical Practice Guidelines and Clinical Practice Recommendations for Diabetes and Chronic Kidney Disease. *Am J Kidney Dis* 49(Suppl. 2):S12–S154, 2007

137. Andersen S, Tarnow L, Rossing P, et al.: Renoprotective effects of angiotensin II receptor blockade in type 1 diabetic patients with diabetic nephropathy. *Kidney International* 57:601–606, 2000
138. Strippoli GF, Craig MC, Schena FP, et al.: Role of blood pressure targets and specific antihypertensive agents used to prevent diabetic nephropathy and delay its progression. *J Am Soc Nephrol* 17:S153–S155, 2006
139. Laffel LM, McGill JB, Gans DJ: The beneficial effect of angiotensin-converting enzyme inhibition with captopril on diabetic nephropathy in normotensive IDDM patients with microalbuminuria. North American Microalbuminuria Study Group. *Am J Medicine* 99:497–504, 1995
140. Mathiesen ER, Hommel E, Giese J, et al.: Efficacy of captopril in postponing nephropathy in normotensive insulin dependent diabetic patients with microalbuminuria. *BMJ* 303:81–87, 1991
141. Jerums G, Allen TJ, Campbell DJ, et al.: Long-term comparison between perindopril and nifedipine in normotensive patients with type 1 diabetes and microalbuminuria. *Am J Kidney Dis* 37:890–899, 2001
142. Bakris GL, Weir MR: Angiotensin-converting enzyme inhibitor-associated elevations in serum creatinine: is this a cause for concern? *Arch Intern Med* 160:685–693, 2000
143. Miyamori I, Yasuhara S, Takeda Y, et al.: Effects of converting enzyme inhibition on split renal function in renovascular hypertension. *Hypertension* 8:415–421, 1986
144. Tobe SW, Clase CM, Gao P, et al.: Cardiovascular and renal outcomes with telmisartan, ramipril, or both in people at high renal risk: results from the ONTARGET and TRANSCEND studies. *Circulation* 123:1098–1107, 2011
145. Angeli F, Reboldi G, Mazzotta G, Poltronieri C, Garofoli M, Ramundo E, Biadetti A, Verdecchia P: Safety and efficacy of aliskiren in the treatment of hypertension and associated clinical conditions. *Curr Drug Saf* 7:76–85, 2012
146. Mauer M, Zinman B, Gardiner R, Suissa S, Sinaiko A, Strand T, et al. Renal and retinal effects of enalapril and losartan in type 1 diabetes. *N Engl J Med* 361(1):40–51, 2009
147. ONTARGET Investigators, Yusuf S, Teo KK, Pogue J, Dyal L, Copland I, Schumacher H, Dagenais G, Sleight P, Anderson C: Telmisartan, ramipril, or both in patients at high risk for vascular events. *N Engl J Med* 358(15):1547–1559, 2008
148. Giorgino F, Laviola L, Cavallo Perin P, et al.: Factors associated with progression to macroalbuminuria in microalbuminuric type 1 diabetic patients: the EURODIAB Prospective Complications Study. *Diabetologia* 47:1020–1028, 2004
149. Araki, S., Haneda M, Sugimoto T, et al.: Factors associated with frequent remission of microalbuminuria in patients with type 2 diabetes mellitus. 54:2983–2987, 2005
150. Perkins BA, Krolewski AS: Early nephropathy in type 1 diabetes: a new perspective on who will and who will not progress. *Curr Diab Rep* 5:455–463, 2005
151. de Boer IH, Rue TC, Cleary PA, Lachin JM, Molitch ME, Steffes MW, Sun W, Zinman B, Brunzell JD, Diabetes Control and Complications Trial/

Epidemiology of Diabetes Interventions and Complications Study Research Group, White NH, Danis RP, Davis MD, Hainsworth D, Hubbard LD, Nathan DM: Long-term renal outcomes of patients with type 1 diabetes mellitus and microalbuminuria: an analysis of the Diabetes Control and Complications Trial/Epidemiology of Diabetes Interventions and Complications cohort. *Arch Intern Med* 171(5):412–420, 2011

152. Perkins BA, Krolewski AS: Early nephropathy in type 1 diabetes: the importance of early renal function decline. *Curr Opin Nephrol Hypertens* 18(3):233–240, 2009

153. Perkins BA, Ficociello LH, Ostrander BE, Silva KH, Weinberg J, Warram JH, Krolewski AS: Microalbuminuria and the risk for early progressive renal function decline in type 1 diabetes. *J Am Soc Nephrol* 18(4):1353–1361, 2007

154. Perkins BA, Nelson RG, Ostrander BE, Blouch KL, Krolewski AS, Myers BD, Warram JH: Detection of renal function decline in patients with diabetes and normal or elevated GFR by serial measurements of serum cystatin C concentration: results of a 4-year follow-up study. *J Am Soc Nephrol* 16(5):1404–1412, 2005

155. Skupien J, Warram JH, Smiles AM, Niewczas MA, Gohda T, Pezzolesi MG, Cantarovich D, Stanton R, Krolewski AS: The early decline in renal function in patients with type 1 diabetes and proteinuria predicts the risk of end-stage renal disease. *Kidney Int* 82:589–597, 2012

156. Perkins BA, Rabbani N, Weston A, Ficociello LH, Adaikalakoteswari A, Niewczas M, Warram J, Krolewski AS, Thornalley P: Serum levels of advanced glycation endproducts and other markers of protein damage in early diabetic nephropathy in type 1 diabetes. *PLoS One* 7(4):e35655, 2012

157. Gohda T, Walker WH, Wolkow P, Lee JE, Warram JH, Krolewski AS, Niewczas MA: Elevated urinary excretion of immunoglobulins in nonproteinuric patients with type 1 diabetes. *Am J Physiol Renal Physiol* 303(1):F157–F162, 2012

158. Ficociello LH, Rosolowsky ET, Niewczas MA, Maselli NJ, Weinberg JM, Aschengrau A, Eckfeldt JH, Stanton RC, Galecki AT, Doria A, Warram JH, Krolewski AS: High-normal serum uric acid increases risk of early progressive renal function loss in type 1 diabetes: results of a 6-year follow-up. *Diabetes Care* 33(6):1337–1343. 2010

159. Gohda T, Niewczas MA, Ficociello LH, Walker WH, Skupien J, Rosetti F, Cullere X, Johnson AC, Crabtree G, Smiles AM, Mayadas TN, Warram JH, Krolewski AS: Circulating TNF receptors 1 and 2 predict stage 3 CKD in type 1 diabetes. *J Am Soc Nephrol* 23(3):516–524, 2012

160. Senior PA, Zeman M, Paty BW, Ryan EA, Shapiro AM. Changes in renal function after clinical islet transplantation: four-year observational study. *Am J Transplant* 7:91–98, 2007

161. Leitao CB, Cure P, Messinger S, et al.: Stable renal function after islet transplantation: importance of patient selection and aggressive clinical management. *Transplantation* 87:681–688, 2009

162. Fioretto P, Steffes MW, Sutherland DE, Goetz FC, Mauer M: Reversal of lesions of diabetic nephropathy after pancreas transplantation. *N Engl J Med* 339:69–75, 1998

163. Handelsman Y, Mechanick JI, Blonde L, et al.: American Association of Clinical Endocrinologists medical guidelines for clinical practice for developing a diabetes mellitus comprehensive care plan. *Endocr Pract* 17(Suppl. 2):S1–S53, 2011.
164. Early Treatment Diabetic Retinopathy Study research group: Photocoagulation for diabetic macular edema. Early Treatment Diabetic Retinopathy Study report number 1. *Arch Ophthalmol* 103(12):1796–1806, 1985
165. Kempen JH, O'Colmain BJ, Leske MC, Haffner SM, Klein R, Moss SE, et al.: The prevalence of diabetic retinopathy among adults in the United States. *Arch Ophthalmol* 122(4):552–563, 2004
166. Roy MS, Klein R, O'Colmain BJ, Klein BE, Moss SE, Kempen JH: The prevalence of diabetic retinopathy among adult type 1 diabetic persons in the United States. *Arch Ophthalmol* 122(4):546–551, 2004
167. Melendez-Ramirez LY, Richards RJ, Cefalu WT: Complications of type 1 diabetes. *Endocrinol Metab Clin North Am* 39(3):625–640, 2010
168. Klein R, Klein BE, Moss SE: Epidemiology of proliferative diabetic retinopathy. *Diabetes Care* 15(12):1875–1891, 1992
169. Klein R, Klein BE, Moss SE, Davis MD, DeMets DL: The Wisconsin epidemiologic study of diabetic retinopathy. IV. Diabetic macular edema. *Ophthalmology* 91(12):1464–1474, 1984
170. Vu HT, Keeffe JE, McCarty CA, Taylor HR: Impact of unilateral and bilateral vision loss on quality of life. *Br J Ophthalmol* 89(3):360–363, 2005
171. Cusick M, Meleth AD, Agron E, Fisher MR, Reed GF, Knatterud GL, et al.: Associations of mortality and diabetes complications in patients with type 1 and type 2 diabetes: early treatment diabetic retinopathy study report no. 27. *Diabetes Care* 28(3):617–625, 2005
172. Klein R, Klein BE, Moss SE, Davis MD, DeMets DL: The Wisconsin epidemiologic study of diabetic retinopathy. II. Prevalence and risk of diabetic retinopathy when age at diagnosis is less than 30 years. *Arch Ophthalmol* 102(4):520–526, 1984
173. Cho YH, Craig ME, Hing S, et al.: Microvascular complications assessment in adolescents with 2- to 5-yr duration of type 1 diabetes from 1990 to 2006. *Pediatric Diabetes* 12(8):682–689, 2011
174. Ferris FL, III: How effective are treatments for diabetic retinopathy? *JAMA* 269(10):1290–1291, 1993
175. Klein R, Klein BE, Moss SE, Davis MD, DeMets DL: The Wisconsin Epidemiologic Study of Diabetic Retinopathy. IX. Four-year incidence and progression of diabetic retinopathy when age at diagnosis is less than 30 years. *Arch Ophthalmol* 107(2):237–243, 1989
176. Klein R, Klein BE, Moss SE, Davis MD, DeMets DL: The Wisconsin Epidemiologic Study of Diabetic Retinopathy. VII. Diabetic nonproliferative retinal lesions. *Ophthalmology* 94(11):1389–1400, 1987
177. Klein R, Moss SE, Klein BE, Davis MD, DeMets DL: The Wisconsin Epidemiologic Study of Diabetic Retinopathy. XI. The incidence of macular edema. *Ophthalmology* 96(10):1501–1510, 1989
178. Younis N, Broadbent DM, Harding SP, Vora JP: Incidence of sight-threatening retinopathy in Type 1 diabetes in a systematic screening programme. *Diabetic Medicine* 20(9):758–765, 2003

179. Younis N, Broadbent DM, Vora JP, Harding SP, Liverpool Diabetic Eye S: Incidence of sight-threatening retinopathy in patients with type 2 diabetes in the Liverpool Diabetic Eye Study: a cohort study. *Lancet* 361(9353):195–200, 2003

180. Maguire A, Chan A, Cusumano J, Hing S, Craig M, Silink M, et al.: The case for biennial retinopathy screening in children and adolescents. *Diabetes Care* 28(3):509–513, 2005

181. Kohner EM, Stratton IM, Aldington SJ, Holman RR, Matthews DR, Group UKPDS: Relationship between the severity of retinopathy and progression to photocoagulation in patients with type 2 diabetes mellitus in the UKPDS (UKPDS 52). *Diabetic Medicine* 18(3):178–184, 2001

182. Klein R: Screening interval for retinopathy in type 2 diabetes. *Lancet* 361(9353):190–191, 2003

183. Antonetti DA, Klein R, Gardner TW: Diabetic retinopathy. *N Engl J Med* 366(13):1227–1239, 2012

184. Hirsch IB, Brownlee M: Beyond hemoglobin A1c—need for additional markers of risk for diabetic microvascular complications. *JAMA* 303(22):2291–2292, 2010

185. Klein R: The epidemiology of diabetic retinopathy. In *Diabetic Retinopathy*. Duh E, Ed. Totowa, NJ, Humana, 2008, p. 67–107.

186. Estacio RO, McFarling E, Biggerstaff S, Jeffers BW, Johnson D, Schrier RW: Overt albuminuria predicts diabetic retinopathy in Hispanics with NIDDM. *Am J Kidney Dis* 31(6):947–953, 1998

187. Hsieh YY, Huang YC, Chang CC, Wang YK, Lin WH, Tsai FJ: Chromosome 15q21-22-related polymorphisms and haplotypes are associated with susceptibility to type-2 diabetic nonproliferative retinopathy. *Genet Test Mol Biomarkers* 16:442–448, 2012

188. West SD, Groves DC, Lipinski HJ, et al.: The prevalence of retinopathy in men with type 2 diabetes and obstructive sleep apnoea. *Diabetic Medicine* 27(4):423–430, 2010

189. Targher G, Bertolini L, Chonchol M, et al.: Non-alcoholic fatty liver disease is independently associated with an increased prevalence of chronic kidney disease and retinopathy in type 1 diabetic patients. *Diabetologia* 53(7):1341–1348, 2010

190. Arnold E, Rivera JC, Thebault S, et al.: High levels of serum prolactin protect against diabetic retinopathy by increasing ocular vasoinhibins. *Diabetes* 59(12):3192–3197, 2010

191. Zietz B, Buechler C, Kobuch K, Neumeier M, Scholmerich J, Schaffler A: Serum levels of adiponectin are associated with diabetic retinopathy and with adiponectin gene mutations in Caucasian patients with diabetes mellitus type 2. *Exp Clin Endocrinol Diabetes* 116(9):532–536, 2008

192. Nguyen TT, Alibrahim E, Islam FM, et al.: Inflammatory, hemostatic, and other novel biomarkers for diabetic retinopathy: the multi-ethnic study of atherosclerosis. *Diabetes Care* 32(9):1704–1709, 2009

193. Kaur H, Donaghue KC, Chan AK, et al.: Vitamin D deficiency is associated with retinopathy in children and adolescents with type 1 diabetes. *Diabetes Care* 34(6):1400–1402, 2011

194. Cappai G, Songini M, Doria A, Cavallerano JD, Lorenzi M: Increased prevalence of proliferative retinopathy in patients with type 1 diabetes who are

deficient in glucose-6-phosphate dehydrogenase. *Diabetologia* 54(6):1539–1542, 2011

195. Photocoagulation treatment of proliferative diabetic retinopathy: the second report of diabetic retinopathy study findings. *Ophthalmology* 85(1):82–106, 1978

196. Ferris F: Early photocoagulation in patients with either type I or type II diabetes. *Transactions of the American Ophthalmological Society* 94:505–537, 1996

197. Buxton MJ, Sculpher MJ, Ferguson BA, Humphreys JE, Altman JF, Spiegelhalter DJ, et al.: Screening for treatable diabetic retinopathy: a comparison of different methods. *Diabetic Medicine* 8(4):371–377, 1991

198. UK Prospective Diabetes Study (UKPDS) Group: Intensive blood-glucose control with sulphonylureas or insulin compared with conventional treatment and risk of complications in patients with type 2 diabetes (UKPDS 33). *Lancet* 352(9131):837–853, 1998

199. UK Prospective Diabetes Study Group: Tight blood pressure control and risk of macrovascular and microvascular complications in type 2 diabetes: UKPDS 38. *BMJ* 317(7160):703–713, 1998

200. Mohamed Q, Gillies MC, Wong TY: Management of diabetic retinopathy: a systematic review. *JAMA* 298(8):902–916, 2007

201. White NH, Sun W, Cleary PA, Danis RP, Davis MD, Hainsworth DP, et al.: Prolonged effect of intensive therapy on the risk of retinopathy complications in patients with type 1 diabetes mellitus: 10 years after the Diabetes Control and Complications Trial. *Arch Ophthalmol* 126(12):1707–1715, 2008

202. Holman RR, Paul SK, Bethel MA, Matthews DR, Neil HA: 10-year follow-up of intensive glucose control in type 2 diabetes. *N Engl J Med* 359(15):1577–1589, 2008

203. DCCT Research Group: Early worsening of diabetic retinopathy in the Diabetes Control and Complications Trial. *Arch Ophthalmol* 116:874–886, 1998

204. Group AS, Group AES, Chew EY, Ambrosius WT, Davis MD, Danis RP, et al.: Effects of medical therapies on retinopathy progression in type 2 diabetes. *N Engl J Med* 363(3):233–244, 2010

205. Beulens JW, Patel A, Vingerling JR, Cruickshank JK, Hughes AD, Stanton A, et al.: Effects of blood pressure lowering and intensive glucose control on the incidence and progression of retinopathy in patients with type 2 diabetes mellitus: a randomised controlled trial. *Diabetologia* 52(10):2027–2036, 2009

206. Chaturvedi N, Porta M, Klein R, Orchard T, Fuller J, Parving HH, et al.: Effect of candesartan on prevention (DIRECT-Prevent 1) and progression (DIRECT-Protect 1) of retinopathy in type 1 diabetes: randomised, placebo-controlled trials. *Lancet* 372(9647):1394–1402, 2008

207. Sjolie AK, Klein R, Porta M, Orchard T, Fuller J, Parving HH, et al.: Effect of candesartan on progression and regression of retinopathy in type 2 diabetes (DIRECT-Protect 2): a randomised placebo-controlled trial. *Lancet* 372(9647):1385–1393, 2008

208. Bergerhoff K, Clar C, Richter B: Aspirin in diabetic retinopathy. A systematic review. *Endocrinology and Metabolism Clinics of North America* 31(3):779–793, 2002

209. Aiello LP, Cahill MT, Wong JS: Systemic considerations in the management of diabetic retinopathy. *Am J Ophthalmol* 132(5):760–776, 2001
210. Early Treatment Diabetic Retinopathy Study Research Group: Effects of aspirin treatment on diabetic retinopathy. ETDRS report number 8. *Ophthalmology* 98(Suppl. 5):S757–S765, 1991
211. Diabetic Retinopathy Vitrectomy Study Group: Early vitrectomy for severe vitreous hemorrhage in diabetic retinopathy. Four-year results of a randomized trial: Diabetic Retinopathy Vitrectomy Study. *Arch Ophthalmol* 108(7):958–964, 1990
212. The Diabetic Retinopathy Vitrectomy Study Research Group: Early vitrectomy for severe proliferative diabetic retinopathy in eyes with useful vision. Results of a randomized trial: Diabetic Retinopathy Vitrectomy Study report 3. *Ophthalmology* 95(10):1307–1320, 1988
213. Nguyen QD, Brown DM, Marcus DM, Boyer DS, Patel S, Feiner L, et al. Ranibizumab for diabetic macular edema: results from 2 phase iii randomized trials: RISE and RIDE. *Ophthalmology* 119(4):789–801, 2012
214. Mitchell P, Bandello F, Schmidt-Erfurth U, Lang GE, Massin P, Schlingemann RO, et al.: The RESTORE study: ranibizumab monotherapy or combined with laser versus laser monotherapy for diabetic macular edema. *Ophthalmology* 118(4):615–625, 2011
215. Pearson PA, Comstock TL, Ip M, Callanan D, Morse LS, Ashton P, et al.: Fluocinolone acetonide intravitreal implant for diabetic macular edema: a 3-year multicenter, randomized, controlled clinical trial. *Ophthalmology* 118(8):1580–1587, 2011
216. Campochiaro PA, Brown DM, Pearson A, Ciulla T, Boyer D, Holz FG, et al.: Long-term benefit of sustained-delivery fluocinolone acetonide vitreous inserts for diabetic macular edema. *Ophthalmology* 118(4):626–635, 2011
217. Ferris FL, III, Davis MD, Aiello LM: Treatment of diabetic retinopathy. *N Engl J Med* 341(9):667–678, 1999
218. Chew EY, Ferris FL, III, Csaky KG, Murphy RP, Agron E, Thompson DJ, et al.: The long-term effects of laser photocoagulation treatment in patients with diabetic retinopathy: the early treatment diabetic retinopathy follow-up study. *Ophthalmology* 110(9):1683–1689, 2003
219. Elman MJ, Bressler NM, Qin H, Beck RW, Ferris FL, III, Friedman SM, et al.: Expanded 2-year follow-up of ranibizumab plus prompt or deferred laser or triamcinolone plus prompt laser for diabetic macular edema. *Ophthalmology* 118(4):609–614, 2011
220. Rajendram R, Fraser-Bell S, Kaines A, Michaelides M, Hamilton RD, Esposti SD, Peto T, Egan C, Bunce C, Leslie RD, Hykin PG: A 2-year prospective randomized controlled trial of intravitreal bevacizumab or laser therapy (BOLT) in the management of diabetic macular edema: 24-month data: report 3. *Arch Ophthalmol* 130:972–979, 2012
221. Smiddy WE, Flynn HW, Jr.: Vitrectomy in the management of diabetic retinopathy. *Survey of Ophthalmology* 43(6):491–507, 1999
222. El-Asrar AM, Al-Mezaine HS, Ola MS: Changing paradigms in the treatment of diabetic retinopathy. *Current Opinion in Ophthalmology* 20(6):532–538, 2009

223. Chew EY, Klein ML, Murphy RP, Remaley NA, Ferris FL, III: Effects of aspirin on vitreous/preretinal hemorrhage in patients with diabetes mellitus. Early Treatment Diabetic Retinopathy Study report no. 20. *Arch Ophthalmol* 113(1):52–55, 1995

224. Chew EY, Benson WE, Remaley NA, Lindley AA, Burton TC, Csaky K, et al.: Results after lens extraction in patients with diabetic retinopathy: Early Treatment Diabetic Retinopathy Study report no. 25. *Arch Ophthalmol* 117(12):1600–1606, 1999

225. Brown JS, Mahmoud TH: Anticoagulation and clinically significant postoperative vitreous hemorrhage in diabetic vitrectomy. *Retina* 31(10):1983–1987, 2011

226. Fonda GE: Optical treatment of residual vision in diabetic retinopathy. *Ophthalmology* 101(1):84–88, 1994

227. Bernbaum M, Albert SG: Referring patients with diabetes and vision loss for rehabilitation: who is responsible? *Diabetes Care* 19(2):175–177, 1996

228. van Dijk HW, Kok PH, Garvin M, et al.: Selective loss of inner retinal layer thickness in type 1 diabetic patients with minimal diabetic retinopathy. *Invest Ophthalmol Vis Sci* 50:3404–3409, 2009

229. van Dijk HW, Verbraak FD, Kok PH, et al.: Decreased retinal ganglion cell layer thickness in patients with type 1 diabetes. *Invest Ophthalmol Vis Sci* 51:3660–3665, 2010

230. Benitez-Aguirre P, Craig ME, Sasongko MB, Jenkins AJ, Wong TY, Wang JJ, Cheung N, Donaghue KC: Retinal vascular geometry predicts incident retinopathy in young people with type 1 diabetes: a prospective cohort study from adolescence. *Diabetes Care* 34:1622–1627, 2011

231. Parravano M, Oddone F, Mineo D, et al.: The role of Humphrey Matrix testing in the early diagnosis of retinopathy in type 1 diabetes. *Br J Ophthalmol* 92:1656–1660, 2008

232. Jackson JR, Scott IU, Quillen DA, Walter LE, Hershey ME, Gardner TW: Inner retinal visual dysfunction is a sensitive marker of nonproliferative diabetic retinopathy. *Br J Ophthalmol* 96:699–703, 2012

233. Harrison WW, Bearse MA Jr, Schneck ME, et al.: Prediction, by retinal location, of the onset of diabetic edema in patients with nonproliferative diabetic retinopathy. *Invest Ophthalmol Vis Sci* 52:6825–6831, 2011

234. Holfort SK, Norgaard K, Jackson GR, et al.: Retinal function in relation to improved glycaemic control in type 1 diabetes. *Diabetologia* 54:1853–1861, 2011

235. Willard AL, Herman IM: Vascular complications and diabetes: current therapies and future challenges. *J Ophthalmol* 209538, 2012. Epub 9 January 2012

236. Sultan MB, Zhou D, Loftus J, Dombi T, Ice KS: A phase 2/3, multicenter, randomized, double-masked, 2-year trial of pegaptanib sodium for the treatment of diabetic macular edema. *Ophthalmology* 118(6):1107–1118, 2011

237. Behl Y, Krothapalli P, Desta T, DiPiazza A, Roy S, Graves DT: Diabetes-enhanced tumor necrosis factor-alpha production promotes apoptosis and the loss of retinal microvascular cells in type 1 and type 2 models of diabetic retinopathy. *Am J Pathol* 172(5):1411–1418, 2008

238. Han JH, Ha SW, Lee IK, Kim BW, Kim JG: High glucose-induced apoptosis in bovine retinal pericytes is associated with transforming growth factor

beta and betaIG-H3: betaIG-H3 induces apoptosis in retinal pericytes by releasing Arg-Gly-Asp peptides. *Clin Experiment Ophthalmol* 38(6):620–628, 2010

239. Wang H, Feng L, Hu JW, Xie CL, Wang F: Characterisation of the vitreous proteome in proliferative diabetic retinopathy. *Proteome Sci* 10(1):1–11, 2012

240. Keech AC, Mitchell P, Summanen PA, et al.: Effect of fenofibrate on the need for laser treatment for diabetic retinopathy (FIELD study): a randomised controlled trial. *Lancet* 370(9600):1687–1697, 2007

241. Wright AD, Dodson PM: Medical management of diabetic retinopathy: fenofibrate and ACCORD Eye studies. *Eye (Lond)* 25(7):843–849, 2011

242. Phipps JA, Clermont AC, Sinha S, Chilcote TJ, Bursell SE, Feener EP: Plasma kallikrein mediates angiotensin II type 1 receptor-stimulated retinal vascular permeability. *Hypertension*53:175–181, 2009

243. Chew EY, Klein ML, Ferris FL, III, Remaley NA, Murphy RP, Chantry K, et al.: Association of elevated serum lipid levels with retinal hard exudate in diabetic retinopathy. Early Treatment Diabetic Retinopathy Study (ETDRS) report no. 22. *Arch Ophthalmol* 114(9):1079–1084, 1996

244. Miljanovic B, Glynn RJ, Nathan DM, Manson JE, Schaumberg DA: A prospective study of serum lipids and risk of diabetic macular edema in type 1 diabetes. *Diabetes* 53(11):2883–2892, 2004

245. Colhoun HM, Betteridge DJ, Durrington PN, Hitman GA, Neil HA, Livingstone SJ, et al.: Primary prevention of cardiovascular disease with atorvastatin in type 2 diabetes in the Collaborative Atorvastatin Diabetes Study (CARDS): multicentre randomised placebo-controlled trial. *Lancet* 364(9435):685–696, 2004

246. Whited JD: Accuracy and reliability of teleophthalmology for diagnosing diabetic retinopathy and macular edema: a review of the literature. *Diabetes Technology and Therapeutics* 8(1):102–111, 2006

17

Pregnancy: Preconception to Postpartum Care

INTRODUCTION

Type 1 diabetes (T1D) complicates ~0.1–0.2% of all pregnancies (ADA Medical Management of Type 1 Diabetes, p. 154, 2008). Education, counseling, and medical care promoting healthy planned pregnancies can reduce maternal and perinatal mortality and morbidity. All women of reproductive age should be informed about the increased pregnancy risks associated with T1D, as good glycemic control and preconception pregnancy planning can mitigate these risks. This chapter discusses T1D and pregnancy and reviews the current standards of care during preconception, pregnancy, and postpartum. It also integrates the latest research findings and summarizes the gaps in clinical research, with the goal of improving future outcomes.

I. Preconception Counseling and Care

Jennifer Wyckoff, MD

INTRODUCTION

The combined risks associated with pregnancy and type 1 diabetes (T1D) can be minimized by optimizing preconception care in women of child-bearing age. The two key components of preconception care are contraception and glycemic control. Comprehensive preconception care covers a larger domain, including education about pregnancy risks, optimizing nutrition, and managing maternal complications and comorbidities, including obesity. Pregnancy planning is essential because the hemoglobin A1C (A1C) at conception predicts pregnancy outcomes.[1–10] High–blood glucose levels during conception and the first trimester are associated with rates of congenital malformations between 4.2% and 13.4% compared with rates of around 2% in control populations.[3,4,11–14] The most commonly reported defects are cardiac and neural tube defects.[4,5,9] Higher A1Cs also are associated with preterm deliveries,[7,10,15–17] spontaneous abortions,[9,12] intrauterine fetal demise,[18] and perinatal mortality.[3–5,7,9] Between 15 and 50% of the elevated perinatal mortality is attributed to congenital malformations with the other most common cause being preterm delivery.[7,19]

PRECONCEPTION CARE

Studies in women with T1D show that preconception care with tight glycemic control improved outcomes, including reduced prevalence of congenital malformations,[20–28] greater gestational age at delivery,[29,30] lower A1C before and during pregnancy,[27–29] lower cesarean delivery rates,[29] and decreased perinatal mortality.[22,24,27] The crucial component to these preconception care models is thought to be optimizing glycemic control before conception. Discontinuing contraception only after the A1C goal has been achieved provides optimal outcomes.[5]

Guerin et al. used a multilevel log normal model derived from a systematic literature review showing an increase of 1.2 in the odds ratio for congenital malformations for every 1 standard deviation above normal in the A1C.[31] Goals for optimal A1C and glycemic targets before pregnancy are discussed later in the chapter.

Unfortunately, many women with T1D do not receive preconception care or do not have planned pregnancies. About 40% of postpartum women with preexisting diabetes report that their pregnancies were unplanned.[32] This failure to obtain preconception care is partly the result of a lack of education. Physicians often omit preconception and contraceptive counseling. In a 2007 retrospective chart review, only 25% documented any discussion of preconception counseling or contraception.[33] In the Translating Research Into Action for Diabetes

DOI: 10.2337/9781580404785ch17s1

(TRIAD) study (http://www.triadstudy.org), a multicenter longitudinal study of diabetes treatments in managed care settings, only 37% of women surveyed recalled receiving family planning advice.[34] In a 2010 survey of teenagers ages 13–19 years with T1D, less than half had discussed birth control with their provider.[35]

Many women with T1D are not aware of the risks and recommendations regarding pregnancy. In a 2006 telephone survey of women (16–20 years) with T1D, only 25% were aware that tight glucose control was needed during pregnancy,[36] only 25% realized that they were at increased risk of complications, and only 10% were aware that preconception counseling was recommended. Furthermore, misinformation is common. In a 2010 survey of teens with T1D, 43% incorrectly believed that birth control was less effective in women with T1D. In a separate study, 6% of women with T1D believed that birth control was dangerous for women with T1D.[36] In addition, some women believed that they have decreased fertility because of diabetes.[37] In a survey of pregnant women with T1D who had not received preconception care, two reasons for not having had preconception care were commonly cited: *1)* women became pregnant faster than expected, and *2)* women believed that diabetes decreased fertility.[37] In a 2010 survey, 50% of 13–19-year-olds with T1D reported having intercourse without any form of birth control.[35]

Even in women with a high level of diabetes education, women do not always choose to plan their pregnancies carefully. In the Diabetes Control and Complications Trial (DCCT), despite strong recommendations regarding preconception care, only 39% of subjects in the conventional arm had preconception care.[11] Women reported that two of the reasons they did not attend preconception counseling were *1)* a desire for a "normal" pregnancy and *2)* logistical barriers (e.g., transportation and so on).[37]

Factors associated with planned pregnancies include higher income, higher education levels, private health insurance, endocrinology care before pregnancy, married, Caucasian, and encouragement from their physician.[32,38] Education about contraception and preconception is recommended for all women of reproductive age with T1D, especially teenagers. Counseling and contraception should not be overlooked in older women and decreased fertility should not be assumed.

Fertility and Contraception

Although fertility generally should be assumed to be normal, there is some evidence for reduced child bearing.[39–41] The data are limited and fertility in women with T1D requires more study.

Counseling women about their contraceptive options and establishing a clear plan is essential. For contraception to be effective, it must suit the woman's lifestyle and be used consistently. This requires a detailed conversation between the physician and the patient. It is prudent to have a plan in place for when a woman suspects an unplanned pregnancy. Emergency contraception should be discussed. Table 17.I.1 lists contraceptive methods and some of the associated considerations.

Table 17.I.1 Contraceptive Methods

Method	Form	Advantages	Disadvantages
Barriers	Condoms Sponges Cervical shields Spermicides	Easily accessible Inexpensive Condoms reduce STD transmission	16–21% failure rates
Progestin Only[42]	Pills Implants Injections	No effect on BP No effect on coagulation	Increase insulin resistance Increase LDL Decrease HDL Injections associated with weight gain
Estrogen–Progestin	Pills Transdermal patches Transvaginal rings[43] Injections	Transvaginal rings showed less coronary artery calcium progression[40]	Estrogen raises BP and increases coagulability Women at risk for stroke and other coagulation events should not use estrogen containing contraceptives (women over 35 year; known vascular disease, severe obesity, microvascular disease, hypertension, or migraine headaches)[42]
Intrauterine Devices (IUD)	Copper IUD Levonorgestrel (LVN) IUD	LVN IUD reduces menstrual blood loss[44] No effect on coagulation, lipids, glucose, or blood pressure Highly effective.	Increased risk of PID in the first 20 days after insertion; risk of PID is higher in nonmonogamous relationships

[a] BP, blood pressure; HDL, high-density lipoprotein; LDL, low-density lipoprotein; PID, pelvic inflammatory disease; STD, sexually transmitted disease.

Nutritional Requirements before Pregnancy

Medical nutrition therapy (MNT), blood glucose monitoring, and an intensive insulin regimen are necessary to optimize glucose management. Meal planning guides, including consistent timing of meals and snacks, should be established or maintained for each patient.[45] Women need folic acid supplementation (600 micrograms/day), vitamin D, and 1,000 mg/day of calcium.[45] The amount of vitamin D that should be supplemented in pregnancy is a current area of research and debate.[46] Prenatal vitamins, containing folic acid, reduce the risk of congenital malformations in infants of mothers with diabetes.[5,45,47]

Obesity

Obesity is increasing in the T1D population and should be addressed preconception.[48] Obesity is associated with increased risk of intrauterine fetal demise,[49,50] preeclampsia,[49,51] perinatal mortality,[49,50] and preterm delivery[49] (among people without diabetes) and therefore must be addressed. Preconception treatment of obesity, both through lifestyle intervention and through bariatric procedures,[52] may reduce those risks. Women who undergo nonadjustable bariatric procedures usually are advised to delay conception until a year postprocedure.[53]

Preconception Diabetes Management

Preconception visits should be scheduled monthly until control is achieved and then at longer intervals. Optimal timing and targets for finger stick blood glucose monitoring are debated.[54] Some groups advocate for 1-h postprandial blood glucose targets, whereas others advocate for 2-h postprandial targets. Data are inadequate about recommended blood glucose targets; however, data suggest that lower A1C levels equate to better pregnancy outcomes. Many patients have difficulty maintaining low postprandial levels without running the risk of hypoglycemia. Postprandial targets are 100–155 mg/dl, with fasting targets 80–110 mg/dl. An A1C <7% and as close to normal as possible without significant hypoglycemia is recommended.[55,56] Well-studied data are lacking, however, about any blood glucose target level except for the clear data suggesting that a lower A1C level equals better outcomes.

Studies suggest that basal–bolus insulin regimens benefit patients with T1D.[57] Women with T1D who are not already treated with a basal–bolus insulin regimen should begin one preconception: either multiple daily injections using an insulin to carbohydrate (I:CHO) ratio regimen and a correction factor or a continuous subcutaneous insulin infusion (CSII) regimen, to reduce peak postprandial glucose.[55,58] Superiority of CSII for T1D in pregnancy has not been proven,[59,60] but some providers feel that CSII may offer benefits.

Insulin generally does not cross the placenta and is thought to be safe in pregnancy. There are theoretic concerns, however, about insulin analog safety in pregnancy. Neutral protamine Hagedorn (NPH) insulin is the standard of care for long-acting insulin in pregnancy. Some insulin analogs, like glargine, have increased affinity for the IGF-1 receptor,[55] which plays an important role in fetal development. This raises concerns about its safety in pregnancy. A recent meta-analysis of studies comparing the safety of insulin glargine to NPH insulin concluded that there was no evidence for adverse outcomes in these short-term studies related to glargine use in pregnancy.[61] Long-term risks of glargine in pregnancy are not known, however. The Food and Drug Administration (FDA) has designated glargine as Class C in pregnancy. Another long-acting insulin analog, detemir, is listed as Class B in pregnancy. A study of the efficacy and safety of detemir in pregnancy has recently been published and supports metabolic noninferiority of basal dosing of insulin detemir compared with NPH insulin.[62] Pregnancy and neonatal outcomes from this study have not yet been published.

Similarly, rapid-acting insulin analogues also have raised concern and been studied to varying degrees. Aspart has been studied in pregnancy in a randomized controlled trial and lispro in an observational study.[63] Both aspart and lispro appeared safe in these studies and are widely used.

PRECONCEPTION COMPLICATIONS

Nephropathy

Diabetic kidney disease is fairly common. In a study of 240 pregnant Danish women with T1D, 11% had microalbuminuria and 5% had overt nephropathy.[64] Kidney disease increases the risk for hypertension, preterm delivery, preeclampsia, intrauterine growth retardation (IUGR), neonatal jaundice, and mechanical ventilation of the infant. Renal disease severity is predictive of adverse outcomes, with increasing proteinuria and creatinine inversely associated with gestational age and birth weight.[65]

Chronic renal insufficiency is related to a high risk of both maternal renal failure and perinatal mortality. In women with significant renal disease (serum creatinine 1.4–2.7 mg/dl), 43% had persistent loss of renal function at 6 months postpartum. Of these pregnancies, 59% were complicated by preterm delivery and 37% by IUGR.[66] Case series support the observation that impaired renal function in pregnancy is associated with poor maternal renal outcomes.[67]

Although renal disease seems to worsen both maternal and perinatal outcomes for women with T1D, pregnancy does not seem to worsen maternal renal outcomes in women without chronic renal insufficiency.[68] The DCCT showed that the number of pregnancies was not associated with increased risks of either microalbuminuria or proteinuria.[69] Preconception assessment should include blood pressure (BP) measurements, serum creatinine, and urine albumin–creatinine ratio.

Retinopathy

Pregnancy may exacerbate retinopathy and macular edema.[70] In women in the DCCT (13–39 years old), 13.3% of eye exams in nonpregnant subjects reported clinically significant progression of retinopathy compared with 17% of eye exams in pregnant participants.[69] DCCT subjects who switched to intensive treatment preconception appeared to have a lower risk of retinopathy progression during pregnancy, but this did not reach statistical significance.[69] Risk factors for retinopathy progression during pregnancy include poor glycemic control before pregnancy,[69,72] rapid improvement of glycemic control,[69,71] previous diabetic retinopathy severity,[71,73] diabetes duration,[72,73] and hypertension.[70,72] In the Diabetes in Early Pregnancy study, retinopathy progression during pregnancy was seen in 10.3% of women with no retinopathy at baseline.[71] Retinopathy progression was seen in 54.8% of women with moderate-to-severe retinopathy at baseline.[71] Pregnancy itself during the DCCT, however, was not associated with an increased risk of significant worsening of retinopathy at the study's end.[69] Similarly, giving birth was not a risk factor for retinopathy in the EURODIAB trial.[74] Preconception care should include a dilated retinal exam performed by a professional diabetic retinopathy specialist. Proliferative diabetic retinopathy should be treated and quiescent for a year before conception.

Blood Pressure

Preconception BP targets are systolic BP <130 mmHg and diastolic BP <80 mmHg.[75] Preconception treatment with angiotensin-converting-enzyme inhibitors (ACE-Is) and angiotensin receptor blockers (ARBs) is controversial. Although a woman using effective contraception is optimizing glycemic control and ACE-Is and ARBs may be safely continued, the timing of discontinuing them for pregnancy is debated. There is strong evidence that ACE-Is and ARBs cause oligohydramnios and renal insufficiency in infants exposed in the second and third trimesters, so these drugs definitely should be stopped as soon as pregnancy is diagnosed.[76] The debate lies in whether they should be discontinued for women who are trying to conceive. A 2006 study suggested that ACE-Is may increase the risk of cardiac and central nervous system malformations in infants exposed in the first trimester;[77] however, recent additional studies of women exposed to either ACE-Is[78] or both ACE-Is and ARBs[79,80] or ARBs alone[80] suggest that they may not be teratogenic. Until this the question of teratogenicity is resolved, in most cases, ACE-Is and ARBs should be discontinued when clearance to conceive is given. During periconception, BP control should be achieved with a calcium channel blocker or β-blocker (labetalol[81] or diltiazem or nifedipine). Methyldopa is another safe alternative. Atenolol has been associated with IUGR, so it is not recommended (see Table 17.II.7 in Section II).[82]

Coronary Artery Disease

Coronary artery disease (CAD) in pregnancy is rare.[83] Most reported cases occurred in the third trimester in women over 33 years old.[83] CAD screening, with an electrocardiogram (ECG) or an exercise echocardiogram, should be considered in patients with significant risk factors other than diabetes alone (e.g., advanced maternal age, chronic renal insufficiency, smoking, hypertension, hyperlipidemia, and a family history of premature CAD). Women with known CAD, who intend to become pregnant, should consult with a cardiologist because of an increased risk of maternal mortality.

Thyroid Disease

Autoimmune thyroid disease occurs in 11% of patients with T1D, with a higher rate in women with T1D,[84] so a common component of preconception care should be optimizing thyroid status. Given the high prevalence, even those patients with no known thyroid disease should have a thyroid stimulating hormone level checked preconception. Screening for other commonly associated autoimmune diseases, like celiac disease and B12 deficiency, could be considered.[54]

Mental Health

Depression is common in T1D, with 29% of adults meeting the lifetime criteria for a major depressive disorder. Eating disorders are also common, with up to 35% of women meeting criteria for subthreshold eating disorders. Both have been associated with poor diabetes control and poor diabetes outcomes.[85] In addition, in the general population, eating disorders have been clearly associated with poor outcomes in pregnancy.[86] There are limited data regarding mental health disorders and outcomes of pregnancy in women with T1D[87] and no data on screening preconception (see chapter 8, for psychosocial recommendations). Further study is needed.

REFERENCES

1. Ray JG, O'Brien TE, Chan WS: Preconception care and the risk of congenital anomalies in the offspring of women with diabetes mellitus: a meta-analysis. *QJM* 94:435–444, 2001
2. Centers for Disease Control and Prevention: Perinatal mortality and congenital malformations in infants born to women with insulin-dependent diabetes mellitus—United States, Canada, and Europe, 1940–1988. *MMWR* 39:363–365, 1990
3. Ricart W, Bach C, Gernandez-Real JM, Sabria J: Major fetal complications in optimised pregestational diabetes mellitus. *Diabetologia* 43:1077–1078, 2000
4. Casson IF, Clarke CA, Howard CV, et al.: Outcomes of pregnancy in insulin dependent diabetic women: results of a five year population cohort study. *BMJ* 315:275–278, 1997
5. Pearson DW, Kernaghan D, Lee R, Penney GC; Scottish Diabetes in Pregnancy Study Group: The relationship between pre-pregnancy care and early pregnancy loss, major congenital anomaly or perinatal death in type I diabetes mellitus. *BJOG* 114:104–107, 2007
6. Clausen TD, Mathiesen E, Ekbom P, Hellmuth E, Mandrup-Poulsen T, Damm P: Poor pregnancy outcome in women with type 2 diabetes. *Diabetes Care* 28:323–328, 2005
7. Jensen DM, Damm P, Moelsted-Pedersen L, et al.: Outcomes in type 1 diabetic pregnancies: a nationwide, population-based study. *Diabetes Care* 27:2819–2823, 2004
8. Suhonen L, Hiilesmaa V, Teramo K: Glycaemic control during early pregnancy and fetal malformations in women with type I diabetes mellitus. *Diabetologia* 43:79–82, 2000
9. Galindo A, Burguillo AG, Azriel S, Fuente Pde L: Outcome of fetuses in women with pregestational diabetes mellitus. *J Perinat Med* 34:323–331, 2006

10. Casson IF: Pregnancy in women with diabetes—after the CEMACH report, what now? *Diabet Med* 23:481–484, 2006

11. Pregnancy outcomes in the Diabetes Control and Complications Trial. *Am J Obstet Gynecol* 174:1343–1353, 1996

12. Greene MF HJ, Cloherty JP, Benacerraf BR, Soeldner JS: First-trimester hemoglobin A1 and risk for major malformation and spontaneous abortion in diabetic pregnancy. *Teratology* 39:225–231, 1989

13. Key TC GR, Moore TR: Predictive value of early pregnancy glycohemoglobin in the insulin-treated diabetic patient. *Am J Obstet Gynecol* 156:1096–1100, 1987

14. Galindo A, Burguillo AG, Azriel S, Fuente Pdl: Outcome of fetuses in women with pregestational diabetes mellitus. *J Perinat Med* 34:323–331, 2006

15. Lepercq J, Coste J, Theau A, Dubois-Laforgue D, Timsit J: Factors associated with preterm delivery in women with type 1 diabetes: a cohort study. *Diabetes Care* 27:2824–2828, 2004

16. Boulot P, Chabbert-Buffet N, d'Ercole C, et al.: French multicentric survey of outcome of pregnancy in women with pregestational diabetes. *Diabetes Care* 26:2990–2993, 2003

17. Evers IM, de Valk HW, Visser GH: Risk of complications of pregnancy in women with type 1 diabetes: nationwide prospective study in the Netherlands. *BMJ* 328:915, 2004

18. Key TC, Giuffrida R, Moore TR: Predictive value of early pregnancy glycohemoglobin in the insulin-treated diabetic patient. *Am J Obstet Gynecol* 156:1096–1100, 1987

19. Cundy T, Gamble G, Neale L, et al.: Differing causes of pregnancy loss in type 1 and type 2 diabetes. *Diabetes Care* 30:2603–2605, 2007

20. Jensen DM, Damm P, Moelsted-Pedersen L, et al.: Outcomes in type 1 diabetic pregnancies: a nationwide, population-based study. *Diabetes Care* 27:2819–2823, 2004

21. Steel JM JF, Hepburn DA, Smith AF: Can prepregnancy care of diabetic women reduce the risk of abnormal babies? *BMJ* 301:1070–1074, 1990

22. Willhoite MB, Bennert HW Jr, Palomaki GE, Zaremba MM, Herman WH, Williams JR, Spear NH: The impact of preconception counseling on pregnancy outcomes. The experience of the Maine Diabetes in Pregnancy Program. *Diabetes Care* 16:450–455, 1993

23. Kitzmiller JL, Gavin LA, Gin GD, Jovanovic-Peterson L, Main EK, Zigrang WD: Preconception care of diabetes. Glycemic control prevents congenital anomalies. *JAMA* 265:731–736, 1991

24. McElvy SS, Miodovnik M, Rosenn B, Khoury J, Siddiqi T, St John Dignan P Tsang RC: A focused preconceptional and early pregnancy program in women with type 1 diabetes reduces perinatal mortality and malformation rates to general population levels. *J Matern-Fetal Med* 9:14–20, 2000

25. Ray JG, O'Brien TE, Chan WS: Preconception care and the risk of congenital anomalies in the offspring of women with diabetes mellitus: a meta-analysis. *QJM* 94:435–444, 2001

26. Evers IM, de Valk HW, Visser GHA: Risk of complications of pregnancy in women with type 1 diabetes: nationwide prospective study in the Netherlands. *BMJ* 328:915, 2004

27. Wahabi H, Alzeidan R, Bawazeer G, Alansari L, Esmaeil S: Preconception care for diabetic women for improving maternal and fetal outcomes: a systematic review and meta-analysis. *BMC Pregnancy and Childbirth* 10:63, 2010

28. Murphy HR, Roland JM, Skinner TC, et al.: Effectiveness of a regional prepregnancy care program in women with type 1 and type 2 diabetes. *Diabetes Care* 33:2514–2520, 2010

29. Gunton JE, Morris J, Boyce S, Kelso I, McElduff A.: Outcome of pregnancy complicated by pre-gestational diabetes—improvement in outcomes. *Aust NZ J Obstet Gynaecol* 42:478–481, 2002

30. Temple RC, Aldridge VJ, Murphy HR.: Prepregnancy care and pregnancy outcomes in women with type 1 diabetes. *Diabetes Care* 29:1744–1749, 2006

31. Guerin A, Nisenbaum R, Ray JG: Use of maternal GHb concentration to estimate the risk of congenital anomalies in the offspring of women with prepregnancy diabetes. *Diabetes Care* 30:1920–1925, 2007

32. Holing EV, Beyer CS, Brown ZA, Connell FA: Why don't women with diabetes plan their pregnancies? *Diabetes Care* 21:889–895, 1998

33. Varughese GI, Chowdhury SR, Warner DP, Barton DM: Preconception care of women attending adult general diabetes clinics—are we doing enough? *Diab Res Clin Pract* 76:142–145, 2007

34. Kim C, Ferrara A, McEwen LN, et al.: Preconception care in managed care: the Translating Research into Action for Diabetes study. *Am J Obstet Gynecol* 192:227–232, 2005

35. Schwarz EB, Sobota M, Charron-Prochownik D.: Perceived access to contraception among adolescents with diabetes: barriers to preventing pregnancy complications. *Diabetes Educ* 36:489–494, 2010

36. Charron-Prochownik D, Sereika SM, Wang S-L, et al.: Reproductive health and preconception counseling awareness in adolescents with diabetes: what they don't know can hurt them. *Diabetes Educ* 32:235–242, 2006

37. Murphy HR, Temple RC, Ball VE, et al.: Personal experiences of women with diabetes who do not attend pre-pregnancy care. *Diabet Med* 27:92–100, 2010

38. Janz NK, Herman WH, Becker MP, et al.: Diabetes and pregnancy: factors associated with seeking pre-conception care. *Diabetes Care* 18:157–165, 1995

39. Jonasson JM, Brismar K, Sparen P, et al.: Fertility in women with type 1 diabetes: a population-based cohort study in Sweden. *Diabetes Care* 30:2271–2276, 2007

40. Snell-Bergeon JK, Dabelea D, Ogden LG, et al.: Reproductive history and hormonal birth control use are associated with coronary calcium progression in women with type 1 diabetes mellitus. *J Clin Endocrinol Metab* 93:2142–2148, 2008

41. Whitworth KW, Baird DD, Stene LC, Skjaerven R, Longnecker MP: Fecundability among women with type 1 and type 2 diabetes in the Norwegian Mother and Child Cohort Study. *Diabetologia* 54:516–522, 2011

42. Kjos SL: Contraception for women with diabetes. In *Diabetes in Women: Pathophysiology and Treatment.* Tsatsoulis A, Wyckoff JA, Brown FM, Eds. New York, Humana, 2009, p. 167–180.

43. Grodnitskaya EE, Grigoryan OR, Klinyshkova EV, Andreeva EN, Melnichenko GA, Dedov, II: Effect on carbohydrate metabolism and analysis of acceptability (menstrual cycle control) of extended regimens of the vaginally inserted hormone-releasing system "NuvaRing" as compared with the standard 21/7 regime in reproductive-age women with type 1 diabetes mellitus. *Gynecol Endocrinol* 26:663–668, 2010

44. Stewart A, Cummins C, Gold L, Jordan R, Phillips W: The effectiveness of the levonorgestrel-releasing intrauterine system in menorrhagia: a systematic review. *BJOG* 108:74–86, 2001

45. Reader D, Thomas AM: Medical nutrition therapy: goals for pregnancy complicated by pre-existing diabetes mellitus. In *Managing Preexisting Diabetes and Pregnancy: Technical Reviews and Consensus Recommendations.* Kitzmiller JL, Jovanovic LB, Brown FM, Coustan DR, Reader D, Eds. Alexandria, VA, American Diabetes Assocation, 2008, p. 15–89

46. De-Regil LM, Palacios C, Ansary A, Kulier R, Pena-Rosas JP: Vitamin D supplementation for women during pregnancy. *Cochrane Database Syst Rev* CD008873, 2012

47. Correa A, Botto L, Liu Y, Mulinare J, Erickson JD: Do multivitamin supplements attenuate the risk for diabetes-associated birth defects? *Pediatrics* 111:1146–1151, 2003

48. Conway B, Miller RG, Costacou T, et al.: Temporal patterns in overweight and obesity in type 1 diabetes. *Diabet Med* 27:398–404, 2010

49. Cnattingius S, Bergstrom R, Lipworth L, Kramer MS: Prepregnancy weight and the risk of adverse pregnancy outcomes. *N Engl J Med* 338:147–152, 1998

50. Kristensen J, Vestergaard M, Wisborg K, Kesmodel U, Secher NJ: Prepregnancy weight and the risk of stillbirth and neonatal death. *BJOG* 112:403–408, 2005

51. Chung JH, Melsop KA, Gilbert WM, Caughey AB, Walker CK, Main EK: Increasing pre-pregnancy body mass index is predictive of a progressive escalation in adverse pregnancy outcomes. *J Matern Fetal Neonatal Med* 9:1635–1639, 2012

52. Dixon JB, Dixon ME, O'Brien PE: Birth outcomes in obese women after laparoscopic adjustable gastric banding. *Obstet Gynecol* 106:965–972, 2005

53. Magdaleno R, Jr., Pereira BG, Chaim EA, Turato ER: Pregnancy after bariatric surgery: a current view of maternal, obstetrical and perinatal challenges. *Arch Gynecol Obstet* 285:559–566, 2012

54. Kitzmiller JL, American Diabetes Association: *Managing Preexisting Diabetes and Pregnancy: Technical Reviews and Consensus Recommendations for Care.* Alexandria, VA, American Diabetes Association, 2008

55. Kitzmiller JL, Block JM, Brown FM, et al.: Managing preexisting diabetes for pregnancy: summary of evidence and consensus recommendations for care. *Diabetes Care* 31:1060–1079, 2008

56. Kitzmiller JL, Buchanan TA, Kjos S, Combs CA, Ratner RE: Pre-conception care of diabetes, congenital malformations, and spontaneous abortions. *Diabetes Care* 19:514–541, 1996

57. Garg S, Ampudia-Blasco FJ, Pfohl M: Rapid-acting insulin analogues in basal-bolus regimens in type 1 diabetes mellitus. *Endocrine Practice* 16:486–505, 2010

58. Kinsley B: Achieving better outcomes in pregnancies complicated by type 1 and type 2 diabetes mellitus. *Clinical Therapeutics* 29(Suppl. D):S153–S160, 2007

59. Mukhopadhyay A, Farrell T, Fraser RB, Ola B: Continuous subcutaneous insulin infusion vs. intensive conventional insulin therapy in pregnant diabetic women: a systematic review and metaanalysis of randomized, controlled trials. *Am J Obstet Gynecol* 197:447–456, 2007

60. Wollitzer AD, Zisser H, Jovanovic L: Insulin pumps and their use in pregnancy. *Diabetes Technol Ther* 12 (Suppl. 1):S33–S36, 2010

61. Pollex E, Moretti ME, Koren G, Feig DS: Safety of insulin glargine use in pregnancy: a systematic review and meta-analysis. *Ann Pharmacother* 45:9–16, 2011

62. Mathiesen ER, Hod M, Ivanisevic M, Duran Garcia S, Brondsted L, Jovanovic L, Damm P, McCance DR, on behalf of the Detemir in Pregnancy Study Group: Maternal efficacy and safety outcomes in a randomized, controlled trial comparing insulin detemir with NPH insulin in 310 pregnant women with type 1 diabetes. *Diabetes Care* 35:2012–2017, 2012

63. de Valk HW, Visser GH: Insulin during pregnancy, labour and delivery. *Best Pract Res Clin Obstet Gynaecol* 25:65–76, 2011

64. Ekbom P, Damm P, Feldt-Rasmussen B, Feldt-Rasmussen U, Molvig J, Mathiesen ER: Pregnancy outcome in type 1 diabetic women with microalbuminuria. *Diabetes Care* 24:1739–1744, 2001

65. Gordon M, Landon MB, Samuels P, Hissrich S, Gabbe SG: Perinatal outcome and long-term follow-up associated with modern management of diabetic nephropathy. *Obstet Gynecol* 87:401–409, 1996

66. Jones DC, Hayslett JP: Outcome of pregnancy in women with moderate or severe renal insufficiency. *N Engl J Med* 335:226–232, 1996

67. Biesenbach GS, H. Zazgornik, J: Influence of pregnancy on progression of diabetic nephropathy and subsequent requirement of renal replacement therapy in female type 1 diabetic patients with impaired renal function. *Nephrol Dial Transplant* 7:105–109, 1992

68. Rossing K, Jacobsen P, Hommel E, et al.: Pregnancy and progression of diabetic nephropathy. *Diabetologia* 45:36–41, 2002

69. The Diabetes Control and Complications Trial Research Group: Effect of pregnancy on microvascular complications in the diabetes control and complications trial. *Diabetes Care* 23:1084–1091, 2000

70. Klein BE MS, Klein R: Effect of pregnancy on progression of diabetic retinopathy. *Diabetes Care* 13:34–40, 1990

71. Chew EY, Mills JL, Metzger BE, Remaley NA, Jovanovic-Peterson L, Knopp RH, Conley M, Rand L, Simpson JL, Holmes LB, et al.: Metabolic control and progression of retinopathy. The Diabetes in Early Pregnancy study. National Institute of Child Health and Human Development Diabetes in Early Pregnancy study. *Diabetes Care* 18:631–637, 1995

72. Rahman W RF, Yassin S, Al-Suleiman SA, Rahman J: Progression of retinopathy during pregnancy in type 1 diabetes mellitus. *Clinical and Experimental Ophthalmology* 35:231–236, 2007
73. Temple RC, Aldridge VA, Sampson MJ, Greenwood RH, Heyburn PJ, Glenn A: Impact of pregnancy on the progression of diabetic retinopathy in type 1 diabetes. *Diabet Med* 18:573–577, 2001
74. Vérier-Mine O, Chaturvedi N, Webb D, Fuller JH: Is pregnancy a risk factor for microvascular complications? The EURODIAB Prospective Complications study. *Diabet Med* 22:1503–1509, 2005
75. Chobanian AV, Bakris GL, Black HR, et al.: Seventh report of the Joint National Committee on Prevention, Detection, Evaluation, and Treatment of High Blood Pressure. *Hypertension* 42:1206–1252, 2003
76. Bos-Thompson M-A, Hillaire-Buys D, Muller F, et al.: Fetal toxic effects of angiotensin II receptor antagonists: case report and follow-up after birth. *Ann Pharmacother* 39:157–161, 2005
77. Cooper WO, Hernandez-Diaz S, Arbogast PG, et al.: Major congenital malformations after first-trimester exposure to ACE inhibitors. *N Engl J Med* 354:2443–2451, 2006
78. Li DK, Yang C, Andrade S, Tavares V, Ferber JR: Maternal exposure to angiotensin converting enzyme inhibitors in the first trimester and risk of malformations in offspring: a retrospective cohort study. *BMJ* 343:d5931, 2011
79. Diav-Citrin O, Shechtman S, Halberstadt Y, et al.: Pregnancy outcome after in utero exposure to angiotensin converting enzyme inhibitors or angiotensin receptor blockers. *Reproductive Toxicology* 31:540–545, 2011
80. Porta M, Hainer JW, Jansson SO, et al.: Exposure to candesartan during the first trimester of pregnancy in type 1 diabetes: experience from the placebo-controlled DIabetic REtinopathy Candesartan Trials. *Diabetologia* 54:1298–1303, 2011
81. Sibai BM, Mabie WC, Shamsa F, Villar MA, Anderson GD: A comparison of no medication versus methyldopa or labetalol in chronic hypertension during pregnancy. *Am J Obstetrics and Gynecology* 162:960–966; discussion 6–7, 1990
82. Butters L, Kennedy S, Rubin PC: Atenolol in essential hypertension during pregnancy. *BMJ* 301:587–589, 1990
83. Roth A, Elkayam U: Acute myocardial infarction associated with pregnancy. *Ann Intern Med* 125:751–762, 1996
84. Duntas LH, Orgiazzi J, Brabant G: The interface between thyroid and diabetes mellitus. *Clinical Endocrinology* 24 Feb 2011. doi: 10.1111/j.1365-2265.2011.04029.x. [Epub ahead of print]
85. Tsatsoulis A, Wyckoff J, Brown FM, eds.: *Diabetes in Women: Pathophysiology and Therapy.* New York, Humana, 2009
86. Pasternak Y, Weintraub AY, Shoham-Vardi I, et al.: Obstetric and perinatal outcomes in women with eating disorders. *J Womens Health* (Larchmt) 21:61–65, 2012
87. Dalfra MG, Nicolucci A, Bisson T, Bonsembiante B, Lapolla A: Quality of life in pregnancy and post-partum: a study in diabetic patients. *Qual Life Res* 21:291–298, 2012

APPENDIX 17.I.A

Preconception Checklist:

1. Achieve optimal glycemic control
2. Supplement with folic acid 600 mcg daily
3. Consult with a registered dietitian familiar with diabetes and pregnancy care (see chapter 10)
4. Exercise (see chapter 11)
5. Develop strong diabetes self-management skills (see chapter 7)
6. Take a dilated retinal exam
7. Treat proliferative diabetic retinopathy or macular edema before conception
8. Screen for nephropathy with serum creatinine or estimated glomerular filtration rate and urine albumin-to-creatinine ratio
9. Thyroid function test screening (thyroid stimulating hormone)
10. Consider coronary artery disease screening, if multiple risk factors
11. Pursue mental health counseling, when indicated

APPENDIX 17.I.B Risk of Major or Minor Anomaly According to Periconceptional A1C

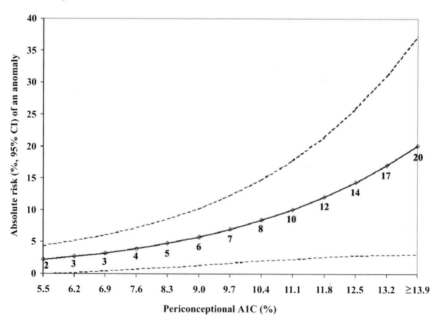

Data are presented as an absolute risk (solid line) ± 95% CIs (dashed lines).

Reprinted from Guerin et al.,[31] with permission from the publisher.

II. Pregnancy

Florence M. Brown, MD

INTRODUCTION

Type 1 diabetes (T1D) profoundly affects the complex physiologic and metabolic changes occurring during pregnancy.[1] In normal pregnancy, the physiology is tightly regulated. In pregnant women with T1D, however, insulin insufficiency causes wide fluctuations in blood glucose levels.

This section reviews optimal glucose management in varying degrees of insulin resistance during pregnancy, describes how pregnancy affects diabetes complications, and explains how to screen for and treat complications and concurrent conditions of diabetes. It also describes how diabetes complicates pregnancy and may affect neonatal outcomes. When possible, the literature reviewed will include studies done in women with T1D. Because of the paucity of research in pregnant T1D women, where necessary, this section extrapolates from various studies performed on pregnant women with type 2 diabetes (T2D), gestational diabetes, pregnant women without diabetes, and nonpregnant women with T1D. An important resource for the reader is the American Diabetes Association's "Managing Preexisting Diabetes for Pregnancy."[2,3] Obstetric management is beyond the scope of this chapter.

The health care team must work closely with the pregnant woman to optimize glucose levels and monitor potential complications. This helps to ensure a more positive outcome for both mother and infant.

INFANTS OF DIABETIC MOTHERS

The insulin insufficiency in T1D causes higher maternal blood glucoses and may result in a surfeit of glucose from the maternal circulation to the fetus. This causes excessive fetal adipose growth and affects anthropomorphic measurements as well as metabolic homeostasis of the fetus. In patients with diabetes, the Pederson hypothesis refers to the transplacental passage of excessive maternal glucose to the fetus, resulting in accretion of fetal fat.[4] In addition to glucose, other factors such as free fatty acids may affect fetal fat accumulation and increase the risk of large for gestational age (LGA) or macrosomia in infants. This is true particularly in pregnancies complicated by obesity.[5]

The long-term impact of excessive fuel to the fetus results in behavioral, anthropometric, and metabolic imprinting and constitutes fuel-mediated teratogenesis,[6] as infants of diabetic mothers are more likely to develop obesity[7] and impaired glucose tolerance as children and adolescents.[8,9] On the other hand, inadequate nutrient supply, possibly related to placental vascular insufficiency[10,11] may result in small for gestational age (SGA) infants.

SGA is common in patients with kidney disease. In one study, SGA was observed in 2, 4, and 45% of T1D patients with normal urinary albumin excretion (UAE), microalbuminuria, and diabetic nephropathy, respectively.[12] SGA consequences may include an adverse cardiometabolic profile as proposed by Barker (1986).[13] Low target blood glucoses may predispose the mother to severe hypoglycemia and its consequences.[14] Therefore, establishing optimal maternal glucose targets and weight gain in pregnancy is critical for the maternal fetal unit but may need to be individualized based on such factors as maternal hypoglycemia unawareness[15] and infant growth patterns in utero.[16,17]

MATERNAL COMPLICATIONS

Attention to maternal complications of diabetes (such as eye or renal disease) is necessary. Pregnancy may lead to exacerbations of these conditions and complications may adversely affect the pregnancy, resulting in greater risk of premature delivery and hypertensive complications.[2,3] The management complexity of T1D in pregnancy requires a team approach to care.[18,19] Complex pregnancy care issues require the following management team for women with T1D: diabetologist or endocrinologist, obstetrician (perinatal specialist), pediatrician or neonatologist, certified diabetes educator, registered dietician, patient and her partner, and any other relevant members of her support system.[18,19]

Interestingly, cases of new-onset T1D may be seen in pregnancy. The insulin resistance of pregnancy in the setting of inadequate β-cell reserve because of autoimmune destruction[20,21] may precipitate new cases of T1D.

INSULIN MANAGEMENT

Continuous Subcutaneous Insulin Infusion vs. Multiple Daily Injections

Excellent glycemic control in the first trimester and continued throughout pregnancy is associated with the lowest frequency of maternal, fetal, and neonatal complications.[3] The role of daily pattern management of insulin with either multiple daily injections (MDI) or continuous subcutaneous insulin infusion (CSII) is to achieve overnight, fasting, and pre- and postprandial targets while minimizing postabsorptive and nocturnal hypoglycemia. A few randomized controlled trials (RCTs) involving small numbers of patients of CSII versus MDI in pregnancy reveal that the outcome measures are not significantly different between the two groups.[22] In a Cochrane review of 23 different RCTs involving 976 nonpregnant subjects using CSII versus MDI, CSII was associated with lower A1C, lower risk of severe hypoglycemia, and improved quality of life.[23] CSII requires commitment and adherence to frequent glucose monitoring, carbohydrate counting, and an ability to implement sick-day rules quickly in the setting of unexplained hyperglycemia or ketonuria to reduce the risk of diabetic ketoacidosis.

Fluctuating Insulin Requirements

During pregnancy, insulin requirements fluctuate (see Table 17.II.1). In the first 9 weeks of gestation, insulin requirements increase. This is followed by a period

Table 17.II.1 Insulin Requirements during Pregnancy

Time Period	Insulin Sensitivity	Insulin Requirements
Early first trimester 0–9 weeks	Decreased	Increasing requirements
Late first and early second trimester 9–16 weeks	Increased	Reduce basal and bolus insulin
16 weeks	Nadir	Low requirements
16–37 weeks	Decreased	Requirements double or triple (from preconception doses); more bolus insulin, higher basal doses at nighttime: daytime basal may be truncated
~37–40 weeks	Increased	Insulin requirements may decrease
Immediately postpartum	Increased	Insulin requirements decrease to ~50% of preconception doses

of decreased insulin requirements with a nadir at ~16 weeks. Insulin requirements then increase sharply from 16 to 37 weeks,[24] often doubling during this time[25] and then decrease in approximately the final month until delivery.[26] Insulin delivery concurrent to mealtime may not adequately match glucose absorption into the blood stream and often results in peak postprandial blood glucose levels that are above target followed by postabsorptive hypoglycemia (see Table 17.II.2). Adjusting the timing of the insulin bolus to 15 min before the meal, if the preprandial glucose is >70 mg/dl with no hypoglycemia symptoms, may decrease the

Table 17.II.2 ADA Standards of Care Targets[2,3]

Target Maternal Glucose[a]	
Fasting	60–99 mg/dl
Peak postprandial	100–129
Mean	<100
Labor and delivery	80–110 mg/dl (mean <100)[52,53]
	Insulin drips + D10 50cc/hr[2]
A1C	Preconception <7% and as close to normal as possible without significant hypoglycemia[2,3] During pregnancy <6%

[a] These represent the mean +2 standard deviation for normal. They are targets, but not everyone can achieve them. There is certainly marked variability, which explains why there is greater incidence of LGA in patients with T1D.

postprandial glucose and reduce postabsorptive hypoglycemia in the setting of controlled carbohydrate intake. More research is needed, however, to evaluate the timing of insulin boluses to meals during pregnancy. During labor and delivery, diabetes is best managed with insulin drips (Table 17.II.3). After delivery, there is marked insulin sensitivity that requires an immediate reduction in insulin dose to ~50% of the preconception doses. Women who breast-feed may continue to have lower basal insulin needs than women who do not breast-feed.[27]

Maternal Hypoglycemia

Hypoglycemia, defined as glucose <50 mg/dl, occurs in 20% of pregnancy days.[28] Severe hypoglycemia occurs in 23–71% of pregnancies in T1D women,[29–32] with most occurring during the first trimester (41 vs. 19% in third trimester)[33] and at night.[30] Most incidences occur in women with hypoglycemia unawareness (35%) compared with those who sense hypoglycemia (19%).[34]

The pathophysiology of hypoglycemia unawareness is related to lower A1C and glucose targets,[14] causing a lower threshold for glucose counterregulation.[35,36] Bjorklund,[37] however, found glucose counter-regulation to be normal in pregnancy, with the exception of growth hormone secretion. During pregnancy, hypoglycemia may occur in patients who reactively dose insulin to address increasing insulin requirements rather than manage dosing by observing glucose patterns. For example giving a supplemental (reactive) bolus correction for an elevated 1-h postprandial blood glucose increases the risk of hypoglycemia from the bolus stacking. Nausea does not appear to be associated with increased hypoglycemia frequency,[31] although review articles speculate that morning sickness in the first trimester causes hypoglycemia. Patients should be mindful of consuming consistent carbs during this time when morning sickness, nausea, or vomiting may lead to carbohydrate avoidance or overindulgence.

Hypoglycemia does not increase the risk of birth defects[30,32,38–40] or fetal death.[30] It does not affect fetal heart rate, breathing, body movement, umbilical artery Doppler wave forms,[41,42] or neonatal intelligence.[43] A catastrophic hypoglycemic event, however, such as a motor vehicle accident, could have profound adverse effects on the mother and, consequently, on the fetus.[44]

The cornerstone of hypoglycemia screening is self-monitoring of blood glucose (SMBG). Women with T1D in pregnancy should test before and after meals, before and after exercise, and periodically in the middle of the night (see Table 17.II.4). Patients should always test blood glucoses before driving. Some women self-test as many as 10–20 times each day. Continuous glucose monitoring (CGM) provides a large data set that may help assess a patient's health risk more accurately.[44] Low glucose alarms may alert patients of hypoglycemia before the onset of symptoms.

Hyperglycemia and Diabetic Ketoacidosis

SMBG and intensive insulin therapies have decreased the prevalence of diabetic ketoacidosis (DKA) in pregnancies from 16.7% in 1960[45] to 1.2–4.1% in the past two decades.[20,46,47] Stillbirth rates have reduced dramatically from 1920

Table 17.II.3 Two Protocols for Insulin Management of Labor and Delivery

	A.	B.
Intravenous Fluids	Intravenous infusion of normal saline is begun. Once active labor begins or glucose levels decrease to <70 mg/dL, infusion is changed to 5% dextrose and delivered at a rate of 100–150 cc/h to achieve a glucose level of ~100 mg/dL (5.6 mM).	BG >130 mg/dL, LR at 125 mL/h BG <130 mg/dL, begin D5LR at 125 mL/h
Initiating insulin	Regular (short-acting) insulin is administered by intravenous infusion at a rate of 1.25 units/h if glucose levels are >100 mg/dL.	Mix 25 units regular insulin in 250 mL normal saline (1U: 10 mL) Algorithm (see Protocol B Algorithm)

Protocol B Algorithm

Maternal Plasma Glucose in mg/dL (mM)	Insulin (units/h)	Individualized Dose
<70 (<3.9)	0.0	
71–90 (3.9–5.0)	0.5	
91–110 (5.1–6.1)	1.0	
111–130 (6.2–7.2)	2.0	
131–150 (7.3–8.3)	3.0	
151–170 (8.4–9.4)	4.0	
171–190 (9.5–10.6)	5.0	
>190 (>10.6)	Check ketones	

The usual dose of intermediate-acting insulin is given at bedtime, but the usual morning dose is withheld. In both protocols, glucose levels are checked hourly using a bedside meter allowing for adjustment in the insulin or glucose infusion rate. Protocols differ in the blood glucose thresholds at which to infuse dextrose-containing solutions and regular short-acting insulin. Many nursing clinicians believe it is simpler to always infuse 5% dextrose, as with perioperative management of diabetic patients.

Data discussed in the text suggests a maternal glucose target <100 mg/dL (<5.6 mM) to minimize neonatal hypoglycemia.

Protocol A is taken from ACOG 05a based on data from Jovanovic 80 and Coustan 04.

Protocol B is taken from Kitzmiller, American Diabetes Association[2] and assumes that many patients with T1D will have a small insulin requirement to remain normoglycemic.

LR, lactated Ringer's solution; D5LR, 5% dextrose lactated Ringer's solution

Reprinted from Kitzmiller, American Diabetes Association[2] with permission from the publisher.

Table 17.II.4 Treating Hypoglycemia in Pregnancy

Blood Glucose or Situation	Treatment
BG <70 mg/dl with symptoms	15 grams of fast-acting carbohydrate every 15 min
BG <50 mg/dl	30 grams of fast-acting carbohydrate every 15 min until BG >70 mg/dl
Unconscious or uncooperative patients	Glucagon emergency kit

when it was 650 in 1,000 births to the current levels of 18–25 in 1,000 births (relative risk 3.6–6.2 compared with normal pregnancies),[48] presumably from improved glycemic control and fetal monitoring (Figure 17.II.1). Excess still-births in pregnancies complicated by diabetes are related to poorly controlled hyperglycemia and congenital malformations. Stillbirths may occur for reasons unrelated to diabetes.

Pathophysiology

DKA occurs at lower glucose levels because of the ketosis-prone state of pregnancy.[46,49] Precipitating factors may include infection, insulin omission, insulin pump infusion problems, use of β-sympathomimetic drugs such as ter-butaline (to prevent preterm labor), or glucocorticoids (to induce fetal lung maturity).[20,50,51] Most cases are avoidable if close attention is paid to glucose

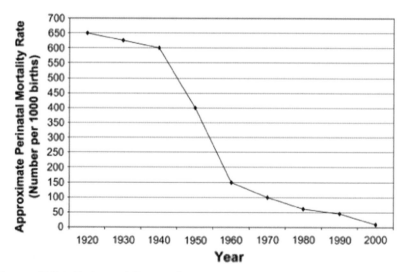

Figure 17.II.1 Estimated Rate of Stillbirth in Diabetic Women: 1920–2000.[48]

Reprinted with permission from the publisher.

monitoring and the use of sick-day rules. Insulin pump–related hyperglycemia should be promptly treated with subcutaneous insulin bolus injection and changing the infusion set.

Maternal and Fetal Outcomes

Neonatal hypoglycemia, macrosomia, and respiratory distress are reduced when average antepartum blood glucoses are <110 mg/dl.[52] The lowest risk of neonatal hypoglycemia occurs when maternal intrapartum glucose is <100 mg/dl.[53] Intrapartum glucose weighs more heavily on the risk of neonatal hypoglycemia than antepartum glucose control.[53,54] Maternal mortality from DKA is rare.[33] Fetal mortality from DKA ranges between 9 and 35%.[46,47,55] Increased stillbirth rates occur in poorly controlled T1D and may be related to fetal hypoxia and acidosis from acute and chronic fetal hyperglycemia.[48]

Patients and providers should have a low threshold for testing urine or serum ketones or electrolytes in patients with more than usual symptoms of nausea, vomiting, abdominal pain, thirst, urination, or persistent and unexplained glucose >200 mg/dl.

DKA treatment is the same as for nonpregnant adults. Poor fetal heart rate variability and late decelerations may reverse with rapid treatment of DKA, and therefore they are not indications for immediate delivery.[20]

COMPLICATIONS OF DIABETES AND CONCURRENT CONDITIONS

Hypertension

Hypertension is a blood pressure >130/80 mmHg. Standards for women with T1D are compiled from information from nonpregnant women with diabetes and pregnant women without diabetes (see Table 17.II.5). Hypertension management ideally starts preconception. For women who present for prenatal care de novo, however, antihypertensive medications that are safe in pregnancy should replace those associated with adverse effects.

Perinatal Outcomes

A randomized controlled study of pregnant hypertensive women (not stated as having diabetes) evaluating tight (target BP <140/90) versus very tight blood pressure control (target BP <130/80 mmHg) demonstrated less severe hypertension, fewer hospitalizations, more advanced gestational age without a difference in preterm delivery or difference in birth weight in the very tight control group.[60] Thus, there is target blood pressure concordance with respect to normative data, with the long-term goal to reduce maternal end organ damage and with improved fetal outcomes. One should avoid targeting blood pressure significantly below the mean, however, because of the potential increased risk of fetal growth restriction and fetal mortality.[61]

Table 17.II.5 Standards of Care and Normative Data

Nonpregnant individuals with diabetes ADA <130/80 mmHg	■ Reduce risk of micro/macrovascular complications based on RCT[56,57]
Pregnant women without diabetes 110–129/65–79 mmHg	■ Normative data (mean + 2 standard deviation) in pregnant women without diabetes ■ Depends on trimester and ethnicity[58,59]
Pregnant women with diabetes 110–129/65–79 mmHg	■ Taking into account above recommendations[2,3]

RCT, randomized controlled trial.

Treatment

Antihypertensives are indicated for the treatment of chronic hypertension (not gestational hypertension or preeclampsia)[62] during pregnancy when the blood pressure is greater than 130/80. RCTs of antihypertensive therapy in pregnancy were reviewed in a Cochrane study[63] and noted in Kitzmiller[2] (see Table 17.II.6 and Table 17.II.7).

Diabetic Nephropathy

UAE rates increase during the normal pregnancy in the third trimester[68] and persist through the first postpartum week.[69,70] Glomerular filtration rate (GFR) increases by 50% above nonpregnant levels.[71]

In uncomplicated T1D, UAE rates are mildly increased above normal physiology but return to normal by 6 weeks after delivery.[72] In patients with diabetic nephropathy, there may be marked increases in UAE with nephrotic range proteinuria in some cases, but postpartum UAE rates usually return to baseline preconception levels.[42,73] Diabetic nephropathy with renal insufficiency, however, confers significant maternal risk (see Table 17.II.8 and Table 17.II.9).[2]

Please refer to Section I: Preconception Counseling and Care for perinatal outcomes.[2]

As preeclampsia presents with proteinuria (300 mg/day) and hypertension (BP >140/90),[62] it may be difficult to distinguish between worsening of diabetic nephropathy, pregnancy-specific transient glomerular and tubular changes, and superimposed preeclampsia. A retrospective cohort study demonstrated increased risk of preterm delivery at 32 weeks in patients with diabetic nephropathy and suboptimal hypertension control based on BP >130/80 versus <130/80 mmHg (38.1 vs. 4.6%), $P < 0.007$.[74] In a small prospective study in women with T1D and microabuminuria or nephropathy, primary methyl dopa (first-line therapy) and/or labetolol or nifedipine to target BP <135/85 and UAE <300 mg/24 h

Table 17.II.6 Randomized, Controlled Trials of Antihypertensive Drug Therapy before 28 Weeks Gestation in Pregnant Women with Chronic Hypertension[a]

Author (year)[b]	Study Group (N)	Comparison Group (N)	Significant Treatment: Maternal	Effects: Infant
Leather, 1968	Methyldopa and bendrofluazide, 23	No drug, 24	Diastolic BP lowered 10 mmHg	Gestation 10 days longer; fetal loss 0 of 23 vs. 5 of 24
Redman, 1976, 1977 Mutch, 1977a,b Cockburn, 1982	Methyldopa, 101	No drug, 107	S/D BP lowered 10/6 mmHg; threefold less signs of late severe hypertension	Reduced midpregnancy loss; BW, SGA NS; infant development NS
Arias, 1979	Thiazide plus methyldopa or hydralazine, 29	No drug, 29	Less late-pregnancy aggravation of hypertension	BW, SGA NS
Sibai, 1984	Thiazide continued, 10	Thiazide stopped by 14 weeks, 10	Much less gain in plasma volume at 26–32 weeks; MAP NS	Perinatal outcome NS
Weitz, 1987	Methyldopa, 13	Placebo, 12	MAP lowered from 108 to 96 mmHg	Gestation 10 days longer; BW NS; SGA 0 of 13 vs. 3 of 12
Butters, 1990	Atenolol, 15	Placebo, 14	Mean diastolic BP 74 vs. 81 in control group	Reduced placental weight and BW; atenolol 10/15 SGA; infant weight NS at 1 year
Sibai, 1990	Methyldopa, 87; labetalol, 86	No drug, 90	Mean systolic BP* 126 vs. 122 vs. 133; mean diastolic BP* 78 vs. 76 vs. 82	Perinatal outcome NS

[a] Mostly stage 1 hypertension

[b] All are English-language publication.

*At 27–29 weeks after ~16 weeks of treatment; percentage of subjects who were African American not stated

BP, blood pressure; BW, birth weight; MAP, mean arterial pressure; N, number; NS, no significant difference; SID, systolic/diastolic; SGA, small for gestational age (<10th percentile)
Reprinted from Kitzmiller, American Diabetes Association[2] with permission from the publisher.

Table 17.II.7 Hypertensive Medications and Recommendations

Agent	Recommendations
Central-acting sympathoplegic: methyl dopa	■ Most studied agent ■ Reduces fetal loss and increases length of gestation compared with placebo
Methyl dopa and labetolol	Labetolol may be more effective than methyl dopa[64] and better tolerated
Calcium channel blockers: Nifedipine and diltiazem	No RCT comparing these agents with other meds, but they are routinely used
ACE-Is and ARBs	Contraindicated in pregnancy*
Diuretics	Usually not prescribed because of concern of reduced plasma volume & utero-placental blood flow[65]
Atenolol and clonidine	Reduce cardiac output & have been associated with fetal growth restriction[66,67]

* Fetopathy associated with ACE-Is and ARBs in the second and third trimesters is well established and consists of intrauterine growth restriction, oligohydramnios, skull defects, infant anuria, renal failure, and death.

ACE-I, angiotensin-converting-enzyme inhibitors; ARB, angiotensin receptor blockers; RCT, randomized controlled trial

Table 17.II.8 Perinatal Outcome in 188 Women with Diabetic Neuropathy Whose Pregnancies Advanced to >20 Weeks Gestation, Grouped by Preserved or Impaired Renal Function in Early Pregnancy

	Preserved Initial Renal Function (*n* = 123)	Impaired Initial Renal function (*n* = 65)*
Delivery <34 weeks	17 (13.8)	29 (44.6)
Fetal growth restriction (<10th %)	17 (13.8)	18 (27.7)
Major congenital malformation	8 (6.5)	5 (7.7)
Stillbirth	2 (1.6)	2 (3.1)
Neonatal death	0	2 (3.1)
Perinatal survival	121 (98.4)	61 (93.8)

Data are *n* (%)

* sCr > 1.2–1.4 mg/dL (>106–125 μM) or CrCl <80 mL/min

Data based on Kitzmiller 81a, Jovanovic 84, Dicker 86, Reece 88, Kimmerle 95, Mackie 96, Purdy 96, Bar 99, Khoury 02.

DN, diabetic nephropathy.

Reprinted from Kitzmiller, American Diabetes Association [2] with permission from the publisher.

Table 17.II.9 Maternal Outcome and Nephropathy

Maternal Outcome	Diabetic Nephropathy and Impaired Renal Function	Diabetic Nephropathy with Intact Renal Function
GFR decline >15%	67%	26.7%
Renal failure after pregnancy	44.7	4.7

GFR, glomerular filtration rate

may improve outcomes.[75] A nondihydropyridine calcium channel blocker (CCB) diltiazem has been shown to reduce urine protein excretion in nonpregnant subjects with T1D[76] and in a small (*n* = 7) study of pregnant women.[77] ACE-Is and ARBs are contraindicated as noted in the section on hypertension. A knowledge gap exists in the treatment of diabetic nephropathy in pregnancy. Multicentered RCTs are needed to evaluate various antihypertensive options.

Retinopathy

Classifying diabetic retinopathy (DR) is the same as in the nonpregnant state and is defined according to the ADA Technical Review and Position Statement on DR.[78,79] (Also see chapter 16, Complications: Detection and Management.)

Table 17.II.10 International Clinical Diabetic Retinopathy Disease Severity Scale

Disease Severity Level	Findings Based upon Dilated Ophthalmoscopy	Frequency of Examinations
No apparent retinopathy	No abnormalities	First and third trimester
Mild NPDR	Microaneurysms only	First and third trimester
Moderate NPDR	More than just microaneurysms, but less than severe NPDR	Each trimester
Severe NPDR	Any of the following, but no proliferative changes: >20 intraretinal hemorrhages in each of 4 quadrants; definite venous beading in ≥2 quadrants; prominent intraretinal vascular/microvascular abnormalities in ≥1 quadrant	Monthly
PDR	≥1 of the following: neovascularization; vitreous/preretinal hemorrhage	Monthly if active; each trimester if previously treated

Based upon Wilkinson 03 and Fong 04b.

NPDR, nonproliferative diabetic retinopathy; PDR, proliferative diabetic retinopathy.

Consider more frequent screening in milder retinopathy at baseline but other strong risk factors.

Reprinted from Kitzmiller, American Diabetes Association[2] with permission from the publisher.

Pregnancy induces a transient worsening of retinopathy (see Table 17.II.10).[80,81] The relationship of angiogenic (vascular endothelial growth factors [VEGF]), inflammatory, vasoactive, and growth (IGF) factors to the worsening of diabetic retinopathy in pregnancy are unclear.[82,83]

The risk factors for progression during pregnancy[2,84] include retinal status at conception,[2] diabetes duration, elevated A1C at conception, rapid normalization of glycemia,[85] hypertension or nephropathy, and preeclampsia.

Optimal screening during pregnancy is approximately every trimester or more frequently depending on the degree of baseline retinopathy or macular edema. Laser therapy is the standard of care based on the Early Treatment Diabetic Retinopathy Study[86] and the Diabetic Retinopathy Study[87] with attention to potential rapid progression in pregnancy. There are no studies of intraocular steroids or anti-VEGF in pregnancy to evaluate risks or benefits of these therapies. Anti-VEGF could potentially adversely affect pregnancy, as anti-VEGF mechanisms may be implicated in preeclampsia.[88]

Neuropathy

Diabetes is a risk factor for hyperemesis.[89] *Gastroparesis* antedating pregnancy may worsen resulting in severe hyperemesis gravidarum.[90] For gastroparesis, metoclopramide appears to be safe in pregnancy,[91] demonstrating no increased risk of congenital malformations, preterm delivery, low birth weight, or perinatal death. Ondansetron has not been studied in RCTs.[92] Intravenous (IV) hydration with diazempam for intractable cases of hyperemesis reduces hospitalizations and improves patient satisfaction.[93] A useful review of the literature around therapeutic options for gastroparesis is provided by Festin.[92]

Carpal tunnel syndrome is more common in pregnant patients with diabetes[94] and may cause discomfort. Wrist splints are a noninvasive treatment of choice. Local dexamethasone injection may be effective in reducing pain and improving the electrophysiologic parameters of the median nerve in patients that do not respond to wrist splinting.[95] Surgery may be necessary for cases that do not resolve postpartum.[96] There are few reports of painful diabetic peripheral neuropathy in pregnancy, but no RCTs regarding treatment.

Cardiovascular Disease

There are only case reports of cardiovascular complications in pregnant women with T1D. The incidence in nonpregnant women with T1D is a function of age and renal status.[97] Pregnancy increases cardiac output, heart rate, and hypercoagulability (prothrombotic state) and therefore may exacerbate any preexisting cardiac disease. If a woman has atypical symptoms, then consider obtaining an electrocardiogram (ECG), transthoracic echocardiogram (ECHO), or exercise ECHO.[98] Acute management of the patient with coronary artery disease (CAD) will not be discussed here, as it is rare. Anginal equivalents, such as dyspnea on exertion and fatigue, may be difficult to distinguish from normal pregnancy symptoms.

To manage the long-term risk factors, it is important to optimize glycemic control.[99] Smoking cessation, blood pressure (see hypertension targets) control, and improving lipid profiles are critical for improving outcomes. Medical nutrition therapy to reduce trans and saturated fats in diet may lower low-density lipoprotein (LDL) cholesterol. Statins are contraindicated during pregnancy, but the risk of inadvertent use appears to be small in studies with small numbers of subjects.[100] Omega-3 fatty acids may reduce hypertriglyceridemia. Aspirin therapy is not indicated for primary prevention in most women of child-bearing age with diabetes.[101]

Hyperlipidemia

In the nonpregnant state, lipid profiles in well-controlled, uncomplicated T1D are not different from nondiabetic patients.[102,103] LDL cholesterol and triglycerides increase, however, in those with albuminuria and retinopathy compared with uncomplicated T1D.[104]

In normal pregnancy, triglycerides may more than double, and total cholesterol and LDL cholesterol levels may increase by 50%. High-density lipoprotein (HDL) cholesterol rises midgestation and then returns to baseline in late gestation.[105] In women with T1D, lipid changes in pregnancy are not so different from normal pregnancies except for a blunting of the normal midtrimester rise of HDL with corresponding lower total cholesterol.[106]

If a preconception lipid panel is not available, then one should be obtained with the baseline prenatal labs.[3] This helps assess cardiovascular risk with the understanding that levels may be higher during pregnancy. It also may identify patients who are at higher risk of hypertriglyceridemia (those with albuminuria and poorly controlled diabetes).

Medical nutrition therapy counseling should advise on a reduction of saturated fats to <7% of energy, the elimination of trans fats, and initiation of moderate exercise (e.g., walking, if not contraindicated). Omega-3 fatty acids in patients with marked hypertriglyceridemia (>1,000 mg/dl) may prevent pancreatitis, although this would be very unusual in the T1D population. The effects of omega-3 fatty acids during pregnancy in reducing childhood obesity,[107,108] allergies,[109,110] preventing preterm births,[111,112] enhancing neonatal neurologic development,[113,114] and reducing maternal depression[115] have been mixed and therefore would not be recommended at this time. The TrialNet omega-3 pilot study results are anticipated in 2013.

Thyroid Disease

Hypothyroidism. In normal pregnancies, human chorionic gonadotropin (hCG) stimulates the thyroid gland to increase thyroid hormone output and suppresses TSH.[116] Estrogen stimulates thyroid-binding globulin, leading to higher levels of total T4.[117] The target reference range for T4 is 1.5 times normal.[118] Plasma volume also increases 30–40%.[119] Increased iodine needs in pregnancy and increased renal clearance of iodine may cause maternal iodine deficiency, especially in iodine-poor regions of the world.[120–122]

In women with T1D, the prevalence of Hashimoto's is quite high (17–31%).[123–125] All women with T1D should be screened for thyroid disease early in pregnancy. Women with Hashimoto's should have TSH levels checked every 4 to 6 weeks. The prevalence of abortion, anemia, gestational hypertension, placental abruption, and postpartum hemorrhages are more frequently seen with overt hypothyroidism than with subclinical hypothyroidism,[121,126–130] but adverse perinatal outcomes were not seen in other studies.[131,132] Cognitive defects have been seen in some offspring evaluations[133–136] but not others.[122,137–139]

For treatment, the *Endocrine Society Practice Guidelines* suggests that if overt hypothyroidism is diagnosed during pregnancy, then thyroid function tests should be normalized as rapidly as possible. T4 dosage should be titrated to rapidly reach and thereafter maintain serum TSH concentrations of 0.1–2.5 µU/ml in the first trimester, 0.2–3 µU/ml in the second trimester, and 0.3–3.0 in the third trimester.[139,140]

Levothyroxine requirements rapidly increase between 6 and 16 weeks of gestation and subsequently plateau after 20 weeks. By 10 weeks of gestation, the levothyroxine dose increases ~30% compared with the baseline dose. By 20 weeks, the dose increases ~50% relative to the baseline dose but remains stable thereafter.[141,142] An effective titration strategy is to advise the patient with hypothyroidism to take two extra pills each week (e.g., nine instead of seven tabs) once they find out that they are pregnant until their first prenatal visit.[141] Postpartum, the L-thyroxine dose usually returns to the baseline preconception dose.

Hyperthyroidism due to Graves' disease. Hyperthyroidism is much less common than hypothyroidism, and the prevalence is not well described. It is more common in patients with T1D than in the general population, however, so women with T1D should be screened early in pregnancy. In cases of hyperthyroidism with unclear etiology, the presence of thyroid receptor antibodies may support the diagnosis of Graves' disease. Thyroid receptor antibodies may be helpful in evaluating disease activity in the fetus of patients with Graves' disease who have been treated previously with radioactive iodine or surgery. Postpartum, the neonate must be monitored when the mother has a history of Graves' disease, regardless of the current status of the mother's disease.

The diagnosis of hyperthyroidism is based on TSH suppression that is below trimester-specific norms (see normal ranges in the section Hypothyroidism) and a total T4 or total T3 that is greater than 1.5 times the normal nonpregnant reference range.[143] This may be distinguished from gestational hyperthyroidism in which the TSH is suppressed but total T4 and T3 are in the normal range for pregnancy.[143] Other less common causes of hyperthyroidism may include a toxic nodule or excessively high hCG levels resulting from molar pregnancy-induced changes.

Pregnancies complicated by Graves' disease may be at increased risk of preterm deliveries[144] or low–birth-weight infants.[145] There are no RCTs for treating hyperthyroidism in pregnancy.[146] Treatment with methimazole (MMI) in the first trimester may result in aplasia cutis (focal absence of the scalp epidermal layer), and treatment with propylthiouracil (PTU) rarely may cause fatal hepatotoxicity. Thus, the American Thyroid Association and the American Association of Clinical Endocrinologists recommend using PTU in the first trimester and methimazole in the second and third trimesters of pregnancy.[143] Thyroidectomy is recommended only in cases in which antithyroid drugs cannot be used. Radioactive iodine (RAI) is contraindicated in pregnancy.

Large for gestational age. Infants >90 percentile of weight for gestational age are considered LGA and those infants >4,000 grams have macrosomia. The incidence of macrosomia varies depending on the study (29%)[147] and (56%),[148] (45%).[33] An LGA incidence of 47% has been noted, with worse LGA in premature infants of T1D mothers (vs. control mothers) and overall a broader bell-shaped curve shifted to the right.[149]

The literature states variable findings for the pathophysiology, and it is probably multifactorial. Infant birth weight may be related to maternal gestational weight gain but not to preconception BMI,[150] although other studies suggest infant weight is related to preconception BMI.[151] After correcting for infant birth and placental weight,[152] maternal weight gain differences in pregnancies complicated by infants with macrosoma (vs. nonmacrosomia) may not be significant.

There is a knowledge gap in the literature about the pathophysiology and treatment of infants with LGA and macrosomia. Causes associated with LGA or macrosomia are poor glycemic control (A1C >7.0%) in the periconception to 12 weeks gestation period,[17] A1C >6.5% in the third trimester,[34] elevated fasting[52] or postprandial blood glucose,[153,154] elevated average daily blood glucose,[155] and episodic elevated postprandial blood glucoses despite normal A1C level.[156]

There is a strong relationship of LGA infants and the future risk of childhood obesity.[157–159] Maternal smoking during pregnancy may increase this risk.[160] LGA and macrosomia are associated with various complications, including neonatal hypoglycemia, metabolic imprinting, cardiomyopathy, immature lung development, and hyperbilirubinemia.

Fetal growth ultrasound with special attention to change in velocity of abdominal circumference growth relative to the biparietal diameter may predict LGA and macrosomia.[17] Recommended treatment is to achieve target glucoses while avoiding clinically significant hypoglycemia, follow target weight gain according to the Institute of Medicine 2009 recommendations,[161] and avoid tobacco use during pregnancy. Despite excellent medical care at many institutions, there continues to be a very high risk of this complication in infants of T1D mothers compared with control offspring.

Preterm Delivery

Preterm delivery is birth before 37 weeks. Prevalence in T1D varies from 21 to 37% (vs. 5.1% in control subjects).[162] In a French study, the prevalence of preterm delivery was 24% with spontaneous preterm delivery occurring in 9% and indicated preterm delivery occurring in 15% of pregnancies complicated by T1D. A1C >7% was associated with spontaneous preterm delivery. A1C >7%, worsening nephropathy, preeclampsia, and nulliparity were risk factors for indicated preterm delivery.[163]

Tocolytics (such as calcium channel blockers), magnesium sulfate, and bedrest are used to treat preterm labor. Several case reports note the onset of severe insulin resistance and DKA in patients treated with terbutaline for tocolysis, so it is best avoided in T1D patients.[164] Steroids (betamethasone or dexamethasone) accelerate fetal organ (including lung) development. Treatment with antenatal corticosteroids is associated with a reduction in neonatal deaths relative risk (RR) 0.69, 95% confidence levels (CI) 0.58–0.81, respiratory distress syndrome (RDS; RR 0.66, 95% CI 0.59–0.73), cerebroventricular hemorrhage (RR 0.54, 95% CI 0.43–0.69), and necrotizing enterocolitis (RR 0.46, 95% CI 0.29–0.74).[165] Insulin doses need to be adjusted in women with T1D treated with steroids. A tested and corrected algorithm for insulin dosing to control blood glucoses, after betamethasone 12 mgs IM and repeated after 24 h, endorses 27, 45, 40, 31, and 11% increases from the baseline insulin dose on days 1 through 5 from the start of betamethasone therapy, respectively.[166]

Tables 17.II.11 and 17.II.12 summarize pregnancy and neonatal complications in patients with T1D compared with nondiabetes pregnancies.

Depression

It is estimated that perinatal depression affects ~10% of women.[167,168] Women with T1D are more likely to experience perinatal depression, which could affect pregnancy outcomes.[169,170] Symptoms that present in pregnancy are similar to those at any other stage in a woman's life, requiring 8 of the 14 symptoms for at least 2 weeks based on American Psychiatric Association's *Diagnostic and Statistical Manual of Mental* Disorders.[171] The exact triggers and hormonal profile of perinatal depression are unknown. It is characterized, however, by dysregulation of the hypothalamic-pituitary-adrenal (HPA) axis.[172,173] Elevations in CRH are associated with classic melancholic depression.[173]

A history of previous depression[174,175] is the strongest risk factor. In addition, black or Hispanic ethnicities, financial hardship, unwanted pregnancy, lack of a partner, and younger maternal age were associated with an increased risk of prenatal depression. These risk factors may be particularly important in women

Table 17.II.11 Pregnancy Complications and Mode of Delivery in T1D and Control Pregnancies

| Outcome Variable | Proportions (%) | | OR (95% CI) for Group Differences | |
	T1D	Nondiabetes	Crude	Adjusted
PIH	1.6	0.87	1.93 (1.50–2.49)	1.53 (1.18–1.99)
Preeclampsia, mild	9.7	2.0	5.37 (4.81–6.00)	4.30 (3.83–4.83)
Preeclampsia, severe	4.3	0.8	5.58 (4.75–6.57)	4.47 (3.77–5.31)
Cesarean section	46	12	5.85 (5.49–6.25)	5.31 (4.97–5.69)
Vacuum extraction/forceps	9.6	6.6	1.48 (1.33–1.66)	1.41 (1.25–1.58)

Data are proportions or OR (95% CI): n = 5,089 for diabetic pregnancies; n = 1,260,207 for control pregnancies. Adjusted OR, OR adjusted for group differences in maternal age, BMI, parity, chronic hypertensive disorder, smoking habits, and ethnicity.

Tables are from Persson, Norman, Hanson[151] reprinted with permission.

Table 17.II.12 Fetal and Neonatal Complications in T1D Pregnancies and the General Obstetric Population

Outcome Variable	Proportions (% if not indicated otherwise)		OR (95% CI) for Group Differences	
	T1D	**Control**	**Crude**	**Adjusted**
Stillbirth	1.5	0.3	4.04 (3.02–5.40)	3.34 (2.46–4.55)
Fetal distress	14	6.2	2.45 (2.24–2.69)	2.34 (2.12–2.58)
Perinatal mortality (‰)	20	4.8	4.02 (3.11–5.20)	3.29 (2.50–4.33)
Neonatal mortality, 0–7 days (‰)	5.1	1.8	2.91 (1.97–4.28)	3.05 (1.68–5.55)
Neonatal mortality, 0–28 days (‰)	7.0	2.2	3.08 (2.02–4.70)	2.67 (1.72–4.16)
Birth <37 weeks gestational age	21	5.1	5.27 (4.88–5.71)	4.86 (4.47–5.28)
Birth <32 weeks gestational age	2.3	0.7	3.58 (2.89–4.44)	3.08 (2.45–3.87)
LGA	31	3.6	12.2 (11.4–13.1)	11.4 (10.6–12.4)
SGA	2.3	2.5	0.80 (0.63–1.02)	0.71 (0.55–0.91)
Major malformations	4.7	1.8	2.70 (2.37–3.08)	2.50 (2.13–2.94)
Apgar score <7 at 5 min	3.1	1.1	2.98 (2.54–3.50)	2.60 (2.14–3.17)
Apgar score <4 at 5 min	0.80	0.30	2.60 (1.79–3.78)	2.39 (1.64–3.51)
Erb palsy*	2.1	0.25	7.91 (5.77–10.8)	6.69 (4.81–9.31)
Respiratory distress syndrome	1.0	0.20	4.88 (3.51–6.81)	4.65 (2.20–9.84)
Respiratory disorders	9.5	2.6	4.02 (3.67–4.42)	3.42 (3.04–3.85)

Data are proportions or OR (95% CI). Adjusted OR, OR adjusted for group differences in maternal age, BMI, parity, chronic hypertensive disorder, smoking habits, and ethnicity.
*Vaginal deliveries only
Tables are from Persson, Norman, Hanson[151] reprinted with permission.

with T1D.[167,168] Stressful life events are also associated with increased risk of prenatal depression.[167,168]

Prenatal depression may lead to inadequate weight gain, underutilization of prenatal care, and increased substance use. In addition, infant outcomes include lower infant birth weight, decreased Apgar scores, prematurity, and smaller head circumference.[176] For women with T1D, who are already at risk of pregnancy complications, such as preterm birth, it may be important to screen for prenatal depression.

The American College of Obstetrics and Gynecology recommends screening for depression during each trimester of pregnancy,[177] but no specific perinatal depression screening tool is endorsed.[178] Many tests can be completed in <10 min and have a specificity ranging from 77% to 100%.[179] Sensitivity may need to be the determining factor for selecting a tool. Several tools are available for use (see chapter 8, Psychosocial Issues in Type 1 Diabetes).[179–182]

There have been no studies of these tools on women with T1D. In general, there is mixed data about the association between selective serotonin reuptake inhibitors (SSRIs) and birth defects in infants.[175,183,184] Two large-scale studies found a slight increase in a variety of congenital malformations in infants exposed to SSRIs, but no consistent pattern was found and the authors concluded that SSRIs should not be considered teratogenic.[185,186]

The exception is a possible association between paroxetine and congenital cardiac malformations, which are higher in women with T1D.[186] This drug has a class D label.[175] Neonatal abstinence syndrome (NAS) is also of some concern when considering neonatal outcomes in infants exposed to SSRIs in utero.[175] Thus, the risks of untreated maternal depression versus fetal exposure must be weighed. The long-term impact of SSRI exposure during pregnancy on the infant is unknown and merits further study.

The following are key areas in which T1D may complicate a pregnancy:

- Renal disease and vascular insufficiency as well as SGA infant[10–12]
- Suboptimal periconception glucose control and the risk of congenital malformations
- Increased risk of macrosomia LGA infant,[33,149] preterm delivery,[163] and stillbirth[48]
- SGA and long-term cardiometabolic risk in the infant of the diabetic mother[13]
- Maternal hypoglycemia unawareness and severe hypoglycemia risk[14] (need to individualize glucose targets)
- Increased monitoring for retinopathy progression[2,3]
- Increase risk of hypertensive complications[42,73]

A summary of pregnancy recommendations is provided in Table 17.II.13.

Table 17.II.13 Summary of Pregnancy Recommendations

Item	Intervention Recommendations
Glycemic Control	Fasting BG/Postprandial BG
Fasting	60–99 mg/dl
Peak postprandial	100–129
Mean	<100
Labor and delivery	80–110 (mean <100)[52,53]; insulin drips + D10 50cc/hr[2]
A1C	Preconception <7%, or as close to normal as possible without significant hypoglycemia[2,3]
	During pregnancy <6%

(Continued)

Table 17.II.13 Summary of Pregnancy Recommendations (Continued)

Item	Intervention Recommendations
Blood pressure	110–129/65–79 mmHg
Hypertension	First line: methyl dopa and labetolol
	Second line: calcium channel blockers
	Note: ACE-I and ARB contraindicated
Nephropathy	Same as hypertension
Retinopathy	Every trimester or more frequently depending on the degree of baseline retinopathy or macular edema
	Consider more frequent screening in milder retinopathy at baseline plus other strong risk factors.
	Laser therapy is the standard of care based on the Early Treatment Diabetic Retinopathy Study
Neuropathy	
Gastroparesis	Metoclopramide[91] *Note:* Ondansetron has not been studied[92]
Intractable hyperemesis	Diazepam IV plus hydration
Carpal tunnel syndrome	First-line therapy: wrist splints (noninvasive) treatment Second-line therapy: local dexamethasone[95] Third-line therapy: surgery, if no resolution postpartum[96]
Peripheral nerve pain	No RCTs evaluating treatment. There is an increased risk of congenital malformations with antiepileptic drugs (AEDs), such as carbamazepine and gabapentine. These drugs may alter later cognitive development in the offspring. *Note:* AEDs, the benefit of treating seizure disorders (life-threatening condition) in pregnancy probably outweighs the risk of using these medications; this is not the case with peripheral neuropathic pain.
Cardiovascular disease	With atypical symptoms, consider ECG, transthoracic ECHO, or exercise ECHO[98]
Lipids	Baseline lipid panel
Hypertriglyceride-mia	Discontinue statins (class X: contraindicated during pregnancy and postpartum) Dietary management Consider omega-3s for high TG

(Continued)

Table 17.II.13 Summary of Pregnancy Recommendations (Continued)

Item	Intervention Recommendations
Thyroid disease	Baseline thyroid panel (if thyroid disease then TSH every 4–6 weeks)
Hypothyroid (Hashimoto's)	Titrate T4 dose to maintain serum TSH: First trimester 0.1–2.5 µU/ml Second trimester 0.2–3.0 Third trimester 0.3–3.0[139,140] Hypothyroidism: two extra pills per week (e.g., nine vs. seven tabs) upon conception until first prenatal visit.[141] Postpartum, L-thyroxine dose usually returns to baseline preconception dose.
Hyperthyroidism (Grave's)	First trimester: PTU Second and third trimesters: methimazole[143] Thyroidectomy when antithyroid drugs cannot be used *Note:* Radioactive iodine (RAI) is contraindicated in pregnancy. Consider TSH receptor antibodies in third trimester of pregnancy (if mother treated w/radioactive iodine or surgery) Postpartum: Monitor free T4 and TSH in the infant cord blood and watch for signs of hyperthyroidism in the first few days of life after maternal antithyroid drugs wear off. Maternal antibodies may persist for 3 months.
Depression	Depression screening in each trimester SSRIs are used after assessment of risks and benefits *Note:* Paroxetine contraindicated (class D)[175]
LGA/Macrosomia	Maternal: Target glucoses while avoiding hypoglycemia Maintain target weight gain[161] Avoid tobacco use Fetal Growth: Special attention to change in velocity of abdominal circumference growth relative to the biparietal diameter (may predict LGA and macrosomia)[17]
Preterm delivery	Preterm labor: tocolytics (e.g., calcium channel blockers, magnesium sulfate) plus bedrest *Note:* Avoid terbutaline (association with DKA and insulin resistance) Antenatal steroids plus insulin adjustment 27, 45, 40, 31, and 11% increases from the baseline insulin dose on days 1 through 5 from the start of betamethasone therapy respectively[166]

ACE-I, angiotensin-converting-enzyme inhibitors; ARB, angiotensin receptor blocker; BG, blood glucose; BP, blood pressure; DKA, diabetic ketoacidosis; ECG, electrocardiogram; ECHO, echocardiogram; LGA, large for gestational age; PTU, propylthiouracil; RCT, randomized controlled trial; SSRI, selective serotonin reuptake inhibitors; TSH, thyroid stimulating hormone

REFERENCES

1. Freinkel N.: Banting lecture 1980. Of pregnancy and progeny. *Diabetes* 29:1023–1035, 1980
2. Kitzmiller JL, American Diabetes Association: *Managing Preexisting Diabetes and Pregnancy: Technical Reviews and Consensus Recommendations for Care*. Alexandria, VA, American Diabetes Association, 2008
3. Kitzmiller JL, Block JM, Brown FM, et al.: Managing preexisting diabetes for pregnancy: summary of evidence and consensus recommendations for care. *Diabetes Care* 31:1060–1079, 2008
4. Pedersen J: *The Pregnant Diabetic and Her Newborn; Problems and Management*. Baltimore, MD, Williams & Wilkins, 1967
5. Catalano PM, Hauguel-De Mouzon S: Is it time to revisit the Pedersen hypothesis in the face of the obesity epidemic? *Am J Obstet Gynecol* 204:479–487, 2011
6. Freinkel N: Diabetic embryopathy and fuel-mediated organ teratogenesis: lessons from animal models. Hormone and metabolic research = Hormonund Stoffwechselforschung. *Hormones et Metabolisme* 20:463–475, 1988
7. Lindsay RS, Nelson SM, Walker JD, et al.: Programming of adiposity in offspring of mothers with type 1 diabetes at age 7 years. *Diabetes Care* 33:1080–1085, 2010
8. Silverman BL, Metzger BE, Cho NH, Loeb CA: Impaired glucose tolerance in adolescent offspring of diabetic mothers. Relationship to fetal hyperinsulinism. *Diabetes Care* 18:611–617, 1995
9. Buinauskiene J, Baliutaviciene D, Zalinkevicius R: Glucose tolerance of 2- to 5-yr-old offspring of diabetic mothers. *Pediatric Diabetes* 5:143–146, 2004
10. Pietryga M, Brazert J, Wender-Ozegowska E, Biczysko R, Dubiel M, Gudmundsson S: Abnormal uterine Doppler is related to vasculopathy in pregestational diabetes mellitus. *Circulation* 112:2496–2500, 2005
11. Zawiejska A, Wender-Ozegowska E, Pietryga M, Brazert J: Maternal endothelial dysfunction and its association with abnormal fetal growth in diabetic pregnancy. *Diabetic Medicine* 28:692–698, 2011
12. Ekbom P, Damm P, Feldt-Rasmussen B, Feldt-Rasmussen U, Molvig J, Mathiesen ER: Pregnancy outcome in type 1 diabetic women with microalbuminuria. *Diabetes Care* 24:1739–1744, 2001
13. Barker DJ, Osmond C: Infant mortality, childhood nutrition, and ischaemic heart disease in England and Wales. *Lancet* 1:1077–1081, 1986
14. The Diabetes Control and Complications Trial Research Group: The effect of intensive treatment of diabetes on the development and progression of long-term complications in insulin-dependent diabetes mellitus. *N Engl J Med* 329:977–986, 1993
15. Rosenn BM, Miodovnik M, Holcberg G, Khoury JC, Siddiqi TA: Hypoglycemia: the price of intensive insulin therapy for pregnant women with insulin-dependent diabetes mellitus. *Obstetrics and Gynecology* 85:417–422, 1995
16. Raychaudhuri K, Maresh MJ: Glycemic control throughout pregnancy and fetal growth in insulin-dependent diabetes. *Obstetrics and Gynecology* 95:190–194, 2000

17. Mulder EJ, Koopman CM, Vermunt JK, de Valk HW, Visser GH: Fetal growth trajectories in type-1 diabetic pregnancy. *Ultrasound in Obstetrics and Gynecology* 36:735–742, 2010
18. Bailey BK, Cardwell MS: A team approach to managing preexisting diabetes complicated by pregnancy. *Diabetes Educator* 22:111–112, 115, 1996
19. Quevedo SF, Coustan DR: Diabetes and pregnancy. Use of an integrated "team" approach provides the necessary comprehensive care. *Rhode Island Medical Journal* 72:129–132, 1989
20. Schneider MB, Umpierrez GE, Ramsey RD, Mabie WC, Bennett KA: Pregnancy complicated by diabetic ketoacidosis: maternal and fetal outcomes. *Diabetes Care* 26:958–959, 2003
21. Sills IN, Rapaport R: New-onset IDDM presenting with diabetic ketoacidosis in a pregnant adolescent. *Diabetes Care* 17:904–905, 1994
22. Farrar D, Tuffnell DJ, West J: Continuous subcutaneous insulin infusion versus multiple daily injections of insulin for pregnant women with diabetes. *Cochrane Database Syst Rev* CD005542, 2007
23. Misso ML, Egberts KJ, Page M, O'Connor D, Shaw J: Continuous subcutaneous insulin infusion (CSII) versus multiple insulin injections for type 1 diabetes mellitus. *Cochrane Database Syst Rev* CD005103, 2010
24. Garcia-Patterson A, Gich I, Amini SB, Catalano PM, de Leiva A, Corcoy R: Insulin requirements throughout pregnancy in women with type 1 diabetes mellitus: three changes of direction. *Diabetologia* 53:446–451, 2010
25. Callesen NF, Ringholm L, Stage E, Damm P, Mathiesen ER: Insulin requirements in type 1 diabetic pregnancy: do twin pregnant women require twice as much insulin as singleton pregnant women? *Diabetes Care* 35:1246–1248, 2012
26. McManus RM, Ryan EA: Insulin requirements in insulin-dependent and insulin-requiring GDM women during final month of pregnancy. *Diabetes Care* 15:1323–1327, 1992
27. Riviello C, Mello G, Jovanovic LG: Breastfeeding and the basal insulin requirement in type 1 diabetic women. *Endocrine Practice* 15:187–193, 2009
28. Sacks DA, Chen W, Greenspoon JS, Wolde-Tsadik G: Should the same glucose values be targeted for type 1 as for type 2 diabetics in pregnancy? *Am J Obstet Gynecol* 177:1113–1119, 1997
29. Heller S, Damm P, Mersebach H, et al.: Hypoglycemia in type 1 diabetic pregnancy: role of preconception insulin aspart treatment in a randomized study. *Diabetes Care* 33:473–477, 2010
30. Kimmerle R, Heinemann L, Delecki A, Berger M: Severe hypoglycemia incidence and predisposing factors in 85 pregnancies of type I diabetic women. *Diabetes Care* 15:1034–1037, 1992
31. Nielsen LR, Pedersen-Bjergaard U, Thorsteinsson B, Johansen M, Damm P, Mathiesen ER: Hypoglycemia in pregnant women with type 1 diabetes: predictors and role of metabolic control. *Diabetes Care* 31:9–14, 2008
32. Rosenn B, Siddiqi TA, Miodovnik M: Normalization of blood glucose in insulin-dependent diabetic pregnancies and the risks of hypoglycemia: a therapeutic dilemma. *Obstetrical & Gynecological Survey* 50:56–61, 1995
33. Evers IM, de Valk HW, Visser GH: Risk of complications of pregnancy in women with type 1 diabetes: nationwide prospective study in the Netherlands. *BMJ* 328:915, 2004

34. Evers IM, ter Braak EW, de Valk HW, van Der Schoot B, Janssen N, Visser GH: Risk indicators predictive for severe hypoglycemia during the first trimester of type 1 diabetic pregnancy. *Diabetes Care* 25:554–559, 2002
35. Diamond MP, Reece EA, Caprio S, et al.: Impairment of counterregulatory hormone responses to hypoglycemia in pregnant women with insulin-dependent diabetes mellitus. *Am J Obstet Gynecol* 166:70–77, 1992
36. Rosenn BM, Miodovnik M, Khoury JC, Siddiqi TA: Deficient counterregulation: a possible risk factor for excessive fetal growth in IDDM pregnancies. *Diabetes Care* 20:872–874, 1997
37. Bjorklund A, Adamson U, Andreasson K, et al.: Hormonal counterregulation and subjective symptoms during induced hypoglycemia in insulin-dependent diabetes mellitus patients during and after pregnancy. *Acta Obstetricia et Gynecologica Scandinavica* 77:625–634, 1998
38. Kitzmiller JL, Gavin LA, Gin GD, Jovanovic-Peterson L, Main EK, Zigrang WD: Preconception care of diabetes. Glycemic control prevents congenital anomalies. *JAMA* 265:731–736, 1991
39. Mills JL, Knopp RH, Simpson JL, et al.: Lack of relation of increased malformation rates in infants of diabetic mothers to glycemic control during organogenesis. *N Engl J Med* 318:671–676, 1988
40. Steel JM, Johnstone FD, Hepburn DA, Smith AF: Can prepregnancy care of diabetic women reduce the risk of abnormal babies? *BMJ* 301:1070–1074, 1990
41. Bjorklund AO, Adamson UK, Almstrom NH, et al.: Effects of hypoglycaemia on fetal heart activity and umbilical artery Doppler velocity waveforms in pregnant women with insulin-dependent diabetes mellitus. *BJOG* 103:413–420, 1996
42. Reece EA, Coustan DR, Hayslett JP, et al.: Diabetic nephropathy: pregnancy performance and fetomaternal outcome. *Am J Obstet Gynecol* 159:56–66, 1988
43. Rizzo T, Metzger BE, Burns WJ, Burns K: Correlations between antepartum maternal metabolism and child intelligence. *N Engl J Med* 325:911–916, 1991
44. Zisser HC, Biersmith MA, Jovanovic LB, Yogev Y, Hod M, Kovatchev BP: Fetal risk assessment in pregnancies complicated by diabetes mellitus. *Journal of Diabetes Science and Technology* 4:1368–1373, 2010
45. Kyle GC: Diabetes and pregnancy. *Ann Intern Med* 59(Suppl. 3):1–82, 1963
46. Cullen MT, Reece EA, Homko CJ, Sivan E: The changing presentations of diabetic ketoacidosis during pregnancy. *Am J Perinatol* 13:449–451, 1996
47. Kilvert JA, Nicholson HO, Wright AD: Ketoacidosis in diabetic pregnancy. *Diabetic Medicine* 10:278–281, 1993
48. Dudley DJ: Diabetic-associated stillbirth: incidence, pathophysiology, and prevention. *Obstetrics and Gynecology Clinics of North America* 34:293–307, ix, 2007
49. Guo RX, Yang LZ, Li LX, Zhao XP: Diabetic ketoacidosis in pregnancy tends to occur at lower blood glucose levels: case-control study and a case report of euglycemic diabetic ketoacidosis in pregnancy. *Journal of Obstetrics and Gynaecology Research* 34:324–330, 2008

50. Bernstein IM, Catalano PM: Ketoacidosis in pregnancy associated with the parenteral administration of terbutaline and betamethasone. A case report. *Journal of Reproductive Medicine* 35:818–820, 1990
51. Lindenbaum C, Menzin A, Ludmir J: Diabetic ketoacidosis in pregnancy resulting from insulin pump failure. A case report. *Journal of Reproductive Medicine* 38:306–308, 1993
52. Landon MB, Gabbe SG, Piana R, Mennuti MT, Main EK: Neonatal morbidity in pregnancy complicated by diabetes mellitus: predictive value of maternal glycemic profiles. *Am J Obstet Gynecol* 156:1089–1095, 1987
53. Curet LB, Izquierdo LA, Gilson GJ, Schneider JM, Perelman R, Converse J: Relative effects of antepartum and intrapartum maternal blood glucose levels on incidence of neonatal hypoglycemia. *J Perinatol* 17:113–115, 1997
54. Taylor R, Lee C, Kyne-Grzebalski D, Marshall SM, Davison JM: Clinical outcomes of pregnancy in women with type 1 diabetes(1). *Obstetrics and Gynecology* 99:537–541, 2002
55. Carroll MA, Yeomans ER: Diabetic ketoacidosis in pregnancy. *Critical Care Medicine* 33:S347–353, 2005
56. Chobanian AV, Bakris GL, Black HR, et al.: Seventh report of the Joint National Committee on Prevention, Detection, Evaluation, and Treatment of High Blood Pressure. *Hypertension* 42:1206–1252, 2003
57. Rabi DM, Daskalopoulou SS, Padwal RS, et al.: The 2011 Canadian Hypertension Education Program recommendations for the management of hypertension: blood pressure measurement, diagnosis, assessment of risk, and therapy. *Canadian Journal of Cardiology* 27:415–433 e1–e2, 2011
58. Ochsenbein-Kolble N, Roos M, Gasser T, Huch R, Huch A, Zimmermann R: Cross sectional study of automated blood pressure measurements throughout pregnancy. *BJOG* 111:319–325, 2004
59. Peterson CM, Jovanovic-Peterson L, Mills JL, et al.: The Diabetes in Early Pregnancy study: changes in cholesterol, triglycerides, body weight, and blood pressure. The National Institute of Child Health and Human Development—the Diabetes in Early Pregnancy study. *Am J Obstet Gynecol* 166:513–518, 1992
60. El Guindy AA, Nabhan AF: A randomized trial of tight vs. less tight control of mild essential and gestational hypertension in pregnancy. *Journal of Perinatal Medicine* 36:413–418, 2008
61. von Dadelszen P, Magee LA: Fall in mean arterial pressure and fetal growth restriction in pregnancy hypertension: an updated metaregression analysis. *JOGC* 24:941–945, 2002
62. ACOG Practice Bulletin: Diagnosis and management of preeclampsia and eclampsia. *International Journal of Gynaecology and Obstetrics* 77:67–75, 2002
63. Abalos E, Duley L, Steyn DW, Henderson-Smart DJ: Antihypertensive drug therapy for mild to moderate hypertension during pregnancy. *Cochrane Database of Syst Rev* CD002252, 2007
64. Sibai BM, Mabie WC, Shamsa F, Villar MA, Anderson GD: A comparison of no medication versus methyldopa or labetalol in chronic hypertension during pregnancy. *Am J Obstetrics and Gynecology* 162:960–966; discussion 6–7, 1990

65. Sibai BM, Grossman RA, Grossman HG: Effects of diuretics on plasma volume in pregnancies with long-term hypertension. *Am J Obstet Gynecol* 150:831–835, 1984
66. Butters L, Kennedy S, Rubin PC: Atenolol in essential hypertension during pregnancy. *BMJ* 301:587–589, 1990
67. Rothberger S, Carr D, Brateng D, Hebert M, Easterling TR: Pharmaco-dynamics of clonidine therapy in pregnancy: a heterogeneous maternal response impacts fetal growth. *American Journal of Hypertension* 23:1234–1240, 2010
68. Waugh J, Bell SC, Kilby MD, et al.: Urinary microalbumin/creatinine ratios: reference range in uncomplicated pregnancy. *Clinical Science* 104:103–107, 2003
69. Hayashi M, Tomobe K, Hirabayashi H, Hoshimoto K, Ohkura T, Inaba N: Increased excretion of N-acetyl-beta-D-glucosaminidase and beta2-microglobulin in gestational week 30. *American Journal of the Medical Sciences* 321:168–172, 2001
70. Taylor AA, Davison JM: Albumin excretion in normal pregnancy. *Am J Obstet Gynecol* 177:1559–1560, 1997
71. Davison JM, Noble MC: Serial changes in 24 hour creatinine clearance during normal menstrual cycles and the first trimester of pregnancy. *BJOC* 88:10–17, 1981
72. McCance DR, Traub AI, Harley JM, Hadden DR, Kennedy L: Urinary albumin excretion in diabetic pregnancy. *Diabetologia* 32:236–239, 1989
73. Kitzmiller JL, Brown ER, Phillippe M, et al.: Diabetic nephropathy and perinatal outcome. *Am J Obstet Gynecol* 141:741–751, 1981
74. Carr DB, Koontz GL, Gardella C, et al.: Diabetic nephropathy in preg-nancy: suboptimal hypertensive control associated with preterm delivery. *American Journal of Hypertension* 19:513–519, 2006
75. Nielsen LR, Damm P, Mathiesen ER: Improved pregnancy outcome in type 1 diabetic women with microalbuminuria or diabetic nephropathy: effect of intensified antihypertensive therapy? *Diabetes Care* 32:38–44, 2009
76. Vivian EM, Rubinstein GB: Pharmacologic management of diabetic nephropathy. *Clinical Therapeutics* 24:1741–1756, discussion 19, 2002
77. Khandelwal M, Kumanova M, Gaughan JP, Reece EA: Role of diltiazem in pregnant women with chronic renal disease. *J Matern Fetal Neonatal Med* 12:408–412, 2002
78. Fong DS, Aiello L, Gardner TW, et al.: Retinopathy in diabetes. *Diabetes Care* 27(Suppl. 1):S84–S87, 2004
79. Fong DS, Aiello LP, Ferris FL, 3rd, Klein R: Diabetic retinopathy. *Diabetes Care* 27:2540–2553, 2004
80. The Diabetes Control and Complications Trial Research Group: Effect of pregnancy on microvascular complications in the diabetes control and com-plications trial. *Diabetes Care* 23:1084–1091, 2000
81. Klein BE, Moss SE, Klein R: Effect of pregnancy on progression of diabetic retinopathy. *Diabetes Care* 13:34–40, 1990
82. Chang LK, Sarraf D: Current and future approaches in the prevention and treatment of diabetic retinopathy. *Clinical Ophthalmology* 2:425–433, 2008

83. Rahman W, Rahman FZ, Yassin S, Al-Suleiman SA, Rahman J: Progression of retinopathy during pregnancy in type 1 diabetes mellitus. *Clinical & Experimental Ophthalmology* 35:231–236, 2007

84. Kaaja R, Loukovaara S: Progression of retinopathy in type 1 diabetic women during pregnancy. *Current Diabetes Reviews* 3:85–93, 2007

85. Chew EY, Mills JL, Metzger BE, et al.: Metabolic control and progression of retinopathy. The Diabetes in Early Pregnancy study. National Institute of Child Health and Human Development Diabetes in Early Pregnancy study. *Diabetes Care* 18:631–637, 1995

86. Early Treatment Diabetic Retinopathy Study Research Group: Early photocoagulation for diabetic retinopathy. ETDRS report number 9. *Ophthalmology* 98:766–785, 1991

87. Diabetic Retinopathy Study Research Group: Photocoagulation treatment of proliferative diabetic retinopathy. Clinical application of Diabetic Retinopathy Study (DRS) findings, DRS report number 8. *Ophthalmology* 88:583–600, 1981

88. Levine RJ, Lam C, Qian C, et al.: Soluble endoglin and other circulating antiangiogenic factors in preeclampsia. *N Engl J Med* 355:992–1005, 2006

89. Roseboom TJ, Ravelli AC, van der Post JA, Painter RC: Maternal characteristics largely explain poor pregnancy outcome after hyperemesis gravidarum. *European Journal of Obstetrics, Gynecology, and Reproductive Biology* 156:56–59, 2011

90. Macleod AF, Smith SA, Sonksen PH, Lowy C: The problem of autonomic neuropathy in diabetic pregnancy. *Diabetic Medicine* 7:80–82, 1990

91. Matok I, Gorodischer R, Koren G, Sheiner E, Wiznitzer A, Levy A: The safety of metoclopramide use in the first trimester of pregnancy. *N Engl J Med* 360:2528–2535, 2009

92. Festin M: Nausea and vomiting in early pregnancy. *Clinical Evidence* 2009 Jun 3;2009. pii: 1405

93. Tasci Y, Demir B, Dilbaz S, Haberal A: Use of diazepam for hyperemesis gravidarum. *J Matern Fetal Neonatal Med* 22:353–356, 2009

94. Stevens JC, Beard CM, O'Fallon WM, Kurland LT: Conditions associated with carpal tunnel syndrome. *Proc Mayo Clinic* 67:541–548, 1992

95. Moghtaderi AR, Moghtaderi N, Loghmani A: Evaluating the effectiveness of local dexamethasone injection in pregnant women with carpal tunnel syndrome. *Journal of Research in Medical Sciences* 16:687–690, 2011

96. Ekman-Ordeberg G, Salgeback S, Ordeberg G: Carpal tunnel syndrome in pregnancy. A prospective study. *Acta Obstetricia et Gynecologica Scandinavica* 66:233–235, 1987

97. Krolewski AS, Kosinski EJ, Warram JH, et al.: Magnitude and determinants of coronary artery disease in juvenile-onset, insulin-dependent diabetes mellitus. *Am J Cardiol* 59:750–755, 1987

98. Raggi P, Bellasi A, Ratti C: Ischemia imaging and plaque imaging in diabetes: complementary tools to improve cardiovascular risk management. *Diabetes Care* 28:2787–2794, 2005

99. Nathan DM, Cleary PA, Backlund JY, et al.: Intensive diabetes treatment and cardiovascular disease in patients with type 1 diabetes. *N Engl J Med* 353:2643–2653, 2005

100. Taguchi N, Rubin ET, Hosokawa A, et al.: Prenatal exposure to HMG-CoA reductase inhibitors: effects on fetal and neonatal outcomes. *Reproductive Toxicology* 26:175–177, 2008
101. Pignone M, Alberts MJ, Colwell JA, et al.: Aspirin for primary prevention of cardiovascular events in people with diabetes: a position statement of the American Diabetes Association, a scientific statement of the American Heart Association, and an expert consensus document of the American College of Cardiology Foundation. *Diabetes Care* 33:1395–1402, 2010
102. Effect of intensive diabetes management on macrovascular events and risk factors in the Diabetes Control and Complications Trial. *Am J Cardiol* 75:894–903, 1995
103. Perez A, Wagner AM, Carreras G, et al.: Prevalence and phenotypic distribution of dyslipidemia in type 1 diabetes mellitus: effect of glycemic control. *Archives of Internal Medicine* 160:2756–2762, 2000
104. Chaturvedi N, Fuller JH, Taskinen MR: Differing associations of lipid and lipoprotein disturbances with the macrovascular and microvascular complications of type 1 diabetes. *Diabetes Care* 24:2071–2077, 2001
105. Knopp RH, Warth MR, Carrol CJ: Lipid metabolism in pregnancy. I. Changes in lipoprotein triglyceride and cholesterol in normal pregnancy and the effects of diabetes mellitus. *J Reprod Med* 10:95–101, 1973
106. Knopp RH, Van Allen MI, McNeely M, et al.: Effect of insulin-dependent diabetes on plasma lipoproteins in diabetic pregnancy. *J Reprod Med* 38:703–710, 1993
107. Muhlhausler BS, Gibson RA, Makrides M: Effect of long-chain polyunsaturated fatty acid supplementation during pregnancy or lactation on infant and child body composition: a systematic review. *American Journal of Clinical Nutrition* 92:857–863, 2010
108. Rytter D, Bech BH, Christensen JH, Schmidt EB, Henriksen TB, Olsen SF: Intake of fish oil during pregnancy and adiposity in 19-y-old offspring: follow-up on a randomized controlled trial. *American Journal of Clinical Nutrition* 94:701–708, 2011
109. Klemens CM, Berman DR, Mozurkewich EL: The effect of perinatal omega-3 fatty acid supplementation on inflammatory markers and allergic diseases: a systematic review. *BJOG* 118:916–925, 2011
110. Klemens CM, Berman DR, Mozurkewich EL: The effect of perinatal omega-3 fatty acid supplementation on inflammatory markers and allergic diseases: a systematic review. *BJOG* 118:916–925, 2011
111. Harper M, Thom E, Klebanoff MA, et al.: Omega-3 fatty acid supplementation to prevent recurrent preterm birth: a randomized controlled trial. *Obstetrics and Gynecology* 115:234–242, 2010
112. Salvig JD, Lamont RF: Evidence regarding an effect of marine n-3 fatty acids on preterm birth: a systematic review and meta-analysis. *Acta Obstetricia et Gynecologica Scandinavica* 90:825–838, 2011
113. Escolano-Margarit MV, Ramos R, Beyer J, et al.: Prenatal DHA status and neurological outcome in children at age 5.5 years are positively associated. *Journal of Nutrition* 141:1216–1223, 2011
114. Smithers LG, Gibson RA, Makrides M: Maternal supplementation with docosahexaenoic acid during pregnancy does not affect early visual

development in the infant: a randomized controlled trial. *American Journal of Clinical Nutrition* 93:1293–1299, 2011

115. Wojcicki JM, Heyman MB: Maternal omega-3 fatty acid supplementation and risk for perinatal maternal depression. *J Matern Fetal Neonatal Med* 24:680–686, 2011

116. Nissim M, Giorda G, Ballabio M, et al.: Maternal thyroid function in early and late pregnancy. *Hormone Research* 36:196–202, 1991

117. Guillaume J, Schussler GC, Goldman J: Components of the total serum thyroid hormone concentrations during pregnancy: high free thyroxine and blunted thyrotropin (TSH) response to TSH-releasing hormone in the first trimester. *J Clin Endocrinol Metab* 60:678–684, 1985

118. Mandel SJ, Spencer CA, Hollowell JG: Are detection and treatment of thyroid insufficiency in pregnancy feasible? *Thyroid* 15:44–53, 2005

119. Peck TM, Arias F: Hematologic changes associated with pregnancy. *Clinical Obstetrics and Gynecology* 22:785–798, 1979

120. de Benoist B, Andersson M, Takkouche B, Egli I: Prevalence of iodine deficiency worldwide. *Lancet* 362:1859–1860, 2003

121. Klubo-Gwiezdzinska J, Burman KD, Van Nostrand D, Wartofsky L: Levothyroxine treatment in pregnancy: indications, efficacy, and therapeutic regimen. *Journal of Thyroid Research* 2011:843591, 2011

122. Behrooz HG, Tohidi M, Mehrabi Y, Behrooz EG, Tehranidoost M, Azizi F: Subclinical hypothyroidism in pregnancy: intellectual development of offspring. *Thyroid* 21:1143–1147, 2011

123. Gray RS, Borsey DQ, Seth J, Herd R, Brown NS, Clarke BF: Prevalence of subclinical thyroid failure in insulin-dependent diabetes. *J Clin Endocrinol Metab* 50:1034–1037, 1980

124. McCanlies E, O'Leary LA, Foley TP, et al.: Hashimoto's thyroiditis and insulin-dependent diabetes mellitus: differences among individuals with and without abnormal thyroid function. *J Clin Endocrinol Metab* 83:1548–1551, 1998

125. Perros P, McCrimmon RJ, Shaw G, Frier BM: Frequency of thyroid dysfunction in diabetic patients: value of annual screening. *Diabetic Medicine* 12:622–627, 1995

126. Abalovich M, Gutierrez S, Alcaraz G, Maccallini G, Garcia A, Levalle O: Overt and subclinical hypothyroidism complicating pregnancy. *Thyroid* 12:63–68, 2002

127. Allan WC, Haddow JE, Palomaki GE, et al.: Maternal thyroid deficiency and pregnancy complications: implications for population screening. *Journal of Medical Screening* 7:127–130, 2000

128. Davis LE, Leveno KJ, Cunningham FG: Hypothyroidism complicating pregnancy. *Obstetrics and Gynecology* 72:108–112, 1988

129. Leung AS, Millar LK, Koonings PP, Montoro M, Mestman JH: Perinatal outcome in hypothyroid pregnancies. *Obstetrics and Gynecology* 81:349–353, 1993

130. Ashoor G, Maiz N, Rotas M, Jawdat F, Nicolaides KH: Maternal thyroid function at 11 to 13 weeks of gestation and subsequent fetal death. *Thyroid* 20:989–993, 2010

131. Cleary-Goldman J, Malone FD, Lambert-Messerlian G, et al.: Maternal thyroid hypofunction and pregnancy outcome. *Obstetrics and Gynecology* 112:85–92, 2008

132. Casey BM, Dashe JS, Spong CY, McIntire DD, Leveno KJ, Cunningham GF: Perinatal significance of isolated maternal hypothyroxinemia identified in the first half of pregnancy. *Obstetrics and Gynecology* 109:1129–1135, 2007

133. Man EB, Brown JF, Serunian SA: Maternal hypothyroxinemia: psychoneurological deficits of progeny. *Annals of Clinical and Laboratory Science* 21:227–239, 1991

134. Man EB, Jones WS, Holden RH, Mellits ED: Thyroid function in human pregnancy. 8. Retardation of progeny aged 7 years; relationships to maternal age and maternal thyroid function. *Am J Obstet Gynecol* 111:905–916, 1971

135. Pop VJ, Brouwers EP, Vader HL, Vulsma T, van Baar AL, de Vijlder JJ: Maternal hypothyroxinaemia during early pregnancy and subsequent child development: a 3-year follow-up study. *Clinical Endocrinology* 59:282–288, 2003

136. Haddow JE, Palomaki GE, Allan WC, et al.: Maternal thyroid deficiency during pregnancy and subsequent neuropsychological development of the child. *N Engl J Med* 341:549–555, 1999

137. Lazarus JH: Screening for thyroid dysfunction in pregnancy: is it worthwhile? *Journal of Thyroid Research* 2011:397012, 2011

138. Lazarus JH, Bestwick JP, Channon S, et al.: Antenatal thyroid screening and childhood cognitive function. *N Engl J Med* 366:493–501, 2012

139. Abalovich M, Amino N, Barbour LA, et al.: Management of thyroid dysfunction during pregnancy and postpartum: an Endocrine Society Clinical Practice Guideline. *J Clin Endocrinol Metab* 92:S1–47, 2007

140. Stagnaro-Green A, Abalovich M, Alexander E, et al.: Guidelines of the American Thyroid Association for the diagnosis and management of thyroid disease during pregnancy and postpartum. *Thyroid* 21:1081–1125, 2011

141. Alexander EK, Marqusee E, Lawrence J, Jarolim P, Fischer GA, Larsen PR: Timing and magnitude of increases in levothyroxine requirements during pregnancy in women with hypothyroidism. *N Engl J Med* 351:241–249, 2004

142. Mandel SJ, Larsen PR, Seely EW, Brent GA: Increased need for thyroxine during pregnancy in women with primary hypothyroidism. *N Engl J Med* 323:91–96, 1990

143. Bahn RS, Burch HB, Cooper DS, et al.: Hyperthyroidism and other causes of thyrotoxicosis: management guidelines of the American Thyroid Association and American Association of Clinical Endocrinologists. *Endocrine Practice* 17:456–520, 2011

144. Stagnaro-Green A: Maternal thyroid disease and preterm delivery. *J Clin Endocrinol Metab* 94:21–25, 2009

145. Phoojaroenchanachai M, Sriussadaporn S, Peerapatdit T, et al.: Effect of maternal hyperthyroidism during late pregnancy on the risk of neonatal low birth weight. *Clin Endocrinol (Oxf)* 54:365–370, 2001

146. Earl R, Crowther CA, Middleton P: Interventions for preventing and treating hyperthyroidism in pregnancy. *Cochrane Database of Syst Rev* CD008633, 2010

147. Al-Agha R, Firth RG, Byrne M, et al.: Outcome of pregnancy in type 1 diabetes mellitus (T1DMP): results from combined diabetes-obstetrical clinics in Dublin in three university teaching hospitals (1995–2006). *Ir J Med Sci* 181:105–109, 2012

148. Aman J, Hansson U, Ostlund I, Wall K, Persson B: Increased fat mass and cardiac septal hypertrophy in newborn infants of mothers with well-controlled diabetes during pregnancy. *Neonatology* 100:147–154, 2011
149. Persson M, Pasupathy D, Hanson U, Norman M: Birth size distribution in 3,705 infants born to mothers with type 1 diabetes: a population-based study. *Diabetes Care* 34:1145–1149, 2011
150. Feghali MN, Khoury JC, Timofeev J, Shveiky D, Driggers RW, Miodovnik M: Asymmetric large for gestational age newborns in pregnancies complicated by diabetes mellitus: is maternal obesity a culprit? *J Matern Fetal Neonatal Med* 25:32–35, 2012
151. Persson M, Norman M, Hanson U: Obstetric and perinatal outcomes in type 1 diabetic pregnancies: a large, population-based study. *Diabetes Care* 32:2005–2009, 2009
152. Lepercq J, Hauguel-De Mouzon S, Timsit J, Catalano PM: Fetal macrosomia and maternal weight gain during pregnancy. *Diabetes Metab* 28:323–328, 2002
153. Combs CA, Gunderson E, Kitzmiller JL, Gavin LA, Main EK: Relationship of fetal macrosomia to maternal postprandial glucose control during pregnancy. *Diabetes Care* 15:1251–1257, 1992
154. Jovanovic-Peterson L, Peterson CM, Reed GF, et al.: Maternal postprandial glucose levels and infant birth weight: the Diabetes in Early Pregnancy study. The National Institute of Child Health and Human Development-Diabetes in Early Pregnancy study. *Am J Obstet Gynecol* 164:103–111, 1991
155. Mello G, Parretti E, Mecacci F, et al.: What degree of maternal metabolic control in women with type 1 diabetes is associated with normal body size and proportions in full-term infants? *Diabetes Care* 23:1494–1498, 2000
156. Kyne-Grzebalski D, Wood L, Marshall SM, Taylor R: Episodic hyperglycaemia in pregnant women with well-controlled type 1 diabetes mellitus: a major potential factor underlying macrosomia. *Diabet Med* 16:702–706, 1999
157. Hummel S, Pfluger M, Kreichauf S, Hummel M, Ziegler AG: Predictors of overweight during childhood in offspring of parents with type 1 diabetes: response to Rodekamp et al. *Diabetes Care* 32:e139, 2009
158. Lamb MM, Dabelea D, Yin X, et al.: Early-life predictors of higher body mass index in healthy children. *Ann Nutr Metab* 56:16–22, 2010
159. Plagemann A, Harder T, Kohlhoff R, Rohde W, Dorner G: Overweight and obesity in infants of mothers with long-term insulin-dependent diabetes or gestational diabetes. *Int J Obes Relat Metab Disord* 21:451–456, 1997
160. Huang JS, Lee TA, Lu MC: Prenatal programming of childhood overweight and obesity. *Matern Child Health J* 11:461–473, 2007
161. Rasmussen KM, Catalano PM, Yaktine AL: New guidelines for weight gain during pregnancy: what obstetrician/gynecologists should know. *Curr Opin Obstet Gynecol* 21:521–526, 2009
162. Murphy HR, Steel SA, Roland JM, et al.: Obstetric and perinatal outcomes in pregnancies complicated by type 1 and type 2 diabetes: influences of glycaemic control, obesity and social disadvantage. *Diabet Med* 28:1060–1067, 2011

163. Lepercq J, Coste J, Theau A, Dubois-Laforgue D, Timsit J: Factors associated with preterm delivery in women with type 1 diabetes: a cohort study. *Diabetes Care* 27:2824–2828, 2004

164. Tibaldi JM, Lorber DL, Nerenberg A: Diabetic ketoacidosis and insulin resistance with subcutaneous terbutaline infusion: a case report. *Am J Obstet Gynecol* 163:509–510, 1990

165. Roberts D, Dalziel S: Antenatal corticosteroids for accelerating fetal lung maturation for women at risk of preterm birth. *Cochrane Database of Syst Rev* CD004454, 2006

166. Mathiesen ER, Christensen AB, Hellmuth E, Hornnes P, Stage E, Damm P: Insulin dose during glucocorticoid treatment for fetal lung maturation in diabetic pregnancy: test of an algorithm [correction of analgoritm]. *Acta Obstet Gynecol Scand* 81:835–839, 2002

167. Ertel KA, Rich-Edwards JW, Koenen KC: Maternal depression in the United States: nationally representative rates and risks. *J Womens Health* (Larchmt) 20:1609–1617, 2011

168. Rich-Edwards JW, Kleinman K, Abrams A, et al.: Sociodemographic predictors of antenatal and postpartum depressive symptoms among women in a medical group practice. *J Epidemiol Community Health* 60:221–227, 2006

169. Kozhimannil KB, Pereira MA, Harlow BL: Association between diabetes and perinatal depression among low-income mothers. *JAMA* 301:842–847, 2009

170. Rasmussen-Torvik LJ, Harlow BL: The association between depression and diabetes in the perinatal period. *Curr Diab Rep* 10:217–223, 2010

171. American Psychiatric Association: Electronic DSM-IV-TR plus [CD-ROM]. In version 1.0. Washington, DC, American Psychiatric Association, 2000

172. Mastorakos G, Ilias I: Maternal and fetal hypothalamic-pituitary-adrenal axes during pregnancy and postpartum. *Ann N Y Acad Sci* 997:136–149, 2003

173. Rich-Edwards JW, Mohllajee AP, Kleinman K, et al.: Elevated midpregnancy corticotropin-releasing hormone is associated with prenatal, but not postpartum, maternal depression. *J Clin Endocrinol Metab* 93:1946–1951, 2008

174. Dietz PM, Williams SB, Callaghan WM, Bachman DJ, Whitlock EP, Hornbrook MC: Clinically identified maternal depression before, during, and after pregnancies ending in live births. *Am J Psychiatry* 164:1515–1520, 2007

175. Dossett EC: Perinatal depression. *Obstet Gynecol Clin North Am* 35:419–434, viii, 2008

176. Marcus SM: Depression during pregnancy: rates, risks and consequences—motherisk update 2008. *Can J Clin Pharmacol* 16:e15–22, 2009

177. Lancaster CA, Gold KJ, Flynn HA, Yoo H, Marcus SM, Davis MM: Risk factors for depressive symptoms during pregnancy: a systematic review. *Am J Obstet Gynecol* 202:5–14, 2010

178. American College of Obstetricians and Gynecologists: Perinatal depression screening: tools for obstetricians-gynecologists. Available from http://mail.ny.acog.org/website/DepressionToolKit.pdf. Accessed 25 October 2012

179. Committee opinion: committee on obstetric practice. Screening for depression during and after pregnancy. The American College of Obstricians and Gynecologists. *Women's Health Care Physicians*, No. 453, 2010.
180. Boyd RC, Le HN, Somberg R: Review of screening instruments for postpartum depression. *Arch Womens Ment Health* 8:141–153, 2005
181. Sharp LK, Lipsky MS: Screening for depression across the lifespan: a review of measures for use in primary care settings. *Am Fam Physician* 66:1001–1008, 2002
182. Spitzer RL, Kroenke K, Williams JB: Validation and utility of a self-report version of PRIME-MD: the PHQ primary care study. Primary care evaluation of mental disorders. Patient health questionnaire. *JAMA* 282:1737–1744, 1999
183. Einarson TR, Einarson A: Newer antidepressants in pregnancy and rates of major malformations: a meta-analysis of prospective comparative studies. *Pharmacoepidemiol Drug Saf* 14:823–827, 2005
184. Wogelius P, Norgaard M, Gislum M, et al.: Maternal use of selective serotonin reuptake inhibitors and risk of congenital malformations. *Epidemiology* 17:701–704, 2006
185. Alwan S, Reefhuis J, Rasmussen SA, Olney RS, Friedman JM: Use of selective serotonin-reuptake inhibitors in pregnancy and the risk of birth defects. *N Engl J Med* 356:2684–2692, 2007
186. Louik C, Lin AE, Werler MM, Hernandez-Diaz S, Mitchell AA: First-trimester use of selective serotonin-reuptake inhibitors and the risk of birth defects. *N Engl J Med* 356:2675–2683, 2007

III. Postnatal Care

Tamarra James-Todd, PhD, MPH

INTRODUCTION

This section provides an overview of and recommendations for the post-natal period for women with type 1 diabetes (T1D) and their infants, primarily focusing on the lactation period, specifically, the breast-feeding benefits to the mother and infant, the impact on T1D, and medication listings.

Breast-feeding is defined as infants who exclusively breast-feed plus those who breast-feed and receive supplementation.[1] Exclusive breast-feeding is defined as an infant's consumption of human milk with no supplements except vitamins, minerals, and medications.[1] The American Academy of Pediatrics (AAP) and the World Health Organization (WHO) provide the most cited breast-feeding recommendations. The AAP recommends exclusive breast-feeding for the first 6 months of life and continued breast-feeding for the first year or as long as the mother and infant would like.[2] The WHO recommends exclusive breast-feeding for 6 months, and breast-feeding with supplementation until 2 years post-delivery.[3] The recommendations to exclusively breast-feed and continue breast-feeding are rooted in its benefits for both mother and child. In women with T1D, these benefits may be particularly important for the long-term health of both mother and child.

OVERALL BREAST-FEEDING RATES

Breast-feeding rates have changed drastically over time. In the 1930s, breast-feeding rates were 80%; however, by the 1970s rates had dropped to 20%.[4] Over the past 30–40 years, breast-feeding rates have increased gradually. In 2006, 74% of women had initiated breast-feeding, with only 44% still breast-feeding by 6 months (see Table 17.III.1).[5]

BREAST-FEEDING BARRIERS

Data suggest that women make their decision about breast-feeding as early as the first trimester of pregnancy. As such, it is important to discuss breast-feeding and its benefits early on in pregnancy to provide needed information to enable balanced decision making. More will be discussed in this section, but specific challenges for T1D women may include issues surrounding balance of their own blood glucose management coupled with infant caregiving needs—specifically balancing good glycemic control with the additional caloric requirements of breast-feeding.[73] Additional barriers are included in Table 17.III.2.

DOI: 10.2337/9781580404785ch17s3

Table 17.III.1 Maternal Benefits of Breast-Feeding

Breast-feeding Benefits to T1D Mother	Breast-Feeding Benefits to Infant
Physiological	

Physiological

- Increased oxytocin, leading to less postpartum bleeding and more rapid uterine involution[6]
- Less maternal weight retention[7–10]
  - May allow for greater insulin sensitivity and better blood glucose (BG) control
  - May reduce future overweight or obesity risk and subsequent risk of obesity-related chronic diseases, such as cardiovascular disease (an inherent risk in many T1D patients)[11–13,a]
- Fewer unintended pregnancies (particularly important for T1D women) because of delayed ovulation from lactational amenhorrea[14–16]
- Increased infant bonding[17]
- Reduced risks of ovarian cancer and premenopausal breast cancer[18–23]
- Improved bone remineralization postpartum,[24] leading to decreased hip fracture risks postmenopause[25]

Financial:

- Reduced maternal anxiety from monetary savings[26]
- Reduced health care costs and reduced employee absenteeism resulting from child illness[27]

Infant column:
- Reduced risk of diarrhea,[29–32] respiratory infections,[33–35] otitis media,[36] bacteremia,[37] bacterial meningitis,[27,38] botulism,[39] urinary tract infection,[40–42,] and necrotizing enterocolitis[43,44]
- Reduced risk of sudden infant death syndrome,[45–48] and studies suggest a reduced risk of Crohn's disease and ulcerative colitis,[49,50] childhood cancers,[51–53] and allergic diseases[54–57]
- Potential increase in cognitive development,[58–60] although evidence is weak[61]
- Reduced future risk of childhood obesity[62–64] and adult chronic disease risk, particularly cardiovascular disease and type 2 diabetes (T2D)[57,65–67]
- Potential reduced risk of developing T1D in breast-fed infant (conflicting evidence)[68–70,b]
- Potential reduced overweight or obesity in childhood if infant breast-fed for at least 2 weeks[71]

[a] Child bearing increases visceral adipose tissue independent of increased body fat, which could lead to an increased risk of cardiovascular disease and lower high-density lipoprotein cholesterol.[28] More research must be done, however, to confirm this potential benefit in women with T1D.

[b] Trial of Type 1 Diabetes Prevention (Trial to Reduce IDDM in the Genetically at Risk [TRIGR]) is currently under way and should provide more definitive evidence for whether breast-feeding (or delay in cow's milk exposure) could result in a reduction in T1D risk in those children at increased risk.[72]

Breast-Feeding in Women with T1D

Breast-feeding rates in women with TID may be lower than in the general population. Although a number of small studies suggest that breast-feeding rates in women with and without diabetes are similar,[75,76] other studies suggest that women with T1D are less likely to breast-feed, likely because of both maternal

Table 17.III.2 Barriers to Breast-Feeding

Sociodemographic	Biomedical and Health Care Related	Psychosocial
■ Return to work ■ Living in an urban area ■ Living in the mid-western or southern region of the U.S. ■ Lower socioeconomic status ■ Single marital status ■ Younger maternal age	■ Cesarean or operative delivery ■ Early introduction to solid foods ■ Formula feeding ■ Limited prenatal education ■ Maternal obesity ■ Maternal smoking during and after pregnancy ■ No prior breast-feeding experience ■ Pacifier introduction in hospital ■ Primiparity	■ Lack of breast-feeding education ■ Low maternal confidence in breast-feeding ■ Low maternal optimism regarding breast-feeding ■ Low maternal self-efficacy in breast-feeding ■ Maternal anxiety during and after pregnancy ■ History of maternal depression, prenatal depression, or postpartum depression ■ Negative maternal attitudes toward breast-feeding

Adapted from Whalen and Cramtom[74]

and infant complications.[77,78] One study showed that initiation of breast-feeding was 77% in women with diabetes compared with 86% in women without diabetes, which reached statistical significance.[78] Another showed that women with T1D were more likely to have a shorter duration of breast-feeding.[79]

A variety of reasons may exist for lower breast-feeding rates among women with T1D. First, complications, such as a Cesarean delivery or a stay in the neonatal intensive care unit, during labor and delivery may result in separation of mother and newborn,[80–82] leading to a delay or infrequent breast-feeding.[79] Both outcomes are more common in women with T1D. Second, biomechanical issues may lead to fewer women with T1D initiating and sustaining breast-feeding. For example, infants of T1D mothers are more likely to have immature latching,[78] making breast-feeding painful for the mother and resulting in less milk consumption for the infant. Even with appropriate latching, women with T1D are more likely to have delayed lactogenesis,[75,83–85] requiring infant supplementation and shorter breast-feeding duration. Third, women with T1D who are breast-feeding may experience more frequent hypoglycemia,[73] causing women to end breast-feeding earlier than recommended.

As mentioned earlier, breast-feeding is beneficial for mothers and infants, but women with T1D may find breast-feeding particularly beneficial to their long-term health. The specific maternal benefits for T1D include the following: increased insulin sensitivity,[73] weight loss[57,86] (may lead to improved cardiovascular health), potentially improved sleep if exclusively breast-feeding,[87] and improved maternal–infant bonding. Because infants of mothers with T1D are at increased risk of developing T1D, breast-feeding could offset some of this increased risk.[68-72]

With these various considerations, providers treating women with T1D in the postpartum period should assess these potential barriers and provide the appropriate support to improve initiation and duration of breast-feeding in this population. Ensuring that mothers and infants are not separated, when not medically necessary, could improve breast-feeding initiation and duration, including early skin-to-skin contact[88,89] and night-time feedings.[90]

MEDICATION USE DURING LACTATION

Certain medications are more commonly used among women with T1D (see Table 17.III.3). When using medications, the following should be taken into consideration during the postpartum period: *1*) impact on milk production and successful breast-feeding and *2*) infant and maternal health risks.

Thyroid[93,94]

The thyroid plays an important role in human lactation, as it regulates prolactin and oxytocin. Women with T1D are more likely to have other autoimmune diseases, such as thyroid disease, and thus the need for thyroid medications in this population is much more common. Hypothyroidism may interfere with breast milk production and therefore should be promptly treated. Levothyroxine is Food and Drug Administration (FDA)–approved for hypothyroid patients during breast-feeding.

The association between hyperthyroidism and breast milk production is less understood. Medications used to treat hyperthyroidism (methimazole and prophythiouracil [PTU]) pass through human breast milk. At high doses, these drugs could block the infant's thyroid gland, resulting in neonatal hypothyroidism, and in significant and long-lasting consequences, such as intellectual and growth retardation.

Methimazole is preferred during breast-feeding.[95] The pediatrician should closely follow infants whose mothers are taking methimazole. If high doses are required, mothers should consider alternative feeding methods to reduce the risk of poor child outcomes.

Lipid Management[73]

The medication risks may outweigh the benefits during the short-term lactation period, potentially making these therapies not justifiable during lactation. The need to use these medications should be considered on a case-by-case basis. Stopping these drugs during lactation should not have a major impact on long-term management of hypercholesterolemia because atherosclerosis is a chronic condition. Lowering maternal cholesterol may affect infant neurodevelopment by lowering milk cholesterol levels. Statins (HMG Co-A reductase inhibitors) are not recommended during breast-feeding, because there are no human studies on breast milk transfer. Atorvastatin is secreted into milk of lactating rats, so

Table 17.III.3 Considerations for Using Medications While Breast-Feeding

Medication[4,91,92]	Lactation	Cautions	Recommendations
Insulins	Safe (large peptides with high molecular weights, small amounts transferred in human breast milk)	None recognized at present by the Food and Drug Administration	Use insulin as clinically appropriate for mother
Antihypertensive Medications			
Angiotensin converting enzyme (ACE) Inhibitors		Premature neonates— contraindicated because of renal toxicity	Premature neonates (≤37 weeks) do not breast-feed ■ Greater than 37 weeks: enalopril, captopril, quinapril, and benazepril compatible with breast-feeding[a] ■ Fosinopril lisinopril, and ramipril—less preferred because of lack of human data and longer half-life.
Angiotensin receptor blockers (ARBs)	Lack of study data on ARB transfer into human breast milk.	Premature neonates: renal toxicity	ARBs should be used in women who cannot tolerate ACE inhibitors, while breast feeding.
Calcium-channel blockers	**Diltiazem:** excreted into human milk; probable compatibility based on limited human studies. **Nifedipine:** excreted into human milk (limited human study data). **Amlodipine:** probably compatible with breast-feeding (no human data confirms compatibility). Likely passes into breast milk (low molecular weight).		AAP classifies both Diltiazem and Nifedipine as breast-feeding compatible.

(Continued)

Table 17.III.3 Considerations for Using Medications While Breast-Feeding (Continued)

Medication[4,91,92]	Lactation	Cautions	Recommendations
ϖϖ-**Blockers** Metoprolol Labetolol Atenolol	**Metoprolol and labetolol:** studies show no adverse outcomes. **Atenolol:** found in infant serum and urine.	β-blockers: concentrated and excreted in breast milk at higher levels than maternal serum levels. Monitor infants for bradycardia, hypotension, and symptoms of α-/β-blockade. No long-term studies. Atenolol: one case study suggested adverse reactions in a nursing infant. Closely monitor if exposed through breast milk.	AAP: Metoprolol and labetolol compatible with breast-feeding. AAP: Atenolol has significant effects in nursing infants, not recommended.
Diuretics Chlorothiazide Bedroflumethiazide Chlorthalidone Hydrochlorothiazide (HCTZ)	**Thiazides:** excreted into breast milk at low concentrations.	Thrombocytopenia may occur in nursing infants (need verification). Chlorothiazide: lactation suppression.	AAP: all thiazides are compatible with breast-feeding.
Centrally Acting Antihypertensives Methyldopa	Excreted in small quantities.	May not control hypertension effectively as other medications.	AAP: compatible with breast-feeding.

[a] This compatibility is due to small observational and case studies in which these drugs were at undetectable levels in human breast milk.

excretion into human milk would be expected.[96] There is little available data on the transfer of fibrates or ezetimbe, so caution should be exercised in using these drugs when breast-feeding. Niacin intake should not exceed the recommended dietary allowance for breast-feeding women (17 mg/day). High doses of niacin required to lower cholesterol could result in hepatotoxicity in infants. In cases in which a woman and her physician determine that treatment of high cholesterol is warranted, use of colesevalam, a bile-acid sequestrant, can be considered because it is minimally absorbed into the gastrointestinal tract and does not enter the bloodstream.

Postpartum Depression

Postpartum depression is fairly common (it affects 10–12% of women)[114] and may affect a greater proportion of T1D women.[97,115] Therefore, women with T1D may need closer monitoring for their increased risk of postpartum depression. Risk factors include pre-pregnancy depression, exposure to violence or other stressful life events, lack of social or financial support, difficult pregnancy or delivery, or neonatal health problems.[97] The etiology of postpartum depression and its relevance to T1D will be explained in greater detail (see chapter 8). This section presents recommendations for drugs and treatment of depression and breast-feeding. If a woman is suffering from her initial episode of depression, the first-line therapies should be paroxetine or sertraline, starting at the lowest dose and increasing slowly.[98] Some antidepressants, such as fluoxetine, exceed acceptable levels in breast milk, according to the American Academy of Pediatrics.[99] Table 17.III.4 summarizes advantages and disadvantages of several medications and vitamins in breast-feeding.

Vitamins

There is some evidence suggesting that individuals with T1D may be deficient in vitamin D, so it is important to ensure that lactating T1D women have adequate levels of vitamin D.[108,109] Several studies suggest that vitamin D deficiency may be associated with increased risk of T1D. Therefore, it is important to ensure that infants of women with T1D have adequate vitamin D levels.[109–111]

Evidence of the use of vitamin A supplementation, especially in women with T1D who choose to breast-feed is lacking.[112] There have been trials with vitamin A that show improvements in infant mortality.

Postpartum Contraception

Ideally, contraceptive methods with no impact on lactation should be used in the postpartum period.[73] For example, the lactational amenorrhea method (LAM) or the natural family planning used with barrier methods are recommended because they do not affect T1D or lactation. Women and their partners or spouses who have completed child-bearing may consider sterilization. Intrauterine devices also have no impact on metabolic status and are highly effective.

Women with T1D[73] must balance highly effective contraceptive methods and also support breast-feeding. For women who use lactational amenorrhea with barrier methods, this is most effective when breast-feeding is exclusive and frequent (at least every 4 h during the day and 6 h at night) without supplementation and <6 months have elapsed since delivery, with no return of menses.

Intrauterine devices (IUDs) are the most effective (99% effective in preventing pregnancy) and reversible contraceptive method. Examples include the Copper T380A IUD and levonorgestrel-releasing intrauterine system. The etongestrel-releasing contraceptive implant is also effective. A trial found no difference in volume or content of breast milk or infant growth.

The second choice methods for postpartum contraception are progestin-only hormonal contraceptives. These drugs, including pills, injections, or implants,

Table 17.III.4 Advantages and Disadvantages for Medications

Medication[98,100]	Advantages	Disadvantages	Recommendations
Antidepressants			
Selective Serotonin Reuptake Inhibitor (SSRI)	Less transmission to breast milk than transplacentally	Isolated adverse events (e.g., infant thrombocytopenia) SSRI impact on neurobehavior in infants and children unclear	AAP: unknown, but may be of concern
Tricyclic Antidepressants (TCA)	Widely used by breast-feeding mothers	Limited data on venlafaxine and buproprion	AAP: unknown, but maybe of concern[101] Doxepin: avoid due to respiratory depression caused in infant[102,103]
Vitamins			
Vitamin A	Problem in low- and middle-income countries		
Vitamin D			Necessary in areas of decreased sun exposure Doses between 4,000 IU and 6,400 IU per day shown to improve hypovitaminosis D without increasing toxicity[104,105]
Omega-3 fatty acids		Maternal mega 3-fatty acids supplementation during lactation did not appear to show improvements in child neurodevelopment, visual acuity, inflammatory makers, or allergic diseases[106,107]	

may affect milk production, especially if given up to 6 weeks postpartum. One study recommended starting progestin-only contraceptives 6 weeks postpartum because of the possibility of slower hepatic metabolism in newborns.

Hormonal contraceptives containing both estrogen and progesterone are not recommended because they risk interfering with milk production due to the dose-dependent reduction in milk supply. A shorter duration of breast-feeding is associated with estrogen and progesterone combined contraceptive use.

If required, emergency contraception should be delayed until at least 6 weeks postpartum. One study suggested discarding breast milk for the first 8 h after taking to limit infant exposure to maximum levonorgestrel through breast milk.

POSTPARTUM WEIGHT RETENTION

The difference between preconception weight and weight at the first year postpartum is defined as postpartum weight retention.[28,113] Excessive postpartum weight retention is defined as weighing >5 kg of the preconception weight at 1 year postpartum. Risk factors for excessive postpartum weight retention include excessive gestational weight gain and prepregnancy overweight or obesity. Women with T1D should be encouraged to return to their prepregnancy weight to better manage their blood glucose levels, as well as reduce their risk of diabetic complications, such as cardiovascular disease.

SLEEP DEPRIVATION[116–120]

Partial sleep deprivation is quite common during the early postpartum period because of infant caregiving. Poor sleep quality and short sleep duration can lead to fatigue and increased weight retention. Poor sleep quality may also affect blood glucose control. Therefore, it is important to evaluate T1D women during this period to ensure they are getting adequate sleep to stabilize blood glucose levels and manage weight during the postpartum.

FUTURE DIRECTIONS AND CONCLUSION

Many studies combine women with T1D and T2D. These two cohorts have significant differences (i.e., demographics, age, BMI, ethnicity, and socioeconomic factors)[121–125] and should be studied separately.

Preconception

1. Strategies to reduce unplanned pregnancies, including improved contraception options and increased education about and access to contraceptive options.
2. Research aimed at developing strategies to improve the A1C at conception through preconception counseling and education, and larger efforts to achieve better A1C control in the adult population.
3. Methods to predict and reduce gestational hypertension and preeclampsia risk.
4. Fertility data in T1D women are extremely limited.
5. Improved forms of contraception.

Pregnancy

1. Treatment of diabetic nephropathy in pregnancy: multicentered randomized controlled trials to evaluate various antihypertensive options are needed.
2. The long-term impact of exposure to selective serotonin reuptake inhibitors during pregnancy on the infant is unknown and merits further study.
3. The pathophysiology, treatment, and prevention of large for gestational age and macrosomia in infants of T1D mothers.
4. More research evaluating insulin dose timing to meals during pregnancy.
5. Impact of hyperlipidemia on pregnancy outcomes.
6. Impact of mood disorders: focused studies with T1D and pregnancy.
7. Pathophysiology and etiology of premature delivery and preterm labor in T1D women.

Postpartum

1. A lack of research exists on medication use during lactation among T1D women, especially for statin use and antidepressants.
2. More research is needed to better understand what affects duration of breast-feeding and whether breast-feeding affects the long-term health of women with T1D. In addition, research is needed to determine how to improve breast-feeding rates either through educational interventions or improved postpartum care in women with T1D.
3. More research should be conducted to determine the impact of postpartum depression on diabetes outcomes during the postpartum period among women with T1D.
4. More research is needed in the areas of postpartum weight retention, postpartum depression, and sleep deprivation on T1D and its subsequent complications.

REFERENCES

1. Data Collection Guide. American Academy of Pediatrics: Breastfeeding residency curriculum. Available at http://www.aap.org/breastfeeding/curriculum/documents/pdf/DataCollectionGuide.pdf. Accessed December 2011
2. Centers for Disease Control and Prevention: Breastfeeding: frequently asked questions. Available at http://www.cdc.gov/breastfeeding/faq/index.htm. Accessed 25 October 2012
3. World Health Organization: Nutrition topics, exclusive breastfeeding. Available at http://www.who.int/nutrition/topics/exclusive_breastfeeding/en. Accessed 25 October 2012
4. Briggs GG, Freeman RK, Yaffe SJ: *Drugs in Pregnancy and Lactation.* 8th ed. Philadelphia, PA, Wolters Kluwer I Lippincott Williams & Wilkins, 2008

5. Centers for Disease Control and Prevention: Breastfeeding among U.S. Children Born 2000–2008. CDC National Immunization Survey. Available from http://www.cdc.gov/breastfeeding/data/nis_data. Accessed 25 October 2012

6. Chua S, Arulkumaran S, Lim I, Selamat N, Ratnam SS: Influence of breastfeeding and nipple stimulation on postpartum uterine activity. *BJOG* 101:804–805, 1994

7. Baker JL, Gamborg M, Heitmann BL, Lissner L, Sorensen TI, Rasmussen KM: Breastfeeding reduces postpartum weight retention. *Am J Clin Nutr* 88:1543–1551, 2008

8. Kac G, Benicio MH, Velasquez-Melendez G, Valente JG, Struchiner CJ: Breastfeeding and postpartum weight retention in a cohort of Brazilian women. *Am J Clin Nutr* 79:487–493, 2004

9. Ostbye T, Krause KM, Swamy GK, Lovelady CA: Effect of breastfeeding on weight retention from one pregnancy to the next: results from the North Carolina WIC program. *Prev Med* 51:368–372, 2010

10. Dewey KG, Heinig MJ, Nommsen LA: Maternal weight-loss patterns during prolonged lactation. *Am J Clin Nutr* 58:162–166, 1993

11. Soedamah-Muthu SS, Fuller JH, Mulnier HE, Raleigh VS, Lawrenson RA, Colhoun HM: All-cause mortality rates in patients with type 1 diabetes mellitus compared with a non-diabetic population from the UK general practice research database, 1992-1999. *Diabetologia* 49:660–666, 2006

12. Swerdlow AJ, Jones ME: Mortality during 25 years of follow-up of a cohort with diabetes. *Int J Epidemiol* 25:1250–1261, 1996

13. Soedamah-Muthu SS, Fuller JH, Mulnier HE, Raleigh VS, Lawrenson RA, Colhoun HM: High risk of cardiovascular disease in patients with type 1 diabetes in the U.K.: a cohort study using the general practice research database. *Diabetes Care* 29:798–804, 2006

14. Gray RH, Campbell OM, Apelo R, et al.: Risk of ovulation during lactation. *Lancet* 335:25–29, 1990

15. Kennedy KI, Visness CM: Contraceptive efficacy of lactational amenorrhoea. *Lancet* 339:227–230, 1992

16. Labbok MH, Colie C: Puerperium and breast-feeding. *Curr Opin Obstet Gynecol* 4:818 825, 1992

17. Leung AK, Sauve RS: Breast is best for babies. *J Natl Med Assoc* 97:1010–1019, 2005

18. Danforth KN, Tworoger SS, Hecht JL, Rosner BA, Colditz GA, Hankinson SE: Breastfeeding and risk of ovarian cancer in two prospective cohorts. *Cancer Causes Control* 18:517–523, 2007

19. Jordan SJ, Green AC, Whiteman DC, Webb PM: Risk factors for benign, borderline and invasive mucinous ovarian tumors: epidemiological evidence of a neoplastic continuum? *Gynecol Oncol* 107:223–230, 2007

20. Nagle CM, Olsen CM, Webb PM, Jordan SJ, Whiteman DC, Green AC: Endometrioid and clear cell ovarian cancers: a comparative analysis of risk factors. *Eur J Cancer* 44:2477–2484, 2008

21. Breast cancer and breastfeeding: collaborative reanalysis of individual data from 47 epidemiological studies in 30 countries, including 50302 women with breast cancer and 96973 women without the disease. *Lancet* 360: 187–195, 2002

22. Bernier MO, Plu-Bureau G, Bossard N, Ayzac L, Thalabard JC: Breastfeeding and risk of breast cancer: a metaanalysis of published studies. *Hum Reprod Update* 6:374–386, 2000

23. Yang L, Jacobsen KH: A systematic review of the association between breastfeeding and breast cancer. *J Womens Health* (Larchmt) 17:1635–1645, 2008

24. Melton LJ, 3rd, Bryant SC, Wahner HW, et al.: Influence of breastfeeding and other reproductive factors on bone mass later in life. *Osteoporos Int* 3:76–83, 1993

25. Cumming RG, Klineberg RJ: Breastfeeding and other reproductive factors and the risk of hip fractures in elderly women. *Int J Epidemiol* 22:684–691, 1993

26. Montgomery DL, Splett PL: Economic benefit of breast-feeding infants enrolled in WIC. *Journal of the American Dietetic Association* 97:379–385, 1997

27. American Academy of Pediatrics Work Group on Breastfeeding: Breastfeeding and the use of human milk. *Pediatrics* 100:1035–1039, 1997

28. Gunderson EP, Sternfeld B, Wellons MF, et al.: Childbearing may increase visceral adipose tissue independent of overall increase in body fat. *Obesity* (Silver Spring) 16:1078–1084, 2008

29. Howie PW, Forsyth JS, Ogston SA, Clark A, Florey CD: Protective effect of breast feeding against infection. *BMJ* 300:11–16, 1990

30. Kovar MG, Serdula MK, Marks JS, Fraser DW: Review of the epidemiologic evidence for an association between infant feeding and infant health. *Pediatrics* 74:615–638, 1984

31. Popkin BM, Adair L, Akin JS, Black R, Briscoe J, Flieger W: Breast-feeding and diarrheal morbidity. *Pediatrics* 86:874–882, 1990

32. Beaudry M, Dufour R, Marcoux S: Relation between infant feeding and infections during the first six months of life. *J Pediatr* 126:191–197, 1995

33. Oddy WH: A review of the effects of breastfeeding on respiratory infections, atopy, and childhood asthma. *J Asthma* 41:605–621, 2004

34. Wright AL, Holberg CJ, Martinez FD, Morgan WJ, Taussig LM: Breast feeding and lower respiratory tract illness in the first year of life. Group Health Medical Associates. *BMJ* 299:946–949, 1989

35. Frank AL, Taber LH, Glezen WP, Kasel GL, Wells CR, Paredes A: Breastfeeding and respiratory virus infection. *Pediatrics* 70:239–245, 1982

36. Abrahams SW, Labbok MH: Breastfeeding and otitis media: a review of recent evidence. *Curr Allergy Asthma Rep* 11:508–512, 2011

37. Hanson LA: Human milk and host defence: immediate and long-term effects. *Acta Paediatr* 88(Suppl.):42–46, 1999

38. Silfverdal SA, Bodin L, Olcen P: Protective effect of breastfeeding: an ecologic study of Haemophilus influenzae meningitis and breastfeeding in a Swedish population. *Int J Epidemiol* 28:152–156, 1999

39. Arnon SS: Breast feeding and toxigenic intestinal infections: missing links in crib death? *Rev Infect Dis* 6(Suppl. 1):S193–S201, 1984

40. Jodal U: Does breast feeding protect against urinary tract infection in the first few months of life? *Pediatr Nephrol* 6:344, 1992

41. Mansour L, Mansour A: Breast feeding protects infants against urinary tract infection. *New Egypt J Med* 8:463–464, 1993
42. Pisacane A, Graziano L, Mazzarella G, Scarpellino B, Zona G: Breast-feeding and urinary tract infection. *J Pediatr* 120:87–89, 1992
43. Lucas A, Cole TJ: Breast milk and neonatal necrotising enterocolitis. *Lancet* 336:1519–1523, 1990
44. Wold AE, Adlerberth I: Breast feeding and the intestinal microflora of the infant—implications for protection against infectious diseases. *Adv Exp Med Biol* 478:77–93, 2000
45. Chapman DJ: New evidence: exclusive breastfeeding and reduced sudden infant death syndrome risk. *J Hum Lact* 27:404–405, 2011
46. Ford RP, Taylor BJ, Mitchell EA, et al.: Breastfeeding and the risk of sudden infant death syndrome. *Int J Epidemiol* 22:885–890, 1993
47. Hauck FR, Thompson JM, Tanabe KO, Moon RY, Vennemann MM: Breastfeeding and reduced risk of sudden infant death syndrome: a meta-analysis. *Pediatrics* 128:103–110, 2011
48. Vennemann MM, Bajanowski T, Brinkmann B, et al.: Does breastfeeding reduce the risk of sudden infant death syndrome? *Pediatrics* 123:e406–410, 2009
49. Klement E, Cohen RV, Boxman J, Joseph A, Reif S: Breastfeeding and risk of inflammatory bowel disease: a systematic review with meta-analysis. *Am J Clin Nutr* 80:1342–1352, 2004
50. Rigas A, Rigas B, Glassman M, et al.: Breast-feeding and maternal smoking in the etiology of Crohn's disease and ulcerative colitis in childhood. *Ann Epidemiol* 3:387–392, 1993
51. Rudant J, Orsi L, Menegaux F, et al.: Childhood acute leukemia, early common infections, and allergy: the ESCALE Study. *Am J Epidemiol* 172:1015–1027, 2010
52. Ortega-Garcia JA, Ferris-Tortajada J, Torres-Cantero AM, et al.: Full breastfeeding and paediatric cancer. *J Paediatr Child Health* 44:10–13, 2008
53. Martin RM, Gunnell D, Owen CG, Smith GD: Breast-feeding and childhood cancer: a systematic review with metaanalysis. *Int J Cancer* 117:1020–1031, 2005
54. Halken S, Host A, Hansen LG, Osterballe O: Effect of an allergy prevention programme on incidence of atopic symptoms in infancy. A prospective study of 159 "high-risk" infants. *Allergy* 47:545–553, 1992
55. Lucas A, Brooke OG, Morley R, Cole TJ, Bamford MF: Early diet of preterm infants and development of allergic or atopic disease: randomised prospective study. *BMJ* 300:837–840, 1990
56. Saarinen UM, Kajosaari M: Breastfeeding as prophylaxis against atopic disease: prospective follow-up study until 17 years old. *Lancet* 346:1065–1069, 1995
57. Stuebe A: The risks of not breastfeeding for mothers and infants. *Rev Obstet Gynecol* 2:222–231, 2009
58. Kramer MS, Aboud F, Mironova E, et al.: Breastfeeding and child cognitive development: new evidence from a large randomized trial. *Arch Gen Psychiatry* 65:578–584, 2008

59. Horwood LJ, Fergusson DM: Breastfeeding and later cognitive and academic outcomes. *Pediatrics* 101:E9, 1998
60. Rao MR, Hediger ML, Levine RJ, Naficy AB, Vik T: Effect of breastfeeding on cognitive development of infants born small for gestational age. *Acta Paediatr* 91:267–274, 2002
61. Jain A, Concato J, Leventhal JM: How good is the evidence linking breastfeeding and intelligence? *Pediatrics* 109:1044–1053, 2002
62. Feig DS, Lipscombe LL, Tomlinson G, Blumer I: Breastfeeding predicts the risk of childhood obesity in a multi-ethnic cohort of women with diabetes. *J Matern Fetal Neonatal Med* 24:511–515, 2011
63. Koletzko B, von Kries R, Closa R, et al.: Can infant feeding choices modulate later obesity risk? *Am J Clin Nutr* 89:1502S–1508S, 2009
64. Ryan AS: Breastfeeding and the risk of childhood obesity. *Coll Antropol* 31:19–28, 2007
65. Horta BL, Bahl R, Martinés JC: Evidence on the long-term effects of breastfeeding: systematic review and meta-analyses. Geneva, World Health Org., Report no. 20071-57,2007
66. Ip S, Chung M, Raman G, et al.: Breastfeeding and maternal and infant health outcomes in developed countries. *Evid Rep Technol Assess* (Full Rep) 2007:1–186, 2007
67. Harder T, Bergmann R, Kallischnigg G, Plagemann A: Duration of breastfeeding and risk of overweight: a meta-analysis. *Am J Epidemiol* 162:397–403, 2005
68. Gerstein HC: Cow's milk exposure and type I diabetes mellitus. A critical overview of the clinical literature. *Diabetes Care* 17:13–19, 1994
69. Norris JM, Scott FW: A meta-analysis of infant diet and insulin-dependent diabetes mellitus: do biases play a role? *Epidemiology* 7:87–92, 1996
70. Kostraba JN, Cruickshanks KJ, Lawler-Heavner J, et al.: Early exposure to cow's milk and solid foods in infancy, genetic predisposition, and risk of IDDM. *Diabetes* 42:288–295, 1993
71. Kreichauf S, Pfluger M, Hummel S, Ziegler AG: [Effect of breastfeeding on the risk of becoming overweight in offspring of mothers with type 1 diabetes]. *Dtsch Med Wochenschr* 133:1173–1177, 2008
72. Akerblom HK, Krischer J, Virtanen SM, et al.: The Trial to Reduce IDDM in the Genetically at Risk (TRIGR) study: recruitment, intervention and follow-up. *Diabetologia* 54:627–633, 2011
73. Tsatsoulis A, Wyckoff J, Brown FM, eds.: *Diabetes in Women: Pathophysiology and Therapy.* New York, Humana, 2009
74. Whalen B, Cramton R: Overcoming barriers to breastfeeding continuation and exclusivity. *Curr Opin Pediatr* 22:655–663, 2010
75. Webster J, Moore K, McMullan A: Breastfeeding outcomes for women with insulin dependent diabetes. *J Hum Lact* 11:195–200, 1995
76. Stage E, Norgard H, Damm P, Mathiesen E: Long-term breast-feeding in women with type 1 diabetes. *Diabetes Care* 29:771–774, 2006
77. Schoen S, Sichert-Hellert W, Hummel S, Ziegler AG, Kersting M: Breastfeeding duration in families with type 1 diabetes compared to non-affected families: results from BABYDIAB and DONALD studies in Germany. *Breastfeeding Medicine* 3:171–175, 2008

78. Hummel S, Winkler C, Schoen S, et al.: Breastfeeding habits in families with type 1 diabetes. *Diabet Med* 24:671–676, 2007
79 Sparud-Lundin C, Wennergren M, Elfvin A, Berg M: Breastfeeding in women with type 1 diabetes: exploration of predictive factors. *Diabetes Care* 34:296–301, 2011
80. Jensen DM, Damm P, Moelsted-Pedersen L, et al.: Outcomes in type 1 diabetic pregnancies: a nationwide, population-based study. *Diabetes Care* 27:2819–2823, 2004
81. Evers IM, de Valk HW, Visser GH: Risk of complications of pregnancy in women with type 1 diabetes: nationwide prospective study in the Netherlands. *BMJ* 328:915, 2004
82. Hawdon JM: Babies born after diabetes in pregnancy: what are the short- and long-term risks and how can we minimise them? *Best Pract Res Clin Obstet Gynaecol* 25:91–104, 2011
83. Neubauer SH, Ferris AM, Chase CG, et al.: Delayed lactogenesis in women with insulin-dependent diabetes mellitus. *Am J Clin Nutr* 58:54–60, 1993
84. Murtaugh MA, Ferris AM, Capacchione CM, Reece EA: Energy intake and glycemia in lactating women with type 1 diabetes. *Journal of the American Dietetic Association* 98:642–648, 1998
85. Hartmann P, Cregan M: Lactogenesis and the effects of insulin-dependent diabetes mellitus and prematurity. *J Nutr* 131:3016S–3020S, 2001
86. Wiklund P, Xu L, Lyytikainen A, et al.: Prolonged breast-feeding protects mothers from later-life obesity and related cardio-metabolic disorders. *Public Health Nutr* 15:67–74, 2012
87. Dorheim SK, Bondevik GT, Eberhard-Gran M, Bjorvatn B: Sleep and depression in postpartum women: a population-based study. *Sleep* 32:847–855, 2009
88. Mahmood I, Jamal M, Khan N: Effect of mother-infant early skin-to-skin contact on breastfeeding status: a randomized controlled trial. *Journal of the College of Physicians and Surgeons—Pakistan* 21:601–605, 2011
89. Moore ER, Anderson GC, Bergman N: Early skin-to-skin contact for mothers and their healthy newborn infants. *Cochrane Database Syst Rev* CD003519, 2007
90. Trevathan WR, Smith EO, McKenna J, eds.: *Evolutionary Medicine and Health, New Perspectives.* New York, Oxford University Press, 2007
91. Ghanem FA, Movahed A: Use of antihypertensive drugs during pregnancy and lactation. *Cardiovasc Ther* 26:38–49, 2008
92. Transfer of drugs and other chemicals into human milk. *Pediatrics* 108:776–789, 2001
93. Bahn RS, Burch HB, Cooper DS, et al.: Hyperthyroidism and other causes of thyrotoxicosis: management guidelines of the American Thyroid Association and American Association of Clinical Endocrinologists. *Endocrine Practice* 17:456–520, 2011
94. Fumarola A, Di Fiore A, Dainelli M, Grani G, Carbotta G, Calvanese A: Therapy of hyperthyroidism in pregnancy and breastfeeding. *Obstet Gynecol Surv* 66:378–385, 2011
95. Food and Drug Administration: Safety. Propylthiouracil Tablets. U.S. Department of Health & Human Services. Available at http://www.fda.gov/Safety/

MedWatch/SafetyInformation/ucm209256.htm. Accessed 25 October 2012

96. Henck JW, Craft WR, Black A, Colgin J, Anderson JA: Pre- and postnatal toxicity of the HMG-CoA reductase inhibitor atorvastatin in rats. *Toxicol Sci* 41:88–99, 1998

97. Kozhimannil KB, Pereira MA, Harlow BL: Association between diabetes and perinatal depression among low-income mothers. *JAMA* 301:842–847, 2009

98. ACOG Practice Bulletin: Clinical management guidelines for obstetrician-gynecologists number 92, April 2008 (replaces practice bulletin number 87, November 2007). Use of psychiatric medications during pregnancy and lactation. *Obstet Gynecol* 111:1001–1020, 2008

99. Berle JO, Spigset O: Antidepressant use during breastfeeding. *Curr Womens Health Review* 7:28–34, 2011

100. Lanza di Scalea T, Wisner KL: Antidepressant medication use during breastfeeding. *Clin Obstet Gynecol* 52:483–497, 2009

101. Boyd RC, Le HN, Somberg R: Review of screening instruments for postpartum depression. *Arch Womens Ment Health* 8:141–153, 2005

102. Frey OR, Scheidt P, von Brenndorff AI: Adverse effects in a newborn infant breast-fed by a mother treated with doxepin. *Ann Pharmacother* 33:690–693, 1999

103. Matheson I, Pande H, Alertsen AR: Respiratory depression caused by N-desmethyldoxepin in breast milk. *Lancet* 2:1124, 1985

104. Hollis BW, Wagner CL: Vitamin D requirements during lactation: high-dose maternal supplementation as therapy to prevent hypovitaminosis D for both the mother and the nursing infant. *Am J Clin Nutr* 80:1752S–1758S, 2004

105. Wagner CL, Hulsey TC, Fanning D, Ebeling M, Hollis BW: High-dose vitamin D3 supplementation in a cohort of breastfeeding mothers and their infants: a 6-month follow-up pilot study. *Breastfeed Med* 1:59–70, 2006

106. Klemens CM, Berman DR, Mozurkewich EL: The effect of perinatal omega-3 fatty acid supplementation on inflammatory markers and allergic diseases: a systematic review. *BJOG* 118:916–925, 2011

107. Dziechciarz P, Horvath A, Szajewska H: Effects of n-3 long-chain polyunsaturated fatty acid supplementation during pregnancy and/or lactation on neurodevelopment and visual function in children: a systematic review of randomized controlled trials. *J Am Coll Nutr* 29:443–454, 2010

108. Azar M, Basu A, Jenkins AJ, et al.: Serum carotenoids and fat-soluble vitamins in women with type 1 diabetes and preeclampsia: a longitudinal study. *Diabetes Care* 34:1258–1264, 2011

109. Takiishi T, Gysemans C, Bouillon R, Mathieu C: Vitamin D and diabetes. *Endocrinol Metab Clin North Am* 39:419–446, table of contents, 2010

110. Wolden-Kirk H, Overbergh L, Christesen HT, Brusgaard K, Mathieu C: Vitamin D and diabetes: its importance for beta cell and immune function. *Mol Cell Endocrinol* 347:106–120, 2011

111. Cooper JD, Smyth DJ, Walker NM, et al.: Inherited variation in vitamin D genes is associated with predisposition to autoimmune disease type 1 diabetes. *Diabetes* 60:1624–1631, 2011

112. Imdad A, Herzer K, Mayo-Wilson E, Yakoob MY, Bhutta ZA: Vitamin A supplementation for preventing morbidity and mortality in children from 6 months to 5 years of age. *Cochrane Database Syst Rev* CD008524, 2010

113. Gunderson EP: Childbearing and obesity in women: weight before, during, and after pregnancy. *Obstet Gynecol Clin North Am* 36:317–332, ix, 2009

114. Gaynes BN, Gavin N, Meltzer-Brody S, et al.: Perinatal depression: prevalence, screening accuracy, and screening outcomes. *Evid Rep Technol Assess* (Summ) 119:1–8, 2005

115. Rasmussen-Torvik LJ, Harlow BL: The association between depression and diabetes in the perinatal period. *Curr Diab Rep* 10:217–223, 2010

116. Hung CH: Predictors of postpartum women's health status. *J Nurs Scholarsh* 36:345–351, 2004

117. Hung CH: Women's postpartum stress, social support, and health status. *West J Nurs Res* 27:148–159, discussion 60–65, 2005

118. Hung CH, Chung HH: The effects of postpartum stress and social support on postpartum women's health status. *J Adv Nurs* 36:676–684, 2001

119. Hung CH, Lin CJ, Stocker J, Yu CY: Predictors of postpartum stress. *J Clin Nurs* 20:666–674, 2011

120. Knutson KL: Impact of sleep and sleep loss on glucose homeostasis and appetite regulation. *Sleep Med Clin* 2:187–197, 2007

121. Clausen TD, Mathiesen E, Ekbom P, Hellmuth E, Mandrup-Poulsen T, Damm P: Poor pregnancy outcome in women with type 2 diabetes. *Diabetes Care* 28:323–328, 2005

122. Cundy T GG, Townend K, Henley P, MacPherson P, Roberts A: Perinatal mortality in type 2 diabetes mellitus. *Diabet Med* 17:33–39, 2000

123. Feig DS, Palda VA: Type 2 diabetes in pregnancy: a growing concern. *Lancet* 359:1690–1692, 2002

124. Diabetes, Pregnancy Group F: French multicentric survey of outcome of pregnancy in women with pregestational diabetes. *Diabetes Care* 26:2990–2993, 2003

125. Hillman N, Herranz L, Vaquero PM, Villarroel A, Fernandez A, Pallardo LF: Is pregnancy outcome worse in type 2 than in type 1 diabetic women? *Diabetes Care* 29:2557–2558, 2006

18

Specific Settings and Populations
I. Inpatient Management and Special Procedures

Kara Hawkins, MD, and Mary Korytkowski, MD

INTRODUCTION

Both children and adults with type 1 diabetes (T1D) are more likely to require hospital admission when compared to those without diabetes.[1] They are also more likely to undergo outpatient medical and surgical procedures that require changes in dietary intake that can affect insulin requirements and glycemic control. In fact, the majority of patients undergoing elective surgical procedures are admitted the morning of the procedure, necessitating adjustments in insulin therapy that are conveyed to and implemented by patients and their family members. It is therefore important that there be protocols and standardized approaches available that guide preoperative and preprocedural insulin adjustments as a way to ensure that glycemic control is maintained during these critical time periods.

Hospitalizations in patients with T1D are often related to acute metabolic complications, such as diabetic ketoacidosis (DKA) or hypoglycemia;[1] chronic diabetes-related complications, such as kidney, heart, or ophthalmologic disorders;[2,3] or general medical or surgical conditions. Approximately 25% of children present in DKA at diagnosis.[4] Severe hypoglycemia occurs at a reported rate of 19 per 100 person-years in children.[5] Adults with T1D experience one severe or disabling hypoglycemic event each year.[6] When hospital admissions do occur, they generally are longer and costlier than for those without diabetes for both children and adults with T1D.[7]

Risk factors for hospital admission include higher outpatient A1C, higher triglyceride levels, significant microalbuminuria, and longer duration of diabetes.[2] Patients with psychiatric disorders and inadequate medical insurance are more likely to have recurrent admissions. Hospitalizations for hyperglycemia related to infection or other nondiabetes illnesses are rare when patients are routinely seen in outpatient settings that provide self-management education and support for "sick-day" management.[4] This suggests that a proportion of hospitalizations are preventable.[8]

Once patients with T1D are admitted to the hospital, they may encounter physicians and nurses who do not appreciate the importance of avoiding interruptions in outpatient insulin therapy. Many hospitals resort to sliding scale insulin (SSI) as the sole method for glycemic management. Use of SSI alone is not recommended as it puts patients with T1D at high risk for both uncontrolled hyperglycemia and hypoglycemia. These glycemic excursions further increase the risk for hospital-acquired infections and prolonged length of stay (LOS).[9–11]

DOI: 10.2337/9781580404785ch18s1

PREPARATION OF THE PATIENT WITH T1D FOR ELECTIVE PROCEDURES OR SURGERY

All patients with T1D require ongoing insulin therapy even when fasting for prolonged periods in preparation for outpatient procedures (e.g., colonoscopy or upper endoscopy) or elective surgery. Insulin dosing the night before and morning of surgery depends on the patient's insulin types, the level of glycemic control, and the plan for glycemic management during the procedure or surgery (i.e., intravenous [IV] insulin infusion). Suggested adjustments to an insulin regimen are outlined in Table 18.I.1.

It is usually safe to administer 70 to 100% of long-acting insulin preparations and 50 to 70% of usual intermediate-acting insulin doses before surgery, depending on the current level of glycemic control.[12] The rationale for the differences in dose adjustments among the different basal insulin preparations is based on their different pharmacokinetic profiles. Patients who use continuous subcutaneous insulin infusions (CSII) may need to continue their usual basal rates or reduce them by up to 30% overnight and the morning of surgery.[13] There are no studies investigating the safety and efficacy of allowing patients to use an insulin pump throughout a surgical procedure. Despite the absence of data, many institutions allow patients to continue to use this form of therapy during short-term outpatient procedures. Careful monitoring of blood glucose (BG)

Table 18.I.1 Guide for Preoperative or Preprocedural Insulin Therapy

	Clear Liquid Diets	NPO Status
Premeal RAA or R insulin	Reduce usual doses by 50% or use carbohydrate counting to calculate doses	Take usual doses up until the time nutritional status changes Discontinue RAA and R once oral intake is discontinued
NPH or insulin detemir	Take 50 to 70 % of usual insulin doses on the evening prior to or morning of the surgical procedure	Take 50 to 70 % of usual insulin doses on the evening prior to or morning of the surgical procedure
Glargine insulin	Take 70 to 100% of usual insulin doses	Take 70 to 100% of usual insulin doses
Premix insulin (70/30, 75/25, 50/50)	Take 50 to 75% of usual doses	Take 1/3 of usual dose as NPH insulin prior to the procedure
Insulin pump therapy	Continue usual basal rates	Continue usual basal rates

NPH, intermediate-acting insulin; NPO, nothing per mouth; R, regular insulin; RAA, rapid-acting insulin analog performed at hourly intervals allows for detection of hypoglycemia or hypergly-cemia with appropriate interventions.

Perioperative Management

Once patients arrive in the procedural suite or preoperative holding area, responsibility for glycemic management is often transferred to hospital person-nel (see Table 18.I.1). Measurement of a capillary or BG on arrival helps identify patients who will require more frequent glucose monitoring or intervention dur-ing the planned procedure. Patients who have glucose levels >150–200 mg/dl may require additional subcutaneous (SC) or IV insulin to avoid further deteriorations in glycemic control during the procedure.[12] Brief surgical procedures or those performed using epidural anesthesia or splanchnic nerve blockade are less likely to be associated with intraoperative increases in cortisol, glucose, free fatty acids, and catecholamine excretion than what occurs with general anesthesia.[14]

IV insulin therapy may be necessary for patients undergoing prolonged surgical procedures with general anesthesia. IV insulin infusion provides the most flexible approach to glycemic control in these situations because it allows for rapid changes in doses.[15,16] If an insulin infusion achieves adequate glycemic control, and the patient is well enough to go to a non–intensive care unit (ICU) setting after recovery from anesthesia, short-acting insulin or rapid-acting insulin analog (RAA) can be administered SC before discontinuation of the IV insulin.[12] Once oral intake is established, the outpatient regimen can be resumed. In the setting of poor appetite with reduced oral intake, prandial doses of insulin can be reduced by ~50%.

For patients treated with insulin pump therapy, IV insulin should be started before or at the time of pump discontinuation as a way to avoid any period of insulin deficiency and risk for uncontrolled hyperglycemia. The use of dextrose (D5 or D10) containing IV fluids can both prevent hypoglycemia and provide substrate for prevention of ketogenesis.[13]

GLYCEMIC GOALS FOR HOSPITALIZED PATIENTS WITH T1D

Recommended glycemic targets for the majority of hospitalized patients with diabetes are to maintain BG values between 100 and 180 mg/dl (Table 18.I.2).[17] Well-controlled patients with near-normal A1C levels in the outpatient setting may be uncomfortable with relaxing their glycemic control to these levels. Cur-rent recommendations allow for individual glycemic goals in the hospital, includ-ing lower BG targets if this can be achieved safely without increasing the risk for severe hypoglycemia. Very young children or older individuals with shorter life expectancy or multiple comorbidities may be treated to a maximal BG of 200 mg/dl to minimize hypoglycemia risk.[18]

Inpatient Glycemic Goals for Children and Geriatric Patients

Inpatient glycemic goals for children and geriatric patients are less established. Some trials in critically ill infants and children suggest an inverse correlation

Table 18.I.2 Glycemic Goals and Recommended Insulin Therapy for Hospitalized Patients with T1D

Population	BG in mg/dl premeal/ random	Insulin
Children ages 0–6 years[a]	100–180 / 110–200	LAA plus RAA for nutrition and correction
Children ages 6–12 years[a]	90–180 / 100–180	LAA plus RAA for nutrition and correction
Adolescents ages 13–19 years[a]	90–130 / 90–150	LAA plus RAA for nutrition and correction
Adults[b]	100–140 / ≤180	LAA plus RAA for nutrition and correction
Adults with multiple comorbidities	≤200	LAA plus RAA for nutrition and correction
Adults with critical illness	140–180	IV insulin infusion

[a] IV insulin infusion recommended in critical illness

IV, intravenous; LAA, long-acting analog; RAA, rapid-acting insulin analog

[b] In adult patients who are well controlled in the outpatient setting, lower BG targets can be attempted if this can be safely achieved.

between severity of hyperglycemia and survival.[19] In one trial performed in infants and children with critical illness–associated hyperglycemia, the use of IV insulin infusions to achieve glycemic targets of 50–79 mg/dl in infants and 70–101 mg/dl in children was associated with improved outcomes when compared to those treated more conventionally.[19] Less than 1% of participants in this trial had diabetes. Another study demonstrated more hypoglycemia and higher mortality in very low birth weight infants treated to achieve a mean BG of 108 mg/dl.[20] The risks of adverse sequelae related to hypoglycemia may be greater among infants and young children who do not have the ability to report hypoglycemic symptoms.[20] Until more data are available, it may be reasonable to adopt the outpatient glycemic goals established by the American Diabetes Association (ADA) for children and adolescents.[21] Others have recommended glycemic targets for critically ill children similar to those for adults.[22] Similar recommendations can be applied to the population of older adults with T1D (Table 18.I.2).

Inpatient Glycemic Management

Noncritical illness. Patients with T1D require combination insulin therapy with long-acting analogs (LAA) or intermediate-acting insulin (NPH) and prandial short-acting (regular) insulin or RAA. It is no longer appropriate to depend on SSI for glycemic management in T1D individuals. This practice results in accelerated hyperglycemia when doses are held for BG below the lower target and in overtreatment when BG levels are higher.

Measuring A1C upon hospital admission helps assess the adequacy of the home insulin regimen and is recommended if an A1C level from the preceding 2–3 months is unavailable. In general, patients who are eating can continue their usual home regimen. In patients who will not be eating for a specified period of time, short-acting insulin or RAA should be held until nutrition is resumed. Correction insulin (also referred to as supplemental insulin) in combination with the basal intermediate or LAA can be provided at intervals of 4–6 h to treat glycemic excursions above 140 mg/dl.[17] Modification of the home insulin regimen may be required to avoid hypoglycemia or prevent hyperglycemia resulting from clinical status changes, illness severity, altered caloric intake or physical activity, and medication use that may affect glycemic control. Many patients can provide useful information in guiding the inpatient insulin regimen based on prior experiences.

Inpatient use of CSII. Many T1D patients use CSII with an insulin pump. Providers must identify whether CSII use in the hospital is safe and appropriate for a patient's clinical situation. Contraindications to inpatient CSII use include altered mental status, suicide risk, critical illness, DKA, patient refusal or preference, or the unavailability of a family member to help the patient if he or she cannot perform self-management.[23] The use of formal protocols for CSII in the hospital has been shown to be effective and safe in guiding the care in appropriately selected patients.[24,25] If hospital personnel cannot support such protocols, it is reasonable to transition a patient to SC injections. The intermediate or long-acting insulin dose is calculated as the total basal insulin dose delivered by the pump device. The prandial insulin dose is based on the usual prandial doses at home. If a patient is unable to provide the dose information, a weight-based calculation for insulin dosing can be made (see the section on insulin therapy).

Critical illness. IV insulin offers the greatest flexibility for glycemic control in the critical care setting. Several published protocols target BG ranges of 110–140 mg/dl and 140–180 mg/dl.[17,26] All IV insulin infusions require careful and frequent BG monitoring to achieve and maintain desired glycemic targets while also avoiding hypoglycemia. At the lower target ranges for BG, some protocols recommend temporary discontinuation of the insulin infusion. These protocols should be modified for patients with T1D to allow for continuous insulin delivery at reduced doses to avert possible untoward increases in BG and DKA.

To ensure uninterrupted insulin treatment when transitioning from IV to SC insulin, all patients with T1D require SC insulin at least 2 h before discontinuation of the IV insulin infusion. The initial dose and distribution of SC insulin is determined by the IV insulin requirement before transition. The clinician must also consider the patient's anticipated nutritional and clinical status and concomitant medications that affect glycemic control, such as vasopressors or steroids.[27]

Glucocorticoid Therapy

Glucocorticoid therapy is one of the most frequent contributors to uncontrolled hyperglycemia in the hospital. Although variability of the therapy depends on the steroid preparation used and dosing interval, postprandial BG is often affected to a greater extent than fasting BG.[28] For example, prednisone has a peak glycemic effect ~8 h following oral administration. Intermediate-acting insulin (NPH) given at the time of a once-daily prednisone dose usually matches the glycemic effect.[29] For patients receiving twice-daily prednisone, an increase in their basal, prandial, and correctional insulin often is necessary. Dexamethasone has a longer half-life and duration of action. Its action profile most closely matches detemir or glargine insulin.[29]

Most patients with T1D are already on insulin therapy at the time glucocorticoids are started, and not all patients experience deterioration in their glycemic control with the use of these agents. Although there are no published guidelines for prevention and management of steroid-associated hyperglycemia, some principles apply. In patients receiving therapy with steroids for the first time, recommendations to increase the frequency of glucose monitoring with instructions to increase prandial or basal insulin doses in the event of hyperglycemia can offset risk for severe hyperglycemia requiring hospitalization. For patients who have a history of steroid-associated hyperglycemia, insulin dose adjustments can be more straightforward. Some guidelines suggest preemptive increases in all insulin doses of 20% or more with the initiation of steroid therapy in these patients. Continued glucose monitoring of capillary glucose levels and close communication with the diabetes health-care team generally is required to guide therapy, however. These principles can be applied to patients who have glucocorticoid therapy prescribed in the outpatient setting as well as in the hospital.

A frequently overlooked important area of management is the downward titration of insulin with the downward titration of glucocorticoid therapy to prevent hypoglycemia. Patients and their families require education regarding the importance of reducing insulin doses with reductions in the doses of steroid therapy.

Use of Enteral or Parenteral Nutrition

There are no randomized controlled trials examining optimal insulin regimens for patients with T1D receiving enteral (EN) or total parenteral nutrition (TPN). For continuous EN, LAAs (glargine or detemir) can be administered once or twice a day in combination with regular insulin every 6 h.[30] Twice-daily LAAs allow for flexible insulin dosing in cases of rapidly changing clinical status. Correction insulin may be used in combination with basal insulin for glycemic excursions >140 mg/dl and may be useful in calculating adjustments to the total daily dose of scheduled insulin. Biphasic 70/30 insulin administered every 6 to 12 h has been shown to achieve desired levels of glycemic control with low risk for hypoglycemia.[31] For patients receiving EN administered over 12–18 h, LAAs or intermediate-acting insulin in combination with short-acting (regular) insulin can be given at the initiation of the nutrition supplement followed by additional doses of scheduled regular insulin at 6 h intervals for the duration of the prandial state. For unexpected interruption of supplemental nutrition, initiation of dextrose-containing IV fluids infused at the same rate can prevent severe hypoglycemic events related to the insulin bolus.

For patients receiving TPN, basal insulin can be used in combination with short-acting insulin given every 6 h or added to the TPN solution. The amount of correction insulin required to maintain glycemic control can be calculated and added to the TPN solution the next day until BG levels are maintained within the desired range without need for excessive doses of correction insulin.

Glucose Monitoring

Reliable and reproducible bedside glucose measurements are essential to ensure the safety of inpatient insulin therapy in patients with T1D. Currently available point of care (POC) bedside meters may vary by 20% when compared with laboratory glucose measures.[32] Many meters provide erroneously high BG results in the setting of anemia (hematocrit [HCT] <25%) and erroneously low values in the setting of polycythemia.[33] In these situations, BG measurement in the central or other clinical laboratory provides accurate results but may not always be feasible outside critical care areas.

Patients may wish to use their own glucose meters when hospitalized. Although this is permissible, these results should be validated against hospital meters, which can be downloaded into a hospital laboratory system.

The timing of bedside BG monitoring is an important component of guiding therapy for patients with T1D. For patients who are eating, BG should be checked no longer than 60 min before meal delivery. BG can be monitored every 6 h for patients receiving EN or TPN or in patients not eating.

TRANSITION FROM INPATIENT TO OUTPATIENT CARE SETTINGS

Hospitalization is an opportunity to provide diabetes self-management education for patients who otherwise may not receive it. Young adults who have had diabetes since childhood may have relied on their parents' knowledge and help with their disease. An admission for an acute complication of diabetes may occur as a result of a knowledge gap in self-management. Assessing such deficiencies in knowledge and addressing them may avert future complications and admissions. Likewise, psychosocial factors interfering with optimal self-management should be sought and discussed with the patient. In the past, patients with newly diagnosed T1D often were kept in the hospital for several days for education in self-management, but most hospitals now discharge patients when they are medically stable and leave the majority of education to be done in the outpatient setting. Because of the many stressors patients undergo during hospitalization, education should focus on any specific knowledge deficiency identified as well as the survival skills of diabetes, including basic meal planning, medication administrations, BG monitoring, hypoglycemia and hyperglycemia detection, and treatment and prevention (Table 18.I.3).[18] Depending on the age of a child, most of these survival skills also need to be taught to a parent or caregiver.

Table 18.I.3 Discharge Planning for Patients with T1D[21]

Discussion topics with written information at discharge	Supplies for discharge
Provider and appointment for diabetes care after discharge	Insulin (vials or pens) Pump/sensor supplies if needed
SMBG instructions	Syringes or pen needles
Insulin doses and timing	BG meter and test strips
Definition, recognition, treatment, and prevention of hyperglycemia and hypoglycemia	Lancets and lancing device
Basic meal planning	Urine ketone strips or blood ketone strips
Sick-day management	Glucose tabs
Proper use and disposal of needles and syringes	Glucagon emergency kit (insulin-treated)
Contact information for diabetes provider	Medical alert bracelet/necklace

SMBG, self-monitoring of blood glucose

Given that hospitalizations are now shorter, referral should be made for continuing education in the outpatient setting for diabetes self-management and nutritional therapy. Instructions should be given for self-monitoring of blood glucose (SMBG), insulin dosing, and when to contact a provider for help. All supplies for SMBG, insulin administration, and hypoglycemia and hyperglycemia treatment should be given at the time of discharge. An outpatient appointment within 1–4 weeks should be arranged before leaving the hospital. Verbally communicated instructions often are inadequate. Several institutions have established formalized, printed discharge instructions for patients.[34] Patients and post–hospital care providers must know that some medications prescribed at the time of hospital discharge (e.g., corticosteroid therapy for pulmonary conditions, octreotide after gastrointestinal surgery) may require adjustments in insulin therapy. Measurement of A1C during the hospital stay can assist in tailoring the glycemic management at time of discharge. A1C <7% usually indicates that the home insulin regimen was adequate and can be resumed at discharge. Patients with elevated A1C values often require intensification of the outpatient insulin regimen, whereas those with a history of severe hypoglycemia may require moderation of their prior regimen.

Whether patients with T1D are admitted for acute or chronic complications of diabetes or for general medical conditions, appropriate management depends on correctly identifying the type of diabetes, and with that, the absolute need for exogenous insulin. Likewise, providers must know that patients with T1D have higher insulin sensitivity and less endogenous insulin production compared to patients with type 2 diabetes; this important difference often requires a change in the insulin-dosing strategy and a heightened awareness for hypoglycemia. Identifying educational needs and limitations to diabetes self-management early in the hospitalization helps target educational interventions. If glycemic control was suboptimal before hospital admission, the opportunity should be seized to intensify or modify the outpatient regimen. Hospital care providers should give clear and complete discharge instructions with referral to outpatient diabetes education and timely follow-up with a diabetes provider.

GAPS ACCORDING TO THE EDITORS

1. There is a need to ensure the proper education and ongoing training of health care providers and hospital personnel on the proper care of patients with T1D of all ages undergoing surgical procedures.
2. Ongoing research is needed to devise strategies to avoid deterioration of glycemic control and ketosis or ketoacidosis during illness and elective or emergent surgical procedures of all patients with T1D.

REFERENCES

1. Donnan PT, Leese GP, Morris AD: Hospitalizations for people with type 1 and type 2 diabetes compared with the nondiabetic population of Tayside, Scotland: a retrospective cohort study of resource use. *Diabetes Care* 23(12):1774–1779, 2000
2. Tomlin AM, Dovey SM, Tilyard MW: Risk factors for hospitalization due to diabetes complications. *Diabetes Research & Clinical Practice* 80(2):244–252, 2008
3. Tomlin AM, Tilyard MW, Dovey SM, Dawson AG: Hospital admissions in diabetic and non-diabetic patients: a case-control study. *Diabetes Research & Clinical Practice* 73(3):260–267, 2006
4. Wolfsdorf J, Glaser N, Sperling MA: Diabetic ketoacidosis in infants, children, and adolescents: A consensus statement from the American Diabetes Association. *Diabetes Care* 29(5):1150–1159, 2006
5. Rewers A, Chase HP, Mackenzie T, et al.: Predictors of acute complications in children with type 1 diabetes. *JAMA* 287(19):2511–2518, 2002
6. Cryer PE: The barrier of hypoglycemia in diabetes. *Diabetes* 57(12):3169–3176, 2008
7. Angus VC, Waugh N: Hospital admission patterns subsequent to diagnosis of type 1 diabetes in children: a systematic review. *BMC Health Services Research* 7:199, 2007
8. Wang J, Imai K, Engelgau MM, Geiss LS, Wen C, Zhang P: Secular trends in diabetes-related preventable hospitalizations in the United States, 1998-2006. *Diabetes Care* 32(7):1213–1217, 2009
9. Clement S, Braithwaite SS, Magee MF, et al.: Management of diabetes and hyperglycemia in hospitals. *Diabetes Care* 27(2):553–591, 2004
10. Capes SE, Hunt D, Malmberg K, Pathak P, Gerstein HC: Stress hyperglycemia and prognosis of stroke in nondiabetic and diabetic patients: a systematic overview. *Stroke* 32(10):2426–2432, 2001

11. Golden SH, Peart-Vigilance C, Kao WH, Brancati FL: Perioperative glycemic control and the risk of infectious complications in a cohort of adults with diabetes. *Diabetes Care* 22(9):1408–14014, 1999
12. DiNardo M, Donihi AC, Forte P, Gieraltowski L, Korytkowski M: Standardized glycemic management and perioperative glycemic outcomes in patients with diabetes mellitus who undergo same-day surgery. *Endocrine Practice* 17(3):404, 2011
13. Glister BC, Vigersky RA: Perioperative management of type 1 diabetes mellitus. *Endocrinology & Metabolism Clinics of North America* 32(2):411–436, 2003
14. Shirasaka C, Tsuji H, Asoh T, Takeuchi Y: Role of the splanchnic nerves in endocrine and metabolic response to abdominal surgery. *British Journal of Surgery* 73(2):142–145, 1986
15. Furnary AP, Zerr KJ, Grunkemeier GL, Starr A: Continuous intravenous insulin infusion reduces the incidence of deep sternal wound infection in diabetic patients after cardiac surgical procedures. *Ann Thorac Surg* 67(2):352–360; discussion 360–362, 1999
16. Akhtar S, Barash PG, Inzucchi SE: Scientific principles and clinical implications of perioperative glucose regulation and control. *Anesthesia & Analgesia* 110(2):478–497, 2010
17. Moghissi ES, Korytkowski MT, DiNardo MM, et al.: American Association of Clinical Endocrinologists and American Diabetes Association consensus statement on inpatient glycemic control. *Diabetes Care* 32(6):1119–1131, 2009
18. Umpierrez GE, Hellman R, Korytkowski MT, et al.: Management of hyperglycemia in hospitalized patients in non-critical care setting: an endocrine society clinical practice guideline. *Journal of Clinical Endocrinology & Metabolism* 97(1):16–38, 2012
19. Vlasselaers D, Milants I, Desmet L, et al.: Intensive insulin therapy for patients in paediatric intensive care: a prospective, randomised controlled study. *Lancet* 373(9663):547–556, 2009
20. Beardsall K, Vanhaesebrouck S, Ogilvy-Stuart AL, et al.: Early insulin therapy in very-low-birth-weight infants. *New England Journal of Medicine* 359(18):1873–1884, 2008
21. American Diabetes Association. Standards of medical care for patients with diabetes mellitus. *Diabetes Care* 35 (Suppl. 1): S11–S63, 2012
22. Tridgell DM, Tridgell AH, Hirsch IB, Tridgell DM, Tridgell AH, Hirsch IB: Inpatient management of adults and children with type 1 diabetes. *Endocrinology & Metabolism Clinics of North America* 39(3):595–608, 2010
23. Nassar AA, Partlow BJ, Boyle ME, Castro JC, Bourgeois PB, Cook CB: Outpatient-to-inpatient transition of insulin pump therapy: successes and continuing challenges. *Journal of Diabetes Science & Technology* 4(4):863–872, 2010
24. Bailon RM, Partlow BJ, Miller-Cage V, Boyle ME, Castro JC, Bourgeois PB, Cook CB: Continuous subcutaneous insulin infusion (insulin pump) therapy can be safely used in the hospital in select patients. *Endocrine Practice* 15:24–29, 2009

25. Noschese ML, DiNardo MM, Donihi AC, et al.: Patient outcomes after implementation of a protocol for inpatient insulin pump therapy. *Endocrine Practice* 15(5):415–424, 2009
26. Reider J, Donihi A, Korytkowski MT, Reider J, Donihi A, Korytkowski MT: Practical implications of the revised guidelines for inpatient glycemic control. *Polskie Archiwum Medycyny Wewnetrznej* 119(12):801–809, 2009
27. Rea RS, Donihi AC, Bobeck M, et al.: Implementing an intravenous insulin infusion protocol in the intensive care unit. *Am J Health Syst Pharm* 64(4):385–395, 2007
28. Iwamoto T, Kagawa Y, Naito Y, Kuzuhara S, Kojima M: Steroid-induced diabetes mellitus and related risk factors in patients with neurologic diseases. *Pharmacotherapy* 24(4):508–514, 2004
29. Clore JN, Thurby-Hay L: Glucocorticoid-induced hyperglycemia. *Endocrine Practice* 15(5):469–474, 2009
30. Korytkowski MT, Salata RJ, Koerbel GL, et al.: Insulin therapy and glycemic control in hospitalized patients with diabetes during enteral nutrition therapy: a randomized controlled clinical trial. *Diabetes Care* 32(4):594–596, 2009
31. Braithwaite SS: Inpatient insulin therapy. *Current Opinion in Endocrinology, Diabetes & Obesity* 15(2):159–166, 2008
32. Scott MG, Bruns DE, Boyd JC, Sacks DB: Tight glucose control in the intensive care unit: are glucose meters up to the task? *Clinical Chemistry* 55(1):18–20, 2009
33. Dungan K, Chapman J, Braithwaite SS, Buse J: Glucose measurement: confounding issues in setting targets for inpatient management. *Diabetes Care* 30(2):403–409, 2007
34. Lauster CD, Gibson JM, DiNella JV, DiNardo M, Korytkowski MT, Donihi AC: Implementation of standardized instructions for insulin at hospital discharge. *Journal of Hospital Medicine* 4(8):E41–E42, 2009

II. Schools

Crystal Crismond Jackson and Janet Silverstein, MD

INTRODUCTION

Managing type 1 diabetes (T1D) in children requires not only the support of family members within the home but also the orchestrated efforts of responsible adults while the child is away from home. Thus, there is a need to ensure the proper education and training of responsible adults to provide care to children with diabetes in a variety of settings, including schools and school-sponsored programs, camps, and child care facilities. This chapter will focus on the school's role in diabetes management of school-age children.

Consideration should be given to the maturity and ability of each child to self-manage their diabetes. Many students are able to handle all or most of their non emergency care without assistance. Others, because of age, development level, or inexperience will need help from school personnel. All children will need help in the event of a diabetes emergency. Schools need to ensure that a school nurse or other trained school personnel is always available, during the school day and at school-sponsored events, to provide necessary care.

LEGAL PROTECTIONS FOR CHILDREN WITH DIABETES

An understanding of federal and state laws that affect school diabetes care and provide protections against unfair treatment of children with disabilities (including diabetes) by their schools and other public facilities will allow health care providers to be effective advocates for their patients and can ensure that their patients are aware of key school advocacy organizations and resources.[1] Federal laws include the Americans with Disabilities Act, Section 504 of the Rehabilitation Act of 1973 (Section 504), and the Individuals with Disabilities Education Act (IDEA).[2] School diabetes care team members are expected to understand these laws and how they affect the school's legal obligation to provide diabetes care in schools.

The Americans with Disabilities Act

The Americans with Disabilities Act prohibits all public and private schools, preschools, day care centers, and camps (except those run by religious institutions) from discriminating against a child with a disability and requires schools to make reasonable changes in its practices and policies to avoid discrimination. Disability is defined as a physical or mental impairment that substantially limits one or more major life activities. Children with diabetes are considered to have a disability in that their β-cells, a key component of the endocrine system, are destroyed and thus are limited in their ability to function adequately without a

DOI: 10.2337/9781580404785ch18s2

special accommodation, i.e., blood glucose (BG) monitoring and administration of insulin. The Americans with Disabilities Act prohibits the consideration of mitigating measures (i.e., use of insulin or other medications) when determining whether a student is substantially limited in a major life activity. For a child with diabetes, this means that they must have an equal opportunity to safely participate in academic and all school-sponsored events, such as field trips and extracurricular activities. This law requires that schools provide necessary health services, such as ensuring that either the school nurse or other trained school personnel are available to administer insulin and glucagon as needed, perform BG checks and act on BG results, recognize and treat hypo- and hyperglycemia, and understand the impact of food intake and physical activity upon BG control. To meet the requirement of federal laws, trained personnel must be available to provide the needed level of care so that students may safely participate in the classroom, field trips, and at school-sponsored events.

Section 504 of the Rehabilitation Act of 1973 (Section 504)

Section 504 applies to public and private schools that receive federal funding assistance. Religious schools may have obligations to provide services and care under this law if the school receives federal financial assistance. The standard of coverage for children under this law is the same as the Americans with Disabilities Act, so children with diabetes are protected against discrimination and unfair treatment. Just as in the Americans with Disabilities Act, Section 504 requires covered schools to identify students with disabilities and provide needed services to enable students with diabetes to safely access and participate in their school activities. These services should be documented in a Section 504 plan.

IDEA

Under IDEA, the federal government provides financial assistance to state and local education agencies for these agencies to provide "free, appropriate education" to qualifying children with disabilities. A student with diabetes is covered if he or she needs special education and related services to benefit from an education. Diabetes itself is not covered by IDEA but it is covered if the diabetes makes it more difficult for the child to learn or if the child has another disability that adversely affects academic progress. Students with diabetes who have adverse events that affect their ability to learn should be entitled to services under this law. Recurrent hypoglycemia or frequent fluctuations in BG levels that may affect the student's ability to concentrate or pay attention are such examples. Children who qualify under this law must be educated in the least restrictive environment possible with other children. Once it has been determined that a student is eligible for services under IDEA, the services should be documented in the student's Individualized Education Program (IEP).

State Laws and Regulations

Most states have laws and regulations that impact school diabetes care. These laws and regulations include nurse practice acts, Good Samaritan laws, education codes, state board of nursing regulations, and others. Many states have laws or regulations that require schools to permit trained school personnel who are not licensed health-care professionals to provide diabetes care, including insulin and glucagon administration; to permit capable students to self-manage their diabetes anywhere, anytime; and to prohibit schools from transferring students with diabetes to a different school to receive care.

Section 504 Plans and IEPs

Before the start of the academic year, parents should be encouraged to contact their child's school principal or 504 coordinator to initiate the process of determining eligibility for services under federal laws. As stated, the student's 504 plan or IEP should document the health services and academic modifications required to meet the needs of the student with diabetes. Although plans should be individualized for each child, every plan should include a provision that the school nurse and trained school personnel will be available to provide care that includes, but is not limited to, BG monitoring, insulin and glucagon administration, and recognition and treatment of hypo- and hyperglycemia. In addition to health services, the student's Section 504 plan or IEP should include provisions for self-care, coverage for field trips and extracurricular activities, and allowance for alternate times to take exams if BG levels are out of range. The plan should also elucidate other academic adjustments as needed.[3]

DIABETES MANAGEMENT AT SCHOOL

Continuous, uninterrupted care is critical for maintaining BG control and minimizing complications. As children spend a substantial amount of time at school ($\geq$6 h per day), it is necessary that the school provide a safe and supportive school environment. A seamless transition from home to school requires diabetes care provisions that include monitoring BG levels throughout the day, insulin administration, and recognition and prompt treatment of hypo- and hyperglycemia. The goal of diabetes management in the school is to provide optimal diabetes care to enable the child to achieve academic success, to fully experience and participate in all school activities, and to support the child's transition to independence. School staff needs to understand how to meet the needs of the individual with diabetes so that they may help and support the student in managing the diabetes with minimal disruption of the child's education. The most effective way to ensure a safe school environment for the students is for the school nurse to lead a team of trained school staff members who volunteer to undergo diabetes specific education and training to aid the child.[4]

Intensive insulin therapy requires the concerted efforts of a small group of school personnel who have custodial responsibility for the student. Achieving optimal BG control demands either multiple daily injections (MDI) of insulin using a syringe or pen or continuous subcutaneous insulin infusion (CSII) via a pump or pod. All insulin regimens require frequent BG monitoring along with careful attention to dietary intake and physical activity. When the school nurse is not available, school personnel, using the student's Diabetes Medical Management

Plan (DMMP) or physician's order, must be trained and prepared to know how to assist the youth in ensuring the correct insulin dose is administered based on food intake, the intensity of physical activity, and BG level. Snacks are likely needed before exercise and extra insulin may be needed before school parties and celebrations that include extra food. It is not surprising that managing diabetes in school-age children with the ever-evolving technology may seem overwhelming to school personnel, but fortunately, there are many comprehensive resources available to educate and train them.

The School Diabetes Care Team

Coordination and collaboration among members of the school diabetes care team is essential for the student's diabetes management. Members of the team, usually led by the school nurse, often include the student and parent, teachers, administrators, 504 coordinators, the guidance counselor, coaches, lunchroom staff, and other school staff members, all of whom may be trained diabetes personnel. This team should have a more in-depth knowledge of diabetes, have specific training on how to implement the student's written care plans, understand hypoglycemia and hyperglycemia effects on behavior, and know the expectations for diabetes management in the classroom. The school health care team needs to communicate frequently to ensure consistent diabetes management. Members should understand the basic physiology of diabetes and the federal laws governing the accommodations for youth with diabetes in the school setting. Each member of the team has specific roles and responsibilities. Information about these specific roles and responsibilities can be found in the National Diabetes Education Program's (NDEP) "Helping the Student with Diabetes Succeed: A Guide for School Personnel."[2] The student's ability to academically thrive and grow in the school environment increases when the school diabetes care team works together to implement the student's written plans.

Training of School Personnel

Although school nurses are primarily responsible for the student's diabetes care, not all schools have a nurse. Even in schools that do have a full-time school nurse, the school nurse cannot be in all places at all times. It is unrealistic to expect school nurses to accompany students with T1D on all field trips and school-sponsored after-school activities. Thus, nonmedical school personnel need to be trained and evaluated for competency in all diabetes tasks, including BG monitoring, insulin and glucagon administration, and recognition and treatment of hypoglycemia and hyperglycemia. The nonmedical personnel may not make medical decisions, but they are expected to carry out the student's DMMP.

The preferred model of school care is one in which the school nurse is the primary care provider with supplemental care being provided by trained school personnel. In states where its nurse practice act does not prohibit nonmedical personnel from performing diabetes-related tasks in schools, the school nurse can provide diabetes training and assess the competency of designated nonmedical school staff. Ideally, each school would have a school nurse and two or three staff trained in diabetes management. The nurse or designee is responsible for performing or supervising all diabetes tasks, including BG monitoring, carbohydrate counting, insulin administration, and treatment of hypoglycemia (including glucagon administration). They should be familiar with insulin pumps and continuous glucose monitors, if needed. Trained school personnel do not make management decisions. Rather, care is provided in accordance with the child's DMMP, physician's orders, or other written care plans. Trained school personnel can help make precise diabetes management easier and more comfortable for children and their parents.

Pediatricians, endocrinologists, and parents need to help schools optimize their child's diabetes management and enable a successful educational experience. For more information about dealing with diabetes in the schools, refer to the NDEP's "Helping the Student with Diabetes Succeed: A Guide for School Personnel."[2] The NDEP Guide recommends the following three levels of training of school personnel:

- **Level 1:** Training all school staff members on recognizing hypoglycemia and hyperglycemia and who to contact for help
- **Level 2:** Training all school staff members who are involved during school, including bus drivers and lunchroom staff, who are responsible for the student with diabetes during school or during school-sponsored extracurricular activities (more in-depth information about diabetes with specific reference to the student); this training includes specific instruction on the student's Quick Reference Diabetes Emergency Plan.
- **Level 3 (highest level):** Training is for school staff designated by the school nurse as trained diabetes personnel or other qualified health care professional who will perform or assist a student with diabetes care tasks, including BG monitoring, insulin and glucagon administration

An excellent resource that school nurses and other health care professional should use for training school staff members is the American Diabetes Association's (ADA's) "Diabetes Care Tasks: What Key Personnel Need to Know."[5]

ROLES AND RESPONSIBILITIES OF SCHOOL DIABETES CARE TEAM MEMBERS

School Nurse

The school nurse is responsible for coordinating the student's diabetes care at school. As the leader of the School Diabetes Care Team, the school nurse's responsibilities include obtaining the student's DMMP to develop the student's written care plans, providing care to the student, coordinating the training of the trained diabetes personnel and other school staff members, and communicating with parents and guardians.

Trained Diabetes Personnel

Trained diabetes personnel can be teachers, school principals, school secretaries, and other school staff members who successfully complete diabetes training so that they may provide the appropriate level of routine and emergency diabetes care in the school setting when the school nurse is not available.

Teacher

Teachers participate in school health meetings that discuss the student's diabetes care and complete the diabetes training needed to implement the student's written plans. The teacher communicates to the student's family and the school health team concerns about the student's diabetes self-management or diabetes-related issues impeding the child's ability to learn.

Other School Staff

All school staff should work with the school health team to implement the student's written plans and should obtain the appropriate level of diabetes training to adequately care for the student's diabetes as determined by the school nurse and school administration. All staff should have a copy of the student's hypoglycemia and hyperglycemia emergency plans (sample plans can be found in the NDEP school guide, pp. 109–112), know how to recognize and treat hypoglycemia, and know whom to contact in the event of a diabetes emergency.

Specific Roles

Physical Education Teacher or Coach

- Should always have BG monitoring equipment and a form of rapid-acting sugar available on-site (e.g., three to four glucose tablets, glucose gel, 4 ounces juice)
- Allow student to check BG before or after physical activity and as needed for symptoms of hypoglycemia
- Recognize hypoglycemia symptoms and administer treatment based on the student's written plans
- Know whom to contact in case of diabetes emergency (e.g., school nurse or designated personnel)

School Psychologist or Counselor

- Should participate in diabetes care team meetings regarding the student and communicate with the family and with the school health team about concerns or progress made by the student
- Be aware of the student's emotional needs and manage issues as they arise
- Work with school personnel to ascertain the student is exposed to a supportive learning environment and is not treated differently than other students
- Promote and encourage compliance with self-care and independence in the diabetes management as developmentally appropriate

Parents and Guardians

Parents and guardians play a critical role in communicating the updated recommendations for their child's diabetes management to the school nurse and his or her team, ensuring that the school has received the signed DMMP and has the needed supplies, medication, and snacks on hand.

Student with Diabetes

The student with diabetes has responsibilities that increase as the child develops and matures. The student needs to identify members of the school health care team (teachers, coaches, or other school personnel) and know who to contact if she or he is not feeling well or is having hypoglycemia symptoms.

HEALTH CARE PLANS

Before the beginning of the school year, or immediately following the diagnosis of diabetes in a school-age child during the academic year, the child's provider should work with the parent or guardian to develop and approve the student's health care plan or physician's orders.

DMMP

The DMMP is completed and approved by the student's personal health care team. (A sample DMMP is provided at the end of this chapter [Appendix 18.II.A],[2] and other written plans may be obtained at www.diabetes.org/safeatschool.[6]) The DMMP is a prescription for the student's diabetes care regimen and should be signed by the student's personal health care team. The DMMP contains the medical orders that are the basis for the student's health care and education plans, such as the Section 504 plan or IEP. The DMMP contains all of the information needed to treat diabetes in school, including, but not limited to, the following information:

- Date of diagnosis
- Insulin types, doses, administration, and timing (correction factor, insulin to carbohydrate [I:C] ratios)
- Frequency and timing of BG monitoring
- Indications for ketone checks
- Glucagon dosing and indications
- Other medications to be given at school
- Meal and snack plan
- Exercise requirements
- Signs, symptoms, and prescribed treatment for hypoglycemia and hyperglycemia
- Student's willingness and ability to self-manage his or her diabetes
- List of diabetes equipment and supplies needed for diabetes management in school
- Emergency contact information
- 72-h disaster or emergency plan

Specific issues in the DMMP include where and when BG monitoring and insulin administration will occur, insulin and medication dosages, provisions for meals and snacks, symptoms and treatment of hypo- and hyperglycemia, and the child's level of self-management skill. The DMMP needs to explicitly state whether the student can independently monitor BG levels, whether the student can monitor BG with supervision, or whether an adult needs to perform BG checks. In addition, the DMMP must state if the student functions independently or requires assistance to determine the carbohydrate content of meals and snacks, calculate I:C ratios and correction insulin doses based on sliding scales.

Individual Health Care Plan (IHP)

The IHP is prepared by the school nurse to translate and implement the DMMP so that medical orders are easily carried out in school. The IHP incorporates assessments of the school environment, the student, and family support, including how to contact parents or guardians, as needed. It outlines diabetes management strategies and the personnel needed at school to best meet the student's health goals as outlined in the DMMP. The nurse reviews the IHP with the student and family before it is implemented. It should be reviewed throughout the school year to reevaluate its utility in ensuring adequate diabetes care and academic progress.

The IHP should list accommodations the student may need to successfully manage diabetes, including timing and dosing of insulin; issues related to BG monitoring, including where to check, when to check, and where supplies should be stored; policies for avoiding penalties for health appointments and illness; and accommodations required during examinations or at other times. The IHP should have a list of trained diabetes personnel with itemized diabetes care tasks and a timeline for their training and supervision. The school nurse should clearly delineate plans to educate other school personnel (e.g., teachers, substitute teachers, bus drivers, physical education instructors, and cafeteria personnel). It should also clearly state the student's responsibility for diabetes-related tasks. See Appendix 18.II.B for a sample IHP (a sample IHP is also in the NDEP school guide, pp. 107–108).[2] In general, elementary school children require diabetes care to be performed by the school nurse or designee, middle school youth can generally perform diabetes self-care with supervision, and high school students may successfully perform diabetes self-care without supervision. All students will need assistance in the event of a diabetes emergency, such as hypoglycemia. Schools should monitor the academic progress of a student who independently manages his or her diabetes at school. Guidelines should be in place for communicating with the family and health care provider.

Emergency Care Plan for Hypoglycemia and Hyperglycemia

The emergency care plan is a single-page summary of the student's symptoms and outlines management of hypoglycemia, hyperglycemia, and ketosis. It includes specific guidelines for checking BG levels, treating hyperglycemia and hypoglycemia, and checking and managing ketones. It may be laminated and should be distributed to all school personnel involved with the child. See Appendix 18.II.B for sample plans.[2]

Diabetes Care Tasks Needed for Successful Management of Diabetes in the Schools

Trained diabetes personnel need instruction in the diabetes tasks noted in the student's DMMP. Table 18.II.1 provides an outline of the required management tasks, which need to be individualized to the particular student's needs.

Table 18.II.1 Diabetes Care Tasks for School Personnel

Diabetes Care Tasks	Signs[a]	Treatment	Outcome If *Not* Treated
Hypoglycemia recognition and treatment	Catecholamine effect (sweating, jitteriness, tachycardia, and palpitations) or neuroglycopenia (behavior change)	■ Concentrated sugar, wait 15 min, recheck, give food if BG adequate (based on DMMP) ■ Know when and how to give glucagon ■ Know when to contact parents or emergency medical services ■ Have all contact information immediately available on emergency plan	Seizure or coma
Hyperglycemia recognition and treatment	■ Polyuria, polydipsia (most common) ■ Difficulty concentrating, headache, or irritability	■ Rapid- or short-acting insulin ■ Dose and frequency should be clearly elucidated on emergency plan to avoid "insulin stacking" and consequent hypoglycemia (see DMMP) ■ Insulin dosing technique (syringe/vial, pens, pumps) ■ Insulin required (DMMP) ■ Ketone checks and when to call parents ■ Correction factor calculations and insulin for hyperglycemia and ketones	Check for ketones. Follow directions for ketones if positive to avoid ketoacidosis.

[a] Varies among individuals but consistent within a given child

OTHER CONSIDERATIONS

Meals

Meal timing and its relationship to physical education are important, as exercise decreases blood glucose whereas food increases blood glucose. Insulin doses and timing often can be adjusted to the student's school schedule in collaboration with the family, the diabetes health-care team, and the school. It is important that the student with diabetes not feel isolated and separated from his or her peers by disruptions in the day to go to the school nurse or office for care. The majority of students now use physiologic insulin replacement either with a basal-bolus regimen or CSII, so it is important that the school nurse or trained diabetes personnel understand carbohydrate counting, I:C ratios, and correction factor calculations or know how to work with the child and family to assist with insulin dosing. Students on fixed-dose regimens usually eat the same carbohydrate content each day. These students frequently require a mid-afternoon snack to avoid hypoglycemia when the insulin peaks.

Extracurricular Activities and Exercise

Exercise has many benefits for youth with diabetes, including increased insulin sensitivity, maintenance of cardiovascular fitness, improved blood glucose control, and positive effects on self-esteem and socialization. Students with diabetes should participate in physical education (PE), but they may need accommodations for PE and extracurricular activities. Checking BG levels before exercise provides an opportunity to give extra carbohydrates to avoid exercise-related hypoglycemia. Criteria for exercise restriction related to hypoglycemia or ketosis should be stated explicitly in the student's DMMP. PE teachers and coaches should be able to recognize and treat signs and symptoms of hypoglycemia and immediately call for help. BG meters and a rapid carbohydrate source (e.g., juice) should be available on site.

Teachers should inform parents about special occasions, such as field trips or parties, as specified in the student's Section 504 plan or IEP, so parents can determine which accommodations the student may need in order to participate in the activity. Occasionally, alternate snacks may need to be provided if the food options do not match the child's needs. Generally, the child with diabetes can partake in all activities with appropriate preparation and planning. The school nurse or trained diabetes personnel should be available to provide needed care to the student for after school activities and field trips. The parent may choose to accompany the student on these occasions, but parental attendance cannot be a requirement for the child's participation. The school nurse or trained school personnel should ascertain that all diabetes supplies accompany the child for the activity.

Common School Diabetes Care Problems

Pediatric providers should be aware of common school diabetes care problems encountered by students with diabetes and be prepared to offer resources and resolution strategies to the parent or guardian. Common problems include the school's failure or refusal to—

- Designate and train school staff members to provide both routine and emergency care when the school nurse is not available
- Administer insulin
- Administer glucagon
- Allow independent and capable students to self-manage their diabetes tasks
- Provide care to student during field trips and extracurricular activities
- Provide carbohydrate content of school meals and other needed nutritional information
- Initiate the process to determine Section 504 or IDEA eligibility
- Continue the enrollment of the student in the school that the student attended before diagnosis without a school nurse or trained personnel and rather assign the child to a different school that has a school nurse
- Allow student to schedule alternative times for academic testing when BG levels are out of target range
- Permit student to enroll because of diabetes

The ADA, through its Safe at School initiative,[6] has an expert team of legal and health care professionals and advocates to guide parents of students who are discriminated against by their schools because of their diabetes. Parents should be encouraged to call the ADA at 1-800-DIABETES to receive a free packet of information and to be referred to ADA's legal advocates who may help provide individual assistance. Additional resources are found at www.diabetes.org/safeatschool.[6]

SCHOOL AND TEACHER EDUCATION RESOURCES

Numerous resources are available for school personnel regarding diabetes education. These include materials from the ADA, Juvenile Diabetes Research Foundation (JDRF), and National Diabetes Education Program (NDEP). The NDEP provides a school guide entitled "Helping the Student with Diabetes Succeed: A Guide for School Personnel,"[2] which explains what school personnel need to know about diabetes, offers online tools, provides information about the federal laws pertaining to students with diabetes in school, and describes actions for school personnel. These resources are available at www.ndep.nih.gov or www.yourdiabetesinfo.org. Additional resources include the NDEP's presentation about "Helping the Student with Diabetes Succeed"[2] and multiple articles in the School Nurse News and the National Association of School Nurse (NASN) journal. The ADA also provides online training and education resources at www.diabetes.org/safeatschool,[6] which includes a two-disc training curriculum with a video entitled "Diabetes Care Tasks at School: What Key Personnel Need to Know"[5] and training resources for school personnel, including "Diabetes Care at School." The JDRF online resources are available at www.jdrf.org and include Resources for School Nurses, School Advisory Toolkit for Families, and a Type 1 Diabetes in School webpage. The Children with Diabetes website[7] also offers education and support for families of children with T1D, including sample 504 plans, chatrooms, and forums in which families can offer advice, ask for help, or share success stories.

COLLEGE

The transition from high school to college can be a difficult time for both parents and the student with diabetes. In most cases, this is the first time the student has complete responsibility for diabetes management. It is also the first time there are no constraints on the emerging young adult regarding social activities, including alcohol ingestion and other risk-taking behaviors, often making diabetes care a low priority. Thus, it is important to ascertain that safeguards are in place to ensure ongoing diabetes care.

Before starting the academic year, the student should speak to the college student's health services to inform them of the student's diabetes. Many colleges have a designated diabetes resource person, usually a nurse, who is responsible for the medical well-being of students with diabetes. This diabetes resource individual should be contacted soon after receipt of the college acceptance packet to arrange a face-to-face meeting, as this individual is the go-to person for all diabetes-related issues. Open dialogue with the health services also provides for timely notification of issues important to the student, for example, when annual flu immunizations become available in the early fall.

Legal protections against discrimination continue beyond high school. Unlike high school, however, the student must be proactive and request accommodations and services from colleges and technical schools. Any special accommodations that might be needed for issues such as hypoglycemia during exams, having a refrigerator in the dorm room, access to the bathroom, and carrying water to class should be discussed and arranged through the college disability services office. Each of the student's professors should be notified that the student has diabetes and be aware of accommodations that may be required. Because this is a time of transition during which parents should be handing over responsibility to the student, the student should be the one requesting the accommodations and services. Students should inquire about the process for evaluation and securing services with the college office of disability services.[8] The American Diabetes Association has written an excellent self-advocacy guide for college students with diabetes: *Going to College with Diabetes: A Self-Advocacy Guide for Students.*

On a related note, the young adult, working with his or her previous pediatric team, must decide if he or she will continue to be followed by the pediatric diabetes team or by a local adult endocrinologist. If the preference is to be followed near the college, the name and contact number of an endocrinologist should be identified before the beginning of the semester and an introductory appointment should be arranged. The new endocrinologist should receive a summary of the student's diabetes history from the pediatric diabetes care team and the student should receive a copy before leaving for school.

Before departure to school, the pediatric team should review recommendations and challenges related to sexually transmitted diseases, contraception, tobacco smoking, alcohol, and recreational drugs. Ongoing support for diabetes management along with efforts at exercise and healthy eating in the context of a structured routine will likely enhance ongoing BG monitoring, adherence to diabetes management and optimal health outcomes while allowing for socialization and development as an independent young adult. Some colleges have support groups that provide an opportunity to share experiences and concerns.[9,10]

The entering college freshman should disclose the diagnosis of diabetes to the new roommate and the dormitory resident advisors (RAs) and make them aware of signs and symptoms of hypoglycemia, hyperglycemia, and ketoacidosis. Sample letters explaining diabetes are available at www.jdrf.org. Lists of needed diabetes supplies for life away from home are available from the pediatric team or websites.[11,12]

Food supplies and glucagon should be placed in a designated place, and the RA and roommate should be aware of the location of this hypoglycemia kit. Roommates and RAs can be educated in glucagon administration and must be aware of how to contact medical emergency services. Typical symptoms of hypoglycemia should be reviewed and the potential impact of the consumption of alcohol should be discussed.

CONCLUSION

Successful management of diabetes involves careful attention to diabetes care tasks in all aspects of the youth's life, including home, school, and extracurricular activities. It is critical that school personnel are trained in proper diabetes management and for families to be aware of available resources. As children grow and mature, the expectations for diabetes self-management change. The parent, diabetes care team, and school nurse must collectively determine the youth's ability to independently manage his or her diabetes in the school setting. Elementary school children are usually completely dependent on trained school staff to provide their care, while most, but not all, high school students can independently manage their diabetes. All college-age youth should be able to independently and responsibly manage their diabetes.

This section of chapter 18 lists resources that provide information about legal accommodations for diabetes in the school, training guides for school staff, sample Section 504 and DMMP plans, and detailed roles of the school staff, the diabetes treatment team, and the parent and child. It includes the tools necessary for parents to handle the challenges involved in providing an optimum arrangement for their child's diabetes care at school. Additionally, tools for the diabetes care team and other health care providers are also included to assist the students navigate the school system and, ultimately, succeed in school.

REFERENCES

1. Siminerio L, Deeb L, Dimmick B, Jackson C: The crucial role of health care professionals in advocating for students with diabetes. *Clinical Diabetes* 30:34–37, 2012
2. National Diabetes Education Program: Helping the Student with Diabetes Succeed: A Guide for School Personnel. NIH Publication 10-5217. Bethesda, MD, NDEP, revised September 2010. Available at www.ndep.nih.gov

3. American Diabetes Association: The legal rights of students with diabetes. Available at http://www.diabetes.org/living-with-diabetes/know-your-rights/for-lawyers/education-materials-for-lawyers/. Accessed 23 October 2012

4. American Diabetes Association: Diabetes care in the school and day care setting. *Diabetes Care* 35(Suppl. 1):S76–S80, 2012

5. American Diabetes Association: Diabetes care tasks: what key personnel need to know. Available at www.diabetes.org/schooltraining. Accessed 23 October 2012

6. American Diabetes Association: Safe at school initiative. Available at www.diabetes.org/safeatschool. Accessed 23 October 2012

7. Children with Diabetes website. Available at www.childrenwithdiabetes.com. Accessed 23 October 2012

8. American Diabetes Association: Going to college with diabetes: a self-advocacy guide for students, 2011. Available from http://www.diabetes.org/living-with-diabetes/parents-and-kids/diabetes-care-at-school/special-considerations/post-secondary-education.html. Accessed 23 October 2012

9. Nicole Johnson website. Available at http://studentswithdiabetes.health.usf.edu. Accessed 23 October 2012

10. College Diabetes Network website. Available at http://collegediabetesnetwork.org. Accessed 23 October 2012

11. Children's Diabetes Foundation website. Available at childrensdiabetes-foundation.org. Accessed 23 October 2012

12. National Diabetes Education Program: Transition module. Available at www.ndep.nih.gov/transitions. Accessed 23 October 2012

APPENDIX 18.II.A

Diabetes Medical Management Plan (DMMP)

This plan should be completed by the student's personal diabetes health care team, including the parents/guardian. It should be reviewed with relevant school staff and copies should be kept in a place that can be accessed easily by the school nurse, trained diabetes personnel, and other authorized personnel.

Date of Plan: _____ This plan is valid for the current school year: _____ - _____

Student's Name: _____ Date of Birth: _____

Date of Diabetes Diagnosis: _____ ☐ type 1 ☐ type 2 ☐ Other_____

School: _____ School Phone Number: _____

Grade: _____ Homeroom Teacher: _____

School Nurse: _____ Phone: _____

CONTACT INFORMATION

Mother/Guardian: _____

Address: _____

Telephone: Home _____ Work _____ Cell: _____

Email Address: _____

Father/Guardian: _____

Address: _____

Telephone: Home _____ Work _____ Cell: _____

Email Address: _____

Student's Physician/Health Care Provider: _____

Address: _____

Telephone: _____

Email Address: _____ Emergency Number: _____

Other Emergency Contacts:

Name: _____ Relationship: _____

Telephone: Home _____ Work _____ Cell: _____

Diabetes Medical Management Plan (DMMP) – Page 2

CHECKING BLOOD GLUCOSE

Target range of blood glucose: ☐ 70–130 mg/dL ☐ 70–180 mg/dL
☐ Other: _____

Check blood glucose level: ☐ Before lunch ☐ _____ Hours after lunch
☐ 2 hours after a correction dose ☐ Mid-morning ☐ Before PE ☐ After PE
☐ Before dismissal ☐ Other:_____
☐ As needed for signs/symptoms of low or high blood glucose
☐ As needed for signs/symptoms of illness
Preferred site of testing: ☐ Fingertip ☐ Forearm ☐ Thigh ☐ Other: _____
Brand/Model of blood glucose meter:_____

Note: The fingertip should always be used to check blood glucose level if hypoglycemia is suspected.

Student's self-care blood glucose checking skills:

☐ Independently checks own blood glucose

☐ May check blood glucose with supervision

☐ Requires school nurse or trained diabetes personnel to check blood glucose

Continuous Glucose Monitor (CGM): ☐ Yes ☐ No
Brand/Model: _____ Alarms set for: ☐ (low) and ☐ (high)

Note: Confirm CGM results with blood glucose meter check before taking action on sensor blood glucose level. If student has symptoms or signs of hypoglycemia, check fingertip blood glucose level regardless of CGM.

HYPOGLYCEMIA TREATMENT

Student's usual symptoms of hypoglycemia (list below):

_____

_____

If exhibiting symptoms of hypoglycemia, OR if blood glucose level is less than
_____mg/dL, give a quick-acting glucose product equal to _____ grams of
carbohydrate.

Recheck blood glucose in 10–15 minutes and repeat treatment if blood glucose level is
less than _____ mg/dL.

Additional treatment: _____

Diabetes Medical Management Plan (DMMP) – Page 3

HYPOGLYCEMIA TREATMENT (Continued)

Follow physical activity and sports orders (see page 7).

- If the student is unable to eat or drink, is unconscious or unresponsive, or is having seizure activity or convulsions (jerking movements), give:
- Glucagon: ☐ 1 mg   ☐ 1/2 mg   Route: ☐ SC   ☐ IM
- Site for glucagon injection: ☐ arm   ☐ thigh   ☐ Other:_____
- Call 911 (Emergency Medical Services) and the student's parents/guardian.
- Contact student's health care provider.

HYPERGLYCEMIA TREATMENT

Student's usual symptoms of hyperglycemia (list below):

_____

_____

Check   ☐ Urine   ☐ Blood for ketones every ____hours when blood glucose levels are above ____mg/dL.

For blood glucose greater than ____mg/dL AND at least ____hours since last insulin dose, give correction dose of insulin (see orders below).

For insulin pump users: see additional information for student with insulin pump.

Give extra water and/or non-sugar-containing drinks (not fruit juices): ____ounces per hour.

Additional treatment for ketones: _____

Follow physical activity and sports orders (see page 7).

- Notify parents/guardian of onset of hyperglycemia.
- If the student has symptoms of a hyperglycemia emergency, including dry mouth, extreme thirst, nausea and vomiting, severe abdominal pain, heavy breathing or shortness of breath, chest pain, increasing sleepiness or lethargy, or depressed level of consciousness: Call 911 (Emergency Medical Services) and the student's parents/guardian.
- Contact student's health care provider.

Tools

Diabetes Medical Management Plan (DMMP) – page 4

INSULIN THERAPY

Insulin delivery device: ☐ syringe   ☐ insulin pen   ☐ insulin pump

Type of insulin therapy at school:
☐ Adjustable Insulin Therapy
☐ Fixed Insulin Therapy
☐ No insulin

Adjustable Insulin Therapy

• **Carbohydrate Coverage/Correction Dose:**

  Name of insulin: _____

• **Carbohydrate Coverage:**

  Insulin-to-Carbohydrate Ratio:

  Lunch: 1 unit of insulin per _____ grams of carbohydrate

  Snack: 1 unit of insulin per _____ grams of carbohydrate

Carbohydrate Dose Calculation Example
$$\frac{\textit{Grams of carbohydrate in meal}}{\textit{Insulin-to-carbohydrate ratio}} = \underline{\quad} \text{ units of insulin}$$

• **Correction Dose:**

Blood Glucose Correction Factor/Insulin Sensitivity Factor = _____

Target blood glucose = _____ mg/dL

Correction Dose Calculation Example
$$\frac{\textit{Actual Blood Glucose–Target Blood Glucose}}{\textit{Blood Glucose Correction Factor/Insulin Sensitivity Factor}} = \underline{\quad} \text{ units of insulin}$$

Correction dose scale (use instead of calculation above to determine insulin correction dose):

Blood glucose _____ to _____ mg/dL give _____units
Blood glucose _____ to _____ mg/dL give _____units
Blood glucose _____ to _____ mg/dL give _____units
Blood glucose _____ to _____ mg/dL give _____units

Diabetes Medical Management Plan (DMMP) – page 5

INSULIN THERAPY (Continued)

When to give insulin:

Lunch

☐ Carbohydrate coverage only

☐ Carbohydrate coverage plus correction dose when blood glucose is greater than _____mg/dL and ____ hours since last insulin dose.

☐ Other: _____

Snack

☐ No coverage for snack

☐ Carbohydrate coverage only

☐ Carbohydrate coverage plus correction dose when blood glucose is greater than _____mg/dL and ____ hours since last insulin dose.

☐ Other: _____

☐ Correction dose only:

For blood glucose greater than _____mg/dL AND at least _____ hours since last insulin dose.

☐ Other: _____

Fixed Insulin Therapy

Name of insulin: _____

☐ ____ Units of insulin given pre-lunch daily

☐ ____ Units of insulin given pre-snack daily

☐ Other: _____

Parental Authorization to Adjust Insulin Dose:

☐ Yes ☐ No Parents/guardian authorization should be obtained before administering a correction dose.

☐ Yes ☐ No Parents/guardian are authorized to increase or decrease correction dose scale within the following range: +/- _____ units of insulin.

☐ Yes ☐ No Parents/guardian are authorized to increase or decrease insulin-to-carbohydrate ratio within the following range: _____ units per prescribed grams of carbohydrate, +/- ____ grams of carbohydrate.

☐ Yes ☐ No Parents/guardian are authorized to increase or decrease fixed insulin dose within the following range: +/- _____ units of insulin.

Diabetes Medical Management Plan (DMMP) – page 6

INSULIN THERAPY (Continued)

Student's self-care insulin administration skills:

☑ Yes ☑ No Independently calculates and gives own injections

☑ Yes ☑ No May calculate/give own injections with supervision

☑ Yes ☑ No Requires school nurse or trained diabetes personnel to calculate/give
injections

ADDITIONAL INFORMATION FOR STUDENT WITH INSULIN PUMP

Brand/Model of pump: _____ Type of insulin in pump: _____

Basal rates during school: _____

Type of infusion set: _____

☑ For blood glucose greater than _____ mg/dL that has not decreased within
_____ hours after correction, consider pump failure or infusion site failure. Notify
parents/guardian.

☑ For infusion site failure: Insert new infusion set and/or replace reservoir.

☑ For suspected pump failure: suspend or remove pump and give insulin by syringe or
pen.

Physical Activity

May disconnect from pump for sports activities ☑ Yes ☑ No

Set a temporary basal rate ☑ Yes ☑ No _____% temporary basal for _____ hours

Suspend pump use ☑ Yes ☑ No

Student's self-care pump skills:	Independent?	
Count carbohydrates	☑ Yes	☑ No
Bolus correct amount for carbohydrates consumed	☑ Yes	☑ No
Calculate and administer correction bolus	☑ Yes	☑ No
Calculate and set basal profiles	☑ Yes	☑ No
Calculate and set temporary basal rate	☑ Yes	☑ No
Change batteries	☑ Yes	☑ No
Disconnect pump	☑ Yes	☑ No
Reconnect pump to infusion set	☑ Yes	☑ No
Prepare reservoir and tubing	☑ Yes	☑ No
Insert infusion set	☑ Yes	☑ No
Troubleshoot alarms and malfunctions	☑ Yes	☑ No

Diabetes Medical Management Plan (DMMP) – page 7

OTHER DIABETES MEDICATIONS

Name: _____ Dose: _____ Route: _____ Times given: _____
Name: _____ Dose: _____ Route: _____ Times given: _____

MEAL PLAN

Meal/Snack	Time	Carbohydrate Content (grams)
Breakfast	_____	_____ to _____
Mid-morning snack	_____	_____ to _____
Lunch	_____	_____ to _____
Mid-afternoon snack	_____	_____ to _____

Other times to give snacks and content/amount:_____

Instructions for when food is provided to the class (e.g., as part of a class party or food sampling event): _____

Special event/party food permitted: ☐ Parents/guardian discretion
☐ Student discretion

Student's self-care nutrition skills:

☐ Yes ☐ No Independently counts carbohydrates

☐ Yes ☐ No May count carbohydrates with supervision

☐ Yes ☐ No Requires school nurse/trained diabetes personnel to count carbohydrates

PHYSICAL ACTIVITY AND SPORTS

A quick-acting source of glucose such as ☐ glucose tabs and/or ☐ sugar-containing juice must be available at the site of physical education activities and sports.

Student should eat ☐ 15 grams ☐ 30 grams of carbohydrate ☐ other_____
☐ before ☐ every 30 minutes during ☐ after vigorous physical activity
☐ other _____

If most recent blood glucose is less than _____ mg/dL, student can participate in physical activity when blood glucose is corrected and above _____ mg/dL.

Avoid physical activity when blood glucose is greater than _____ mg/dL or if urine/blood ketones are moderate to large.

(Additional information for student on insulin pump is in the insulin section on page 6.)

Diabetes Medical Management Plan (DMMP) – page 8

DISASTER PLAN

To prepare for an unplanned disaster or emergency (72 HOURS), obtain emergency
supply kit from parent/guardian.

☐ Continue to follow orders contained in this DMMP.

☐ Additional insulin orders as follows: _____

☐ Other: _____

SIGNATURES

This Diabetes Medical Management Plan has been approved by:

_____

Student's Physician/Health Care Provider   Date

I, (parent/guardian:) _____ give permission to the school nurse

or another qualified health care professional or trained diabetes personnel of

(school:) _____ to perform and carry out the diabetes care

tasks as outlined in (student:) _____'s Diabetes Medical Management

Plan. I also consent to the release of the information contained in this Diabetes Medical

Management Plan to all school staff members and other adults who have responsibility

for my child and who may need to know this information to maintain my child's health

and safety. I also give permission to the school nurse or another qualified health care

professional to contact my child's physician/health care provider.

_____

Acknowledged and received by:

_____

Student's Parent/Guardian   Date

_____

Student's Parent/Guardian   Date

_____

School Nurse/Other Qualified Health Care Personnel   Date

APPENDIX 18.II.B

Sample Template

Individualized Health Care Plan (IHP)

Student: _____

Grade: _____

Dates: _____

School Year: _____

IHP Completed by and Date: _____

IHP Review Dates: _____

Nursing Assessment Review: _____

Nursing Assessment Completed by and Date: _____

Nursing Diagnosis	Sample Interventions and Activities	Date Implemented	Sample Outcome Indicator	Date Evaluated
Managing Potential Diabetes Emergencies (risk for unstable blood glucose)	Establish and document student's routine for maintaining blood glucose within goal range including while at school: **Blood Glucose Monitoring** • Where to check blood glucose: ❑ Classroom ❑ Health room ❑ Other • When to check blood glucose: ❑ Before breakfast ❑ Mid-morning ❑ Before lunch ❑ After lunch ❑ Before snack ❑ Before PE ❑ After PE ❑ 2 hours after correction dose ❑ Before dismissal ❑ As needed ❑ Other: _____ • Student Self-Care Skills: ❑ Independent ❑ Supervision ❑ Full assistance • Brand/model of BG meter: _____ • Brand/model of CGM: _____		**Blood glucose remains in goal range** Percentage of Time 0% 25% 50% 75% 100% 1 2 3 4 5	

Sample Template

Individualized Health Care Plan (IHP) (Continued)

Nursing Diagnosis	Sample Interventions and Activities	Date Implemented	Sample Outcome Indicator	Date Evaluated
Supporting the Independent Student (effective therapeutic regimen management)	**Hypoglycemia Management** **STUDENT WILL:** • Check blood glucose when hypoglycemia suspected • Treat hypoglycemia (follow Diabetes Emergency Care Plan) • Take action following a hypoglycemia episode: _____ • Keep quick-acting glucose product to treat on the spot Type: _____ Location: _____ • Routinely monitor hypoglycemia trends r/t class schedule (e.g., time of PE, scheduled lunch, recess) and insulin dosing • Report and consult with parents/guardian, school nurse, HCP, and school personnel as appropriate		**Monitors Blood Glucose** (records, reports, and correctly responds to results) Never Demonstrated / Consistently Demonstrated 1 2 3 4 5	
Supporting Positive Coping Skills (readiness for enhanced coping)	**Environmental Management** • Ensure confidentiality • Discuss with parents/guardian and student preference about who should know student's coping status at school • Collaborate with parents/guardian and school personnel to meet student's coping needs • Collaborate with school personnel to create an accepting and understanding environment		**Readiness to Learn** Severely Compromised / Not Compromised 1 2 3 4 5	

Hypoglycemia Emergency Care Plan
(For Low Blood Glucose)

Student's Name: _____

Grade/Teacher: _____

Date of Plan: _____

Emergency Contact Information

Mother/Guardian: _____

Email address: _____ Home phone: _____

Work phone: _____ Cell: _____

Father/Guardian: _____

Email address: _____ Home phone: _____

Work phone: _____ Cell: _____

Health Care Provider: _____

Phone number: _____

School Nurse: _____

Contact number(s): _____

Trained Diabetes Personnel: _____

Contact number(s): _____

The student should never be left alone, or sent anywhere alone, or with another student, when experiencing hypoglycemia.

Causes of Hypoglycemia	Onset of Hypoglycemia
• Too much insulin • Missing or delaying meals or snacks • Not eating enough food (carbohydrates) • Getting extra, intense, or unplanned physical activity • Being ill, particularly with gastrointestinal illness	• Sudden—symptoms may progress rapidly

Tools

Hypoglycemia Symptoms		
Circle student's usual symptoms.		
Mild to Moderate		Severe
• Shaky or jittery	• Uncoordinated	• Inability to eat or drink
• Sweaty	• Irritable or nervous	• Unconscious
• Hungry	• Argumentative	• Unresponsive
• Pale	• Combative	• Seizure activity or convulsions (jerking movements)
• Headache	• Changed personality	
• Blurry vision	• Changed behavior	
• Sleepy	• Inability to concentrate	
• Dizzy	• Weak	
• Confused	• Lethargic	
• Disoriented	• Other:_____	

Actions for Treating Hypoglycemia
Notify School Nurse or Trained Diabetes Personnel as soon as you observe symptoms. If possible, check blood glucose (sugar) at fingertip. Treat for hypoglycemia if blood glucose level is less than ____mg/dL. **WHEN IN DOUBT, ALWAYS TREAT FOR HYPOGLYCEMIA AS SPECIFIED BELOW.**

Treatment for Mild to Moderate Hypoglycemia	Treatment for Severe Hypoglycemia

• Provide quick-acting glucose (sugar) product equal to _____ grams of carbohydrates. Examples of 15 grams of carbohydrates include:
   ○ 3 or 4 glucose tablets
   ○ 1 tube of glucose gel
   ○ 4 ounces of fruit juice (not low-calorie or reduced sugar)
   ○ 6 ounces of soda (½ can) (not low-calorie or reduced sugar)
• Wait 10 to 15 minutes.
• Recheck blood glucose level.
• Repeat quick-acting glucose product if blood glucose level is less than_____ mg/dL.
• Contact the student's parents/guardian.
	• Position the student on his or her side.
	• Do not attempt to give anything by mouth.
	• Administer glucagon: _____ mg at _____ site.
	• While treating, have another person call 911 (Emergency Medical Services).
	• Contact the student's parents/guardian.
	• Stay with the student until Emergency Medical Services arrive.
	• Notify student's health care provider.

Hyperglycemia Emergency Care Plan
(For High Blood Glucose)

Student's Name: _____

Grade/Teacher: _____

Date of Plan: _____

Emergency Contact Information

Mother/Guardian: _____

Email address: _____ Home phone: _____

Work phone: _____ Cell: _____

Father/Guardian: _____

Email address: _____ Home phone: _____

Work phone: _____ Cell: _____

Health Care Provider: _____

Phone number: _____

School Nurse: _____

Contact number(s): _____

Trained Diabetes Personnel: _____

Contact number(s): _____

Causes of Hyperglycemia	Onset of Hyperglycemia
• Too little insulin or other glucose-lowering medication • Food intake that has not been covered adequately by insulin • Decreased physical activity • Illness • Infection • Injury • Severe physical or emotional stress • Pump malfunction	• Over several hours or days

Hyperglycemia Signs	Hyperglycemia Emergency Symptoms
	(Diabetic Ketoacidosis, DKA, which is associated with hyperglycemia, ketosis, and dehydration)
Circle student's usual signs and symptoms.	
• Increased thirst and/or dry mouth • Frequent or increased urination • Change in appetite and nausea • Blurry vision • Fatigue • Other: _____	• Dry mouth, extreme thirst, and dehydration • Nausea and vomiting • Severe abdominal pain • Fruity breath • Heavy breathing or shortness of breath • Chest pain • Increasing sleepiness or lethargy • Depressed level of consciousness

Actions for Treating Hyperglycemia	
Notify School Nurse or Trained Diabetes Personnel as soon as you observe symptoms.	
Treatment for Hyperglycemia	Treatment for Hyperglycemia Emergency
• Check the blood glucose level: _____ mg/dL. • Check urine or blood for ketones if blood glucose levels are greater than: _____ mg/dL. • If student uses a pump, check to see if pump is connected properly and functioning. • Administer supplemental insulin dose:_____. • Give extra water or non-sugar-containing drinks (not fruit juices): _____ ounces per hour. • Allow free and unrestricted access to the restroom. • Recheck blood glucose every 2 hours to determine if decreasing to target range of _____ mg/dL. • Restrict participation in physical activity if blood glucose is greater than _____ mg/dL and if ketones are moderate to large. • Notify parents/guardian if ketones are present.	• Call parents/guardian, student's health care provider, and 911 (Emergency Medical Services) right away. • Stay with the student until Emergency Medical Services arrive.

III. Diabetes Camp

Janet Silverstein, MD

Before the development of specialized diabetes camps, parents were concerned that camp personnel were not adequately trained in diabetes management and would not know how to deal with diabetes emergencies, such as ketones and hypoglycemia, so children with type 1 diabetes (T1D) often did not attend these camps. Since the first diabetes camp was started in 1925, the number of diabetes camping experiences has increased so that now almost every state and many countries have specialized camps for children and adolescents with diabetes. Approximately 30,000 children attended these camps in 2011, with an additional 16,000 attending one of the 180 camps in countries other than North America.[1]

Diabetes camps have the same goals as other camps, but in addition, they attempt to teach campers to be more independent in their diabetes management, to share experiences and encouragement with others, to recognize that diabetes should not limit them, and, most important, to enjoy the camping experience. Children are reminded that they are not "diabetics" and are not defined by their diabetes: they are children who happen to have diabetes. On the other hand, children also receive validation that diabetes care takes a lot of effort, and it is expected that the campers will ask for help and support. These goals are not achieved with formal educational programs, but rather they are incorporated into camping activities and informal cabin rap sessions with trained personnel. Campers practice carbohydrate counting at mealtime and, based on their level of maturity, may participate in determining insulin doses.

Camps have various structures. Some diabetes camps use a medical model, in which medical professionals supervise the diabetes care. Other camps train counselors to teach and supervise insulin administration, determine premeal insulin doses based on the campers' camp correction factors and carbohydrate ratios, and check for ketones based on an algorithm given to them during precamp training sessions. Rounds are made daily by the cabin medical team member (physician, diabetes educator, or other heath care professional) to discuss each camper's blood glucose (BG) levels and to adjust insulin doses as needed. Rounds typically are done again at bedtime to determine who needs to have BG values checked at night between 1:00 and 3:00 a.m. and who may need extra snacks to prevent hypoglycemia. Good diabetes practices are modeled at camp. Frequent BG monitoring, recording, and reviewing glucose data and having older campers participate in suggesting insulin doses are incorporated into the daily camp routine with the hope that some of these activities will carry over to improved diabetes management at home.

GOALS OF CAMP

Many youth with diabetes do not know any other children with diabetes who are their own age; they may feel isolated and angry or depressed about having

DOI: 10.2337/9781580404785ch18s3

the disease. Diabetes camp provides a safe environment with trained personnel to allow the camper to feel comforted and supported by staff and other youth with the same medical issues. And because camps offer challenging activities, youth learn that they are not limited by their disease. Goals for campers are as follows:

- Cope more effectively with diabetes
- Encourage confidence and provide support
- Decrease sense of isolation and share experiences with other youth with diabetes
- Incorporate self-management approaches for greater independence, including
  - Carbohydrate counting
  - Exercise management
- Learn about hypoglycemia prevention and treatment
- Gain exposure to diabetes technologies, including pumps and sensors

Other potential opportunities at camp include performing diabetes research with appropriate institutional review and approval and parental consent and youth assent.

PRECAMP PREPARATION

Before camp, parents, the diabetes care team, diabetes camp staff, and camp medical staff complete a variety of tasks.

Parents

- Complete medical history form (including information about diabetes-related hospitalizations, emergency department visits, allergies [including food allergies and celiac disease], medications, immunization records, and psychological or other medical issues)
- Provide recent (2 weeks) data on BG values and insulin doses for camp medical staff to determine whether the insulin dose needs to be adjusted during camp, as high activity levels in the camp setting often require a reduction in dosage

Diabetes Care Team

- Send information on current and past treatments with information about ongoing management, including insulin regimen and last A1C value

Diabetes Camp Staff

- Complete medical intake form on camper arrival
- Educate counselors on signs and symptoms of hypoglycemia, timing of hypoglycemia, and other issues needing to be addressed (e.g. celiac disease)

Camp Medical Staff

- Complete medical intake form on camper arrival
- Review medical history and BG values and confirm insulin dose adjustments
- Ensure that camp nurses have all nondiabetes medications other than asthma inhalers and epinephrine pens to administer during the camp session

RECORDKEEPING

The medical staff should develop protocols for BG testing that includes times to review complete records of BG, ketones, and insulin doses. Plans for hypoglycemia treatment and ketone testing should be established, and medical staff should document and review events at least once a day, and optimally twice daily. Usually campers have middle-of-the-night BG checks on the first full day of camp. Those with bedtime BG values <100 mg/dl require an extra snack or possible reductions in overnight basal rates delivered by pump or long-acting insulin dose injected at bedtime. In addition, campers with frequent hypoglycemia during the day, low BG levels on previous nights, and low BG levels before dinner or bedtime require middle-of-the-night glucose monitoring. There should be a protocol for measuring ketones (blood or urine depending on the camp's protocol) for high BG levels for those taking insulin by injection and for those using insulin pumps.

FOOD AT CAMP

Camp food is served in various ways at different camps: individualized meal trays for each camper, cafeteria style with fixed amounts of food given to each camper, and family style. Mealtime is a teachable moment, during which healthy food choices and portion sizes are emphasized. The carbohydrate content of all foods, including food served in a salad bar, should be posted. It is helpful to have a sample plate with the correct portion sizes. Campers, with the supervision of a counselor, can calculate the carbohydrate grams ingested and the correct insulin bolus. Insulin administration timing is difficult at camp. Some camps serve family-style meals and have insulin administered immediately after the child has eaten because of the difficulty of predicting how much the camper will eat, whereas others, especially those camps offering fixed-carbohydrate meals, give the insulin before the meal. It is preferable that prandial insulin be administered before eating unless there is preprandial hypoglycemia because of the expected delay in insulin action with current formulations of rapid-acting insulins.

INSULIN PUMPS AND WATER SPORTS

Insulin pumps during swimming or boating are challenging. It is necessary to disconnect most pumps when in the water for a prolonged period of time. Given the numerous pumps, campers need to properly label their pump before removal. BG levels are obtained before disconnecting and hourly while the pump is disconnected. In most cases, a correction dose of insulin is given if the BG is too high based on the camper's insulin plan and the pump waterfront protocol. Campers who consistently develop hypoglycemia during swimming need to have the insulin dose adjusted or given proper treatment (e.g., 15–30 g of carbohydrates as snack, juice, and so on) before entering the water.

OCCUPATIONAL SAFETY AND HEALTH ASSOCIATION AND UNIVERSAL PRECAUTIONS

All camp staff and counselors must be aware of Occupational Safety and Health Association (OSHA) guidelines, Clinical Laboratory Improvement Amendments (CLIA), and state regulations. Universal precautions include the following:

- Wearing gloves for all procedures involving blood
- Disposal of blood-soaked materials in red bags
- Disposal of sharps (pen needles, lancets, syringes, pump insertion sets) in sharps boxes
- No sharing of insulin pens, syringes, or lancing devices
- New Centers for Disease Control and Prevention (CDC) rules regarding sharing of meters

  o Whenever possible, all campers should have their own meters
  o If not possible, it is recommended that meters be cleaned and disinfected after every use to prevent cross-contamination[2]

Additional precautions include the following:

- Use retractable single unit lancets to avoid blood touching a shared machine and to decrease the likelihood of a contaminated needle stick by another camper or staff member
- Red bags and sharps boxes should be easily accessible and located in each cabin, in the infirmary, the dining hall and, ideally, at all activity sites
- Campers should place their own sharps in the sharps containers to decrease the likelihood of another camper or a counselor getting stuck by a contaminated needle or lancet
- Protocols to deal with needle sticks from contaminated sharps should be in place
- Insulin pens should be clearly labeled with the camper's name
- All meters should be calibrated at the start of camp and at intervals, as indicated by the specific meter, during the camp session using a control solution or strip
- Diluted bleach and a sponge should be available in each cabin or at BG testing sites and the testing table should be sponged down after each blood test

CAMP STAFF

It takes a village to staff a diabetes camp, including a medical director, usually a pediatric endocrinologist, other physicians with an expertise in diabetes, a registered dietitian, nurses, diabetes educators, psychologists or social workers, and, in some camps, pediatric or family practice residents and medical students. In other camps, the residents and medical students serve as counselors. Each individual at camp should have a clearly defined role. All staff should have a unified approach to diabetes management at camp, and written protocols should be available (e.g., dealing with pumps at the waterfront, treatment of hypoglycemia, treatment of elevated ketone levels, and snacking at bedtime).

Camp counselors serve as role models for the campers. An ideal counselor would be knowledgeable about T1D, mature, empathetic, and able to handle stressful situations. Counselors serve as surrogate parents in many respects and are the front-line staff to recognize symptoms of hypoglycemia, illness, or psychological issues. Because of this, diabetes camps provide an excellent environment for training the next generation of health care providers in diabetes management. Recruitment of counselors who are contemplating or studying a career related to medicine, nursing, nutrition, pharmacy, psychology, or social work can provide personnel with expertise in diabetes when they enter the workforce and, thus, provide better care for patients. In addition, young adults with diabetes who successfully manage their diabetes are excellent role models for the campers and often provide advice that campers accept because of this mutual experience. Regardless, all counselors, even those with diabetes, must have extensive training before camp begins and be highly competent. Following are the necessary camp counselor competencies:

- Recognition and treatment of hypoglycemia with juice or low-dose glucagon, depending on the mental status of the camper and the ability to swallow
- Knowing when to test for ketones and to let medical staff know whenever ketones are present, especially important for campers using the insulin pump
- Knowing when to bring the camper to the infirmary
- Knowing who is at risk and who to check for nocturnal hypoglycemia
- Knowledge of diabetes tasks, including insulin administration, BG monitoring, and changing insulin pump sites and settings
- An understanding of carbohydrate counting and calculation of boluses
- Knowledge on how to be a good counselor (e.g., recognize signs of physical/sexual abuse and reporting when suspicious about abuse; manage disruptive or non-participating campers; recognize signs of depression)
- An understanding of group and peer-to-peer interaction, reinforcing positive behaviors and connections

STUDIES ON BENEFITS OF DIABETES CAMPS

Studies on the efficacy of diabetes camps in improving metabolic control, adherence to diabetes treatment regimens, knowledge, and self-esteem are difficult to interpret, as few of these studies describe the camping experience and even fewer provide long-term outcome data. A meta-analyses of studies done in the camp setting highlights these shortcomings.[3] Despite these limitations, several studies have reviewed the effect of diabetes camps on glycemic control but with conflicting results. It is likely that the duration of camp is too short to allow for significant decreases in A1C, as the life span of a red blood cell is 120 days. Fructosamine is a much more accurate assessment of recent change in glycemia, and studies of fructosamine levels give a truer assessment of short-term glycemic changes.

Improved glucose control during camp, however, is not one of the primary goals of the camping experience. It is hoped that the durable effects on coping, self-esteem, attitude about having diabetes, diabetes knowledge, and independence in managing the disease will result in sustained improvement in glycemic control after the camp sessions end. Not surprisingly, most U.S. studies found no change in A1C values at the beginning of camp compared with the end of a 2-week camp. One study found a significant decrease in glycosylated serum proteins[4] and another U.S. study found significantly improved serum fructosamine levels among those campers in poor control at the beginning of camp.[5] On the other hand, another study found a nonsignificant decrease in A1C but a slight increase in glycosylated serum proteins, thought to be secondary to lowering of the insulin dose and increase in food intake.[6]

DIABETES KNOWLEDGE AND INDEPENDENT MANAGEMENT SKILLS

All studies assessing diabetes knowledge found improved knowledge at the end of camp compared to when the child entered camp. Yet, there is a lack of consensus as to the age at which knowledge accrual is best and at what ages children learn which concepts. A questionnaire administered to 93 campers ages 10–15 years at the beginning and end of a 2-week camp session found that campers 12–15 years of age had significant improvement in their test scores, whereas the younger campers did not demonstrate improved scores.[7] Other studies found children of all ages improve knowledge at the end of camp but that the things they retain differ by age-group. One study found children 9–10 years old increased their knowledge about everything except diet, whereas those older than 10 years of age primarily learned about diet. In general, children who had been to camp before had greater baseline knowledge than those who had never attended camp, but even the veteran campers continued to accrue new information at each camp session.[8] A 12-month follow-up study indicated that the increased knowledge obtained at camp persisted.[9]

Six months after the camp session ended, 87% of parents felt their children had increased knowledge about diabetes care and had improved diabetes self-management skills.[10] Studies on diabetes education, however, repeatedly have shown that improved knowledge does not necessarily translate to improved self-care behaviors. A more recent study did not find many changes 3 months after camp ended, but they did find that younger campers gained more independence in diabetes-related tasks, such as BG monitoring, drawing up insulin, and insulin injections, and that older campers had better problem-solving skills with regard to their diabetes management.[11]

SELF-ESTEEM, QUALITY OF LIFE, AND COPING

Two studies using the Child Attitude toward Illness Scale found a significant improvement in their attitude following a camp experience.[12,13] In addition, campers felt they had more control over their diabetes than matched youth with T1D who did not attend camp. Perhaps most important, though, is a study looking at child and parent satisfaction with meeting the goals they had set for themselves for camp. These goals were as follows:

- Meeting and befriending other children with diabetes
- Gaining knowledge in diabetes self-management
- Having fun

Patients and their parents were given a questionnaire at a 6-month postcamp meeting. All campers and 98% of the parents thought the camp was valuable, both parents and campers felt that it was easier to cope with diabetes after attending the camp, and many campers stated they had more self-esteem and more confidence in their ability to handle diabetes because of what they had learned at camp and because of the support they felt they had received from the medical team and from their new friends who also have diabetes.[14]

SPECIAL CAMPING PROGRAMS

Many camps provide special programs, especially for the adolescent camper. Some of these programs focus on sports and give the camper more independence in their management than is provided in a more traditional camping environment. But, as is true in all diabetes camp settings, all campers need close supervision, as the responsibility for the well-being of every camper lies with the camp staff.

OTHER CAMPING PROGRAMS

In addition to the residential camping programs, many programs run day and weekend camps. These camps (e.g., family weekends, grandparent weekends, and bring-a-friend weekends) require the same staff training, background checks, and attention to safe medical practice as the residential camps. Family weekends allow families, including siblings, to come together for educational sessions and to share potential solutions of common issues with each other. Registered dietitians and psychologists, as well as diabetes educators and physicians, often attend these weekends and have separate sessions with the campers, siblings, and parents.

Bring-a-friend weekends are designed to help youth with diabetes feel less isolated by inviting a friend without diabetes to spend a weekend with them. Education sessions are interspersed with fun activities for the friends. Other programs include teen weekends, largely for middle school students, and weekends for elementary school youth. A sibling may attend instead of a friend, but parents cannot attend. The intent is to expose the friends to the daily management issues for the youth with diabetes and to teach the friends how they may best support their friend. Evaluations have been overwhelmingly positive, with campers feeling more comfortable that their friend knows how to aid them (i.e., with hypoglycemia, for example), and the friends feel more comfortable supporting their friends with diabetes and encouraging their friends to care for themselves.[15]

GAPS ACCORDING TO THE EDITORS

1. There remains an ongoing need to demonstrate the impact of camping on medical, behavioral, and emotional outcomes of youth with T1D.
2. The increasing intensity of diabetes management in youth with T1D demands efficient and cost-effective ways to implement management safely and uniformly for youth at camp with avoidance of severe hypoglycemia and hyperglycemia.
3. Diabetes camps require extraordinary resources to ensure optimal medical supervision; there is a need to identify sustainable funding sources to provide for camping experiences for all youth with T1D who want to participate, independent of a family's ability to pay.

REFERENCES

1. American Diabetes Association: Clinical practice recommendations—2012. *Diabetes Care* 35 (Suppl. 1):S1–S110, 201
2. Centers for Disease Control and Prevention: Infection prevention during blood glucose monitoring and insulin administration, 7 August 2011. Available at http://www.cdc.gov/injectionsafety/blood-glucose-monitoring.html. Accessed 26 October 2012
3. Maslow GR, Lobato D: Diabetes summer camps: history, safety, and outcomes. *Pediatric Diabetes* 10(4):278–288, 2008
4. Strickland AL, McFarland KF, Murtiashaw MH, Tharpe SR, Baynes JW: Changes in blood protein glycosylation during a diabetes summer camp. *Diabetes Care* 7:183–185, 1984
5. Post EM, Moore JD, Ihrke J, Aisenberg J: Fructosamine levels demonstrate improved glycemic control for some children attending a diabetes summer camp. *Pediatric Diabetes* 1:204–208, 2000
6. Spevack M, Johnson SB, Silverstein J: The effect of summer camp on patient adherence and glycemic control. In *Advances in Child Health Psychology*. Johnsom SB, Ed. Gainesville, FL, University of Florida Press, 1991, p. 285–292
7. Dorchy H, Loeb H, Morzin MJ, Lemiere B, Ernould C: Vacation camps: goals and needs. *Pediatr Adolesc Endocrinol* 10:161–165, 1982
8. Karaguzel G, Bircan I, Erisir S, Bundak R: Metabolic control and educational status in children with type 1 diabetes: effects of a summer camp and intensive insulin treatment. *Acta Diabetol* 42:156–161, 2005
9. Harkavy J, Johnson SB, Silverstein, J, Spillar R, McCallum M, Rosenbloom A: Who learns what at summer diabetes camps? *Journal of Pediatric Psychology* 8(2):143–153, 1983
10. Lebovitz FL, Ellis GJ III, Skyler JS. Performance of technical skills of diabetes management: increased independence after a camp experience. *Diabetes Care* 1:23–26, 1978
11. Hunter HL, Rosnov DL, Koontz D, Roberts M: Camping programs for children with chronic illness as a modality for recreation, treatment, and

evaluation: an example of a mission-based program evaluation of a diabetes camp. *J Clin Psychol Med Settings* 13:67–80, 2006

12. Keeter EL, Linehan MS: Affecting children's attitudes toward diabetes through camp. *Nurse Practice* 18:25–26, 1993

13. Briery BG, Rabian B: Psychosocial changes associated with participation in a pediatric summer camp. *J Pediatr Psychol* 24:183–190, 1999

14. Santiprabhop J, Likitmaskul S, Kiattisakthavee P, et al.: Glycemic control and the psychosocial benefits gained by patients with type 1 diabetes mellitus attending the diabetes camp. *Patient Education and Counseling* 73(1): 60–66, 2008

15. Lehmkuhl H, Merlo L, Devine K, Gaines J, Storch, E, Silverstein J, Geffken G: Perceptions of type 1 diabetes among affected youth and their peers. *J Clin Psychol Med Settings* 16:209–215, 2009

IV. Diabetes in the Workplace

Pamela Allweiss, MD, MPH

T he workplace can present challenges to both employees with diabetes and their employers and requires awareness of several issues, such as reasonable accommodations on the job for managing one's diabetes and strategies to keep people with diabetes healthy and productive. To provide the most complete overview, this section of chapter 18 does not differentiate between individuals with type 1 (T1D) and type 2 diabetes. Specific jobs, such as becoming a firefighter, law enforcement officer, or an interstate truck driver, may have separate regulations regarding insulin therapy and should be handled on a case-by-case basis. This section offers a broad perspective and resources to assist both the employer and employee to accomplish these goals.

BACKGROUND

Diabetes is one of the most common and costly chronic diseases affecting people in the U.S. at this time and, unfortunately, public health experts expect it to become even more prevalent in coming years.[1] By 2034, scientists project the number of people with diagnosed and undiagnosed diabetes will increase from 26 million (in 2010) to 44 million, and annual diabetes-related spending will increase to $336 billion (in 2007 dollars).[2,3] Hospitalizations, outpatient clinical care, medicines, and other expenses make up the direct medical costs. Indirect costs related to diabetes, however, such as absenteeism, presenteeism (being at work but with reduced productivity), short-term disability, and other indirect expenses made up about one-third of the overall cost.[4] In fact, >30% of employer costs associated with employees who have diabetes can be attributed to medical-related absences or disability.[5–11] Combining costs related to absenteeism, costs for medicines, claims for short-term disability, and other direct medical expenditures make diabetes the third most costly physical health condition for employers.[5,10]

EMPLOYMENT AND EDUCATION LEVELS IN YOUNG ADULTS WITH DIABETES

Although the crux of this section of the chapter revolves around integrating capable people with diabetes into the workforce, these same people may have experienced similar challenges in the school setting. For people in the U.S. with or without diabetes, lower educational and income levels are associated with poorer overall health and, in people with diabetes, they are associated with a greater chance of having diabetes-related complications.[12] This does not apply to each individual, but it does point out the need to raise the education and income standards for people with diabetes as one path toward better health outcomes.

DOI: 10.2337/9781580404785ch18s4 **579**

Schools, in partnership with other public agencies, should consider seeking out and identifying interventions to initiate progress in these areas.[13]

These earlier-in-life issues related to education and health may reduce the likelihood that some of these people ever become qualified to apply for certain professional positions.[14] Specifically, people with diabetes are ~6% more likely to drop out of high school, 4% to 6% less likely to attend college,[13] and 50% less likely to graduate college[15] than their peers without diabetes. At least in part because of these factors, people with diabetes will make ~$160,000 less in average lifetime earnings than people who do not have diabetes.

PLACEMENT OF PEOPLE WITH DIABETES IN THE WORKPLACE

Given the high percentage of people in the U.S. who have or are at risk for diabetes, the pool of potential employees contain many people with or at risk for diabetes. As a result, many employers may need to eventually address the potential challenges that people with diabetes sometimes face. This likely will require employers to collaborate with employees to develop individual strategies as necessary. This collaboration should result in employees with diabetes being able to care for their diabetes-related needs, but at the same time being able to be productive. With small allowances for accommodation for diabetes self-management, most people with diabetes are as productive as employees without diabetes.

Job placement issues can be a balancing act; current and potential employees have certain rights, and employers have certain requirements that also must be considered. This section provides a general outline of these rights and requirements and suggests resources from which readers can find out more detailed information.

The American Diabetes Association (ADA) has stated its position on employment as follows: "Any person with diabetes, whether insulin [treated] or non–insulin [treated], should be eligible for any employment for which he/she is otherwise qualified." The ADA has also issued guidelines reflective of the Americans with Disabilities Act Amendments Act of 2009 (ADAAA), including the following two, of which both employers and job candidates should be aware during the hiring process.[16]

- An employer may not ask about an individual's health status regardless of the type of job *before* making a job offer but may require a medical examination *after* an offer of employment has been made and before the job begins.
- The job offer may be contingent on the results of the medical examination and an employer may withdraw an offer from an applicant with diabetes only if it becomes clear that the person cannot do the essential functions of the job or would pose a direct threat to health or safety.

Other points in the guidelines cover rights and limitations related to workplace accommodations, fitness-for-duty examinations, requests for medical information, individualized assessments, and recordkeeping. The complete guidelines can be found on the ADA's website under Living with Diabetes/Employment Examinations.

INDIVIDUALIZED ASSESSMENT

Unfortunately, in the past, some people with diabetes were denied employment for certain jobs just on the basis of their condition. Under the original Americans with Disabilities Act, based on court rulings, diabetes was not considered a disability. The ADAAA, however, specifies that people with diabetes be covered under the act because diabetes constitutes a substantial limitation on endocrine system functioning.

Diabetes affects each person differently. He or she may or may not suffer health complications, such as retinopathy (eye damage), nephropathy (kidney disease), or neuropathy (nerve damage), or may experience them at different levels of severity. The activities required to manage diabetes and complications also vary widely among individuals. For many people, having diabetes is not a barrier to fully performing the job.

Doubts persist among some employers about the ability of individuals with diabetes to safely and effectively perform certain jobs. Some of these worries may be dispelled through education. When deemed necessary, employers do have the right to make "[a] job offer contingent on the results of [a] medical examination." But, if an employer does request a medical exam for a person already offered a position, he or she "may withdraw [the] offer from an applicant with diabetes only if it becomes clear that the person cannot do the essential functions of the job or would pose a direct threat to health or safety."[17]

As legal protection for people with diabetes who are required to undergo a medical examination, the ADAAA introduced the concept of *individualized assessment*. This provision requires that a person with diabetes should be assessed as an individual, not as one in a generalized group of "people with diabetes," to determine whether or not that individual can safely and effectively perform the particular duties of the specific position offered.[17]

CONSIDERATIONS

Most people with diabetes can safely and successfully perform most jobs, but individual assessment is necessary for certain jobs because not *all* people (including those without diabetes) can do *all* jobs. One element needed to make an individual assessment is a description of the specific job. For example, is it a desk job or a physically active one? If physically active, what type of activity is involved? Is it episodic, fairly constant, or is there a pattern to the physical activity? Is shift work involved? Are there any potential hazards inherent in performing the job? Does it involve driving or handling heavy equipment? Is the person working at heights? Is he or she working alone or around others? Is special clothing, including footwear, required? The answers to these questions and many others may affect the ability of anyone, including a person with diabetes, to safely and effectively complete the job.

For a person with diabetes, an example of a relevant factor might be whether performing one or more requirements of the job (e.g., lifting heavy packages, physical activity) affect the individual's blood glucose level. If so, the individual may need to make adjustments to his or her usual diabetes control activities. Also, might the person's diabetic complications limit his or her ability to perform all of the essential required tasks? For example, if a person has a diabetes-related condition called *autonomic neuropathy with postural hypotension*, a job requiring work on a ladder might be inadvisable.

In addition to these individual considerations, a limited number of professions require a person with diabetes to take certain training or have a special license or certification. Law enforcement, firefighting agencies, and all trucking companies, for example, require a person with diabetes to meet certain requirements relevant to the nature of the specific job.[18–20]

REASONABLE ACCOMMODATIONS

Language in the ADAAA specifies that most employers provide "reasonable accommodations" to enable a person with diabetes to safely and successfully perform the job, unless doing so would place an "undue burden" on the employer. Accommodations must be individually tailored, such as providing a special computer monitor for a person with vision problems. The employer must allow time away from the job, whether leaving the workplace for a doctor visit or just leaving the desk to perform a glucose test. The ADA provides a more extensive list of employer obligations to provide reasonable accommodation for an employee with diabetes.[16]

GUIDANCE FOR PEOPLE WITH DIABETES IN THE WORKPLACE

Responsibility for caring for one's diabetes in the workplace (and elsewhere) also falls on the individual. Among these personal responsibilities are having all necessary diabetes supplies (e.g., testing strips, medications) on hand, eating healthfully to control one's diabetes, and becoming aware of all safety issues and regulations. Doing so benefits both the employee and employer as better glucose control has been linked to greater productivity.[21]

In addition, it is helpful for people with diabetes to be aware of possible comorbidities, such as hypertension and high cholesterol, as well as certain mental health disorders, like depression. For some people, job-related stress can increase the chances of such conditions developing.

Many resources can help people with diabetes to learn about their condition and to help them improve their self-management skills. Some employers provide an employee wellness program; taking advantage of this service may provide resources to help the employee with diabetes maintain physical and mental health. Other resources in the public domain also help people with diabetes on the job. The National Diabetes Education Program provides information on some of these resources.[22]

Finally, an employee with diabetes is not obligated to reveal his or her diagnosis to supervisors or fellow employees. If he or she is comfortable enough to do so, however, talking about one's experiences can help educate others and dispel misinformation about the realities of living with diabetes.[23]

CONCLUSION

This section of the chapter on people with diabetes in the workplace provides an overview of both practical and legal considerations related to the workplace.

The broad message is that employers and employees with diabetes need to work together to find solutions to common problems and to better educate themselves about the rights and obligations related to people with diabetes in the workplace.

GAPS ACCORDING TO THE EDITORS

1. There is a need to ensure equal education opportunities for youth with T1D to maximize their future earning potential.
2. Ongoing advocacy is needed to support employment of people with T1D in various work environments.

Acknowledgment: The author appreciates the editorial assistance of Tony Pearson-Clarke, CDC Division of Diabetes Translation.

Disclaimer: The findings and conclusions in this chapter are those of the author and do not necessarily represent the official position of the Centers for Disease Control and Prevention.

REFERENCES

1. Centers for Disease Control and Prevention: National Diabetes Fact Sheet: National Estimates and General Information on Diabetes and Prediabetes in the United States, 2011. Atlanta, GA, U.S. Department of Health and Human Services, Centers for Disease Control and Prevention, 2011
2. Boyle J, Thompson T, Gregg E, Barker L, Williamson D: Projection of the year 2050 burden of diabetes in the US adult population: dynamic modeling of incidence, mortality, and prediabetes prevalence. *Popul Health Metr* 8:29–41, 2010
3. Huang ES, Basu A, O'Grady M, Capretta JC: Projecting the future diabetes population size and related costs for the U.S. *Diabetes Care* 32(12):2225–2229, 2009
4. American Diabetes Association: Economic costs of diabetes in the U.S. in 2007. *Diabetes Care* 31(3):596–615, 2008
5. Goetzel RZ, Long SR, Ozminkowski RJ, Hawking K, Wang S, Lynch W: Health, absence, disability, and presenteeism cost estimates of certain physical and mental health conditions affecting U.S. employers. *J Occup Environ Med* 46:398–412, 2004
6. Goetzel RZ, Hawkins K, Ozminkowski RJ, Wang S: The health and productivity cost burden of the "top 10" physical and mental health conditions affecting six large U.S. employers in 1999. *J Occup Environ Med* 45:5–14, 2003
7. Ramsey, S, Summers KH, Leong SA, Birnbaum HG, Kemner JE, Greenberg P: Productivity and medical costs of diabetes in a large employer population. *Diabetes Care* 25:23–29, 2002
8. Ng YC, Jacobs P, Johnson J: Productivity losses associated with diabetes in the U.S. *Diabetes Care* 24:257–261, 2001
9. Tuncelli K, Bradley C, Nerenz D, Williams L, Pladevall M, Lafata J: The impact of diabetes on employment and work productivity. *Diabetes Care* 28:2662–2667, 2005

10. Thorpe KE, Florence CS, Joski P: Which medical conditions account for the rise in health care spending? *Health Aff (Millwood)* July–Dec:W4-437–445, 2004

11. Vijan S, Hayward R, Langa K: The impact of diabetes on workforce participation: results from a national household sample. *Health Serv Res* 39(6 Pt 1): 1653–1670, 2004

12. Secrest A, Costacou T, Gutelius B, Miller R, Songer T, Orchard T: Associations between socioeconomic status and major complications in type 1 diabetes: the Pittsburgh Epidemiology of Diabetes Complication (EDC) study. *Ann Epidemiol* 21:374–381, 2011

13. Fletcher J, Richards M: Diabetes's "health shock" to schooling and earnings: increased dropout rates and lower wages and employment in young adults. *Health Affairs* 31:27–34, 2012

14. Milton B, Holland P, Whitehead M: The social and economic consequences of childhood-onset type 1 diabetes mellitus across the lifecourse: a systematic review. *Diabet Med* 23(8):821–829, 2006

15. Maslow G, Haydon A, McRee AL, Ford C, Halpern C: Growing up with a chronic illness: Social success, educational/vocational distress. *J Adolesc Health* 49:206–212, 2011

16. American Diabetes Association: Diabetes and employment. *Diabetes Care* 35(Suppl. 1):S94–S98, 2012

17. American Diabetes Association: Diabetes and employment. *Diabetes Care* 34 (Suppl. 1):S82–S86, 2011

18. American Diabetes Association: Diabetes and driving. *Diabetes Care* 35 (Suppl. 1):S81–S86, 2012

19. Allweiss P: Diabetes in law enforcement officers. *Clin Occup Envrion Med* 3:571–594, 2003

20. National Fire Protection Association: NFPA 1582: standard on comprehensive occupational medical program for fire departments. Available at http://www.nfpa.org/aboutthecodes/AboutTheCodes.asp?DocNum=1582&cookie%5Ftest=1. Accessed 10 June 2012

21. Testa MA, Simonson DC: Health economic benefits and quality of life during improved glycemic control in patients with type 2 diabetes mellitus: a randomized, controlled, double-blind trial. *JAMA* 280:1490–1496, 1998

22. National Diabetes Education Program website. Available at www.diabetes atwork.org. Accessed 10 June 2012

23. Hieronymus L: Diabetes on the job. *Diabetes Self Manag* 28(5):8,10–2,15, 2011

V. Nursing Home and Geriatric Populations

Medha N. Munshi, MD

INTRODUCTION

Diabetes is a burgeoning problem in older adults affecting 10.9 million (26.9%) people over the age of 65 years.[1] Although the exact prevalence of type 1 diabetes (T1D) in this age-group is not known, it accounts for 5–10% of all diagnosed cases of diabetes in adults. With improved understanding of pathophysiology of disease and comprehensive care, patients with diabetes are living longer. Thus, even though management of T1D is traditionally focused on caring for children and young adults, health care providers are going to see an increasing number of older adults with T1D in their practices. The primary management goal in older adults remains the same as with all T1D individuals: achieving optimal glycemic control for their age and life expectancy and preventing acute and chronic complications associated with this disease. An additional goal in the older population is to prevent treatment-related complications, especially hypoglycemia, which can be more harmful than the disease itself. A better understanding of the unique presentation and disease course in older T1D patients is warranted to enable us to care for this vulnerable population.

In recent years, with the help of small studies and subanalysis of large studies, we have developed a better understanding of differences between presentation and management of type 2 diabetes (T2D) in older compared to younger adults. There is a paucity of information, however, on older adults with T1D. Therefore, part of the information presented in this section of chapter 18 is extrapolated from management of individuals with T2D and based on clinical expertise.

STANDARD OF CARE

At both ends of the life spectrum, in pediatrics and in geriatrics, there are significant differences in patient–disease interactions. Older patients with diabetes are a distinctly different population compared to younger adults. Special considerations involved in care of older adults with diabetes are shown in Table 18.V.1. This is due to their heterogeneity (clinical, functional, and psychosocial), the presence of coexisting medical conditions that interfere with self-care, and unique factors affecting goal setting.[2] When the same diabetes management criteria and strategies used in younger adults are applied to the elderly without considering their special challenges, there is an increased risk of nonadherence to treatment, complications related to treatment (e.g., hypoglycemia and falls), and poor glycemic control. Standard of care to manage older adults with T2D is primarily based on expert opinions.[3] There are no published guidelines for care of older T1D.

DOI: 10.2337/9781580404785ch18s5

Table 18.V.1 Special Considerations for Diabetes Management in Older Adults

Category	Considerations	Barriers and Conditions
Patient-specific considerations	– Assess for clinical, functional, and psychosocial barriers periodically. They may interfere with patients' ability to perform complex tasks for self-care.	Barriers include – Cognitive dysfunction – Depression – Physical disabilities, such as vision loss, hearing loss, gait and balance problems, difficulty performing daily activities – Polypharmacy leading to side effects, drug–drug interactions – Lack of social support system, transportation, difficulty navigating medical establishment – Financial problems with medical care
Goal-setting considerations	– Complications of hypoglycemia may be more harmful to some elderly than hyperglycemia with increasing age. – A1C measurement might be affected by other variables and may not match level of glycemia.	Common conditions affecting A1C measurement in elderly include – Anemia and other conditions affecting red cell span – Renal insufficiency, dialysis, erythropoietin therapy
Treatment strategy–related considerations	– Patients may not be able to continue complex treatment strategies they have followed for many years because of added comorbidities. – Frequent errors and wide excursions in glucose levels may suggest difficulty coping with complex regimen. – Simplified regimens and greater supervision and caregiver involvement can reduce errors and stress in patients unable to cope with complexity.	

Goal-Setting

As patients with T1D age, they develop diabetes-related and diabetes-unrelated comorbid conditions. These comorbidities are often accompanied by functional decline. Functional decline can further lead to loss of independence, increased caregiver needs, and decreased quality of life.[4] The complex interaction of these conditions may interfere with the patient's ability to execute routine tasks previously performed for decades, such as rigorous glucose monitoring, complex insulin dose management, pump operation, or dietary compliance. Although many older adults with T1D continue to successfully mange their diabetes, it is important to watch for warning signs, such as sudden decline in glycemic control, coping difficulties, or multiple errors in medications or insulin regimen, which may manifest as a change in diabetes control with significant hypoglycemia or hyperglycemia. These issues suggest that the patient is experiencing difficulty performing self-care. These are the warning signs for clinicians to alter their strategies, liberalize the A1C, and set individual self-monitoring of blood glucose (SMBG) goals to avoid hypoglycemia and its complications.

Recently a cross-sectional study characterizing the rate of complications in patients with T1D with duration of diabetes >50 years (mean age 67.5±7.5 years) showed unusually few complications, including retinopathy, neuropathy, nephropathy, and cardiovascular diseases.[5] In addition, glycemic control (A1C) was not associated with risk of complications in this population. Although the exact mechanism for this finding is unclear, this long-surviving population is thought to have protective factors against diabetes complications. Another observational study showed higher prevalence of macrovascular diseases and hypertension in older T1D.[6] More studies are needed to better understand this phenomenon. These studies suggest, however, that tight glycemic control may not benefit older patients with T1D with long duration of disease. These findings are especially important for those patients who have high risk of hypoglycemia.

COMORBIDITIES IN OLDER ADULTS

Cognitive Dysfunction

Aging T1D patients are often burdened with medical, functional, and psychosocial comorbidities that make self-care difficult. Cognitive dysfunction, depression, physical disabilities, polypharmacy, and chronic pain are well documented as frequent comorbidities in older patients with diabetes.[3] Cognitive dysfunction in older T2D individuals is manifested as deficits in psychomotor efficiency, global cognition, episodic memory, semantic memory, and working memory.[7–9] In particular, executive functioning,[10] mediated by the frontal lobe, affects such behaviors as problem solving, planning, organization, insight, reasoning, and attention. Thus, even subtle executive dysfunction may interfere with a patient's ability to follow a complex regimen and may lead to insulin dosing errors, inability to operate complex devices such as an insulin pump or continuous glucose monitor, or difficulty performing complicated tasks such as carbohydrate counting. There are some small studies specifically looking at cognitive function in T1D. One study assessing cognitive function in older adults with T1D (mean age 61±6 years) showed more self-reported cognitive and depressive symptoms.[11] They did not differ, however, in performance on objective cognitive function tests when compared to age-matched controls. Another study evaluating the effect of chronic hyperglycemia on cognitive functions in adults with T1D (>45 years of age) found no independent effect of chronic hyperglycemia on cognitive changes.[12]

Recently, a small longitudinal study that followed 36 patients with T1D (mean age 60±6 years; median follow-up = 4.1 years) did not show any greater cognitive decline in T1D individuals compared to age-matched controls.[13] In this study, however, the subgroup with one or more cardiovascular or hypoglycemic events was more likely to develop cognitive decline. The data linking cognitive dysfunction to T1D are not as robust as those linking T2D to cognitive dysfunction. Nonetheless, aging independently also increases risk of cognitive dysfunction and thus screening for subtle cognitive and executive dysfunction is important in all older patients with diabetes because of its impact on self-care abilities.

Depression

The relationship between diabetes and depression has been studied extensively. A recent meta-analysis showed that there is inadequate evidence to conclude that prevalence of depression is different in adult patients with T1D (ages 21–43 years) compared to the general population.[14] although the study did not include older adults. Other smaller studies have shown that depression in adults with T1D is associated with metabolic syndrome[15] and subclinical carotid atherosclerosis in men.[16] Various studies on depression in older adults with T2D have shown associations with poor glycemic control, decreased adherence to treatment strategies, and increased functional disability and mortality.[17–19] It is not clear exactly how aging affects depression in individuals with T1D. It is important, however, to be aware of the relationship among diabetes, depression, and self-care abilities. Short screening tools can be used to screen for depression in clinical settings.

Polypharmacy

Polypharmacy is a challenging aspect of caring for older adults with multiple chronic diseases. In older patients with T1D, complex insulin regimens are frequently needed to achieve glycemic control. In addition, more medications are needed for other comorbidities and to control cardiovascular risk factors associated with diabetes. Taking multiple daily medications can increase complexity because of nonadherence, drug–drug interactions, side effects, and errors leading to catastrophic consequences. Older patients may have multiple medical providers for different diseases and medication reconciliation at each visit is an important part of managing older patients with T1D.

Functionality and Falls

Older people with diabetes are at increased risk of falls because of lower limb dysfunction, cardiovascular disease, polypharmacy, and impaired balance.[20,21] In addition, they have reduced physical function and health status, and therefore they are more likely to use mobility aids (such as a cane or a walker). Other self-care barriers seen frequently in older adults with diabetes include vision impairment (resulting from cataracts, macular degeneration, and diabetic retinopathy), hearing loss, and chronic pain. The increased number of disabilities lead to difficulties performing activities of daily living (ADLs include bathing, grooming, toileting, transferring, feeding, continence) and instrumental activities of daily living (IADLs include managing finances, arranging transportation, medication management, shopping, cooking, use of telephone, and so on). In addition to issues related to driving with diabetes, other barriers to driving safely in older adults include decreased range of movements in limbs and neck due to arthritis, decreased vision and hearing acuity, slower reflexes, and cognitive dysfunction. Thus, older patients with T1D may suffer loss of independence and need more caregiver support. Goals of glycemic control and other cardiovascular risk factors may need to be adjusted to accommodate change in overall health in such situations. Issues pertaining to driving in T1D are not different from those in younger patients with T1D. Additional burden of comorbidities and its impact on driving skills with aging should be considered periodically. As many of the barriers to optimal diabetes management develop gradually with subtle presentations, it is important to periodically assess older individuals with T1D for physical, social, and emotional or cognitive dysfunctions.

HYPOGLYCEMIA

Risk of hypoglycemia should be the main consideration when establishing glycemic goals in older adults.[22] The outcome of even mild hypoglycemia can be devastating and may lead to cardiac and cerebrovascular events, progression of dementia, injurious falls, emergency department visits, and hospitalizations.[23–25] The decline in overall functioning may even lead to institutionalization. Although these findings have not been replicated in older adults with T1D specifically, the comorbidities associated with poor outcomes are likely to be age dependent and may affect older patients with both T1D and T2D. In older patients with T1D, reduction in the autonomic warning symptoms of hypoglycemia may lead to hypoglycemic unawareness. Neuroglycopenic symptoms such as dizziness, weakness, delirium, or confusion frequently can be misconstrued as secondary medical conditions such as transient ischemic attack (TIA), dementia, or orthostatic hypotension and may go unrecognized. Patients with cognitive dysfunction may forget to report or treat hypoglycemia appropriately. Older care partners may be unable to provide hypoglycemia treatment support. Finally, some older patients are afraid of the adverse effects of hypoglycemia (e.g., falling and confusion) and overtreat lows, leading to widely fluctuating blood glucose readings. Paradoxically, some older adults with T1D are less concerned about hypoglycemic risks as they are accustomed to them, which leads to frequent episodes. In these older patients, appropriate and repeated education is needed as the hypoglycemic consequences may be more deleterious than that of hyperglycemia.

Most experts recommend a liberal goal for A1C to avoid hypoglycemia in vulnerable patients. A small study evaluating risk of hypoglycemia in older adults with poorly controlled diabetes (A1C >8%) showed that 65% of study subjects had ≥1 episode of glucose <70 mg/dl on continuous glucose monitoring (CGM) and 46% of these episode showed glucose <50 mg/dl. In this study, 30% of the subjects had T1D.[26] Thus, higher A1C values frequently suggest wide fluctuations of glucose levels and do not reflect lower risk of hypoglycemia. In another study assessing the use of C-peptide to simplify the regimen in older adults with T2D, less complex regimens resulted in lower hypoglycemia risk without deterioration of A1C levels.[27] Results of these studies suggest that simply liberal-izing A1C goals are insufficient to avoid hypoglycemia. The best way to lower the risk of hypoglycemia is to prescribe a diabetes treatment regimen that is individualized and suitable to the patient's coping ability. In addition, the care goals should be reassessed at frequent intervals because the health status may change rapidly in older adults, and the risk-to-benefit ratio of tight glycemic control can quickly change.

MULTIDISCIPLINARY TEAM APPROACH

It has been well established that optimal diabetes management in all patients requires input from a team that consists of an endocrinologist, a diabetes educa-tor, a nutritionist, an exercise physiologist, and a psychologist. Because of the clinical, functional, and psychosocial diversity, older adults benefit from services of additional disciplines beyond the traditional teams; this may include a clini-cal pharmacist, physical and occupational therapist, and rehabilitation services.[28] Primary care physicians play an important role in the care of older adults by coordinating the various aspects of care and managing the multiple comorbidi-ties. Caregivers also are an important part of the team caring for older adults who are not able to perform self-care by themselves. Commonly found barriers and strategies used to overcome them are shown in Table 18.V.2.

Caregiver Support

As with pediatric diabetes management, social support systems and care-giver availability are critical in caring for older adults. Diabetes education and treatment plans need to be flexible because strategies frequently change as a result of new obstacles or a decline in the individual's support structure. For example, visiting nurses and home physical therapy might be available for homebound patients or posthospitalization for a short time; however, delirium and deconditioning may last longer in frail patients with T1D who may need a simplified insulin regimen and more support from educators. Finances may dictate whether or not an older individual can afford personal care. Family sup-port might be less robust in geriatric compared to pediatric patients as many older adults live alone.

Long-Term Care

Diabetes (of all types) is highly prevalent in long-term care facilities. A recent cross-sectional national survey showed that in nursing homes, diabetes increased from 16.9% in 1995 to 26.4% in 2004 in male residents and from 16.1 to 22.2% in female residents.[29] The prevalence of T1D in nursing home residents is not currently known, but one can safely assume that it has increased with longer life expectancies. The American Medical Directors Association has published guidelines describing the principles of diabetes management in nursing homes; however, most recommendations are for T2D and are based on expert opinions and extrapolation from other populations.

Table 18.V.2 Common Barriers and Strategies in Older Adults with Diabetes

Barriers	Strategies
Difficulty coping with self-care because of multiple comorbidities	Referral to geriatrician, neurologist, psychiatrist for overall health assessment and improvement strategies
Medication errors	– Careful assessment of all medications, including over-the-counter drugs – Remove unnecessary medications – Assess medication adherence – Suggest aids such as a pill box
Insulin dose errors	– Screen for cognitive dysfunction especially executive dysfunction – Check for vision impairment
Falls, gait, and balance problems	– Encourage different exercises, including aerobic training, resistance training, gait and balance training – Consider referral to physical therapist – Help patient to find safe venue to exercise, such as senior centers or indoor gym (outside walking might be dangerous in weather that is too hot or too cold)
Recent hospitalization	– Communicate with visiting nurse regarding glycemic goals and need for adjustment in insulin dose – Watch for sudden but reversible decline in cognitive function (delirium) after hospitalization or acute illness that can increase risk of errors in insulin dosing
Hearing impairment	– Referral to audiologist – May present as depression as patient seem uninterested in surroundings
Vision impairment	– Regular follow-up with ophthalmologist
Difficulty performing activities of daily living, such as meal preparation and transportation	– Community services such as meals-on-wheels deliver free meals once a day – Rides are available at lower cost for patients who are unable to use public transportation. – Faith-based organizations provide companions, shopping services, and prepared meals in some communities – Senior centers provide variety of support system in individual communities.

As nursing home residents are known to have greater comorbidities and functional disabilities, the risks and benefits of tight glycemic control and various medications should be considered carefully. The risk of treatment-related complications, primarily hypoglycemia, is much higher than the benefits of tight glycemic control, and a prudent approach is to aim for the best glycemic control possible without exposing the patient to hypoglycemic risks. It is important to educate nursing home staff on diabetes management as they become the caregiver for the residents. This education should include unique challenges facing patients with T1D as compared to commonly seen T2D, an overview of the different insulins, interaction between insulin and carbohydrate content of the meals, and hypoglycemic recognition and treatment.

PRACTICAL ISSUES IN CARING FOR OLDER ADULTS WITH T1D

Older patients with T1D are unique in that they have survived many decades with a very complex disease. These patients are usually comfortable managing their disease and feel strongly about controlling their hyperglycemia. On the other hand, they do develop age-related diseases and impairments that may interfere with complex management. The chronic complications of diabetes that develop over time, such as retinopathy, gastropathy, peripheral and autonomic neuropathy, peripheral vascular disease, and vascular dementia can all lead to increased functional disability and difficulty performing self-care. These patients make errors in insulin dosing, meal planning, or insulin and meal timing that is due to newly developed disabilities rather than lack of knowledge. These errors lead to great frustration on the part of the patients and caregivers. It is common to see frequent hypoglycemic episodes in older patients with T1D who are not as concerned about these episodes as they were in childhood. The consequences of hypoglycemia and aging are serious, however. It is difficult for some of these patients who have had T1D for >50–60 years to now learn that hypoglycemia can be more harmful for them then hyperglycemia. Repeated education and patience is required on the part of medical providers and caregiver while patients try to change the behavior that originally led to their successful management of diabetes and long survival.

Health care providers need to be reminded that the measurement of A1C may not be accurate in some older patients, especially if they have conditions that change red blood cell life span (e.g., anemia, transfusions, hemoglobinopahies), severe renal or hepatic diseases, or recent hospitalizations. This issue is especially important in the nursing home population. In such instances, finger-stick glucose readings are more reliable for making treatment changes than A1C.

FUTURE CLINICAL RESEARCH

The fundamental challenge for making diabetes-related treatment decisions among older adults with T1D is the lack of clinical trial data. Future studies in this population should focus on the risks and benefits of tight glycemic control: the best treatment strategies for those with multiple comorbidities, including depression and quality of life; the role of exercise and nutrition; and the impact of hypoglycemia. Surveillance data differentiating the type of diabetes in the older population will also be important.

CONCLUSION

As we successfully manage younger patients with T1D, we will be seeing an increased number of older adults with this disease. Managing T1D is truly a partnership between the patient and his or her provider. At this stage, patients know their disease and management strategies well. The role of the provider is to continue to support the patients in their effort. As the individuals age, medical providers need to watch carefully for age-related barriers and help the patient adjust their goals and strategies to achieve successful aging and the best possible quality of life.

GAPS ACCORDING TO THE EDITORS

1. There is a need to understand the risks and benefits of intensive glycemic control in older patients.
2. There is a need to study approaches to preventing severe hypoglycemia in elderly patients.
3. There is a need to ensure the proper training and education of health care workers who provide care to older patients with diabetes across multiple locales, in the home, in the hospital, in nursing facilities, and elsewhere.
4. Additional studies are needed to understand the psychosocial needs of older patients with T1D.

REFERENCES

1. Centers for Disease Control and Prevention U.S. Department of Health and Human Services CfDCaP: National Diabetes Fact Sheet: National Estimates and General Information on Diabetes and Prediabetes in the United States, 2011. Atlanta, GA, CDC, 2011
2. Munshi M: Managing the "geriatric syndrome" in patients with type 2 diabetes. *Consult Pharm* 23(Suppl. B):12–16, 2008
3. Brown AF, Mangione CM, Saliba D, Sarkisian CA: Guidelines for improving the care of the older person with diabetes mellitus. *J Am Geriatr Soc* 51:S265–S280, 2003
4. Gregg EW, Mangione CM, Cauley JA, et al.: Diabetes and incidence of functional disability in older women. *Diabetes Care* 25:61–67, 2002
5. Sun JK, Keenan HA, Cavallerano JD, Asztalos BF, Schaefer EJ, Sell DR, Strauch CM, Monnier VM, Doria A, Aiello LP, King GL: Protection from retinopathy and other complications in patients with type 1 diabetes of

extreme duration: the Joslin 50-year medalist study. *Diabetes Care* 34:968–974, 2011

6. Weinstock RS, Dubose SN, Aleppo GM, Beck RW, Bergenstal RM, Goland RS, Hirsch IB, Liljenquist DR, Odegard PS, Peters AL: Characteristics of older adults with type 1 diabetes: data from the T1D exchange (abstract). *Diabetes* 61:A357, 2012

7. Arvanitakis Z, Wilson RS, Bienias JL, Evans DA, Bennett DA: Diabetes mellitus and risk of Alzheimer disease and decline in cognitive function. *Arch Neurol* 61:661–666, 2004

8. Hassing LB, Hofer SM, Nilsson SE, Berg S, Pedersen NL, McClearn G, Johansson B: Comorbid type 2 diabetes mellitus and hypertension exacerbates cognitive decline: evidence from a longitudinal study. *Age Ageing* 33:355–361, 2004

9. Kuo H-K, Jones RN, Milberg WP, Tennstedt S, Talbot L, Morris JN, Lipsitz LA: Effect of blood pressure and diabetes mellitus on cognitive and physical functions in older adults: a longitudinal analysis of the advanced cognitive training for independent and vital elderly cohort. *J Am Geriatr Soc* 53:1154–1161, 2005

10. Gregg EW, Yaffe K, Cauley JA, Rolka DB, Blackwell TL, Venkat Narayan KM, Cummings SR: Is diabetes associated with cognitive impairment and cognitive decline among older women? Study of osteoporotic fractures research group. *Arch Intern Med* 160:174–180, 2000

11. Brands AM, Biessels GJ, de Haan EH, Kappelle LJ, Kessels RP: The effects of type 1 diabetes on cognitive performance: a meta-analysis. *Diabetes Care* 28:726–735, 2005

12. Johnston H, McCrimmon R, Petrie J, Astell A: An estimate of lifetime cognitive change and its relationship with diabetes health in older adults with type 1 diabetes: preliminary results. *Behav Neurol* 23:165–167, 2010

13. Duinkerken E, Brands AM, van den Berg E, Henselmans JM, Hoogma RP, Biessels GJ: Cognition in older patients with type 1 diabetes mellitus: a longitudinal study. *J Am Geriatr Soc* 59:563–565, 2011

14. Barnard KD, Skinner TC, Peveler R: The prevalence of co-morbid depression in adults with type 1 diabetes: systematic literature review. *Diabet Med* 23:445–448, 2006

15. Ahola AJ, Thorn LM, Saraheimo M, Forsblom C, Groop PH: Depression is associated with the metabolic syndrome among patients with type 1 diabetes. *Ann Med* 42:495–501, 2010

16. Spitzer C, Völzke H, Barnow S, Krohn U, Wallaschofski H, Lüdemann J, John U, Freyberger HJ, W. Kerner W, Grabe HJ: Association between depression and subclinical carotid atherosclerosis in patients with type 1 diabetes. *Diabet Med* 25:349–354, 2008

17. Ciechanowski PS, Katon WJ, Russo JE: Depression and diabetes: impact of depressive symptoms on adherence, function, and costs. *Arch Intern Med* 160:3278–3285, 2000

18. Lin EHB, Katon W, Von Korff M, Rutter C, Simon GE, Oliver M, Ciechanowski P, Ludman EJ, Bush T, Young B: Relationship of depression and diabetes self-care, medication adherence, and preventive care. *Diabetes Care* 27:2154–2160, 2004

19. Zhang X, Norris SL, Gregg EW, Cheng YJ, Beckles G, Kahn HS: Depressive symptoms and mortality among persons with and without diabetes. *Am J Epidemiol* 161:652–660, 2005
20. Volpato S, Leveille SG, Blaum C, Fried LP, Guralnik JM: Risk factors for falls in older disabled women with diabetes: the women's health and aging study. *J Gerontol A Biol Sci Med Sci* 60:1539–1545, 2005
21. Schwartz AV, Hillier TA, Sellmeyer DE, Resnick HE, Gregg E, Ensrud KE, Schreiner PJ, Margolis KL, Cauley JA, Nevitt MC, Black DM, Cummings SR: Older women with diabetes have a higher risk of falls: a prospective study. *Diabetes Care* 25:1749–1754, 2002
22. Shorr RI, Ray WA, Daugherty JR, Griffin MR: Incidence and risk factors for serious hypoglycemia in older persons using insulin or sulfonylureas. *Arch Intern Med* 157:1681–1686, 1997
23. Desouza C, Salazar H, Cheong B, Murgo J, Fonseca V: Association of hypoglycemia and cardiac ischemia: a study based on continuous monitoring. *Diabetes Care* 26:1485–1489, 2003
24. Frier BM: How hypoglycaemia can affect the life of a person with diabetes. *Diabetes Metab Res Rev* 24:87–92, 2008
25. Frier BM: Epidemiology, short and long-term consequences of hypoglycaemia. *Diabetes Nutr Metab* 15:378–384; discussion 84–85, 2002
26. Munshi MN, Segal AR, Suhl E, Staum E, Desrochers L, Sternthal A, Giusti J, McCartney R, Lee Y, Bonsignore P, Weinger K: Frequent hypoglycemia among elderly patients with poor glycemic control. *Arch Intern Med* 171:362–364, 2011
27. Munshi MN, Hayes M, Sternthal A, Ayres D: Use of serum C-peptide level to simplify diabetes treatment regimens in older adults. *Am J Med* 122:395–397, 2009
28. Elbert S, Huang PJ, Munshi MN: Multidisciplinary approach for the treatment of diabetes in the elderly. *Aging Health* 5:207–216, 2009
29. Zhang X, Decker FH, Luo H, Geiss LS, Pearson WS, Saaddine JB, Gregg EW, Albright, A: Trends in the prevalence and comorbidities of diabetes mellitus in nursing home residents in the United States: 1995–2004. *J Am Geriatr Soc* 58:724–730, 2010

VI. Special Population Groups

William C. Hsu, MD

TYPE 1 DIABETES (T1D) IN ETHNIC MINORITIES

Minorities now make up ~35% of the population in the U.S., according to U.S. Census 2010, and 2011 was the first year in which the majority of newborns were infants born from racial and minority parents. Thus, much of the nation's demographic change is seen among children. For example in California, minorities make up 72% of those under age 15 years. The tremendous diversity in language, cultural, and dietary preferences in the nation's demographic makeup has a profound impact on disease incidence, health behavior, glycemic control, and diabetes-related complications. In addition, rates of T1D and progression of β-cell failure likely are influenced by racial and ethnic background (genetics) as well as environmental factors that, in turn, are influenced by race and ethnicity. There is a need for additional understanding of the unique pathophysiology in different populations and for more data that are population based, disaggregated, and granular with respect to specific minority populations, especially among the smaller subgroups. Such information will help inform and influence health outcomes, research funding, and health-care policies.

BURDEN OF DISEASE

According to the SEARCH study, a national multicenter study funded by the Centers for Disease Control and Prevention (CDC) and National Institutes of Health (NIH) aimed at understanding more about diabetes among children and young adults in the U.S., minority youth generally have lower rates of new cases of T1D compared to non-Hispanic white youth. Specifically, the prevalence (per 1,000) of T1D was 0.57 (95% CI 0.47–0.69) and for those ages 10–19 years 2.04 (CI 1.85–2.26) among African American youth ages 0–9 years. Among African American youth ages 0–9 years, annual T1D incidence (per 100,000) was 15.7 (13.7–17.9) and for those ages 10–19 years 15.7 (13.8–17.8).[1] Recent data published in 2012 and presented at the annual scientific meetings of the American Diabetes Association confirm the increased prevalence of T1D in American youth under the age of 20 years, with rates increasing 23% between 2001 and 2009 among all racial and ethnic groups except for American Indians.[2]

Among Hispanic American youth, T1D was more prevalent than type 2 diabetes (T2D) except among female youth ages 15–19 years for whom the incidence of T2D exceeded that of T1D.[3] In contrast, the SEARCH database for Navajo showed that among adolescents ages 15–19 years, 1 in 359 Navajo youth had diabetes in 2001 and 1 in 2,542 developed diabetes annually. The vast

596

DOI: 10.2337/9781580404785ch18s6

majority of diabetes among Navajo youth with diabetes is T2D.[4] Similarly for Asian American and Pacific Islanders youth, the rate of new cases was greater for T2D than for T1D. The incidence of T1D for youth ages 0–9 years was 6.4 per 100,000 person-years and 7.4% per 100,000 person-years for youth ages 10–19 years.[5]

PATHOPHYSIOLOGY

The fundamental pathophysiology of T1D involving β-cell destruction is by and large similar across different ethnicity. There are important variations, however, in presentation that can present diagnostic challenges.

For example, in 1994 a report described a cohort of 21 African Americans adults from Brooklyn, New York, who presented initially with ketoacidosis but actually had T2D confirmed by resolution to insulin independence, absence of anti-islet antibodies, and low prevalence of common human leukocyte antigen (HLA) genotypes typically associated with T1D. Their presentation was characterized by acute and severely defective insulin secretion with insulin resistance and less suppression of glucagon without evidence for autoimmunity.[6] There is a similar sample of patients who have been characterized in Houston, Texas,[7] with recurrent diabetic ketoacidosis (DKA). Such a clinical constellation could easily lead to a misdiagnosis of T1D especially among younger individuals. Accurate diagnosis is important because, following initiation of insulin treatment, some insulin secretory capacity is recovered and ketoacidosis generally does not recur, thus allowing these patients to be treated without insulin therapy.[8]

On the other hand, the current epidemic of overweight and obesity in the pediatric and adult populations may lead to an incorrect diagnosis of T2D in the setting of hyperglycemia with or without ketosis, especially among racial and ethnic minority groups. Recent data suggest that ~10% of pediatric patients with T2D clinically diagnosed by pediatric specialists have positive IA2 or GAD antibodies, confirming the presence of β-cell autoimmunity.[9] The SEARCH for Diabetes in Youth study suggests an approach to correctly diagnosing diabetes based on the presence or absence of β-cell autoimmunity and the presence or absence of insulin resistance noted by elevated C-peptide levels.[10]

As another example, T1D occurs much less frequently among Asian descendants.[11] The pathophysiology for T1D remains poorly understood in this population as only a fraction of affected individuals have DR3/4 and DQB1 HLA haplotypes[12] with <50% possessing anti-islet autoantibody positivity.[13] Among siblings, however, who have these genotypes, there is an increased rate of developing T1D.[14] Therefore, because of these features, T1D can be difficult to differentiate from T2D in this population as T2D tends to present at younger ages and with lower BMI.[15] It can be distinguished by differences in insulin sensitivity, serum adiponectin, free fatty acid, high-density lipoprotein (HDL) concentrations, and truncal fat.[16] In contrast, Native Hawaiians and Pacific Islanders with T1D were more likely to be obese, with a mean BMI of 26 vs. 20 kg/m2 for Asian Americans.[5] Confirming the diagnosis of T1D in patients with adult onset diabetes, especially in racial and ethnic minority groups and other underserved populations, requires that providers consider T1D in the differential diagnosis and assess antibody status, presenting ketoacidosis and other metabolic factors.

GLYCEMIC CONTROL AND ITS DETERMINANTS FOR ETHNIC DISPARITIES

Children and young adults from racial and ethnic minority groups have an increased risk for developing ketoacidosis.[17] After diagnosis, minority youths with T1D continue to experience glycemic disparities compared with their white non-Hispanic counterparts.[18] For example, in African American and Hispanic American youths, high A1C levels, defined as ≥9.5, were common among youth age 15 years or older.[1] In addition, Navajo youth with T1D have poor glycemic control, high prevalence of unhealthy behaviors, and evidence of severely depressed mood.[4]

It is unclear, however, whether ethnicity in itself is an independent risk factor for poor glycemic control. Possible explanations may include linguistic barriers in the immigrant communities,[19] lack of access to adequate health care,[20] and lack of socioeconomic resources, with more than one-third of African American youth with T1D having household annual incomes of <$25,000 and 50% living in one-parent households. Recent data collected from the Type 1 Diabetes Exchange and presented at the American Diabetes Association meetings in 2012 demonstrate that socioeconomic status does not account for the racial and ethnic disparities that exist in the penetration of insulin pump therapy and in glycemic outcomes that are apparent in racial and ethnic minority groups.[21,22] Similarly, data from Texas Children's Hospital in Houston also report higher rates of depression, poorer glycemic control, and more rehospitalization for DKA following the diagnosis of T1D in African American youth.[23]

Some have attributed the higher hemoglobin A1C levels in minority population to an underlying biologic basis, that is, a faster glycation rate[24] or possible differences in red cell survival.[25] More recent study has shown that glycated albumin, fructosamine, and 1,5-anhydroglucitol levels parallel differences between African Americans and Caucasians in A1C values, suggesting racial differences in hemoglobin glycation and erythrocyte turnover are not likely to be reasons to explain racial disparities in these serum markers.[26]

DEVELOPING CULTURAL EFFECTIVENESS IN DIABETES CARE

The debate regarding biologic versus social determinants of disparities according to race and ethnicity in diabetes care and outcomes continues to rage on; however, taking cultural factors into treatment consideration is critical to successfully managing diabetes. Culture is a set of shared values, beliefs, goals, and practices that characterizes a particular group of people. It encompasses gender, age, language, faith, immigration history, and socioeconomic level, and it has far-reaching impact. Culture helps shape patient's explanatory models for disease, which, in turn, influences their perceptions about specific treatments and ultimately affects medication adherence. Furthermore, dietary habits, provider–patient relationships, and utilization of support system may be heavily dependent on cultural perspectives held by patients.[27]

According to the American Medical Association:

> Cultural competence is the knowledge and interpersonal skills that allow providers to understand, appreciate, and work with individuals from cultures other than their own. It involves an awareness and acceptance of cultural differences; self-awareness; knowledge of patient's culture; and adaptation of skills.[28]

Although diabetes knowledge and the acquisition of management skills are necessary, they are not sufficient unless taught in a culturally sensitive manner. The diabetes treatment team should display motivation to achieve cultural competency that arises from an attitude of openness, respect, and desire to learn from patients and families with the ultimate goal of supporting them to modify their behaviors for healthful outcomes. Some states, such as New Jersey and California, require cultural competency training in the form of continuing medical education for maintenance of physician licensure. Dozen of other states are currently considering the need for similar requirements while others oppose this approach, raising the concern that such requirements may burden physicians with such mandated training. Independent as to whether such training becomes a requirement, it is apparent that patients and families with T1D will respond best to care and education that are delivered in a culturally sensitive manner by a caring and responsive multidisciplinary team.

There is census that cultural competency training raises clinicians' awareness of racial disparities among minority patients.[29,30] Additional research is needed to determine whether cultural competency training leads to improvements in A1C. Indeed, there are complex issues related to health disparities, and cultural competency is likely one component.[31] Future research should focus approaches to cultural competency training and how such training can improve care and health outcomes as well as potentially reduce costs.

GAPS ACCORDING TO THE EDITORS

1. There is a need to understand the occurrence of T1D in racial and ethnic minority groups and other underserved populations across the life span.
2. Studies are needed to assess if the onset and progression of β-cell autoimmunity and β-cell failure differ according to race and ethnicity.
3. Diabetes multidisciplinary teams require ongoing training to understand the unique cultural needs of racial and ethnic minority groups in order to optimize health care delivery, improve glycemic control, and prevent complications.
4. There appears to be substantial disparity in diabetes health care delivery as evidenced by the disproportionate penetration of insulin pump therapy in non-Hispanic Caucasians with T1D. Additional research is needed to identify approaches to reduce these disparities and improve health outcomes in racial and ethnic minorities and underserved populations with T1D.

REFERENCES

1. Mayer-Davis EJ, Beyer J, Bell RA, Dabelea D, D'Agostino, Jr. R, Imperatore G, Lawrence JM, Liese AD, Liu L, Marcovina S, Rodriguez B: Diabetes in African American youth: prevalence, incidence, and clinical characteristics: the SEARCH for Diabetes in Youth Study. *Diabetes Care* 32:S112–S122, 2009

2. Mayer-Davis EJ, Dabelea D, Talton JW, Hamman RF, Divers J, Badaru A, Crume TL, Dolan LM, Imperatore G, Lawrence JM, Liese AD, Linder B, Saydah S, the Search for Diabetes in Youth Study Group: Increase in prevalence of type 1 diabetes from the SEARCH for Diabetes in Youth study: 2001 to 2009. Abstract #1248. *Diabetes* 61:A322, 2012

3. Lawrence JM, Mayer-Davis EJ, Reynolds K, Beyer J, Pettitt DJ, D'Agostino, Jr. RB, Marcovina SM, Imperatore G, Hamman RF, the SEARCH for Diabetes in Youth Study Group: Diabetes in Hispanic American youth: prevalence, incidence, demographics, and clinical characteristics: the SEARCH for Diabetes in Youth study. *Diabetes Care* 32:S123–S132, 2009

4. Dabelea D, DeGroat J, Sorrelman C, Glass M, Percy CA, Avery C, Hu D, D'Agostino, Jr. RB, Beyer J, Imperatore G, Testaverde L, Klingensmith G, Hamman RF: Diabetes in Navajo youth: prevalence, incidence, and clinical characteristics: the SEARCH for Diabetes in Youth study. *Diabetes Care* 32:S141–S147, 2009

5. Liu LL, Yi JP, Beyer J, Mayer-Davis EJ, Dolan LM, Dabelea DM, Lawrence JM, Rodriguez BL, Marcovina SM, Waitzfelder BE, Fujimoto WY: Type 1 and type 2 diabetes in Asian and Pacific Islander U.S. youth: the SEARCH for Diabetes in Youth study. *Diabetes Care* 32:S133–S140, 2009

6. Banerji MA, Chaiken RL, Huey H, Tuomi T, Norin AJ, Mackay IR, Rowley MJ, Zimmet PZ, Lebovitz HE: GAD antibody negative NIDDM in adult black subjects with diabetic ketoacidosis and increased frequency of human leukocyte antigen DR3 and DR4. *Diabetes* 43:741–745, 1994

7. Balasubramanyam A, Garza G, Rodriguez L, Hampe C, Gaur L, Lernmark A, Maldonado M: Accuracy and predictive value of classification schemes for ketosis-prone diabetes. *Diabetes Care* 29 (12):2575–2579, 2006

8. Banerji MA: Impaired beta-cell and alpha-cell function in African-American children with type 2 diabetes mellitus—"Flatbush diabetes." *J Pediatr Endocrinol Metab* 15(Suppl. 1):493–501, 2002

9. Klingensmith GJ, Pyle L, Arslanian S, Copeland KC, Cuttler L, Kaufman F, Laffel L, Marcovina S, Tollefsen SE, Weinstock RS, Linder B, for the TODAY Study Group: The presence of GAD and IA-2 antibodies in youth with a type 2 diabetes phenotype: results from the TODAY study. *Diabetes Care* 33:1970–1975, 2010

10. SEARCH for Diabetes in Youth Study Group, Liese AD, D'Agostino RB Jr, Hamman RF, Kilgo PD, Lawrence JM, Liu LL, Loots B, Linder B, Marcovina S, Rodriguez B, Standiford D, Williams DE: The burden of diabetes mellitus among US youth: prevalence estimates from the SEARCH for Diabetes in Youth Study. *Pediatrics* 118:1510–1518, 2006

11. International Diabetes Federation: *IDF Diabetes Atlas.* 5th ed. Brussels, Belgium, International Diabetes Federation, 2011 Available at http://www.idf.org/diabetesatlas. Accessed 26 October 2012

12. Rewers M, Bugawan TL, Norris JM, Blair A, Beaty B, Hoffman M, McDuffie RS, Hamman RF, Klinensmith G, Eisenbarth GS, Erlich HA: Newborn screening for HLA markers associated with IDDM: Diabetes Autoimmunity Study in the Young (DAISY). *Diabetolgia* 39:807–812, 1996

13. Li JKY, Chan JCN, Zimmet PZ, Rowley MJ, Mackay IR, Cockram CS: Young Chinese adults with new onset of diabetic ketoacidosis: clinical course, autoimmune status and progression of pancreatic beta-cell function. *Diabetic Medicine* 17:295–298, 2000

14. Ikegami H, Kawabata Y, Noso S, Fujisawa T, Ogihara T: Genetics of type 1 diabetics in Asian and Caucasian populations. *Diabetes Research and Clinical Practice* 77:S116–S121, 2007

15. Hsu WC, Boyko EJ, Fujimoto WY, Kanaya A, Karmally W, Karter A, King GL, Look M, Maskarinec G, Misra R, Tavake-Pasi F, Arakaki R: Pathophysiologic differences among Asians, Native Hawaiians, and other Pacific Islanders and treatment implications. *Diabetes Care* 35:1189–1198, 2012

16. Hsu WC, Okeke E, Cheung S, Keenan H, Tsui T, Cheng K, King GL: A cross-sectional characterization of insulin resistance by phenotype and insulin clamp in East Asian Americans with type 1 and type 2 diabetes. *PLoS One* 6:e28311, 2011

17. Usher-Smith JA, Thompson MJ, Sharp SJ, Walter FM: Factors associated with the presence of diabetic ketoacidosis at diagnosis of diabetes in children and young adults: a systematic review. *British Medical Journal* 343:d4092, 2011

18. Gallegos-Macias AR, Macias SR, Kaufman E, Skipper B, Kalishman N: Relationship between glycemic control, ethnicity and socioeconomic status in Hispanic and white non-Hispanic youths with type 1 diabetes mellitus. *Pediatric Diabetes* 4:19–23, 2003

19. Hsu WC, Cheung S, Ong E, Wong K, Lin S, Leon K, Weinger K, King GL: Identification of linguistic barriers to diabetes knowledge and glycemic control in Chinese Americans with diabetes. *Diabetes Care* 29:415–416, 2006

20. Weech-Maldonado R, Morales LS, Spritzer K, Elliott M, Hays RD: Racial and ethnic differences in parents' assessments of pediatric care in Medicaid managed care. *Health Services Research* 36:575–594, 2001

21. Klingensmith GJ, Miller KM, Beck RW, Cruz E, Laffel LM, Lipman TH, Schatz DA, Tamborlane WV, Willi SM: Racial disparities in insulin pump therapy and hemoglobin A1C (A1C) among T1D exchange participants. Poster 1377-P. *ADA 2012 Scientific Sessions* 61(Suppl. 1), 2012

22. Cortina S, Repaske DR, Hood KK: Sociodemographic and psychosocial factors associated with continuous subcutaneous insulin infusion in adolescents with type 1 diabetes. *Pediatric Diabetes* 11:337–344, 2010

23. Schwartz DD, Cline VD, Axelrad ME, Anderson BJ: Feasibility, acceptability, and predictive validity of a psychosocial screening program for children and youth newly diagnosed with type 1 diabetes. *Diabetes Care* 34(2):326–331, 2011

24. Cohen RM: Does one size fit all? *Diabetes Care* 30:2756–2758, 2007

25. Herman WH, Cohen RM: Racial and ethnic differences in the relationship between HbA1C and blood glucose: implications for the diagnosis of diabetes. *J Clin Endocrinol Metab* 97:1067–1072, 2012

26. Selvin E, Steffes MW, Ballantyne CM, Hoogeveen RC, Coresh J, Brancati FL: Racial differences in glycemic markers: a cross-sectional analysis of community-based data. *Annals of Internal Medicine* 154:303–309, 2011

27. Hsu WC, Yoon HH, Gavin JR 3rd, Wright EE Jr, Cabellero AE, Tenzer P: Building cultural competency for improved diabetes care: introduction and overview. *J Fam Pract* 56(9 Suppl. Building):S11–S14, 2007

28. American Medical Association: *Cultural Competence Compendium*. Chicago, American Medical Association, 1999

29. Kutob RM, Senf JH, Harris, Jr. JM: Teaching culturally effective diabetes care: results of a randomized controlled trial. *Family Medicine* 41:167–174, 2009

30. Sequist TD, Ayanian JZ, Marshall R, Fitzmaurice GM, Safran DG: Primary-care clinician perceptions of racial disparities in diabetes care. *Journal of General Internal Medicine* 23:678–684, 2008

31. Sequist TD, Fitzmaurice GM, Marshall R, Shaykevich S, Marston A, Safran DG, Ayanian JZ: Cultural competency training and performance reports to improve diabetes care for black patients: a cluster randomized, controlled trial. *Annals of Internal Medicine* 152:40–46, 2010

VII. Developing Countries

Hussain Mahmud, MD, and Mary Korytkowski, MD

Type 1 diabetes (T1D) increasingly is being recognized as a global public health challenge because of its rising incidence, chronicity, and the burden it places on already overstretched public health systems, especially in developing countries. There is paucity of published literature from developing countries pertaining specifically to T1D. In the following text, if the information is not clearly stated to refer to T1D, it can be assumed that it relates to both T1D and type 2 diabetes.

EPIDEMIOLOGY

A rapid increase in the incidence of T1D has been a global phenomenon during the past few decades. World Health Organization's DIAMOND project, which collects standardized incidence data worldwide, reported a statistically significant increase in the incidence of T1D in all continents except for South and Central America between 1990 and 1999. Wide variation in incidence rates exists between different populations, with lower incidence in developing countries (China and Venezuela had the lowest incidence rate of 0.1 per 100,000 people per year) compared to the industrial countries (Finland and Sardinia had the highest incidence rate of 37 per 100,000 people per year at the end of the twentieth century).[1] By 2005, the age-standardized incidence rate of T1D had increased to 64.2 per 100,000 people per year in Finnish children.[2] Other studies report incidences ranging from 1.5 to 2.1 per 100,000 people per year in Tanzania and Ethiopia.[3,4] These studies, however, based their estimates on previously diagnosed cases rather than population screening. Misdiagnosis and high mortality within communities may leave many cases unaccounted.

The peak age of onset in sub-Saharan Africa has been noted to be a decade later than in the Western Hemisphere countries.[3] The prevalence of autoantibodies is also less common when compared to Western Hemisphere countries. For example, in one study, 30 to 44% of patients with T1D from Cameroon and South Africa were GAD positive at diagnosis compared to ~70% in Western Hemisphere populations.[5,6]

The rising incidence of T1D worldwide has been attributed to a complex interplay between genetic predisposition and environmental factors such as diet, micronutrients, infectious agents, psychological stress, chemicals, and toxins that lead to breakdown of self-tolerance and increase in autoimmunity. Interestingly, a transmigratory effect has been noted among immigrant populations who move from low- to high-incidence areas.[7] This highlights the role of environmental triggers. For example, the incidence of T1D among

DOI: 10.2337/9781580404785ch18s7

South Asian children residing in Yorkshire was 14.7 per 100,000 compared to the estimated incidence of 0.5 per 100,000 in Pakistan. This incidence, however, is still considerably lower than the observed rate of 21.5 per 100,000 among non–South Asians in the same county.[7]

There is considerable variability in the presentation of insulin-dependent diabetes in developing countries. Clinicians should recognize the following variant forms of diabetes because of their impact on long-term management. Some older or middle-age patients who are often obese can present with diabetic ketoacidosis (DKA) as the first manifestation of diabetes. Ketosis-prone type 2 diabetes (also referred to as atypical or Flatbush diabetes) can be considered as the etiology, particularly in patients who have a decline in their insulin requirement over time.[8] Ketosis-prone diabetes has been reported across almost all populations studied, including minorities in the U.S. (African Americans, Hispanics), immigrant populations in Europe, Africans, and Asians.[8]

The existence of malnutrition-related diabetes mellitus (previously referred to as tropical diabetes) as a separate disease entity has been debated. These patients tend to have a later peak age of onset (25–29 years), male preponderance, history of childhood malnutrition, and a disadvantaged socioeconomic background. Typically these patients have severe symptoms (emaciation, polyuria, polydipsia, and weakness) but are not sufficiently insulinopenic to develop ketoacidosis.[4]

Fulminant T1D is another diabetes variant described in Asian countries. It is characterized by rapid progression of severe hyperglycemia resulting in severe DKA. The progression of disease from normal β-cell mass to almost complete β-cell destruction occurs within a few days, rarely exceeding a week.[9]

BARRIERS TO DIABETES CARE

The challenges to provide adequate diabetes care in the developing world are unique. With few exceptions, health care systems in developing countries are primarily designed around the needs for acute rather than chronic care. The organizational structure for providing chronic disease management is nonexistent. The "double burden of disease" in developing countries is attributed to the continued high prevalence of infectious diseases such as HIV/AIDS, tuberculosis, and malaria, in concert with the emerging epidemic of noncommunicable diseases, such as diabetes, hypertension, and cardiovascular disease usually associated with industrial countries. With limited health care budgets, diabetes management costs have to compete with other health care priorities, such as combating infectious diseases.

Access to health care also presents a significant barrier to the delivery of chronic disease management. In a study conducted in Ethiopia, the prevalence of insulin-dependent diabetes was five times greater in urban than rural areas.[4] This suggests either migration of individuals from rural to urban areas once a chronic disease is diagnosed, sampling bias, or limited access to health care in rural areas due to disproportionate distribution of health facilities, poverty, lack of roads, and means of transport. In addition, potential cases can be missed because of underdiagnosis of T1D and misclassification of causes of death in rural areas.

Economic factors pose a major barrier to the delivery of adequate diabetes care delivery in developing countries. Insulin remains an expensive drug with an estimated annual cost of ~40 times the annual allotment for public sector spending for pharmaceutical supplies in resource-limited countries.[10] In countries where insulin access is not guaranteed by the public health system, care of a child with T1D may consume up to 65% of a family's annual household health expenditure.[11] A rapid assessment protocol to assess insulin access was developed by Beran et al.,[10] who reported the following problems with insulin supply: poor quantification of need, failure to take advantage of less expensive insulin preparations, and erratic delivery of insulin even in hospital settings. Insulin was found to be consistently available in only 20% of the hospitals studied in Mozambique.[10] International organizations, such as the International Diabetes Federation's (IDF) Life for a Child (LFAC), are working with insulin manufacturers and local health care delivery systems to help ensure insulin availability.

The International Insulin Foundation recently published a position statement encouraging the use of lower cost animal based or biosynthetic human insulin preparations as a way to improve insulin availability and reduce barriers to insulin use in developing countries.[12] The high cost of analog insulins and the associated pen devices can result in severe limitations to the numbers of people who can receive insulin therapy in resource poor countries.

Logistical problems and maintenance of appropriate temperatures during insulin delivery and storage to prevent degradation and decreased efficacy of insulin products pose significant challenges, especially in rural areas. In one study, insulin syringes and diagnostic supplies such as urine and blood reagent test strips were found to be either in short supply or entirely unavailable in the majority of hospitals surveyed in sub–Saharan Africa. None of the 99 patients with T1D enrolled in a Tanzanian study had the ability to monitor their glucose levels at home. Hospitals were also unable to routinely perform urine or blood glucose testing.[13]

Limited expertise of health care workers in the management of insulin dependent patients also presents a significant challenge in the struggle to achieve adequate levels of glycemic control, which in developing countries can be based more on symptoms of hyperglycemia and hypoglycemia rather than measures of hemoglobin A1C. Because T1D is relatively uncommon or often does not come to attention of medical professionals in these regions, the lack of familiarity and tools for proper diagnosis often can lead to missed diagnosis. DKA may be misdiagnosed as cerebral malaria or other more prevalent conditions, contributing to an unacceptably high mortality rate.[14]

Lack of knowledge among health care workers coupled with a deficiency of organized health care information systems results in poor understanding of their condition by patients. Misconceptions about diet and insulin use affect glycemic control contributing to the development of diabetes-related complications. In many societies, traditional healers form an integral part of the health care system. This can often affect patients' health beliefs and lead to decreased access to effective care. Reluctance to initiate insulin therapy secondary to perceived fear and anxiety of injections, inconvenience, and interference with work and social activities has been reported in developing as well as industrial countries and cultures.[15]

COMPLICATIONS

The acute metabolic complications of diabetes including DKA and hypoglycemia are quite common. A Tanzanian survey estimated that 89% of children with T1D had experienced DKA in the preceding six months.[13] In developing countries, DKA may have a mortality rate of 10–30% because of lack of insulin, delayed presentation, or secondary infections,[16,17] Hypoglycemia was reported by 55% of the participants with insulin-treated diabetes in the preceding 6 months in the Tanzanian study.[13] Severe diabetes associated infections continue to pose a significant challenge and contribute to both diabetes morbidity and mortality. Besides severe foot infections and resulting gangrene, diabetes also contributes to hand infections, tuberculosis, and mucormycosis.[18,19]

The estimated prevalence of chronic diabetes-related complications varies according to T1D duration, glycemic control, population, diagnostic facilities, and genetic or ethnic factors. Complications can occur very early in the setting of poor glycemic control. The Tanzanian study reported prevalence of retinopathy and microalbuminuria at 25.8% and 29.9%, respectively, among prepubertal children with T1D.[13]

In Africa, diabetes accounts for 25% of patients in dialysis units, where renal replacement is both expensive and often not widely available.[20] In India, retinopathy was seen in 77.3%, nephropathy in 12.1%, and neuropathy in 21.4% of those with T1D for >15 years duration.[21] In Africa and India, >80% of foot ulcers occurring in patients with diabetes are neuropathic rather than vascular in origin.[22] Ethnic variation in diabetes complications between different populations needs more study as it will allow better allocation of resources for population-based screening of complications.

MORTALITY

Mortality rates in T1D vary widely depending on access to health care and ability to identify direct cause. Beran et al. estimated life expectancy to vary from 0.6 years for a child in rural Mozambique to 27 years for an adult living in Lusaka, the capital city of Zambia.[10] Twenty-year survival rates in T1D were found to be 57% in Soweto, South Africa, and 63% in Addis Ababa, Ethiopia.[23,24] The major cause of mortality in the Soweto cohort was renal failure; however, acute metabolic emergencies, especially DKA and infections remain important causes of mortality.

COST-EFFECTIVENESS OF INTERVENTIONS AND PRIORITIES

T1D is an expensive disease, especially when the cost of complications is considered. The IDF estimated that in 2010, the national funding for the health care of people with diabetes in Africa was US$112 per person per year, which amounts to ~7% of the national health budget.[25] As a result, patients and their families may have to spend significant proportions of their income on treatment, an expenditure that may not be sustainable. In a review of potential solutions to the global burden of diabetes care, three interventions were identified as cost saving, effective, and feasible. These included achieving A1C <9%, blood pressure <160/95 mmHg, and foot care in people with ulcers.[26] The challenge is achieving even these limited objectives. Other interventions considered as standard of care in industrial countries, such as annual eye examinations or use of ACE inhibitors would incur costs of US$400–1,000 per quality adjusted life year (QALY), which are lower priorities when resources are limited. Intensification of therapy to achieve A1C <8%, screening for microalbuminuria and treatment of hyperlipidemia were deemed to be priority level III interventions as these incur costs of >US$2,500 per QALY.[26] Further research to find cost-effective solutions tailored to the developing world's setting should be prioritized.

POTENTIAL SOLUTIONS AND FILLING THE GAPS

It is important that the future of T1D care include efforts that address the challenges that have been identified. Regional and country-specific data on diabetes incidence, prevalence, access to care, morbidity, mortality, and costs would enable informed and judicious prioritization of available health funding. International agencies and civil societies could be involved in establishing peer educational experiences that allow shared discussion forums to promote development of feasible and cost-effective strategies. Efforts should include increased community awareness to avoid potential mortality from missed doses. Data are needed on the frequency of such occurrences.

International organizations can also play a major role in improving the care of T1D in developing countries. Novo Nordisk's LEAD initiative and IDF's Life for a Child program are examples of external efforts to mitigate some of the costs associated with delivering diabetes care.[27,28] Local solutions for practical problems such as storage of insulin (in areas where refrigeration is not available) with use of clay pots are an example of one cost-effective intervention.[29] Finally, sustainable and cost-neutral local strategies, including nurse-led patient education groups, health worker training, and development of practice guidelines to deliver protocol-based diabetes care, need to be developed and incorporated in national health policies.

REFERENCES

1. DIAMOND Project Group: Incidence and trends of childhood type 1 diabetes worldwide 1990–1999. *Diabet Med* 23(8):857–866, 2006
2. Harjutsalo V, Sjöberg L, Tuomilehto J: Time trends in the incidence of type 1 diabetes in Finnish children: a cohort study. *Lancet* 371(9626):1777–1782, 2008
3. Swai AB, Lutale JL, McLarty DG: Prospective study of incidence of juvenile diabetes mellitus over 10 years in Dar es Salaam, Tanzania. *BMJ* 306(6892):1570–1572, 1993
4. Alemu S, Dessie A, Seid E, Bard E, Lee PT, Trimble ER, Phillips DI, Parry EH: Insulin-requiring diabetes in rural Ethiopia: should we reopen the case for malnutrition-related diabetes? *Diabetologia* 52(9):1842–1845, 2009

5. Panz VR, Kalk WJ, Zouvanis M, Joffe BI: Distribution of autoantibodies to glutamic acid decarboxylase across the spectrum of diabetes mellitus seen in South Africa. *Diabet Med* 17(7):524–527, 2000
6. Bonifacio E, Genovese S, Braghi S, Bazzigaluppi E, Lampasona V, Bingley PJ, Rogge L, Pastore MR, Bognetti E, Bottazzo GF: Islet autoantibody markers in IDDM: risk assessment strategies yielding high sensitivity. *Diabetologia* 38(7):816–822, 1995
7. Harron KL, McKinney PA, Feltbower RG, Bodansky HJ, Norman PD, Campbell FM, Parslow RC: Incidence rate trends in childhood type 1 diabetes in Yorkshire, UK 1978–2007: effects of deprivation and age at diagnosis in the South Asian and non-South Asian populations. *Diabet Med* 28(12):1508–1513, 2011
8. Umpierrez GE, Smiley D, Kitabchi AE: Narrative review: ketosis-prone type 2 diabetes mellitus. *Ann Intern Med* 144(5):350–357, 2006
9. Su XF, Fu LY, Wu JD, Xu XH, Li HQ, Sun R, Ye L, Lee KO, Ma JH: Fulminant type 1 diabetes mellitus: a study of nine cases. *Diabetes Technol Ther* 14:325–329, 2011
10. Beran D, Yudkin JS, de Courten M: Access to care for patients with insulin-requiring diabetes in developing countries: case studies of Mozambique and Zambia. *Diabetes Care* 28(9):2136–2140, 2005
11. Elrayah H, Eltom M, Bedri A, Belal A, Rosling H, Ostenson CG: Economic burden on families of childhood type 1 diabetes in urban Sudan. *Diabetes Res Clin Pract* 70(2):159–165, 2005
12. Gill GV, Yudkin JS, Keen H, Beran D: The insulin dilemma in resource-limited countries: a way forward? *Diabetologia* 54:19–24, 2011
13. Majaliwa ES, Munubhi E, Ramaiya K, Mpembeni R, Sanyiwa A, Mohn A, Chiarelli F: Survey on acute and chronic complications in children and adolescents with type 1 diabetes at Muhimbili National Hospital in Dar es Salaam, Tanzania. *Diabetes Care* 30(9):2187–2192, 2007
14. Rwiza HT, Swai AB, McLarty DG: Failure to diagnose diabetic ketoacidosis in Tanzania. *Diabet Med* 3(2):181–183, 1986
15. Ahmed US, Junaidi B, Ali AW, Akhter O, Salahuddin M, Akhter J: Barriers in initiating insulin therapy in a South Asian Muslim community. *Diabet Med* 27(2):169–174, 2010
16. Elmehdawi RR, Elmagerhei HM: Profile of diabetic ketoacidosis at a teaching hospital in Benghazi, Libyan Arab Jamahiriya. *East Mediterr Health J* 16(3):292–299, 2010
17. Mbugua PK, Otieno CF, Kayima JK, Amayo AA, McLigeyo SO: Diabetic ketoacidosis: clinical presentation and precipitating factors at Kenyatta National Hospital, Nairobi. *East Afr Med J* 82(Suppl. 12):S191–S196, 2005
18. Gill GV, Famuyiwa OO, Rolfe M, Archibald LK: Serious hand sepsis and diabetes mellitus: specific tropical syndrome with western counterparts. *Diabet Med* 15(10):858–862, 1998
19. Baldé NM, Camara A, Camara LM, Diallo MM, Kaké A, Bah-Sow OY: Associated tuberculosis and diabetes in Conakry, Guinea: prevalence and clinical characteristics. *Int J Tuberc Lung Dis* 10(9):1036–1040, 2006
20. Naicker S: End-stage renal disease in sub-Saharan Africa. *Ethn Dis* 19(Suppl. 1):S1-13-5, 2009

21. Amutha A, Datta M, Unnikrishnan IR, Anjana RM, Rema M, Venkat Narayan KM, Mohan V: Clinical profile of diabetes in the young seen between 1992 and 2009 at a specialist diabetes centre in south India. *Prim Care Diabetes* 5(4):223–229, 2011

22. Morbach S, Lutale JK, Viswanathan V, Möllenberg J, Ochs HR, Rajashekar S, Ramachandran A, Abbas ZG: Regional differences in risk factors and clinical presentation of diabetic foot lesions. *Diabet Med* 21(1):91–95, 2004

23. Gill GV, Huddle KR, Monkoe G: Long-term (20 years) outcome and mortality of type 1 diabetic patients in Soweto, South Africa. *Diabet Med* 22(12):1642–1646, 2005

24. Lester FT: Clinical features, complications and mortality in type 1 (insulin-dependent) diabetic patients in Addis Ababa, Ethiopia, 1976–1990. *Q J Med* 83(301):389–399, 1992

25. Zhang P, Zhang X, Brown J, Vistisen D, Sicree R, Shaw J, Nichols G: Global healthcare expenditure on diabetes for 2010 and 2030. *Diabetes Res Clin Pract.* 87(3):293–301, 2010

26. Narayan KMV, Zhang P, Kanaya AM, Williams DE, Engelgau MM, Imperatore G, Ramachandran A: Diabetes: the pandemic and potential solutions. In *Disease Control Priorities in Developing Countries.* 2nd ed. Jamison DT, Breman JG, Measham AR, Alleyne G, Claeson M, Evans DB, Jha P, Mills A, Musgrove P, Eds. Washington, DC, World Bank, 2006, Chapter 30

27. Novo Nordisk Sustainability Report 2003. Novo Nordisk, Bagsværd, 2003

28. Callister LC: The global pediatric diabetes problem. *MCN Am J Matern Child Nurs* 36:66, 2011

29. Vimalavathini R, Gitanjali B: Effect of temperature on the potency & pharmacological action of insulin. *Indian J Med Res* 130(2):166–169, 2009

Index